OXFORD PAPERBACK REFERENCE

Concise Medical Dictionary

Concise Medical Dictionary

SECOND EDITION

OXFORD UNIVERSITY PRESS

Oxford University Press, Walton Street, Oxford OX2 6DP

Oxford New York Toronto
Delhi Bombay Calcutta Madras Karachi
Petaling Jaya Singapore Hong Kong Tokyo
Nairobi Dar es Salaam Cape Town
Melbourne Auckland

and associated companies in
Berlin Ibadan

Oxford is a trade mark of Oxford University Press

© Market House Books Ltd. 1980, 1985

First edition published by arrangement with
Transworld Publishers 1980
Second Edition 1985
First issued as an
Oxford University Press paperback 1987
Reprinted 1987, 1988 (with corrections), 1989 (twice)

British Library Cataloguing in Publication Data
Concise medical dictionary.—2nd ed.—
(Oxford Medical publications)
1. Medicine—Dictionaries
I. Martin, E. A.
610'.3'21   R125
ISBN 0–19–281991–7

Printed in Great Britain by
Richard Clay Ltd.
Bungay, Suffolk

Preface

This dictionary – an entirely new compilation – provides full coverage of all the important items and concepts used in medicine today. Written by a distinguished team of practising specialists and medical writers, it is intended primarily for workers in the paramedical fields: nurses, pharmacists, physiotherapists, speech therapists, social workers, hospital secretaries, administrators, technicians, and so on. It will also be invaluable for medical students and practising doctors. Each entry contains a basic definition, followed – where appropriate – by a more detailed explanation or description. A feature of the dictionary is that the articles are written in clear and concise English without the use of unnecessary technical jargon. For this reason the book will also be of both interest and value to the general reader who needs a home medical dictionary.

The dictionary defines terms in anatomy, physiology, bio-chemistry, and pharmacology, as well as in all the major medical and surgical specialities. Its coverage of psychology and psychiatry, community medicine, and dentistry is unusually comprehensive. To make room for this additional material, many of the more obscure and obsolescent terms found in the larger medical dictionaries have been omitted. The inclusion of these terms in a dictionary reflecting the practice of modern medicine is of questionable value, and their meanings can be readily derived from definitions of the medical prefixes and suffixes, which are included in this book. To avoid cluttering the entry list with derivative words (e.g. adjectives of nouns that are defined), these words are listed at the end of the definitions of the words from which they are derived. Where necessary, articles are supplemented by clear and fully labelled line drawings. An asterisk against a word used in a definition indicates that this term has its own entry in the dictionary and that additional information can be found there. Some entries simply refer the reader to another entry, indicating either that they are synonyms or that they – together with related terms – are most conveniently explained in one of the dictionary's longer articles. Synonyms are shown in brackets after the defined term.

Editor

Elizabeth A. Martin MA

Contributors and Advisors

J. A. D. Anderson MA, MD, FFCM

John Andrewartha BSc, MSc, PhD

Lionel Bender BSc

John R. Bennett MD, FRCP

Stuart Anthony Bentley MB, BS

Bruce M. Bryant MB, ChB, MRCP

Frank Coffin FRCS, FDS

Robert E. Coleman

Patrick Collins MD, MRCP

J. A. Cullen BSc, MSc

H. L. Dalrymple BSc, MSc

W. J. Dinning FRCS, MRCP

Ivan T. Draper MB, ChB, FRCPEd

J. C. Gingell MB, BCh, FRCSEd, FRCS

Alan Howe BSc, PhD

Alan Isaacs BSc, PhD, DIC

Mark Lambert BSc

Anne Lockhart MIBiol, MIHE, Cert. Ed.

Dermod MacCarthy MD, FRCP, DCH

Gordon Macpherson MB, BS

M. A. Openshaw BSc, DPhil

T. R. Pitt Ford PhD, BDS, FDS

D. L. Phillips FRCOG, FRCR

Walter D. Ryder BSc, PhD

Dr John R. Sewell MA, MB, MRCP

Dr Tony Smith MA, BM, BCh

Eric Taylor MA, MB, MRCP, MRCPsych

John Timson BSc, PhD, FLS, MIBiol

H. R. H. Tripp MA, MSc, PhD

Sandra V. Vellucci BSc, PhD, MIBiol

William F. Whimster MRCP, MRCPath

David M. H. Williams MA

A

a- (an-) *prefix denoting* absence of; lacking; not. Examples: *amastia* (absence of breasts); *amorphic* (lacking definite form); *atoxic* (not poisonous).

ab- *prefix denoting* away from. Example: *abembryonic* (away from or opposite the embryo).

abarticulation *n.* **1.** the dislocation of a joint. **2.** a synovial joint (*see* diarthrosis).

abasia *n.* an inability to walk for which no physical cause can be identified. *See also* astasia.

abdomen *n.* the part of the body cavity below the chest (*see* thorax), from which it is separated by the *dia-phragm. The abdomen contains the organs of digestion – stomach, liver, intestines, etc. – and excretion – kidneys, bladder, etc.; in women it also contains the ovaries and womb. The regions of the abdomen are shown in the illustration. —**abdominal** *adj.*

abdomin- (abdomino-) *combining form denoting* the abdomen. Examples: *abdominalgia* (pain in the abdomen); *abdominothoracic* (relating to the abdomen and thorax).

abdominoscopy *n. see* laparoscopy.

abducens nerve the sixth *cranial nerve (VI), which supplies the lateral rectus muscle of each eyeball, responsible for turning the eye outwards.

abduct *vb.* to move a limb or any other part away from the midline of the body. —**abduction** *n.*

abductor *n.* any muscle that moves one part of the body away from another or from the midline of the body.

aberrant *adj.* abnormal: usually applied to a blood vessel or nerve that does not follow its normal course.

abiotrophy *n.* degeneration or loss of function without apparent cause; for example, *retinal abiotrophy* is progressive degeneration of the retina leading to impaired vision, occurring in genetic disorders such as *retinitis pigmentosa.

ablatio *n. see* abruptio, detached retina (ablatio retinae).

ablation *n.* the removal of tissue, a part of the body, or an abnormal growth, usually by cutting.

ablepharia *n.* absence of or reduction in the size of the eyelids.

Regions of the abdomen

1

ablepsia *n.* an obsolete term for *blindness.

abortifacient *n.* a drug that induces abortion or miscarriage.

abortion *n.* the expulsion or removal of an embryo or fetus from the womb at a stage of pregnancy when it is incapable of independent survival (i.e. at any time between conception and the 28th week of pregnancy). In *threatened* abortion there is abdominal pain and bleeding from the womb but the fetus is still alive; once the fetus is dead abortion becomes *inevitable*. It is *incomplete* so long as the womb still contains some of the fetus or its membranes. Abortion may be *spontaneous* (a miscarriage) or it may be *induced* for medical or social reasons (termination of pregnancy). The *abortion rate* (the number of pregnancies lost per 1000 conceptions) is impossible to calculate precisely but is generally reckoned to be between one fifth and one third.

Induction or attempted induction of abortion are both criminal offences in Britain unless carried out within the terms of the Abortion Act. Two doctors have to agree that termination of pregnancy is necessary and the operation must be performed in an approved hospital or clinic. Methods in current use include vacuum *aspiration of the products of conception through a thin cannula; *dilatation and curettage; opening the womb through an abdominal incision (hysterotomy); or the use of *prostaglandins or other drugs to induce premature labour. Termination carries little risk early in pregnancy, but complications are more likely after the 13th week.

abortus *n.* a fetus, weighing less than 500 g, that is expelled from the mother's body either dead or incapable of surviving.

ABO system *see* blood group.

abrasion *n.* **1.** a graze: a minor wound in which the surface of the skin or a mucous membrane is worn away by rubbing or scraping. **2.** the wearing of the teeth, particularly at the necks by overvigorous brushing. **3.** any rubbing or scraping action that produces surface wear.

abreaction *n.* the release of strong emotion associated with a buried memory. While this can happen spontaneously, it is usually deliberately produced by a therapist using psychotherapy, hypnosis, or drugs such as amphetamines or barbiturates. The technique is used as a treatment for hysteria, anxiety state, and other neurotic conditions, especially when they are thought to be caused by *repression of memories or emotions.

abruptio (ablatio) *n.* separation. In *abruptio placentae (ablatio placentae)* the placenta separates from the lining of the womb before the usual time. Bleeding and pain are experienced at the point of separation, and the womb undergoes constant contraction. Severe cases involve shock. The condition is often associated with high blood pressure or *pre-eclampsia. If the neck of the womb is firm and undilated, a live fetus may be delivered by *Caesarean section.

abscess *n.* a localized collection of pus anywhere in the body, surrounded and walled off by damaged and inflamed tissues. A *boil is an example of an abscess within the skin. The usual cause is local bacterial infection, often by staphylococci, that the body's defences have failed to overcome. In a *cold abscess*, sometimes due to tubercle organisms, there is swelling, but little pain or inflammation (as in acute abscesses). Antibiotics, aided by surgical incision to release pus where necessary, are the usual forms of treatment.

abscission *n.* removal of tissue by cutting.

Absidia *n.* a genus of fungi that sometimes cause disease in man (*see* phycomycosis).

absorption *n.* (in physiology) the uptake of fluids or other substances by the tissues of the body. Digested food is absorbed into the blood and lymph from the alimentary canal. Most absorption of food occurs in the small intestine – in the jejunum and ileum – although alcohol is readily absorbed from the stomach. The small intestine is lined with minute finger-like processes (*see* villus), which greatly increase its surface area and therefore the speed at which absorption can take place. *See also* assimilation, digestion.

abulia *n.* absence or impairment of will power. The individual still has desires but they are not put into action; initiative and energy are lacking. It is commonly a symptom of *schizophrenia.

acalculia *n.* an acquired inability to make simple mathematical calculations. It is a symptom of disease in the *parietal lobe of the brain. *See* Gerstmann's syndrome.

acantha *n.* **1.** a spine projecting from a *vertebra. **2.** the *backbone.

acanthion *n.* the tip of the spine formed where projecting processes of the upper jaw bones (maxillae) meet at the front of the face.

acanthosis *n.* generalized thickening of the innermost (prickle-cell) layer of the *epidermis, with abnormal multiplication and increase in the number of cells. In *acanthosis nigricans* dark warty growths occur, especially in skin folds such as the groin, armpits, and mouth. It is usually a sign of internal cancer.

acapnia *n.* a condition in which there is an abnormally low concentration of carbon dioxide in the blood. This may be caused by breathing that is exceptionally deep in relation to the physical activity of the individual.

acariasis *n.* an infestation of mites and ticks and the symptoms, for example allergy and dermatitis, that their presence may provoke.

acaricide *n.* any chemical agent used for destroying mites and ticks.

acarid *n.* a *mite or *tick.

Acarina *n.* the group of arthropods that includes the *mites and *ticks.

Acarus (Tyroglyphus) *n.* a genus of mites. The flour mite, *A. siro* (*T. farinae*), is nonparasitic, but its presence in flour can cause a severe allergic dermatitis in flour-mill workers.

acatalasia *n.* an inborn lack of the enzyme *catalase, leading to recurrent infections of the gums (gingivitis) and mouth. It is most common in the Japanese.

acceptor *n.* (in biochemistry) a substance that helps to bring about oxidation of a reduced *substrate by accepting hydrogen ions.

accessory nerve (spinal accessory nerve) the eleventh *cranial nerve (XI), which arises from two roots, cranial and spinal. Fibres from the cranial root travel with the nerve for only a short distance before branching to join the vagus and then forming the recurrent laryngeal nerve, which supplies the internal laryngeal muscles. Fibres from the spinal root supply the sternomastoid and trapezius muscles, in the neck region (front and back).

accommodation *n.* adjustment of the shape of the lens to change the focus of the eye. When the ciliary muscle (*see* ciliary body) is relaxed, suspensory ligaments attached to the ciliary body and holding the lens in position are stretched, which causes the lens to be flattened. The eye is then able to focus on distant objects. To focus the eye on near objects the ciliary muscles contract and the tension in the ligaments is thus lowered, allowing the lens to become rounder.

accommodation reaction (convergence reaction) the constriction of the pupil that occurs when an individual focuses on a near object.

accouchement *n.* delivery of a baby.

acentric *n.* (in genetics) a chromosome or fragment of a chromosome that has no *centromere. Since acentrics cannot attach to the *spindle they are usually lost during cell division. They are often found in cells damaged by radiation. —**acentric** *adj.*

acephalus *n.* a fetus without a head.

acervulus cerebri a collection of granules of calcium-containing material that is sometimes found within the *pineal body as its calcification proceeds (normally after the 17th year): 'brain sand'.

acetabulum (cotyloid cavity) *n.* either of the two deep sockets, one on each side of the *hip bone, into which the head of the thigh bone (femur) fits.

acetanilide *n.* a drug that relieves pain and reduces fever. Since it can cause haemolytic anaemia and prolonged use may lead to *habituation, it has largely been replaced by safer analgesics.

acetarsol *n.* an arsenic-containing drug administered by mouth for the treatment of amoebic dysentery, yaws, and *Vincent's angina; as vaginal tablets for vaginitis; and as a rectal *suppository for *proctitis. Possible side-effects include skin rashes (after oral administration) and local irritation (with vaginal tablets).

acetazolamide *n.* a *diuretic used in the treatment of glaucoma to reduce the pressure inside the eyeball. Side-effects include drowsiness and numbness and tingling of the hands and feet. Trade names: **Acetazide**, **Diamox**.

acetoacetic acid an organic acid produced in large amounts by the liver under metabolic conditions associated with a high rate of fatty acid oxidation (for example, in starvation). The acetoacetic acid thus formed is subsequently converted to acetone and excreted. *See also* ketone.

acetohexamide *n.* a drug that reduces the level of blood sugar, used in the treatment of *diabetes mellitus. It is administered by mouth; side-effects include headache, dizziness, and nervousness. *See also* tolbutamide, chlorpropamide.

acetone *n.* an organic compound that is an intermediate in many bacterial fermentations and is produced by fatty acid oxidation. In certain abnormal conditions (for example, starvation) acetone and other *ketones may accumulate in the blood (*see* ketosis). Acetone is a volatile liquid that is miscible with both fats and water and therefore of great value as a solvent. It is used in chromatography and in the preparation of tissues for enzyme extraction.

acetone body (ketone body) *see* ketone.

acetonuria *n.* *see* ketonuria.

acetylcholine *n.* the acetic acid ester of the organic base choline: the *neurotransmitter released at the synapses of parasympathetic nerves and at *neuromuscular junctions. After relaying a nerve impulse, acetylcholine is rapidly broken down by the enzyme *cholinesterase. *Atropine and curare cause muscular paralysis by blocking the action of acetylcholine at muscle membranes; *physostigmine prolongs the activity of acetylcholine by blocking cholinesterase.

acetylcysteine *n.* a drug used to break down thick mucous secretions. It is administered as an aerosol, primarily for the treatment of respiratory diseases, such as bronchitis, and cystic fibrosis. Side-effects may include spasm of the bronchial muscles, nausea, vomiting, and fever.

acetylsalicylic acid *see* aspirin.

achalasia (cardiospasm) *n.* a condition in which the normal muscular activity of the oesophagus (gullet) is disturbed, which delays the passage of swallowed material. It may occur at any age: symptoms include difficulty in swallowing liquids and solids, slowly increasing over years; sometimes regurgitation of undigested food; and occasionally severe chest pain caused by spasm of the oesophagus. Diagnosis is by a barium X-ray examination. Treatment is by forceful stretching of the tight lower end of the oesophagus (cardia) or by surgical splitting of the muscular ring in that area (*cardiomyotomy*).

Achilles tendon the tendon of the muscles of the calf of the leg (the *gastrocnemius and soleus muscles), situated at the back of the ankle and attached to the calcaneus (heel bone).

achlorhydria *n.* absence of hydrochloric acid in the stomach. Achlorhydria that persists despite large doses of histamine is associated with atrophy of the lining (mucosa) of the stomach. In this condition there is usually an absence of secretion of *intrinsic factor, which will lead to *pernicious anaemia. In some people, however, achlorhydria is not associated with any disease, produces no ill-effects, and needs no treatment.

acholia *n.* absence or deficiency of bile secretion or failure of the bile to enter the alimentary canal (for example, because of an obstructed bile duct).

acholuria *n.* absence of the *bile pigments from the urine, which occurs in some forms of jaundice (*acholuric jaundice*). —**acholuric** *adj.*

achondroplasia *n.* an inherited disorder in which the bones of the arms and legs fail to grow to normal size due to a defect in both cartilage and bone. It results in a type of *dwarfism characterized by short limbs, a normal-sized head and body, and normal intelligence. —**achondroplastic** *adj.*

achromatic *adj.* without colour.

achromatic lenses lenses specially designed for use in the eyepieces of microscopes and other scientific instruments. They give clear images, unblurred by the coloured fringes that are produced with ordinary lenses (caused by splitting of the light into different wavelengths).

achromatopsia *n.* the inability to perceive colour. Such complete *colour blindness is very rare and is usually associated with poor *visual acuity; it is usually determined by hereditary factors.

achylia *n.* absence of secretion. The term is usually applied to a nonsecreting stomach (*achylia gastrica*) whose lining (mucosa) is atrophied (*see* achlorhydria).

acidaemia *n.* a condition of abnormally high blood acidity. This may result from an increase in the concentration of acidic substances and/or a decrease in the level of alkaline substances in the blood. *See also* acidosis. *Compare* alkalaemia.

acid-base balance the balance between the amount of carbonic acid and bicarbonate in the blood, which must be maintained at a constant ratio of 1:20 in order to keep the hydrogen ion concentration of the plasma at a constant value (pH 7.4). Any alteration in this ratio will disturb the acid-base balance of the blood and tissues and cause either *acidosis or *alkalosis. The lungs and the kidneys play an important role in the regulation of the acid-base balance.

acid-etch technique a technique for bonding resin-based restorative materials to the enamel of teeth. A porous surface is created by applying phosphoric acid for approximately one minute.

acid-fast *adj.* **1.** describing bacteria that have been stained and continue to hold the stain after treatment with an acidic solution. For example, tuberculosis bacteria are acid-fast when stained with a *carbol fuchsin preparation. **2.** describing a stain that is not removed from a specimen by washing with an acidic solution.

acidophil (acidophilic) *adj.* **1.** (in histology) describing tissues, cells, or parts of cells that stain with acid dyes (such as eosin). **2.** (in bacteriology) describing bacteria that grow well in acid media.

acidosis *n.* a condition in which the acidity of body fluids and tissues is abnormally high. This arises because of a failure of the mechanisms responsible for maintaining a balance between acids and alkalis in the blood (*see* acid-base balance). In *gaseous acidosis* more than the normal amount of carbon dioxide is retained in the body, as in drowning. In *renal acidosis*, kidney failure results in excessive loss of bicarbonate or retention of phosphoric and sulphuric acids. Patients with diabetes mellitus suffer from a form of acidosis in which sodium, potassium, and *ketone bodies are lost in the urine.

acinus *n.* (*pl.* **acini**) **1.** a small sac or cavity surrounded by the secretory cells of a gland. Some authorities regard the term as synonymous with *alveolus, but others distinguish an acinus by the possession of a narrow passage (lumen) leading from the sac. **2.** (in the lung) the tissue supplied with air by one terminal *bronchiole. *Emphysema is classified by the part of the acinus involved (i.e. *centriacinar*, *panacinar*, or *periacinar*). —**acinous** *adj.*

aclasis *n. see* diaphysial aclasis.

acne *n.* a skin disorder in which the sebaceous glands become inflamed. The commonest variety, *acne vulgaris*, generally starts in adolescence and is caused by overactivity of the sebaceous glands. The sebum produced by the glands cannot escape because the hair follicles become blocked by a *keratin plug and a pustule forms, with fluid leaking into the surrounding tissue. The keratin plug turns black, forming the familiar blackhead. Acne vulgaris occurs mainly on the face, chest, and back; it is usually mild, disappearing in adulthood, but can be severe and chronic, causing infected cysts and scarring of the skin. The course of this condition may be helped by regular washing, the removal of blackheads, and sometimes the use of antibiotics. There are many other varieties of acne, some being caused by contact with chemical substances (such as tar). *See also* rosacea.

aconite *n.* the dried roots of the herbaceous plant *Aconitum napellus* (monkshood or wolfbane), containing three *analgesic substances: *aconine*, *aconitine*, and *picraconitine*. Aconite was formerly used to prepare liniments for muscular pains and a tincture for toothache, but is regarded as too toxic for use today.

acoustic *adj.* of or relating to sound or the sense of hearing.

acoustic holography a technique of building up a three-dimensional picture of structures within the body using *ultrasound waves. Two separate sound sources cause ultrasound waves to be transmitted through and reflected from the organs being examined. The interference patterns produced on a liquid surface are illuminated by laser light and photographed to form a *hologram*.

acoustic nerve *see* vestibulocochlear nerve.

acquired *adj.* describing a condition or disorder contracted after birth and not attributable to hereditary causes. *Compare* congenital.

acquired immunodeficiency syndrome *see* AIDS.

acrania *n.* congenital absence of the skull, either partial or complete, due to a developmental defect.

acriflavine *n.* a dye used as an antiseptic on skin and mucous membranes and to disinfect contaminated wounds. It may cause sensitivity of the skin to sunlight.

acro- *prefix denoting* **1.** extremity; tip. Example: *acrohypothermy* (abnormal coldness of the extremities (hands and feet)). **2.** height; promontory. Example: *acrophobia* (morbid dread of heights). **3.** extreme; intense. Example: *acromania* (an extreme degree of mania).

acrocentric *n.* a chromosome in which the *centromere is situated at or very near one end. —**acrocentric** *adj.*

acrocyanosis *n.* bluish-purple discoloration of the hands and feet due to slow circulation of the blood through the small vessels in the skin.

acrodermatitis *n.* inflammation of the skin of the feet or hands. A diffuse chronic variety produces swelling and reddening of the affected areas, followed by atrophy. The cause is unknown and there is no treatment.

acrodynia *n. see* pink disease.

acromegaly *n.* increase in size of the hands, feet, and the face due to excessive production of *growth hormone (somatotrophin) by a tumour of the anterior pituitary gland. The tumour can be treated with X-rays or surgically removed. *See also* gigantism.

acromion *n.* an oblong process at the top of the spine of the *scapula, part of which articulates with the clavicle (collar bone) to form the *acromioclavicular joint.* —**acromial** *adj.*

acroparaesthesiae *n.* a tingling sensation in the hands and feet.

acrosclerosis *n.* a skin disease thought to be a type of generalized *scleroderma. It also has features of *Raynaud's disease, with the hands, face, and feet being mainly affected.

acrosome *n.* the caplike structure on the front end of a spermatozoon. It breaks down just before fertilization, releasing a number of enzymes that assist penetration between the follicle cells that still surround the ovum.

acrylic resin one of a group of polymeric materials used for making denture teeth, denture bases, and formerly as a dental filling material.

ACTH (adrenocorticotrophic hormone, adrenocorticotrophin, corticotrophin) a hormone synthesized and stored in the anterior pituitary gland, large amounts of which are released in response to any form of stress. ACTH controls the secretion of *corticosteroid hormones from the adrenal gland. It is administered by injection to test adrenal function and to treat conditions such as rheumatic diseases (especially in children) and asthma.

actin *n.* a protein, found in muscle, that plays an important role in the process of contraction. *See* striated muscle.

Actinobacillus *n.* a genus of Gram-negative nonmotile aerobic bacteria that are characteristically spherical or rodlike in shape but occasionally grow into branching filaments. Actinobacilli cause disease in animals. The species *A. mallei* causes *glanders, an infection of horses that can be transmitted to man.

Actinomyces *n.* a genus of Gram-positive nonmotile fungus-like bacteria that cause disease in animals and man. The species *A. israeli* is the causative organism of human *actinomycosis.

actinomycin *n.* a *cytotoxic drug, produced by *Streptomyces* bacteria, that inhibits the growth of cancer cells. There are two forms, both of which are administered by injection. Actinomycin C may damage bone marrow. Actinomycin D may cause nausea, vomiting, diarrhoea, blood disorders, and bone-marrow damage.

actinomycosis *n.* a noncontagious disease caused by the bacterium *Actinomyces israeli*, which most commonly affects the jaw but may also affect the lungs, brain, or intestines. The bacterium is normally present in the mouth but it may become pathogenic following an *apical abscess or extraction of a tooth. It is characterized by multiple sinuses that open onto the skin. Treatment is by drainage of pus and a prolonged course of antibiotics.

actinotherapy *n.* the treatment of disorders with *infrared or *ultraviolet radiation.

action potential the change in voltage that occurs across the membrane of a nerve or muscle cell when a *nerve impulse is triggered. It is due to the passage of charged particles across the membrane (*see* depolarization) and is an observable manifestation of the passage of an impulse.

active transport (in biochemistry) an energy-dependent process in which certain substances (including ions, some drugs, and amino acids) are able to cross cell membranes against a concentration gradient. The process is inhibited by substances that interfere with cellular metabolism (e.g. high doses of digitalis).

actomyosin *n.* a protein complex formed in muscle between actin and myosin during the process of contraction. *See* striated muscle.

acupuncture *n.* a traditional Chinese system of healing in which symptoms are relieved by thin metal needles inserted into selected points beneath the skin. The needles are stimulated either by rotation or, more recently, by an electric current. Recent hypotheses suggest that the needling activates deep sensory nerves, which cause the pituitary and midbrain to release *endorphins – the brain's natural pain-killers. Acupuncture is widely used in the Far East for the relief of pain and in China itself has become an alternative to anaesthesia for some major operations. Acupuncturists in the West may be medically qualified but many are not.

acute *adj.* **1.** describing a disease of rapid onset, severe symptoms, and brief duration. *Compare* chronic. **2.** describing any intense symptom, such as severe pain.

acute abdomen an emergency surgical condition caused by damage to one or more abdominal organs following injury or disease. The patient is in severe pain and often in shock. Perforation of a peptic ulcer or a severely infected appendix, or rupture of the liver or spleen following a crushing injury, all produce an acute abdomen requiring urgent treatment.

acute rheumatism *see* rheumatic fever.

acyclovir *n.* an antiviral drug that inhibits DNA synthesis in cells infected by *herpesviruses. Administered by mouth or intravenously, it is useful in patients whose immune systems are disturbed and also possibly in the treatment of genital herpes and herpes encephalitis.

ad- *prefix denoting* towards or near. Examples: *adaxial* (towards the main axis); *adoral* (towards or near the mouth).

adamantinoma *n.* an obsolete term for an *ameloblastoma.

Adam's apple (laryngeal prominence) a projection, lying just under the skin, of the thyroid cartilage of the *larynx.

Adams-Stokes syndrome *see* Stokes-Adams syndrome.

adaptation *n.* the phenomenon in which a sense organ shows a gradually diminishing response to continuous or repetitive stimulation. The nose, for example, may become adapted to the stimulus of an odour that is continuously present so that in time it ceases to report its presence. Similarly, the adaptation of touch receptors in the skin means that the presence of clothes can be forgotten a few minutes after they have been put on.

addiction *n.* a state of *dependence produced by the habitual taking of any of certain drugs. Strictly speaking, the term implies the state of physical dependence induced by such drugs as morphine, heroin, and alcohol, but it is also used for the state of psychological dependence, produced by drugs such as barbiturates. Treatment is aimed at gradual withdrawal of the drug and eventually total abstention. *See also* alcoholism, tolerance.

Addison's disease a syndrome due to inadequate secretion of corticosteroid hormones by the *adrenal glands, sometimes as a result of tuberculous infection. Symptoms include weakness, loss of energy, low blood pressure, and dark pigmentation of the skin. Formerly fatal, the disease is now curable by replacement hormone therapy.

adduct *vb.* to move a limb or any other part towards the midline of the body. —**adduction** *n.*

adductor *n.* any muscle that moves one part of the body towards another or towards the midline of the body.

aden- (adeno-) *prefix denoting* a gland or glands. Examples: *adenalgia* (pain in); *adenogenesis* (development of); *adenopathy* (disease of).

adenine *n.* one of the nitrogen-containing bases (*see* purine) that occurs in the nucleic acids DNA and RNA. *See also* ATP.

adenine arabinoside a compound with antiviral activity, particularly against *herpesviruses. It is also active against tumours but its clinical use is restricted by its toxicity.

adenitis *n.* inflammation of a gland or group of glands. For example, *mesenteric adenitis* affects the lymph glands (nodes) in the membranous support of the intestines (the mesentery); *cervical adenitis* affects the lymph glands in the neck.

adenocarcinoma *n.* a malignant epithelial tumour arising from the glandular structures, which are constituent parts of most organs of the body. The term is also applied to tumours showing a glandular growth pattern. These tumours may be subclassified according to the substances that they produce, for example *mucus-secreting* and *serous adenocarcinomas*, or to the microscopical arrangement of their cells into patterns, for example *papillary* and *follicular adenocarcinomas*. They may be solid or cystic (*cystadenocarcinomas*). Each organ may produce tumours showing a variety of histological types; for example, the ovary may produce both mucinous and serous cystadenocarcinomas.

adenohypophysis *n.* the anterior lobe of the *pituitary gland.

adenoidectomy *n.* surgical removal of the *adenoids, commonly combined with tonsillectomy in a child who suffers recurrent sore throats and difficulty in breathing through the nose.

adenoids (pharyngeal tonsils) *n.* the collection of lymphatic tissue at the rear of the nose. Enlargement of the adenoids from recurrent throat infections may cause obstruction to breathing through the nose (*see* adenoidectomy).

adenoma *n.* a benign tumour of epithelial origin that is derived from glandular tissue or exhibits clearly defined glandular structures. Adenomas may become malignant (*see* adenocarcinoma). Some show recognizable tissue elements, such as fibrous tissue (*fibroadenomas*), while others, such as bronchial adenomas, produce active compounds giving rise to clinical syndromes (*see* argentaffinoma). Tumours in certain organs, including the pituitary gland, are often classified by their histological staining affinities, for example *eosinophil*, *basophil*, and *chromophobe adenomas*.

adenosine *n.* a compound containing adenine and the sugar ribose: it occurs in ATP. *See also* nucleoside.

adenosine diphosphate *see* ADP.

adenosine monophosphate *see* AMP.

adenosine triphosphate *see* ATP.

adenosis *n.* (*pl.* **adenoses**) 1. excessive growth or development of glands. 2. any disease of a gland, especially of a lymph gland (node).

adenovirus *n.* one of a group of DNA-containing viruses causing latent infections of the upper respiratory tract that produce symptoms resembling those of the common cold.

adhesion *n.* 1. the union of two normally separate surfaces, such as the moving surfaces of joints, by fibrous connective tissue developing in an inflamed or damaged region. (The fibrous tissue itself is also called an adhesion.) Adhesion between loops of intestine may occur following abdominal surgery, possibly obstructing the alimentary canal. If the pericardial sac is affected by adhesion, the movements of the heart may be restricted. 2. a healing process in which the edges of a wound fit together. In *primary adhesion* there is very little *granulation tissue; in *secondary adhesion* the two edges are joined together by granulation tissue.

adiadochokinesis *n.* *see* dysdiadochokinesis.

Adie's syndrome (Holmes-Adie syndrome) an abnormality of the pupils of the eyes, often affecting only one eye. At rest the affected pupil is larger than the normal one; it reacts slowly to light and the response on convergence of the eyes is also slow. Eventually the affected pupil will constrict much more completely than its fellow. One or more tendon reflexes may be absent. The condition is almost entirely restricted to women.

adipocere *n.* a waxlike substance, consisting mainly of fatty acids, into which the soft tissues of the body can be converted after death. This usually occurs when the body is buried in damp earth or is submerged in water. Adipocere delays post-mortem decomposition and is a spontaneous form of preservation without mummification.

adipose tissue fibrous *connective tissue packed with masses of fat cells. It forms a thick layer under the skin and occurs around the kidneys and in the buttocks. It serves both as an insulating layer and an energy store; food in excess of requirements is converted into fats and stored within these cells.

adiposis (liposis) *n.* the presence of abnormally large accumulations of fat in the body. The condition may arise from overeating, hormone irregularities, or a metabolic disorder. In *adiposis dolorosa*, a condition affecting women more commonly than men, painful fatty swellings are associated with defects in the nervous system. *See also* obesity.

aditus *n.* an anatomical opening or passage; for example, the opening of the tympanic cavity (middle ear) to the air spaces of the mastoid process.

adjuvant *n.* any substance used in conjunction with another to enhance its activity. Aluminium salts are used as adjuvants in the preparation of vaccines from the toxins of diphtheria and tetanus: by keeping the toxins in precipitated form, the salts increase the efficacy of the toxins as antigens.

adnexa *pl. n.* adjoining parts. For example, the *uterine adnexa* are the Fallopian tubes and ovaries (which adjoin the womb).

ADP (adenosine diphosphate) a compound containing adenine, ribose, and two phosphate groups. ADP occurs in cells and is involved in processes requiring the transfer of energy (*see* ATP).

adrenal glands (suprarenal glands) two triangular *endocrine glands, each of which covers the superior surface of a kidney. Each gland has two parts, the *medulla* and *cortex*. The medulla forms the grey core of the gland; it consists mainly of *chromaffin tissue and is stimulated by the sympathetic nervous system to produce *adrenaline and *noradrenaline. The cortex is a yellowish tissue surrounding the medulla. It is derived embryologically from mesoderm and is stimulated by pituitary hormones (principally *ACTH) to produce three kinds of *corticosteroid hormones, which affect carbohydrate metabolism (e.g. *cortisol), electrolyte metabolism (e.g. *aldosterone), and the sex glands (oestrogens and androgens).

adrenaline (epinephrine) *n.* an important hormone secreted by the medulla of the adrenal gland. It has the function of preparing the body for 'fright, flight, or fight' and has widespread effects on circulation, the muscles, and sugar metabolism. The action of the heart is increased, the rate and depth of breathing are increased,

and the metabolic rate is raised; the force of muscular contraction improves and the onset of muscular fatigue is delayed. At the same time the blood supply to the bladder and intestines is reduced, their muscular walls relax, and the sphincters contract. *Sympathetic nerves were originally thought to act by releasing adrenaline at their endings, and were therefore called *adrenergic* nerves. In fact the main substance released is the related substance *noradrenaline, which also forms a portion of the adrenal secretion.

Adrenaline given by injection is valuable for the relief of bronchial asthma, because it relaxes constricted airways. It is also used during surgery to reduce blood loss by constricting vessels in the skin.

adrenergic *adj.* describing nerve fibres that release *noradrenaline as a neurotransmitter. *Compare* cholinergic.

adrenocorticotrophic hormone (adrenocorticotrophin) *see* ACTH.

adrenogenital syndrome precocious sexual development and apparent masculinization in girls, caused by overproduction of hormones by the adrenal cortex in infancy.

adrenolytic *adj.* inhibiting the activity of *adrenergic nerves. Adrenolytic activity is opposite to that of *adrenaline.

advancement *n.* the detachment by surgery of a muscle or tendon from its normal attachment site and its reattachment at a more advanced (anterior) point. The technique is used, for example, in the treatment of squint or in repositioning the womb.

adventitia (tunica adventitia) *n.* **1.** the outer coat of the wall of a *vein or *artery. It consists of loose connective tissue and networks of small blood vessels, which nourish the walls. **2.** the outer covering of various other organs or parts.

adventitious *adj.* **1.** occurring in a place other than the usual one. **2.** relating to the adventitia.

Aëdes *n.* a genus of widely distributed mosquitoes occurring throughout the tropics and subtropics. Most species are black with distinct white or silvery-yellow markings on the legs and thorax. *Aëdes* species are not only important as vectors of *dengue, *yellow fever, *filariasis, and Group B viruses causing encephalitis but also constitute a serious biting nuisance. *A. aegypti* is the principal vector of dengue and yellow fever.

aegophony *n. see* vocal resonance.

-aemia *suffix denoting* a specified condition of the blood. Example: *hyperglycaemia* (excess sugar in the blood).

aer- (aero-) *prefix denoting* air or gas. Examples: *aerogastria* (gas in the stomach); *aerogenesis* (production of gas).

aerobe *n.* any organism, especially a microbe, that requires the presence of free oxygen for life and growth. *See also* anaerobe, microaerophilic.

aerobic *adj.* **1.** of or relating to aerobes: requiring free oxygen for life and growth. **2.** describing a type of cellular *respiration in which foodstuffs (carbohydrates) are completely oxidized by atmospheric oxygen, with the production of maximum chemical energy from the foodstuffs.

aerodontalgia *n.* pain in the teeth due to change in atmospheric pressure during air travel or the ascent of a mountain.

aeroneurosis *n.* a syndrome of anxiety, agitation, and insomnia found in pilots flying unpressurized aircraft and attributed to *anoxia.

aerophagy *n.* the swallowing of air. This may be done voluntarily to stimulate belching, accidentally during rapid eating or drinking, or unconsciously as a habit. Voluntary aerophagy is used to permit oesophageal speech after surgical removal of the larynx (usually for cancer).

aerosol *n.* a suspension of extremely small liquid or solid particles (about 0.001 mm diameter) in the air. Drugs in aerosol form may be administered by inhalation.

aetiology (etiology) *n.* **1.** the study or science of the causes of disease. **2.** the cause of a specific disease.

afebrile *adj.* without, or not showing any signs of, a fever.

affect *n.* (in psychiatry) a wave of emotion or the emotion associated with a particular idea. —**affective** *adj.*

afferent *adj.* **1.** designating nerves or neurones that convey impulses from sense organs and other receptors to the brain or spinal cord, i.e. any sensory nerve or neurone. **2.** designating blood vessels that feed a capillary network in an organ or part. **3.** designating lymphatic vessels that enter a lymph node. *Compare* efferent.

afibrinogenaemia *n.* complete absence of the coagulation factor *fibrinogen in the blood. *Compare* hypofibrinogenaemia.

aflatoxin *n.* a poisonous substance produced in the spores of the fungus *Aspergillus flavus*, which infects peanuts. The toxin is known to produce cancer in certain animals and is suspected of being the cause of liver cancers in human beings living in warm and humid regions of the world, where stored nuts and cereals are contaminated by the fungus.

afterbirth *n.* the placenta, umbilical cord, and ruptured membranes associated with the fetus, which normally become detached from the womb and expelled within a few hours of birth.

after care long-term surveillance as an adjunct or supplement to formal medical treatment of those who are chronically sick or handicapped. After care includes the provision of special aids and the adaptation of homes to improve daily living.

after-image *n.* an impression of an image that is registered by the brain for a brief moment after an object is removed from in front of the eye, or after the eye is closed.

after-pains *pl. n.* pains in the womb during the first few days after childbirth, caused by contraction of the womb muscles as its nonpregnant dimensions are restored. After-pains can be relieved by the use of such drugs as aspirin.

agalactia *n.* absence or abnormally low production of milk in a woman who has just given birth.

agammaglobulinaemia *n.* a total deficiency of the plasma protein *gamma globulin. *Compare* hypogammaglobulinaemia.

agar *n.* an extract of certain seaweeds that forms a gel suitable for the solidification of liquid bacteriological *culture media. *Blood agar* is nutrient agar containing 5–10% horse blood, used for the cultivation of certain bacteria or for detecting haemolytic (blood-destroying) activity.

Age Concern (in Britain) a voluntary agency with particular interest in the problems of the aged.

agenesis *n.* absence of an organ, usually due to total failure of its development in the embryo.

agglutination (clumping) *n.* the sticking together, by serum antibodies called *agglutinins*, of such microscopic antigenic particles as red blood cells or bacteria so that they form visible clumps. Any substance that stimulates the body to produce an agglutinin is called an *agglutinogen*. Agglutination is a specific reaction; in the laboratory, sera containing different known agglutinins provide an invaluable means of identifying unknown bacteria. When blood of different groups is mixed, agglutination occurs because serum contains natural antibodies (*isoagglutinins*) that attack red cells of a foreign group, whether previously encountered or not. This is not the same process as occurs in *blood coagulation.

agglutinin *n.* an antibody that brings about the *agglutination of bacteria, blood cells, or other antigenic particles.

agglutinogen *n.* any antigen that provokes formation of an agglutinin in the serum and is therefore likely to be involved in *agglutination.

aglossia *n.* congenital absence of the tongue.

agnathia *n.* congenital absence of the lower jaw, either partial or complete.

agnosia *n.* a disorder of the brain whereby the patient cannot interpret sensations correctly although the sense organs and nerves conducting sensation to the brain are functioning normally. It is due to a disorder of the *association areas in the parietal lobes. In *auditory agnosia* the patient can hear but cannot interpret sounds (including speech). A patient with *tactile agnosia* (*astereognosis*) retains normal sensation in his hands but cannot recognize three-dimensional objects by touch alone. In *visual agnosia* the patient can see but cannot interpret symbols, including letters (*see* alexia).

agonal *adj.* describing or relating to the phenomena, such as cessation of breathing or change in the ECG or EEG, that are associated with the moment of death.

agonist (prime mover) *n.* a muscle whose active contraction causes movement of a part of the body. Contraction of an agonist is associated with relaxation of its *antagonist.

agoraphobia *n.* a morbid fear of public places and/or of open spaces. *See also* phobia.

agranulocytosis *n.* a disorder in which there is a severe acute deficiency of certain blood cells (*neutrophils) as a result of damage to the bone marrow by toxic drugs or chemicals. It is characterized by fever, with ulceration of the mouth and throat, and rapidly leads to prostration and death. Treatment is by administration of antibiotics in large quantities. When feasible, transfusion of white blood cells may be life-saving.

agraphia (dysgraphia) *n.* an acquired inability to write, although the strength and coordination of the hand remain normal. It is related to the disorders of language and it is caused by disease in the *parietal lobe of the brain. *See* Gerstmann's syndrome.

agromania *n.* a pathologically strong impulse to live alone in open country.

ague *n. see* malaria.

AID *see* artificial insemination.

AIDS (acquired immunodeficiency syndrome) a viral disease characterized by loss of the cell-mediated immune response due to decreased numbers of certain T-lymphocytes. After a long incubation period (up to several years), the patient suffers fever, weight loss, and enlargement of the lymph nodes, eventually succumbing to life-threatening infections (e.g. a severe pneumonia caused by the normally harmless protozoan *Pneumocystis carinii*) or cancers, particularly *Kaposi's sarcoma. The viruses, principally HIV (human immunodeficiency virus), are transmitted in blood, semen, and vaginal fluid, and in western countries AIDS is most prevalent among male homosexuals, haemophiliacs who

have received transfusions of infected blood, and intravenous drug users sharing needles.

AIH *see* artificial insemination.

ainhum *n.* loss of one or more toes due to slow growth of a fibrous band around the toe that eventually causes a spontaneous amputation. The condition is found in negroes and is associated with going barefoot.

air bed a bed with a mattress whose upper surface is perforated with thousands of holes, through which air is forced under pressure. The patient is thus supported, like a hovercraft, on a cushion of air. This type of bed is invaluable for the treatment of patients with large areas of burns.

air embolism an air lock that obstructs the outflow of blood from the right ventricle of the heart. Air may gain access to the circulation as a result of surgery, injury, or intravenous infusions. The patient experiences breathlessness and chest discomfort and develops acute heart failure. Tipping the patient head down, lying on the left side, may move the air lock.

air sickness *see* travel sickness.

akinesia *n.* a loss of normal muscular tonicity or responsiveness. In *akinetic epilepsy* there is a sudden loss of muscular tonicity, making the patient fall with momentary loss of consciousness. *Akinetic mutism* is a state of complete physical unresponsiveness although the patient's eyes remain open and appear to follow movements. It is a consequence of damage to the base of the brain. —**akinetic** *adj.*

ala *n.* (*pl.* **alae**) (in anatomy) a winglike structure; for example, either of the two lateral flared portions of the external nose or the winglike part of the ilium.

alactasia *n.* absence or deficiency of the enzyme lactase, which is essential for the digestion of milk sugar (lactose).

All babies have lactase in their intestines, but the enzyme disappears during childhood in about 10% of northern Europeans, 40% of Greeks and Italians, and 80% of Africans and Asians. Alactasia causes symptoms only if the diet regularly includes raw milk, when the undigested lactose causes diarrhoea and abdominal pain.

alanine n. see amino acid.

alastrim n. a mild form of smallpox, causing only a sparse rash and low-grade fever. Medical name: **variola minor**.

Albers-Schönberg disease see osteopetrosis.

albinism n. the inherited absence of pigmentation in the skin, hair, and eyes (see albino).

albino n. an individual lacking the normal body pigment (melanin). Albinos have white hair and pink skin and eyes. The pink colour is produced by blood in underlying blood vessels, which are normally masked by pigment.

albumin n. a protein that is soluble in water and coagulated by heat. An example is serum albumin, which is found in blood plasma and is important for the maintenance of plasma volume. Albumin is synthesized in the liver; the inability to synthesize it is a prominent feature of chronic liver disease (*cirrhosis).

albuminuria (proteinuria) n. the presence of serum albumin, serum globulin, or other serum proteins in the urine. This may be associated with kidney or heart disease. Albuminuria is not always associated with disease: it may occur after strenuous exercise or after a long period of standing (orthostatic albuminuria).

albumose n. a substance, intermediate between albumin and peptones, produced during the digestion of proteins by pepsin and other endopeptidases (see peptidase).

alcaptonuria (alkaptonuria) n. congenital absence of an enzyme, homogentisic acid oxidase, that is essential for the normal breakdown of the amino acids tyrosine and phenylalanine. Accumulation of *homogentisic acid causes dark brown discoloration of the skin and eyes (ochronosis) and progressive damage to the joints, especially of the spine. The gene responsible for the condition is recessive, so that a child is affected only if both parents are carriers of the defective gene.

alcohol n. any of a class of organic compounds formed when a hydroxyl group (–OH) is substituted for a hydrogen atom in a hydrocarbon. The alcohol in alcoholic drinks is ethyl alcohol (ethanol), which has the formula C_2H_5OH. It is produced by the fermentation of sugar by yeast. 'Pure' alcohol contains not less than 94.9% by volume of ethyl alcohol. It is obtained by distillation. A solution of 70% alcohol can be used as a preservative or antiseptic. When taken into the body ethyl alcohol depresses activity of the central nervous system (see also alcoholism). *Methyl alcohol (methanol) is extremely poisonous.

Alcoholics Anonymous a voluntary agency of self help that is organized and operated locally among those with alcoholic dependency and has national and international support. Members are expected to admit to their drink problems, discuss these openly and frankly at the regular meetings of the group, and also to take part in efficient family support schemes to help those members who have lapses.

alcoholism n. the syndrome due to physical *dependence on alcohol, such that sudden deprivation may cause withdrawal symptoms – tremor, anxiety, hallucinations, and delusions (see delirium tremens). The risk of alcoholism for an individual and its incidence in a society depend on the amount drunk. Countries such as France, where heavy drinking is socially acceptable, have the highest incidence. Usually several years' heavy drinking is needed for addiction to develop, but the range is from one to 40 years. Alcoholism impairs intellectual function, physical skills, memory, and judgment: social skills, such as conversation, are preserved until a late stage. Heavy consumption of alcohol also causes *cardiomyopathy, peripheral *neuritis, *cirrhosis of the liver, and enteritis. Treatment is usually given in a psychiatric hospital, where the alcoholic is first 'dried out' and then helped to understand the psychological pressures that led to his heavy drinking. Drugs such as *disulfiram (Antabuse), which cause vomiting if alcohol is taken, may help in treatment.

Aldomet n. see methyldopa.

aldosterone n. a steroid hormone (see corticosteroid) that is synthesized and released by the adrenal cortex and acts on the kidney to regulate salt (potassium and sodium) and water balance. It may be given by injection as replacement therapy when the adrenal cortex secretes insufficient amounts of the hormone and also to treat shock.

aldosteronism n. overproduction of aldosterone, one of the hormones secreted by the adrenal cortex, leading to abnormalities in the amounts of sodium, potassium, and water in the body. It is one cause of raised blood pressure (hypertension).

Aleppo boil see oriental sore.

aleukaemic adj. describing a stage of *leukaemia in which there is no increase in the number of white cells in the blood. The stage is almost invariably followed by one in which excessive numbers of white cells are produced, as typical in leukaemia.

alexia n. an acquired inability to read. It is due to disease in the left hemisphere of the brain in a right-handed person. In agnosic alexia (word blindness) the patient cannot read because he is unable to identify the letters and words, but he retains the ability to write and his speech is normal. This is a form of *agnosia. A patient with aphasic alexia (visual asymbolia) can neither read nor write and often has an accompanying disorder of speech. This is a form of *aphasia. See also dyslexia.

alexin n. a former name for the serum component now called *complement.

alexithymia n. a lack of psychological understanding of one's own emotions and moods. It is considered by some psychiatrists to be a way in which people develop *psychosomatic symptoms.

algesimeter n. a piece of equipment for determining the sensitivity of the skin to various touch stimuli, especially those causing pain.

-algia suffix denoting pain. Example: neuralgia (pain in a nerve).

algid adj. cold: usually describing the cold clammy skin associated with certain forms of malaria.

alienation n. (in psychiatry) **1.** the experience that one's thoughts are under the control of somebody else, or that other people participate in one's thinking. It is a symptom of *schizophrenia. **2.** insanity.

alimentary canal the long passage through which food passes to be digested and absorbed (see illustration). It extends from the mouth to the anus and each region is specialized for a different stage in the processing of food, from mechanical breakdown in the mouth to chemical *digestion and *absorption in the stomach and small intestine and finally to faeces formation and storage in the colon and rectum.

alizarin (alizarin carmine) *n.* an orange-red dye derived from coal tar and originally isolated from the plant madder (*Rubia tinctorum*). Alizarin is insoluble in water but dissolves in alkalis, alcohol, and ether. It is used as a pH indicator and as a histochemical reagent for calcium, thallium, titanium, and zirconium.

alkalaemia *n.* abnormally high blood alkalinity. This may be caused by an increase in the concentration of alkaline substances and/or a decrease in that of acidic substances in the blood. *See also* alkalosis. *Compare* acidaemia.

alkaloid *n.* one of a diverse group of nitrogen-containing substances that are produced by plants and have potent effects on body function. Many alkaloids are important drugs, including *morphine, *quinine, *atropine, and *codeine.

alkalosis *n.* a condition in which the alkalinity of body fluids and tissues is abnormally high. This arises because of a failure of the mechanisms that usually maintain a balance between alkalis and acids in the arterial blood (*see* acid-base balance). Alkalosis may be associated with loss of acid through vomiting or with excessive sodium bicarbonate intake. Breathing that is abnormally deep in relation to the amount of physical exercise may lead to *respiratory alkalosis*. Alkalosis may produce symptoms of muscular weakness or cramp.

alkaptonuria *n. see* alcaptonuria.

allantois *n.* the membranous sac that develops as an outgrowth of the embryonic hindgut. Its outer (mesodermal)

The alimentary canal

layer carries blood vessels to the *placenta and so forms part of the *umbilical cord. Its cavity is small and becomes reduced further in size during fetal development (see urachus). —**allantoic** adj.

allele (allelomorph) n. one of two or more alternative forms of a *gene, only one of which can be present in a chromosome. Two alleles of a particular gene occupy the same relative positions on a pair of *homologous chromosomes. If the two alleles are the same, the individual is *homozygous for the gene; if they are different he is *heterozygous. See also dominant. —**allelic** adj.

allelomorph n. see allele.

allergen n. any *antigen that causes *allergy in a hypersensitive person. Allergens are diverse and affect different tissues and organs. Pollens, fur, feathers, mould, and dust may cause hay fever; house mites have been implicated in some forms of asthma; drugs, dyes, cosmetics, and a host of other chemicals can cause rashes and dermatitis; some food allergies may cause diarrhoea or constipation or simulate acute bacterial food poisoning. When a patient's allergen has been identified, it may be possible to attempt *desensitization to alleviate or prevent allergic attacks. —**allergenic** adj.

allergy n. a disorder in which the body becomes hypersensitive to particular antigens (called *allergens), which provoke characteristic symptoms whenever they are subsequently encountered, whether inhaled, ingested, injected, or otherwise contacted. Normally antibodies in the bloodstream and tissues react with and destroy specific antigens without further trouble. In an allergic person, however, the reaction of allergen with tissue-bound antibody (*reagin) also leads, as a side-effect, to cell damage, release of *histamine and *serotonin, inflammation, and all the symp-

toms of the particular allergy. Different allergies afflict different tissues and may have either local or general effects, varying from asthma and hay fever to severe dermatitis or gastroenteritis or extremely serious shock (see anaphylaxis). —**allergic** adj.

allograft n. see homograft.

alloisoleucine n. one of the isomers of the amino acid isoleucine.

allopathy n. (in homeopathic medicine) the orthodox system of medicine, in which the use of drugs is directed to producing effects in the body that will directly oppose and so alleviate the symptoms of a disease. Compare homeopathy.

allopurinol n. a drug used in the treatment of chronic gout. It acts by reducing the level of uric acid in tissues and blood. It is administered by mouth; side-effects include nausea, vomiting, diarrhoea, headache, fever, stomach pains, and skin rashes. Occasionally, nerve damage and enlargement of the liver may occur.

alloxan n. a *pyrimidine derivative that has been used to induce diabetes in experimental animals as it destroys the cells of the pancreatic islets of Langerhans that produce insulin.

allylestrenol (allyloestrenol) n. a synthetic female sex hormone (see progestogen) used in the treatment of abnormal bleeding from the womb and threatened abortion. It is administered by mouth. Trade name: **Gestanin**.

almoner n. a former name for a *medical social worker.

alopecia (baldness) n. absence of hair from areas where it normally grows. Alopecia may be hereditary (the usual progressive loss of scalp hair in men); it may be due to disease or injury, or it can occur in old age. Alopecia areata is a condition of unknown origin in which hair falls out in patches.

aloxiprin *n.* a compound made from aluminium oxide and *aspirin. Its actions and uses are similar to those of aspirin, but it is said to be more stable and less liable to cause irritation and bleeding of the stomach.

alpha-fetoprotein (afp) *n.* a protein formed in the liver of the fetus and present in the *amniotic fluid in small amounts. In *anencephaly and *spina bifida the amount of afp in the fluid is greatly increased in the first six months of pregnancy, and this can be detected by *amniocentesis. As there is a 1 in 20 chance of recurrence after one child with these defects and a 1 in 10 chance or higher after two affected babies, amniocentesis early in the second trimester of the next pregnancy is advisable, with a view to termination if the afp level is abnormally high.

alprenolol *n.* a drug used to treat arrhythmia and angina of the heart and to reduce high blood pressure (*see* beta blocker). Its actions and uses are similar to those of *propranolol, but it is less likely to affect respiratory function.

ALS 1. *see* antilymphocytic serum. 2. amyotrophic lateral sclerosis. *See* motor neurone disease.

altitude sickness (mountain sickness) the condition that results from unaccustomed exposure to a high altitude (4500 m or more above sea level). Reduced atmospheric pressure and shortage of oxygen cause deep rapid breathing (*hyperventilation), which lowers the concentration of carbon dioxide in the blood (*see* alkalosis). Symptoms include nausea, exhaustion, and anxiety. In severe cases there may be acute shortness of breath due to fluid collecting in the lungs (pulmonary *oedema), which requires treatment by diuretics and return to a lower altitude.

aluminium hydroxide a safe slow-acting antacid and *laxative. It is administered by mouth as a gel in the treatment of indigestion, gastric and duodenal ulcers, and reflux *oesophagitis.

alveolitis *n.* inflammation of an *alveolus or alveoli. Chronic inflammation of the walls of the lung alveoli is usually caused by inhaled inorganic dusts (*see* pneumoconiosis) or organic dusts (*see* farmer's lung). It is sometimes associated with rheumatoid arthritis or systemic sclerosis. The condition progresses slowly to the state of fibrosis, emphysema, and bronchiectasis known as *honeycomb lung*. Alveolitis can be controlled with corticosteroid therapy.

alveolus *n.* (*pl.* **alveoli**) 1. (in the *lung) a blind-ended air sac of microscopic size. About 30 alveoli open out of each *alveolar duct*, which leads from a respiratory *bronchiole. The *alveolar walls*, which separate alveoli, contain capillaries. The alveoli are lined by a single layer of *pneumocytes, which thus form a very thin layer between air and blood so that exchange of oxygen and carbon dioxide is normally rapid and complete. Children are born with about 20 million alveoli. The adult number of about 300 million is reached around the age of eight. 2. the part of the upper or lower jawbone that supports the roots of the teeth (*see also* mandible, maxilla). After tooth extraction it is largely absorbed. 3. the sac of a *racemose gland (*see also* acinus). 4. any other small cavity, depression, or sac. —**alveolar** *adj.*

alveus *n.* a cavity, groove, or canal. The *alveus hippocampi* is the bundle of nerve fibres in the brain forming a depression in which the hippocampus lies.

Alzheimer's disease a progressive form of *dementia occurring in middle age, for which there is no treatment. It is associated with diffuse degeneration of the brain. *Compare* Pick's disease.

amalgam *n.* any of a group of alloys containing mercury. In dentistry amalgam fillings are made by mixing a silver-tin alloy with mercury.

Amanita *n.* a genus of fungi that contains several species of poisonous toadstools, including *A. phalloides* (death cap), *A. pantherina* (panther cap), and *A. muscaria* (fly agaric). They produce toxins that cause abdominal pain, violent vomiting, and continuous diarrhoea. In the absence of treatment death occurs in approximately 50% of cases, due to severe liver damage.

amantadine *n.* an antiviral drug that probably acts by preventing the penetration of the virus into the host cell. It is used in the treatment of influenza infections and parkinsonism. Common side-effects include nervousness, loss of muscular coordination, and insomnia. Trade name: **Symmetrel**.

amaurosis *n.* partial or complete blindness. For example, *amaurosis fugax* is a condition in which loss of vision is transient. —**amaurotic** *adj.*

amaurotic familial idiocy *see* Tay-Sachs disease.

ambivalence *n.* (in psychology) the condition of holding opposite feelings (such as love and hate) for the same person or object. Excessive and prevalent ambivalence was thought by Bleuler to be a feature of schizophrenia.

Amblyomma *n.* a genus of hard *ticks, several species of which are responsible for transmitting tick *typhus. The bite of this tick can also give rise to a serious and sometimes fatal paralysis.

amblyopia *n.* poor sight, not due to any detectable disease of the eyeball or visual system. In practice this strict definition is not always obeyed. For example, in *toxic amblyopia*, caused by tobacco, alcohol, certain other drugs, and vitamin deficiency, there is a disorder of the *optic nerve. The commonest type is *amblyopia ex anopsia*, in which factors such as squint (*see* strabismus), cataract, and other abnormalities of the optics of the eye (*see* refraction) impair its normal use in early childhood by preventing the formation of a clear image on the retina.

amblyoscope (orthoptoscope, synoptophore) *n.* an instrument for measuring the angle of a squint and assessing the degree to which a person uses both eyes together. It consists of two L-shaped tubes, the short arms of which are joined by a hinge so that the long arms point away from each other. The subject looks into the short end and each eye sees, via a system of mirrors and lenses, a different picture, which is placed at the other end of each tube. If a squint is present, the tubes may be adjusted so that the short arms line up with the direction of each eye.

ambutonium *n.* a drug with actions similar to those of *atropine. It is given by mouth to treat indigestion and peptic ulcer.

amelia *n.* congenital total absence of the arms or legs due to a developmental defect. It is one of the fetal abnormalities induced by the drug *thalidomide taken early in pregnancy. *See also* phocomelia.

ameloblast *n.* a cell that forms the enamel of a tooth and disappears before tooth eruption.

ameloblastoma *n.* a locally malignant tumour in the jaw. It is considered to develop from ameloblasts although it does not contain enamel. The term *adamantinoma*, formerly used for this tumour, is now no longer in use as it suggests (incorrectly) a growth that is as hard as enamel.

amelogenesis *n.* the formation of enamel by *ameloblasts, which is completed before tooth eruption. *Amelogenesis imperfecta* is a hereditary condition in which enamel formation is disturbed.

The teeth have an unusual surface but are not more prone to decay.

amenorrhoea *n.* the absence or stopping of the menstrual periods. It is normal for the periods to be absent before puberty, during pregnancy and milk secretion, and after the end of the reproductive period (*see* menopause). In *primary amenorrhoea* the menstrual periods fail to appear at puberty, often because of a congenital defect (e.g. *Turner's syndrome). In *secondary amenorrhoea* the menstrual periods stop after establishment at puberty, for a great variety of reasons including disorders of the hypothalamus (a part of the brain), deficiency of ovarian hormone, *pituitary or thyroid gland deficiency, diabetes, mental disturbance, depression, anorexia nervosa, change of surroundings, and removal of the womb or ovaries.

amentia *n.* failure of development of the intellectual faculties. *See* subnormality.

amethocaine *n.* a potent local anaesthetic. It is applied to skin or mucous membranes for eye, ear, nose and throat surgery, but it has also been employed for *spinal anaesthesia.

ametropia *n.* any abnormality of *refraction of the eye, resulting in blurring of the image formed on the retina. *See* astigmatism, hypermetropia, myopia. *Compare* emmetropia.

amiloride *n.* a *diuretic that causes the increased excretion of sodium and chloride. It may produce dizziness and weakness and its continued use may lead to an excessive concentration of potassium in the blood. Trade name: **Midamor**.

aminacrine *n.* an antiseptic with the same actions and uses as *acriflavine. Unlike acriflavine, it does not cause staining.

amino acid an organic compound containing an amino group (–NH₂) and a carboxyl group (–COOH). Amino acids are fundamental constituents of all *proteins. Breakdown of proteins found in the body yields the following amino acids: alanine, arginine, asparagine, aspartic acid, cysteine, cystine, glutamic acid, glutamine, glycine, histidine, isoleucine, leucine, lysine, methionine, phenylalanine, proline, serine, threonine, tryptophan, tyrosine, and valine. Some of these amino acids can be synthesized by the body; others, the *essential amino acids, must be obtained from protein in the diet. Certain amino acids present in the body are not found in proteins; these include *citrulline, *ornithine, *taurine, and *gamma-aminobutyric acid.

aminobenzoic acid *see* para-aminobenzoic acid.

aminoglutethimide *n.* a drug used in the treatment of advanced breast cancer. It inhibits synthesis of adrenal steroids (medical adrenalectomy) and the peripheral conversion of androgens to oestrogens. It is administered by mouth, usually with corticosteroid replacement therapy. Side-effects, which are largely dose-related, include drowsiness, dizziness, and a transient skin rash. Trade name: **Orimeten**.

aminophylline *n.* a drug that relaxes smooth muscle and stimulates respiration. It is widely used to dilate the air passages in the treatment of asthma and emphysema, to dilate the coronary arteries in angina pectoris, and as a *diuretic, particularly in cases of *oedema. Administered by injection or in suppositories, it may cause nausea, vomiting, dizziness, and fast heart rate. *See also* theophylline.

amitosis *n.* division of the nucleus of a cell by a process, not involving *mitosis, in which the nucleus is constricted into two.

amitriptyline *n.* a tricyclic *antidepressant drug that has a mild tranquillizing action. Common side-effects include drowsiness, dizziness, numbness, and tingling of limbs. Trade names: **Elatrol, Tryptizol**.

amnesia *n.* total or partial loss of memory following physical injury, disease, drugs, or psychological trauma (*see* confabulation, fugue, repression). *Anterograde amnesia* is loss of memory for events following some trauma; *retrograde amnesia* is loss of memory for events preceding the trauma. Some patients experience both types.

amniocentesis *n.* withdrawal of a sample of the fluid (amniotic fluid) surrounding an embryo in the womb by piercing the amniotic sac through the abdominal wall. As the amniotic fluid contains cells from the embryo (mostly shed from the skin), cell cultures enable chromosome patterns to be studied so that *prenatal diagnosis of chromosomal abnormalities (such as *Down's syndrome) can be made. Metabolic errors and other diseases, such as *spina bifida, can also be diagnosed prenatally from the biochemistry of the cells or that of the fluid (*see* alpha-fetoprotein). Although the risks of amniocentesis, in skilled hands, are extremely low, there is no point in undertaking it unless the parents agree to a termination of the pregnancy if a serious abnormality is discovered. The tests must be completed by the 16th week.
Amniocentesis can also be used in the later weeks of pregnancy to assess the severity of fetal (Rh) haemolytic disease and, by measuring lecithin compounds, the risk of the baby developing the *respiratory distress syndrome.

amniography *n.* the making of X-ray pictures (*amniograms*) of the amniotic sac, which enables the placenta and umbilical cord to be visualized.

amnion *n.* the membrane that forms initially over the dorsal part of the embryo but soon expands to enclose it completely within the *amniotic cavity. It expands outwards and fuses with the chorion, obliterating virtually all the intervening cavity. The double membrane (*amniochorion*) normally ruptures at birth. —**amniotic** *adj.*

amnioscopy *n.* examination of the inside of the amniotic sac by means of an instrument (*amnioscope*) that is passed through the abdominal wall. This allows the developing infant within the cavity to be viewed directly. *Cervical amnioscopy*, performed late in pregnancy, enables the amniotic sac to be inspected through the neck of the womb, using a different instrument. When transilluminated, its fluid volume can be appraised without puncture and any meconium observed.

amniotic cavity the fluid-filled cavity between the embryo and the *amnion. It forms initially within the inner cell mass of the *blastocyst and later expands over the back of the embryo, eventually enclosing it completely. *See also* amniotic fluid.

amniotic fluid the fluid contained within the *amniotic cavity. It surrounds the growing fetus, protecting it from external pressure. The fluid is initially secreted from the *amnion and is later supplemented by urine from the fetal kidneys. Some of the fluid is swallowed by the fetus and absorbed through its intestine. *See also* amniocentesis.

amniotomy *n.* the artificial puncturing of the membranes surrounding the baby in the womb by means of a special instrument (*amniotome*). Labour generally follows naturally, but in some cases it must be started artificially by additional measures.

amodiaquine *n.* an antimalarial drug with effects and uses similar to those of *chloroquine. It has also been used for the treatment of lupus erythematosus, leprosy, and rheumatoid arthritis. Doses used to treat malaria have almost no side-effects, but prolonged use may cause blue-grey deposits on the cornea of the eye, fingernails, and hard palate.

amoeba *n.* (*pl.* **amoebae**) any single-celled microscopic animal of jelly-like consistency and irregular and constantly changing shape. Found in water, soil and other damp environments, they move and feed by means of flowing extensions of the body (*see* pseudopodium). Some amoebae cause disease in man (*see* Entamoeba). *See also* Protozoa. —**amoebic** *adj.*

amoebiasis *n. see* dysentery.

amoebocyte *n.* a cell that moves by sending out processes of its protoplasm in the same way as an amoeba.

amoeboma *n.* a tumour that occurs in the rectum or caecum of the large intestine and is caused by the parasite *Entamoeba histolytica*, a protozoan that invades and destroys the walls of the gut. Tumours may ulcerate and become infected with pus-forming (pyogenic) bacteria, causing severe inflammation of the bowel wall. The tumours usually harden and may even obstruct the bowel.

amok *n.* a sudden outburst of furious and murderous aggression, directed indiscriminately at everybody in the vicinity. It is encountered only in certain cultures, such as that of the Malays.

AMP (adenosine monophosphate) a compound containing adenine, ribose, and one phosphate group. AMP occurs in cells and is involved in processes requiring the transfer of energy (*see* ATP).

ampere *n.* the basic *SI unit of electric current. It is equal to the current flowing through a conductor of resistance 1 ohm when a potential differ-

ence of 1 volt is applied between its ends. The formal definition of the ampere is the current that when passed through two parallel conductors of infinite length and negligible cross section, placed 1 metre apart in a vacuum, produces a force of 2×10^{-7} newton per square metre between them. Symbol: A.

amphetamine *n.* a *sympathomimetic drug that has a *marked stimulant action on the central nervous system. It alleviates fatigue and produces a feeling of mental alertness and well-being. The drug has been used in the treatment of *narcolepsy, mild depressive neuroses, and obesity. It is administered by mouth; side-effects include insomnia and restlessness. *Tolerance of amphetamine develops rapidly, and prolonged use may lead to *dependence.

amphiarthrosis *n.* a slightly movable joint in which the bony surfaces are separated by fibrocartilage (*see* symphysis) or hyaline cartilage (*see* synchondrosis).

amphoric breath sounds *see* breath sounds.

amphotericin *n.* an *antibiotic, derived from the bacterium *Streptomyces griseus*, used to treat deep-seated fungal infections; it is inactive against bacteria and viruses. It can be administered by mouth, but is usually given by intravenous injection. Common side-effects include headache, fever, muscle pains, and diarrhoea. In some cases kidney damage may occur.

ampicillin *n.* an *antibiotic used to treat a variety of infections, including those of the urinary, respiratory, biliary, and intestinal tracts. It is inactivated by *penicillinase and therefore cannot be used against organisms producing this enzyme. It is given by mouth or injection; side-effects include nausea, vomiting, and diarrhoea, and some allergic reactions may occur.

ampoule

Trade names: **Amcill, Penbritin, Polycillin, Principen**.

ampoule (ampule) *n.* a sealed glass or plastic capsule containing one dose of a drug in the form of a sterile solution for injection.

ampulla *n.* (*pl.* **ampullae**) an enlarged or dilated ending of a tube or canal. The semicircular canals of the inner ear are expanded into ampullae at the point where they join the vestibule. The *ampulla of Vater* is the dilated part of the common bile duct where it is joined by the pancreatic duct.

amputation *n.* the removal of a limb, part of a limb, or any other portion of the body (such as a breast). The term is customarily modified by an adjective showing the particular type of amputation. Once a common operation in surgery, it is now usually performed only in cases of severe injury to limbs or, particularly in elderly people, when circulation to a limb is inadequate and gangrene develops. In planning an amputation the surgeon takes account of the patient's work and the type of artificial part (prothesis) that will be fitted.

amygdala (amygdaloid nucleus) *n.* one of the *basal ganglia: a roughly almond-shaped mass of grey matter deep inside each cerebral hemisphere. It has extensive connections with the olfactory system and sends fibres to the hypothalamus; its functions are apparently concerned with mood, feeling, instinct, and possibly memory for recent events.

amylase *n.* an enzyme that occurs in saliva and pancreatic juice and aids the digestion of starch, which it breaks down into glucose, maltose, and dextrins. Amylase will also hydrolyse *glycogen to yield glucose, maltose, and dextrins.

amyl nitrite a drug that relaxes smooth muscle, especially that of blood vessels. Given by inhalation, amyl nitrite is used mainly in the treatment of angina pectoris. It is rapidly absorbed and acts quickly, producing a fall in arterial blood pressure. Side-effects include flushing, faintness, and headache. High doses may cause restlessness, vomiting, and blue coloration of the skin.

amylobarbitone *n.* an intermediate-acting *barbiturate, administered by mouth as a *hypnotic in the treatment of insomnia, as a preoperative sedative, and to treat for anxiety. It is also injected intravenously to produce mental relaxation before psychoanalysis. Prolonged use may lead to *dependence and overdosage has serious toxic effects (*see* barbiturism). Trade names: **Amytal, Amobarbital**.

amyloid *n.* a *glycoprotein, resembling starch, that is deposited in the internal organs in amyloidosis.

amyloidosis *n.* infiltration of the liver, kidneys, spleen, and other tissues with amyloid, a starchlike substance. In *primary amyloidosis* the disorder arises without any apparent cause; *secondary amyloidosis* occurs as a late complication of such chronic infections as tuberculosis or leprosy and also in *Hodgkin's disease. Amyloidosis is also very common in the genetic disease familial Mediterranean fever (*see* polyserositis).

amylopectin *n. see* starch.

amylose *n. see* starch.

amyotonia congenita (floppy baby syndrome) a disorder, present at birth, in which the child's muscles are weak and floppy. A gradual spontaneous improvement occurs and the child's progress is thereafter normal. It must be distinguished from the hypotonic form of *cerebral palsy, infantile *motor neurone disease, and congenital myopathy, which are usually progressive.

amyotrophy *n.* a progressive loss of muscle bulk associated with weakness of these muscles. It is caused by disease of the nerve that activates the affected muscle. Amyotrophy is a feature of any chronic *neuropathy and it may be the most prominent neurological symptom of diabetes mellitus and meningovascular syphilis. A combination of amyotrophy and spasticity characterizes *motor neurone disease.

an- *prefix. see* a-.

anabolic *adj.* promoting tissue growth by increasing the metabolic processes involved in protein synthesis. Anabolic agents are usually synthetic male sex hormones (*see* androgen); they include *ethyloestrenol, *methandienone, nandrolone, norethandrolone, oxymesterone, and stanolone. They are used to help weight gain in underweight patients, such as the elderly and those with serious illnesses, and to strengthen the bones in osteoporosis. Some anabolic steroids cause virilization in women and liver damage.

anabolism *n.* the synthesis of complex molecules, such as proteins and fats, from simpler ones by living things. *See also* anabolic, metabolism.

anacidity *n.* a deficiency or abnormal absence of acid in the body fluids.

anacrotism *n.* the condition in which there is an abnormal curve in the ascending line of a pulse tracing. It may be seen in cases of aortic stenosis. —**anacrotic** *adj.*

anaemia *n.* a reduction in the quantity of the oxygen-carrying pigment *haemoglobin in the blood. The main symptoms are excessive tiredness and fatiguability, breathlessness on exertion, pallor, and poor resistance to infection. There are many causes of anaemia. It may be due to loss of blood (*haemorrhagic anaemia*), resulting from an accident, operation, etc., or from chronic bleeding, as from an ulcer or haemor-

rhoids. *Iron-deficiency anaemia* results from lack of iron, which is necessary for the production of haemoglobin (*see* sideropenia). *Haemolytic anaemias* result from the increased destruction of red blood cells (which contain the pigment). This can be caused by toxic chemicals; *autoimmunity; the action of parasites, especially in *malaria; or conditions such as *thalassaemia and *sickle-cell disease, associated with abnormal forms of haemoglobin, or *spherocytosis, which is associated with abnormal red blood cells. (*See also* haemolytic disease of the newborn.) Anaemia can also be caused by the impaired production of red blood cells, as in *leukaemia (when red-cell production in the bone marrow is suppressed) or *pernicious anaemia.
Anaemias can be classified on the basis of the size of the red cells, which may be large (*macrocytic anaemias*), small (*microcytic anaemias*), or normal-sized (*normocytic anaemias*). (*See also* macrocytosis, microcytosis.) The treatment of anaemia depends on the cause. —**anaemic** *adj.*

anaerobe *n.* any organism, especially a microbe, that is able to live and grow in the absence of free oxygen. A *facultative anaerobe* is a microorganism that grows best in the presence of oxygen but is capable of some growth in its absence. An *obligate anaerobe* can grow only in the absence of free oxygen. *Compare* aerobe, microaerophilic.

anaerobic *adj.* **1.** of or relating to anaerobes. **2.** describing a type of cellular respiration in which foodstuffs (usually carbohydrates) are never completely oxidized because molecular oxygen is not used. *Fermentation is an example of anaerobic respiration.

anaesthesia *n.* loss of feeling or sensation in a part or all of the body. Anaesthesia of a part of the body may occur as a result of injury to or disease of a nerve; for example in leprosy. The term is usually applied, however, to the medical technique of reducing or abolishing an individual's sensation of pain to enable surgery to be performed. This is effected by administering drugs (*see* anaesthetic) or by the use of other methods, such as *acupuncture or hypnosis.

General anaesthesia is total unconsciousness, usually achieved by administering a combination of injections and gases (the latter are inhaled through a mask). It is induced for such major operations as removal of the stomach or a lung. Recently, anaesthesia has been used in combination with artificial lowering of the body temperature (hypothermia) in certain complex operations, such as cardiac surgery. *Local anaesthesia* abolishes pain in a limited area of the body and is used for minor operations, particularly many dental procedures. It may be achieved by injections of substances such as lignocaine (commonly used in dentistry) close to a local nerve, which deadens the tissues supplied by that nerve. Local anaesthesia may be combined with intravenous sedation. An appropriate injection into the spinal column produces *spinal anaesthesia in the lower limbs or abdomen.

anaesthetic 1. *n.* an agent that reduces or abolishes sensation, affecting either the whole body (*general anaesthetic*) or a particular region (*local anaesthetic*). General anaesthetics, used for surgical procedures, depress activity of the central nervous system, producing loss of consciousness. *Anaesthesia is induced by short-acting *barbiturates (such as thiopentone) and maintained by inhalation anaesthetics (such as *halothane). Local anaesthetics inhibit conduction of impulses in sensory nerves in the region where they are injected or applied; they include *cocaine and *lignocaine. **2.** *adj.* reducing or abolishing sensation.

anaesthetist *n.* a medically qualified doctor who administers an anaesthetic to induce unconsciousness in a patient before a surgical operation.

anákhré *n. see* goundou.

anal *adj.* of, relating to, or affecting the anus; for example an anal *fissure or an anal *fistula.

analeptic *n.* a drug that restores consciousness to a patient in a coma or faint; for example, *ethamivan or *nalorphine. Analeptics stimulate the central nervous system to counteract the effects of large doses of narcotic drugs, which depress the central nervous system.

analgesia *n.* reduced sensibility to pain, without loss of consciousness and without the sense of touch necessarily being affected. The condition may arise accidentally, if nerves are diseased or damaged, or be induced deliberately by the use of pain-killing drugs (*see* analgesic). Strictly speaking, local *anaesthesia should be called *local analgesia*. *See also* relative analgesia.

analgesic 1. *n.* a drug that relieves pain. Mild analgesics, such as *aspirin and *paracetamol, are used for the relief of headache, toothache, and mild rheumatic pain. More potent *narcotic analgesics*, such as *morphine and *pethidine, are used only to relieve severe pain since these drugs may produce *dependence and *tolerance. Some analgesics, including aspirin, *ibuprofen, *indomethacin, and *phenylbutazone, also reduce fever and inflammation and are used in rheumatic conditions. **2.** *adj.* relieving pain.

analogous *adj.* describing organs or parts that have similar functions in different organisms although they do not have the same evolutionary origin or development. *Compare* homologous.

analysand *n.* a person undergoing *psychoanalysis.

analysis *n.* (in psychology) any means of understanding complex mental processes or experiences. There are several systems of analysis used by different schools of psychology; for example, *psychoanalysis; transactional analysis,* in which people's relationships are explained in psychoanalytic terms; and *functional analysis,* in which a particular kind of behaviour is thoroughly described with reference to its frequency, its antecedents, and its consequences.

anamnesis *n.* memory, particularly the recollection by a patient of the symptoms that he noticed at the time when his disease was first contracted.

anankastic *adj.* describing a collection of long-standing personality traits, including stubbornness, meanness, an over-meticulous concern to be accurate in small details, a disposition to check things unnecessarily, severe feelings of insecurity about personal worth, and an excessive tendency to doubt evident facts. *See* personality disorder, obsession.

anaphase *n.* the third stage of *mitosis and of each division of *meiosis. In mitosis and anaphase II of meiosis the chromatids separate, becoming daughter chromosomes, and move apart along the spindle fibres towards opposite ends of the cell. In anaphase I of meiosis the pairs of homologous chromosomes separate from each other. *See* disjunction.

anaphylaxis *n.* an abnormal reaction to a particular *antigen, in which histamine is released from tissues and causes either local or widespread symptoms. An allergic attack (*see* allergy) is an example of localized anaphylaxis. Rarer, but much more serious, is *anaphylactic shock*: an extreme and generalized allergic reaction in which widespread histamine release causes swelling (oedema), constriction of the bronchioles, heart failure, circulatory collapse, and sometimes death. —**anaphylactic** *adj.*

anaplasia *n.* a loss of normal cell characteristics or differentiation, which may be to such a degree that it is impossible to define the origin of the cells. Anaplasia is typical of malignant tumours.

anasarca *n.* massive swelling of the legs, trunk, and genitalia due to retention of fluid (*oedema): found in congestive heart failure and some forms of renal failure.

anastomosis *n.* **1.** (in anatomy) a communication between two blood vessels without any intervening capillary network. *See* arteriovenous anastomosis. **2.** (in surgery) an artificial connection between two tubular organs or parts, especially between two normally separate parts of the intestine. *See also* shunt.

anatomy *n.* the study of the structure of living organisms. In medicine it refers to the study of the form and gross structure of the various parts of the human body. The term *morphology* is sometimes used synonymously with anatomy but it is usually used for *comparative anatomy*: the study of differences in form between species. *See also* cytology, histology, physiology. —**anatomical** *adj.* —**anatomist** *n.*

anatoxin *n.* a former name for *toxoid.

anconeus *n.* a muscle behind the elbow that assists in extending the forearm.

Ancylostoma (Ankylostoma) *n.* a genus of small parasitic nematodes (*see* hookworm) that inhabit the small intestine and are widely distributed in Europe, America, Asia, and Africa. The worms suck blood from the gut wall, to which they are attached by means of cutting teeth. Man is the principal and optimum host for *A. duodenale.*

ancylostomiasis *n.* an infestation of the small intestine by the parasitic hookworm *Ancylostoma duodenale*. *See* hookworm disease.

andr- (andro-) *prefix denoting* man or the male sex. Example: *androphobia* (morbid fear of).

androblastoma (arrhenoblastoma) *n.* a tumour of the ovary, composed of Sertoli cells, Leydig cells, or both. It can produce male or female hormones and may give rise to *masculinization; in children it may cause precocious puberty. Up to 30% of these tumours are malignant, but probably as many as 85% of all cases are cured by surgery alone.

androgen *n.* one of a group of steroid hormones, including *testosterone* and *androsterone*, that stimulate the development of male sex organs and male secondary sexual characteristics (e.g. beard growth, deepening of the voice, and muscle development). The principal source of these hormones is the testis (production being stimulated by *luteinizing hormone) but they are also secreted by the adrenal cortex and ovaries in small amounts. In women excessive production of androgens gives rise to *masculinization.

Naturally occurring and synthetic androgens are used in replacement therapy (to treat such conditions as delayed puberty in adolescent boys, *hypogonadism, and impotence due to testicular insufficiency); as *anabolic agents; and in the treatment of breast cancer. Side-effects include salt and water retention, increased bone growth, and masculinization in women. Androgens should not be used in patients with cancer of the prostate gland or in pregnant women. —**androgenic** *adj.*

androsterone *n.* a steroid hormone (*see* androgen) that is synthesized and released by the testes and is responsible for controlling male sexual development.

anencephaly *n.* partial or complete absence of the bones of the rear of the skull and of the cerebral hemispheres of the brain. It occurs as a developmental defect and is not compatible with life for more than a few hours. It is often associated with other defects of the nervous system, such as *spina bifida. Tests for anencephaly can be made early in pregnancy in women from families with a history of the condition (*see* amniocentesis, alpha-fetoprotein).

anergy *n.* **1.** lack of response to a specific antigen or allergen. **2.** lack of energy. —**anergic** *adj.*

aneuploidy *n.* the condition in which the chromosome number of a cell is not an exact multiple of the normal basic (haploid) number. *See* monosomy, trisomy; *compare* euploidy. —**aneuploid** *adj.*, *n.*

aneurin *n. see* vitamin B_1.

aneurysm *n.* a balloon-like swelling in the wall of an artery. This may be due to degenerative disease or syphilitic infection, which damages the muscular coats of the vessel, or it may be the result of congenital deficiency in the muscular wall. An *aortic aneurysm* may develop anywhere in the aorta. A *dissecting aneurysm* usually affects the first part of the aorta and results from a degenerative condition of its muscular coat. This weakness predisposes to a tear in the lining of the aorta, which allows blood to enter the wall and track along (dissect) the muscular coat. A dissecting aneurysm may rupture or it may compress the blood vessels arising from the aorta and produce infarction (localized necrosis) in the organs they supply. The patient complains of severe chest pain that has a tearing quality and often spreads to the back or abdomen. Surgical repair may help in some cases. A *ventricular aneurysm* may develop in the wall of the left ventricle after myocardial infarction. A segment of myocardium becomes replaced by scar tissue, which expands to form an aneurysmal sac. Heart failure may result or thrombosis within the aneurysm may act as a source of embolism.

Most aneurysms within the brain are congenital: there is a risk that they may burst, causing a *subarachnoid haemorrhage. *Charcot-Bouchard aneurysms* are small aneurysms found on tiny arteries within the brain of elderly and hypertensive subjects. These aneurysms may rupture, causing cerebral haemorrhage. *See also* arteriovenous aneurysm. —**aneurysmal** *adj.*

angi- (angio-) *prefix denoting* blood or lymph vessels. Examples: *angiectasis* (abnormal dilation of); *angiopathy* (disease of); *angiotomy* (cutting of).

angiitis (vasculitis) *n.* a patchy inflammation of the walls of small blood vessels. It may result from a variety of conditions, including *polyarteritis nodosa, acute nephritis, and serum sickness. Symptoms include skin rashes, arthritis, purpura, and kidney failure. In some cases treatment with cortisone derivatives may be beneficial.

angina *n.* a sense of suffocation or suffocating pain. *See* angina pectoris, Ludwig's angina.

angina pectoris pain in the centre of the chest, which is induced by exercise and relieved by rest and may spread to the jaws and arms. Angina pectoris occurs when the demand for blood by the heart exceeds the supply of the coronary arteries and it usually results from coronary artery *atheroma. It may be prevented or relieved by such drugs as *glyceryl trinitrate and *propranolol. If drug treatment proves ineffective, *coronary angioplasty or *coronary bypass grafting may be required, the former being less invasive than the latter.

angiocardiography *n.* X-ray examination of the chambers of the heart after introducing a *radio-opaque contrast medium into the blood in the heart.

The contrast medium (e.g. Cardioconray) is injected directly into the atria, ventricles, or great vessels of the heart by means of a slim sterile flexible tube (*cardiac catheter*), which is manipulated into position from an accessible point, such as a vein or artery in a limb (*see* (cardiac) catheterization). Its progress through the heart is followed by a rapid series of X-ray films or by the use of cine film (*cineangiocardiography). The X-ray is called an *angiocardiogram*. Angiocardiography is an important aid in diagnosing and planning the surgical repair of heart defects.

angiography *n.* X-ray examination of blood vessels. A dye that is opaque to X-rays is injected into the artery and a rapid series of X-ray films is taken (*see* arteriography). *Fluorescein angiography* is a common method of investigation in ophthalmology. *Fluorescein sodium is injected into a vein in the arm, from which it circulates throughout the body. Light of an appropriate wavelength is shone into the eye, causing the dye in the retinal blood vessels to fluoresce. This allows the circulation through the retinal blood vessels to be observed and photographed.

angioid *adj.* resembling a blood vessel.

angiokeratoma *n.* a localized collection of thin-walled blood vessels covered by a cap of warty material. It is most often seen as an isolated malformation in the genital skin of the elderly or on the hands and feet of children. It is not malignant and its cause is unknown. Angiokeratomas may be removed surgically. Multiple angiokeratomas affecting the viscera and skin are seen as a rare inherited and fatal disease (*Fabry's disease*).

angiology *n.* the branch of medicine concerned with the structure, function, and diseases of blood vessels.

angioma (arteriovenous malformation) *n.* a knot of distended blood vessels overlying and compressing the surface of the brain. It commonly causes epilepsy and less often one of the vessels may burst, causing a *subarachnoid haemorrhage. It may be associated with a purple birthmark on the face: this is called the *Sturge-Weber syndrome. See also* haemangioma, lymphangioma.

angioneurotic oedema an allergic condition producing transient or persistent swelling of areas of skin accompanied by itching, which may be severe. It is caused by *allergy to food substances, drugs, or other allergens or it may be precipitated by heat, cold, or emotional factors. *See also* urticaria.

angiospasm *n. see* Raynaud's disease.

angiotensin *n.* a protein in the blood, derived from a plasma protein and released by the action of an enzyme (*renin) from the kidneys, that causes an increase in the output of *aldosterone from the adrenal cortex. Angiotensin is also capable of causing constriction of blood vessels, thus raising blood pressure.

angle *n.* **1.** (in anatomy) a corner. For example, the *angle of the eye* is the outer or inner corner of the eye; the *angle of the mouth* is the site where the upper and lower lips join on either side. **2.** the degree of divergence of two lines or planes that meet each other; the space between two such lines. The *carrying angle* is the obtuse angle formed between the forearm and the upper arm when the forearm is fully extended and the hand is supinated.

angstrom *n.* a unit of length equal to one ten millionth of a millimetre (10^{-10} m). It is not a recommended *SI unit but is sometimes used to express wavelengths and interatomic distances: the *nanometre (1 nm = 10 Å) is now the preferred unit. Symbol Å.

anhidrotic 1. *n.* any drug that inhibits the secretion of sweat, such as *para-sympatholytic drugs. **2.** *adj.* inhibiting sweating.

anhydraemia *n.* a decrease in the proportion of water, and therefore plasma, in the blood.

anhydrase *n.* an enzyme that catalyses the removal of water from a compound.

anidrosis (anhidrosis) *n.* the abnormal absence of sweating, accompanying disease or occurring as a congenital defect.

anileridine *n.* a synthetic narcotic analgesic drug, given by mouth or by injection to relieve pain or support anaesthesia. It has the same uses, actions, and toxic effects as *morphine. Drug *dependence, with marked withdrawal symptoms, is easily produced by repeated administration. Trade name: **Leritine**.

anima *n.* (in Jungian psychology) an *archetype that is the feminine component of a male's personality.

animus *n.* the *archetype that is the masculine component of a female's personality.

aniridia *n.* congenital absence of the iris (of the eye).

aniseikonia *n.* a condition in which the image of an object differs markedly in size or shape in each eye.

anisocytosis *n.* an excessive variation in size between individual red blood cells. Anisocytosis may be noted on microscopical examination of a blood film; from this a graph of the numbers of cells of different sizes may be drawn. Anisocytosis may be a feature of almost any disease affecting the blood.

anisomelia *n.* a difference in size or shape between the arms or the legs.

anisometropia *n.* the condition in which the power of *refraction in one eye differs markedly from that in the other.

ankle *n.* **1.** the hinge joint between the leg and the foot. It consists of the *talus (ankle bone), which projects into a socket formed by the lower ends of the *tibia and *fibula. **2.** the whole region of the ankle joint, including the *tarsus and the lower parts of the tibia and fibula.

ankylosing spondylitis *see* spondylitis.

ankylosis *n.* fusion of the bones across a joint space, either by bony tissue (*bony ankylosis*) or by shortening of connecting fibrous tissue (*fibrous ankylosis*). Ankylosis is a complication of prolonged joint inflammation, as may occur in chronic infection (e.g. tuberculosis) or rheumatic disease (e.g. ankylosing *spondylitis).

Ankylostoma *n.* *see* Ancylostoma.

annulus *n.* (in anatomy) a circular opening or ring-shaped structure. —**annular** *adj.*

anodontia *n.* absence of the teeth because they have failed to develop. It is more common for only a few teeth to fail to develop (*see* hypodontia).

anodyne *n.* any treatment or drug that soothes and eases pain.

anomalopia *n.* *Obsolete.* defective colour vision (*see* colour blindness).

anomaloscope *n.* an instrument for testing colour discrimination. By adjusting the controls of the instrument the subject has to produce a mixture of red and green light to match a yellow light. The matching is done on a brightly illuminated disc viewed down a telescope.

anomalous pulmonary venous drainage a congenital abnormality in which the pulmonary veins enter the right atrium or vena cava instead of draining normally into the left atrium. The features are those of an atrial *septal defect.

anomaly *n.* any deviation from the normal, especially a congenital or developmental defect.

anomia *n.* **1.** a form of *aphasia in which the patient is unable to give the names of objects, although retaining an understanding of their use and the ability to put words together into speech. **2.** absence of respect for laws and established customs, which is a feature of *psychopathy.

anonychia *n.* congenital absence of one or more nails.

Anopheles *n.* a genus of widely distributed mosquitoes, occurring in tropical and temperate regions, with some 350 species. The malarial parasite (*see* Plasmodium) is transmitted to man solely through the bite of female *Anopheles* mosquitoes. Some species of *Anopheles* may transmit the parasites of bancroftian *filariasis.

anorchism *n.* congenital absence of one or both testes.

anorexia *n.* loss of appetite.

anorexia nervosa a psychological illness, most common in female adolescents, in which the patients have no desire to eat; eating may, in fact, be abhorrent to them. The problem often starts with a simple desire to lose weight, which then becomes an obsession. The result is severe loss of weight and sometimes even death from starvation. The cause of the illness is complicated – problems within the family and rejection of adult sexuality are often factors involved. Patients must usually be treated by *psychotherapy.

anosmia *n.* a loss of the sense of smell. This is most often due to a head cold but it may be caused by a fracture through the anterior fossa of the skull or a frontal brain tumour.

anovular (anovulatory) *adj.* not associated with the development and release of a female germ cell (ovum) in the ovary, as in *anovular menstruation*.

anoxaemia *n.* a condition in which there is less than the normal concentration of oxygen in the blood. *See also* anoxia, hypoxaemia.

anoxia *n.* a condition in which the tissues of the body receive inadequate amounts of oxygen. This may result from low atmospheric pressure at high altitudes; a shortage of circulating blood, red blood cells, or haemoglobin; or disordered blood flow, such as occurs in heart failure. It can also result from insufficient oxygen reaching the blood in the lungs due to poor breathing movements or because disease, such as pneumonia, is reducing the effective surface area of lung tissue. *See also* hypoxia. —**anoxic** *adj.*

ansa *n.* (in anatomy) a loop; for example, the *ansa hypoglossi* is the loop formed by the descending branch of the hypoglossal nerve.

ansiform *adj.* (in anatomy) shaped like a loop. The term is applied to certain lobules of the cerebellum.

ant- (anti-) *prefix denoting* opposed to; counteracting; relieving. Examples: *antarthritic* (relieving arthritis); *antibacterial* (destroying or stopping the growth of bacteria).

Antabuse *n. see* disulfiram.

antacid *n.* a drug that neutralizes the hydrochloric acid secreted in the digestive juices of the stomach. Antacids, which include aluminium hydroxide, calcium carbonate, magnesium hydroxide, and sodium bicarbonate, are used to relieve pain and discomfort in disorders of the digestive system, including peptic ulcer.

antagonist *n.* **1.** a muscle whose action (contraction) opposes that of another muscle (called the *agonist* or *prime mover*). Antagonists relax to allow the agonists to effect movement. **2.** a drug or other substance with opposite action to that of another drug or natural body chemical, which it inhibits. Examples are the *antimetabolites. —**antagonism** *n.*

antazoline *n.* a short-acting *antihistamine drug, given by mouth to relieve the symptoms of allergic reactions. It is less irritating than the other antihistamines, but it produces their characteristic side-effects, such as drowsiness, dizziness, and incoordination.

ante- *prefix denoting* before. Examples: *antenatal* (before birth); *anteprandial* (before meals).

anteflexion *n.* the abnormal bending forward of an organ, especially the bending of the body of the womb towards the front.

ante mortem before death. *Compare* post mortem.

antenatal diagnosis *see* prenatal diagnosis.

Antepar *n. see* piperazine.

antepartum *adj.* occurring before the onset of labour.

anterior *adj.* **1.** describing or relating to the front (ventral) portion of the body or limbs. **2.** describing the front part of any organ.

anteversion *n.* the normal forward inclination of the womb.

anthelmintic **1.** *n.* any drug or chemical agent used to destroy parasitic worms (helminths), e.g. tapeworms, roundworms, and flukes, and/or remove them from the body. Anthelmintics include *dichlorophen, *mepacrine, and *piperazine. **2.** *adj.* having the power to destroy or eliminate helminths.

anthracosis *n.* a lung disease – a form of *pneumoconiosis – caused by coal dust. It affects mainly coal miners but also other exposed workers, such as lightermen, if the lungs' capacity to accommodate and remove the particles is exceeded.

anthracycline *n.* any of 500 or so antibiotics synthesized or isolated from species of *Streptomyces.* *Doxorubicin is the most important member of this group of compounds, which have wide activity against tumours.

anthrax *n.* an acute infectious disease of farm animals caused by the bacterium *Bacillus anthracis*, which can be transmitted to man by contact with animal hair, hides, or excrement. In man the disease attacks either the lungs, causing pneumonia (*woolsorter's disease*), or the skin, producing severe ulceration (known as *malignant pustule*). Untreated anthrax can be fatal but administration of large doses of penicillin or tetracycline is usually effective.

anthrop- (anthropo-) *prefix denoting* the human race. Examples: *anthropogenesis* (origin and development of); *anthropoid* (resembling); *anthropology* (science of).

anthropometry *n.* the taking of measurements of the human body or its parts. Comparisons can then be made between individuals of different sexes, ages, and races to determine the difference between normal and abnormal development. —**anthropometric** *adj.*

anthropozoonosis *n.* a disease that is transmissible from an animal to man, or vice versa, under natural conditions. Diseases that are found primarily in animals and sometimes affect man include *anthrax, *rabies, and *leptospirosis.

antibiotic *n.* a substance, produced by or derived from a microorganism, that destroys or inhibits the growth of other microorganisms. Antibiotics are used to treat infections caused by organisms that are sensitive to them, usually bacteria or fungi. They may alter the normal microbial content of the body (e.g. in the intestine, lungs, bladder) by destroying one or more groups of harmless organisms, which may result in infections due to overgrowth of resistant organisms. These side-effects are most likely to occur with *broad-spectrum antibiotics* (those active against a wide variety of organisms). Resistance may also develop in the microorganisms being treated (for example, through incorrect dosage), and some antibiotics may cause allergic reactions. Antibiotics should not be used for minor infections, which will clear up unaided. *See also* cephalosporin, chloramphenicol, penicillin, streptomycin, tetracycline.

antibody *n.* a special kind of blood protein that is synthesized in lymphoid tissue in response to the presence of a particular *antigen and circulates in the plasma to attack the antigen and render it harmless. The production of specific antibodies against antigens as diverse as invading bacteria, inhaled pollen grains, and foreign red blood cells is the basis of both *immunity and *allergy. Antibody formation is also responsible for tissue or organ rejection following transplantation. Chemically, antibodies are proteins of the globulin type; they are classified according to their structure and function (*see* immunoglobulin).

anticholinergic *adj.* inhibiting the action of *acetylcholine. *Parasympatholytic drugs are anticholinergic.

anticholinesterase *n.* any substance that inhibits the action of *cholinesterase, the enzyme responsible for the breakdown of the neurotransmitter acetylcholine, and therefore allows acetylcholine to continue transmitting nerve impulses. Drugs with anticholinesterase activity include *neostigmine and *physostigmine; their uses include the diagnosis and treatment of *my-

anticoagulant

asthenia gravis. *See also* parasympathomimetic.

anticoagulant *n.* an agent that prevents the clotting of blood. The natural anticoagulant *heparin directly interferes with blood clotting and is active both within the body and against a sample of blood in a test tube. Synthetic drugs, such as *dicoumarol, *phenindione, and *warfarin, are effective only within the body, since they act by affecting blood *coagulation factors. They take longer to act than heparin. Anticoagulants are used to prevent the formation of blood clots or to break up clots in blood vessels in such conditions as thrombosis and embolism. Incorrect dosage may result in haemorrhage.

anticonvulsant *n.* a drug that prevents or reduces the severity of fits (convulsions) in various types of epilepsy. The choice of anticonvulsant is dictated by the type of fit and the patient's response. Some anticonvulsants, such as *sodium valproate, are used to treat all types of epileptic fits. Others are used specifically for petit mal (e.g. *ethosuximide and *troxidone) or for focal and grand mal epilepsy (e.g. *phenytoin, *primidone, *carbamazepine). The dosage must be adjusted carefully as individuals vary in their response to these drugs and side-effects may be troublesome.

antidepressant *n.* a drug that alleviates the symptoms of depression. The most widely prescribed antidepressants are a group of drugs with a basic chemical structure of three benzene rings, called *tricyclic antidepressants*, which include *amitriptyline and *imipramine. These drugs are useful in treating a variety of different depressive symptoms. Side-effects commonly include dry mouth, blurred vision, constipation, drowsiness, and difficulty in urination. The other main group of antidepressants are the *MAO inhibitors, which have more severe side-effects.

antidiuretic hormone (ADH) *see* vasopressin.

antidote *n.* a drug that counteracts the effects of a poison. For example, *dimercaprol is an antidote to arsenic, mercury, and other heavy metals.

antidromic *adj.* describing impulses travelling 'the wrong way' in a nerve fibre. This is rare but may happen in shingles, when the irritation caused by the virus in the spinal canal initiates impulses that travel outwards in normally afferent nerves. The area of skin that the sensory nerves supply (usually a strip on the trunk) becomes painfully blistered. Antidromic impulses cannot pass *synapses, which work in one direction only.

antiemetic *n.* a drug that prevents vomiting. Various drugs have this effect, including some *antihistamines (e.g. cyclizine, promethazine) and *anticholinergic drugs. They are used for such conditions as motion sickness and vertigo and to counteract nausea and vomiting caused by other drugs.

antigen *n.* any substance that the body regards as foreign or potentially dangerous and against which it produces an *antibody. Antigens are usually proteins, but simple substances, even metals, may become antigenic by combining with and modifying the body's own proteins. These are called *haptens*. —**antigenic** *adj.*

antihelix (anthelix) *n.* the curved inner ridge of the *pinna of the ear.

antihistamine *n.* a drug that inhibits some of the effects of *histamine in the body, in particular its role in allergic reactions. Examples are *chlorpheniramine, *diphenhydramine, and *mepyramine. Antihistamines are used mainly for the relief of hay fever, pruritus (itching), rhinitis, urticaria (nettle rash), and other allergic reactions. Many antihistamines, e.g. *cyclizine and *promethazine, also have strong *antiemetic activity and are used to prevent motion sickness. The most common side-effect of antihistamines is drowsiness and because of this they are sometimes used to promote sleep. Other side-effects include dizziness, blurred vision, tremors, digestive upsets, and lack of muscular coordination.

antiketogenic *n.* an agent that prevents formation of *ketones in the body.

antilymphocytic serum (ALS) an *antiserum, containing antibodies that suppress lymphocytic activity, prepared by injecting an animal with lymphocytes. ALS may be given to a patient to prevent the immune reaction that causes tissue rejection following transplantation of such organs as kidneys. Administration naturally also impairs other immunity mechanisms, making infection a serious hazard.

antimetabolite *n.* a drug that interferes with the normal metabolic processes within cells by combining with the enzymes responsible for them. Some drugs used in the treatment of cancer, e.g. *fluorouracil, *methotrexate, and *mercaptopurine, are antimetabolites that prevent cell growth by interfering with enzyme reactions essential for nucleic acid synthesis. Side-effects of antimetabolites can be severe, involving blood cell disorders and digestive disturbances. *See also* cytotoxic drug.

antimitotic *n.* a drug that inhibits cell division and growth, e.g. *procarbazine. The drugs used to treat cancer are mainly antimitotics. *See also* antimetabolite, cytotoxic drug.

antimony potassium tartrate (tartar emetic) a toxic and irritating salt of antimony. It is administered (usually by slow intravenous injection) for the treatment of *schistosomiasis and *leishmaniasis but may produce severe side-effects, particularly vomiting; it should not be used in patients with heart, kidney, or liver disease. A salt with similar effects and uses is *antimony sodium tartrate*.

antimutagen *n.* a substance that can either reduce the spontaneous production of mutations or prevent or reverse the action of a *mutagen.

antimycotic *n.* a drug active against fungi. Antimycotics are used to treat fungal infections; they include *griseofulvin and *nystatin.

antiperistalsis *n.* a wave of contraction in the alimentary canal that passes in an oral (i.e. upward or backwards) direction (*compare* peristalsis). It was formerly thought that antiperistalsis occurred in vomiting but modern physiological studies indicate that it never takes place in man.

antipruritic *n.* an agent that relieves itching (*pruritus). Examples are *calamine and *crotamiton, applied in creams or lotions, and some *antihistamine drugs, used if the itching is due to an allergy.

antipyretic *n.* a drug that reduces fever by lowering the body temperature. Several analgesic drugs have antipyretic activity, including *aspirin, *mefanamic acid, *paracetamol, and *phenylbutazone.

antisepsis *n.* the elimination of bacteria, fungi, viruses, and other microorganisms that cause disease by the use of chemical or physical methods.

antiseptic *n.* a chemical that destroys or inhibits the growth of disease-causing bacteria and other microorganisms and is sufficiently nontoxic to be applied to the skin or mucous membranes to cleanse wounds and prevent infections or to be used internally to treat infections of the intestine and bladder.

Examples are *crystal violet, *dequalinium, and *hexamine.

antiserum *n.* (*pl.* **antisera**) a serum that contains antibodies against antigens of a particular kind; it may be injected to treat, or give temporary protection (passive *immunity) against, specific diseases. Antisera are prepared in large quantities in such animals as horses. In the laboratory, they are used to identify unknown organisms responsible for infection (*see* agglutination).

antispasmodic *n.* a drug that relieves spasm of smooth muscle. *See* spasmolytic.

antitoxin *n.* an antibody produced by the body to counteract a toxin formed by invading bacteria or from any other source.

antitragus *n.* a small projection of cartilage above the lobe of the ear, opposite the tragus. *See* pinna.

antitussive *n.* a drug, such as *dextromethorphan or *pholcodine, that suppresses coughing, possibly by reducing the activity of the cough centre in the brain and by depressing respiration. Some analgesic drugs also have antitussive activity, e.g. *codeine, diamorphine (*see* heroin), and *methadone.

antivenene (antivenin) *n.* an *antiserum containing antibodies against specific poisons in the venom of such an animal as a snake, spider, or scorpion.

antrectomy *n.* **1.** surgical removal of the bony walls of an *antrum. *See* antrostomy. **2.** a surgical operation in which a part of the stomach (the antrum) is removed. Most secretions of acid, pepsin, and the hormone gastrin occur in the antrum and the operation is used (usually combined with *vagotomy) in the treatment of peptic ulcers.

antroscope *n.* an *endoscope that can be introduced into the stomach via the oesophagus to obtain a view of the pyloric antrum, the region of the stomach wall near the pyloric sphincter.

antrostomy *n.* a surgical operation to produce a permanent or semipermanent artificial opening to an *antrum in a bone, so providing drainage for any fluid. The operation is sometimes carried out to treat infection of the *paranasal sinuses.

antrum *n.* **1.** a cavity, especially a cavity in a bone. The *mastoid* (or *tympanic*) *antrum* is the space connecting the air cells of the *mastoid process with the chamber of the inner ear. **2.** the part of the *stomach adjoining the pylorus (*pyloric antrum*).

anuria *n.* failure of the kidneys to produce urine. This can occur in a variety of conditions that produce a sustained drop in blood pressure. Urgent assessment is required to differentiate lack of production of urine from an obstruction to the flow of urine from the kidneys, which can readily be relieved. Anuria is associated with increasing *uraemia and may require *haemodialysis.

anus *n.* the opening at the lower end of the alimentary canal, through which the faeces are discharged. It opens out from the *anal canal*, below the rectum, and is guarded by two sphincters. The anus is closed except during defecation. —**anal** *adj.*

anvil *n.* (in anatomy) *see* incus.

anxiety *n.* generalized pervasive *fear. *Anxiety state* is a form of neurosis in which anxiety dominates the patient's life. It can be treated with psychotherapy, behaviour therapy, and tranquillizing drugs.

aorta *n.* (*pl.* **aortae** or **aortas**) the main artery of the body, from which all others derive. It arises from the left ventricle (*ascending aorta*), arches over the top of the heart (*see* aortic arch) and descends in front of the backbone (*descending aorta*), giving off large and small branches and finally dividing to form the right and left *iliac arteries. The part of the descending aorta from the aortic arch to the diaphragm is called the *thoracic aorta*; the part below the diaphragm is the *abdominal aorta*. —**aortic** *adj.*

aortic arch that part of the aorta that extends from the ascending aorta, upward over the heart and then backward and down as far as the fourth thoracic vertebra. *Stretch receptors in its outer wall monitor blood pressure and form part of the system maintaining this at a constant level.

aortic regurgitation reflux of blood from the aorta into the left ventricle during diastole. Aortic regurgitation most commonly follows scarring of the aortic valve as a result of previous acute rheumatic fever, but it may also result from other conditions, such as syphilis or dissecting aneurysm. Mild cases are symptom-free, but patients more severely affected develop breathlessness, angina pectoris, and enlargement of the heart; all have a diastolic murmur. A badly affected valve may be replaced surgically with a prosthesis.

aortic stenosis narrowing of the opening of the aortic valve due to fusion of the cusps that comprise the valve. It may result from previous rheumatic fever, or from calcification and scarring in a valve that has two cusps instead of the normal three, or it may be congenital. Aortic stenosis obstructs the flow of blood from the left ventricle to the aorta during systole. Breathlessness on effort, angina pectoris, and fainting may follow. The patient has a systolic murmur. When symptoms develop the valve should be replaced surgically with a mechanical prosthesis (such as a Starr-Edwards ball-cage valve) or with an aortic valve graft.

aortic valve a valve in the heart, lying between the left ventricle and the aorta. It consists of three pockets, shaped like half-moons, that prevent blood returning to the ventricle from the aorta. *See also* semilunar valve.

aortitis *n.* inflammation of the aorta, which most commonly occurs as a late complication of syphilis. Aortitis principally affects the ascending thoracic aorta and may result in the formation of an aneurysm and obstruction to the coronary blood flow. Chest pain may occur from pressure on surrounding structures or from the reduced blood supply to the heart. *Aortic regurgitation may be found. The syphilitic infection is treated with penicillin but surgical repair to the aortic aneurysm or valve may be needed.

aortography *n.* X-ray examination of the aorta, which involves the injection into it of a *radio-opaque contrast medium, after which a series of X-rays is taken (*see* angiocardiography). Aortography is undertaken to reveal the extent and site of diseases such as atheromatous obstruction or aneurysm; it is an essential aid to the planning of surgical treatment.

aperient *n.* a mild *laxative.

apex *n.* the tip or summit of an organ; for example the heart or lung. The apex of a *tooth is the tip of the root, where there is a small hole (the *apical foramen*) through which vessels and nerves pass from the pulp to the periapical tissues. —**apical** *adj.*

apex beat the impact of the heart against the chest wall during *systole. It can be felt or heard to the left of the breastbone, in the space between the fifth and sixth ribs.

Apgar score a method of rapidly assessing the general state of a baby immediately after birth. A maximum of 2 points is given for each of the following signs: type of breathing, heart rate, colour, muscle tone, and response to stimuli. Thus an infant scoring 10 points at 60 minutes after delivery would be in optimum condition. When the score is low, the test is repeated at intervals as a guide to progress.

aphakia *n.* absence of the lens of the eye: the state of the eye after a cataract has been removed.

aphasia (dysphasia) *n.* a disorder of language affecting the generation of speech and its understanding and not simply a disorder of articulation (*see* dyslalia). It is caused by disease in the left half of the brain (the dominant hemisphere) in a right-handed person. It is commonly accompanied by difficulties in reading and writing. —**aphasic** *adj.*

aphonia *n.* absence of or loss of the voice through disease of the larynx or mouth: if loss of speech is due to a defect in the brain the disorder is *aphasia.

aphrenia *n.* failure of development of the intellectual faculties. *See* subnormality.

aphrodisiac *n.* an agent that stimulates sexual excitement.

aphtha *n.* (*pl.* **aphthae**) a small ulcer, occurring singly or in groups in the mouth as white or red spots. Their cause is unknown and only palliative treatment is available. —**aphthous** *adj.*

apical abscess an abscess in the bone around the apex of a tooth. An acute abscess is extremely painful, causing swelling of the jaw and sometimes also the face. It invariably results from death and infection of the pulp of the tooth. Treatment is drainage and *root treatment or extraction of the tooth.

apicectomy *n.* (in dentistry) surgical removal of the apex of the root of a tooth. It is carried out when *root treatment cannot be done or has failed.

aplasia *n.* total or partial failure of development of an organ or tissue. *See also* agenesis. —**aplastic** *adj.*

apneusis *n.* a state in which prolonged inhalation occurs. It occurs when the appropriate inhibitory influences are prevented from reaching the inspiratory centre of the brain.

apnoea *n.* temporary cessation of breathing from any cause. Attacks of apnoea are common in newborn babies and should be taken seriously although they do not necessarily indicate serious illness. —**apnoeic** *adj.*

apocrine *adj.* **1.** describing sweat glands that occur only in hairy parts of the body, especially the armpit and groin. These glands develop in the hair follicles and appear after puberty has been reached. The strong odours associated with sweating result from the action of bacteria on the sweat produced by apocrine glands. *Compare* eccrine. **2.** describing a type of gland that loses part of its protoplasm when secreting. *See* secretion.

apomorphine *n.* an *emetic that produces its effect by direct action on the vomiting centre in the brain. It is given by subcutaneous injection and acts within a few minutes. It is employed in the treatment of poisoning by noncorrosive substances that have been taken by mouth. In nonemetic (lower) dosage, apomorphine has sedative, hypnotic, and expectorant actions.

aponeurosis *n.* a thin but strong fibrous sheet of tissue that replaces a *tendon in muscles that are flat and sheetlike and have a wide area of attachment (e.g. to bones). —**aponeurotic** *adj.*

apophysis *n.* **1.** a projection from a bone. **2.** a projection of any other part, e.g. of the brain (*apophysis cerebri*: the *pineal body).

apophysitis *n.* inflammation of one or more of the synovial joints between the posterior arches of the vertebrae (*apophyseal joints*). This may occur in rheumatoid arthritis or ankylosing *spondylitis and causes pain. It contributes to partial dislocation (subluxation) of the vertebrae in arthritis and to rigidity of the spine (due to fusion of the joints) in ankylosing spondylitis.

apoplexy *n. see* stroke.

appendectomy *n.* the usual US term for *appendicectomy.

appendicectomy *n.* surgical removal of the vermiform appendix. *See also* appendicitis.

appendicitis *n.* inflammation of the vermiform *appendix. *Acute appendicitis*, which has become common this century, usually affects young people. The chief symptom is abdominal pain, first central and later (with tenderness) in the right lower abdomen, over the appendix. Unusual positions of the appendix may cause pain in different sites, leading to difficulty in diagnosis. Vomiting and diarrhoea sometimes occur, but fever is slight. If not treated by surgical removal (appendicectomy) the condition usually progresses to cause an abscess or generalized *peritonitis. Conditions that mimic appendicitis include mesenteric *lymphadenitis, acute ileitis (*see* Crohn's disease), *pyelonephritis, and pneumonia. *Chronic appendicitis* was a popular diagnosis 20–50 years ago to explain recurrent pains in the lower abdomen. It is rare, and appendicectomy will not usually cure such pains.

appendicostomy *n.* an operation in which the vermiform appendix is brought through the abdominal wall and opened in order to drain or decompress the intestine. It is now rarely performed, *ileostomy, *caecostomy, or *colostomy being preferred.

appendicular *adj.* **1.** relating to or affecting the vermiform appendix. **2.** relating to the limbs: the *appendicular skeleton* comprises the bones of the limbs.

appendix (vermiform appendix) *n.* the short thin blind-ended tube, 7–10 cm long, that is attached to the end of the caecum (a pouch at the start of the large intestine). It has no known function in man and is liable to become infected and inflamed, especially in young adults (*see* appendicitis).

apperception *n.* (in psychology) the process by which the qualities of an object, situation, etc., perceived by an individual are correlated with his/her preexisting knowledge.

applicator *n.* any device used to apply medication or treatment to a particular part of the body.

apposition *n.* the state of two structures, such as parts of the body, being in close contact. For example, the fingers are brought into apposition when the fist is clenched, and the eyelids when the eyes are closed.

apraxia (dyspraxia) *n.* an inability to make skilled movements with accuracy. This is a disorder of the *cerebral cortex resulting in the patient's inability to organize the movements rather than clumsiness due to weakness, sensory loss, or disease of the *cerebellum. It is most often caused by disease of the *parietal lobes of the brain and sometimes by disease of the frontal lobes.

aproctia *n.* congenital absence of the anus or its opening. *See* imperforate anus.

aprosexia *n.* inability to fix the attention on any subject, due to poor eyesight, defective hearing, or mental weakness.

apyrexia *n.* the absence of fever.

aqueduct *n.* (in anatomy) a canal containing fluid. For example, the *aqueduct of the midbrain* (*cerebral aqueduct, aqueduct of Sylvius*) connects the third and fourth *ventricles.

aqueous humour the watery fluid that fills the chamber of the *eye immediately behind the cornea and in front of the lens. It is continually being formed – chiefly by capillaries of the ciliary processes – and it drains away into Schlemm's canal, at the junction of the cornea and sclera.

arachidonic acid *see* essential fatty acid.

arachnidism *n.* poisoning from the bite of a spider. Toxins from the less venomous species of spider cause only local pain, redness, and swelling. Toxins from more venomous species, such as the black widow (*Lactrodectus mactans*), cause muscular pains, convulsions, nausea, and paralysis.

arachnodactyly *n.* abnormally long and slender fingers: usually associated with excessive height and congenital defects of the heart and eyes in *Marfan's syndrome.

arachnoid (arachnoid mater) *n.* the middle of the three membranes covering the brain and spinal cord (*see* meninges), which has a fine, almost cobweb-like, texture. Between it and the pia mater within lies the subarachnoid space, containing cerebrospinal fluid and large blood vessels; the membrane itself has no blood supply.

arachnoid villus one of the thin-walled projections outwards of the arachnoid membrane into the blood-filled sinuses of the dura, acting as a one-way valve for the flow of cerebrospinal fluid from the subarachnoid space into the bloodstream. Large villi, known as *arachnoid granulations* (or *Pacchionian bodies*), are found in the region of the superior sagittal sinus.

They may be so distended as to cause pitting of the adjacent bone.

arbor *n.* (in anatomy) a treelike structure. *Arbor vitae* is the treelike outline of white matter seen in sections of the cerebellum; it also refers to the treelike appearance of the inner folds of the neck of the womb.

arbovirus *n.* one of a group of RNA-containing viruses that are transmitted from animals to man by insects (i.e. arthropods; hence *ar*thropod-*bo*rne viruses) and cause diseases resulting in encephalitis or serious fever, such as dengue and yellow fever.

arc-eye *n.* a painful condition of the eyes caused by damage to the surface of the cornea by ultraviolet light from arc welding. It usually resolves if the eyes are padded for 24 hours. It is similar to *snow blindness and the condition caused by overexposure of the eye to sun-tanning lamps.

arch- (arche-, archi-, archo-) *prefix denoting* first; beginning; primitive; ancestral. Example: *archinephron* (first-formed embryonic kidney).

archenteron *n.* a cavity that forms in the very early embryo as the result of gastrulation (*see* gastrula). In man it forms a tubular cavity, the *archenteric canal*, which connects the amniotic cavity with the yolk sac. —**archenteric** *adj.*

archetype *n.* (in Jungian psychology) an inherited idea or mode of thought supposed to be present in the *unconscious mind and to derive from the experience of the whole human race, not from the life experience of the individual.

archipallium *n.* the *hippocampal formation of the cerebrum. The term is seldom used.

arcus *n.* (in anatomy) an arch; for example the *arcus aortae* (*aortic arch).

arcus senilis a greyish line in the periphery of the cornea, concentric with the edge but separated from it by a clear zone. It begins above and below but may become a continuous ring. It consists of an infiltration of fatty material and is common in the elderly. When it occurs in younger people it may indicate abnormal fat metabolism, but there is great racial variation in its incidence. It never affects vision.

areola *n.* **1.** the brownish or pink ring of tissue surrounding the nipple of the breast. **2.** the part of the iris that surrounds the pupil of the eye. **3.** a small space in a tissue. —**areolar** *adj.*

areolar tissue loose *connective tissue consisting of a meshwork of collagen, elastic tissue, and reticular fibres interspersed with numerous connective tissue cells. It binds the skin to underlying muscles and forms a link between organs while allowing a high degree of relative movement.

Argasidae *n. see* tick.

argentaffin cells cells that stain readily with silver salts. Such cells occur, for example, in the crypts of Lieberkühn in the intestine.

argentaffinoma (carcinoid) *n.* a tumour of the *argentaffin cells in the glands of the intestine. Argentaffinomas typically occur in the tip of the appendix and are among the commonest tumours of the small intestine. They may also occur in the rectum and other parts of the digestive tract and in the bronchial tree (*bronchial carcinoid adenoma*). Argentaffinomas sometimes produce 5-hydroxytryptamine (serotonin), prostaglandins, and other physiologically active substances, which are inactivated in the liver. If the tumour has spread to the liver excess amounts of these substances are released into the systemic circulation and the *carcinoid syndrome* results – flushing, headache, diarrhoea, asthma-like attacks, and in some cases damage to the right side of the heart.

arginine *n.* an *amino acid that plays an important role in the formation of *urea by the liver.

Argyll Robertson pupil a disorder of the eyes, common to several diseases of the central nervous system, in which the *pupillary (light) reflex is absent. Although the pupils contract normally for near vision, they fail to contract in bright light.

argyria *n.* a form of silver poisoning in which the skin becomes dark bluish-grey due to the accumulation of the metal in the tissues. The mucous membranes and internal organs are also affected. Argyria is now rare, due to the decline in the use of silver compounds in medicine and industry (except the photographic industry).

ariboflavinosis *n.* the group of symptoms caused by deficiency of riboflavin (vitamin B_2). These symptoms include inflammation of the tongue and lips and sores in the corners of the mouth.

Arnold-Chiari malformation a congenital disorder in which there is distortion of the base of the skull with protrusion of the lower brainstem and parts of the cerebellum through the opening for the spinal cord at the base of the skull. It is commonly associated with *neural tube defects and *hydrocephalus.

arousal *n.* **1.** a state of alertness and of high responsiveness to stimuli. It is produced by strong motivation, by anxiety, and by a stimulating environment. **2.** physiological activation of the *cerebral cortex by centres lower in the brain, such as the *reticular activating system, resulting in wakefulness and alertness. It is hypothesized that unduly high or low degrees of arousal lead to neuropsychiatric problems, such as *narcolepsy and *mania.

arrhenoblastoma

arrhenoblastoma *n. see* androblastoma.

arrhythmia *n.* any deviation from the normal rhythm (sinus rhythm) of the heart. The natural pacemaker of the heart (the sinoatrial node), which lies in the wall of the right atrium, controls the rate and rhythm of the whole heart under the influence of the autonomic nervous system. It generates electrical impulses that spread to the atria and ventricles, via specialized conducting tissues, and cause them to contract normally. Arrhythmias result from a disturbance of the generation or conduction of these impulses and may be intermittent or continuous. They include *ectopic beats (extrasystoles), ectopic *tachycardias, *fibrillation, and *heart block (which is often associated with slow heart rates). Symptoms include palpitations, breathlessness, and chest pain. In more serious arrhythmias the *Stokes-Adams syndrome or *cardiac arrest may occur. Arrhythmias may result from most heart diseases but they also occur without apparent cause.

arsenic *n.* a poisonous greyish metallic element producing the symptoms of nausea, vomiting, diarrhoea, cramps, convulsions, and coma when ingested in large doses. Drugs used as antidotes to arsenic poisoning include *dimercaprol. Arsenic was formerly readily available in the form of rat poison and in fly-papers and was the poisoner's first choice during the 19th century, its presence in a body being then difficult to detect. Today detection is relatively simple. Arsenic was formerly used in medicine, the most important arsenical drugs being *arsphenamine* (*Salvarsan*) and *neoarsphenamine*, used in the treatment of syphilis and dangerous parasitic diseases. Symbol: As.

artefact *n. see* artifact.

arter- (arteri-, arterio-) *prefix denoting* an artery. Examples: *arteriopathy* (disease of); *arteriorrhaphy* (suture of);

arteriovenous (relating to arteries and veins).

arteriectomy *n.* surgical excision of an artery or part of an artery. This may be performed as a diagnostic procedure (for example, to take an arterial biopsy in the diagnosis of arteritis) or during reconstruction of a blocked artery when the blocked segment is replaced by a synthetic graft.

arteriogram *n.* a tracing of the wave form of an arterial pulse. This can be made directly, by means of an arterial needle puncture and pressure recording, or indirectly, by a recorder placed on the skin over an artery. The tracing may be recorded on a paper strip or on a screen (oscilloscope). Some heart defects produce characteristic pulse wave forms.

arteriography *n.* X-ray examination of an artery that has been outlined by the injection of a *radio-opaque contrast medium. The major uses of arteriography are to demonstrate the site and extent of atheroma, especially in the coronary arteries (*coronary angiography*) and leg arteries (*femoral angiography*), and to reveal the site of aneurysms within the skull or cerebral tumours (*carotid* and *vertebral artery angiography*).

arteriole *n.* a small branch of an *artery, leading into many smaller vessels – the *capillaries. By their constriction and dilation, under the regulation of the sympathetic nervous system, arterioles are the principal controllers of blood flow and pressure.

arteriolitis *n.* inflammation of the arterioles (the smallest arteries), which may complicate severe hypertension. This produces *necrotizing arteriolitis*, which may result in kidney failure. A similar condition may affect the lung in pulmonary hypertension.

42

arterioplasty *n.* surgical reconstruction of an artery; for example, in the treatment of *aneurysms.

arteriosclerosis *n.* an imprecise term used for any of several conditions affecting the arteries. The term is often used as a synonym for atherosclerosis (*see* atheroma). It may also be used for *Mönckeberg's degeneration*, in which calcium is deposited in the arteries as part of the ageing process, and *arteriolarsclerosis*, in which the walls of small arteries become thickened due to ageing or hypertension.

arteriotomy *n.* an incision into, or a needle puncture of, the wall of an artery. This is most often performed as a diagnostic procedure in the course of *arteriography or cardiac *catheterization. It may also be required to remove an embolus (*see* embolectomy).

arteriovenous anastomosis a thick-walled blood vessel that connects an arteriole directly with a venule, thus bypassing the capillaries. Arteriovenous anastomoses are commonly found in the skin of the lips, nose, ears, hands and feet; their muscular walls can constrict to reduce blood flow or dilate to allow blood through to these areas.

arteriovenous aneurysm a direct communication between an artery and vein, without an intervening capillary bed. It can occur as a congenital abnormality or it may be acquired following injury or surgery. It may affect the limbs, lungs, or viscera and may be single or multiple. If the connection is large, the short-circuiting of blood may produce heart failure. Large isolated arteriovenous aneurysms may be closed surgically.

arteriovenous malformation *see* angioma.

arteritis *n.* an inflammatory disease affecting the muscular walls of the arteries. It may be part of a *collagen disease or it may be due to an infection, such as syphilis. The affected vessels are swollen and tender and may become blocked. *Temporal* or *giant-cell arteritis* occurs in the elderly and most commonly affects the arteries of the scalp. The patient complains of severe headache, and blindness may result from thrombosis of the arteries to the eyes. Treatment with cortisone derivatives is rapidly effective.

artery *n.* a blood vessel carrying blood away from the heart. All arteries except the *pulmonary artery carry oxygenated blood. The walls of arteries contain smooth muscle fibres (see illustration), which contract or relax under the control of the sympathetic nervous system. *See also* aorta, arteriole.

Transverse section through an artery

arthr- (arthro-) *prefix denoting* a joint. Examples: *arthrology* (science of); *arthrosclerosis* (stiffening or hardening of).

arthralgia *n.* pain in a joint, without swelling or other signs of arthritis. *Compare* arthritis.

arthrectomy *n.* surgical excision of a joint. It is usually performed on a painful joint that has ceased to function, as may result from intractable infection.

arthritis *n.* inflammation of one or more joints, characterized by swelling, warmth, redness of the overlying skin, pain, and restriction of motion. Over 80 diseases may cause arthritis, including *rheumatoid arthritis, *osteoarthritis, *gout, *tuberculosis, and other infections. Diagnosis is assisted by examina-

The principal arteries of the body

tion of the pattern of distribution of affected joints, X-rays, blood tests, and examination of synovial fluid obtained by *aspiration of a swollen joint. *Mono-* or *oligo-arthritis* is inflammation of one joint, *pauciarthritis* of a few, and *polyarthritis* of many joints, either simultaneously or in sequence. Any disease involving the synovial membranes or causing degeneration of cartilage may cause arthritis. Treatment of arthritis depends on the cause, but aspirin and similar analgesics are often used to suppress inflammation, and hence reduce pain and swelling. *See also* psoriatic arthritis, haemarthrosis, pyarthrosis, hydrarthrosis. —**arthritic** *adj.*

arthrodesis *n.* fusion of bones across a joint space by surgical means, which eliminates movement. This operation is performed when a joint is very painful, highly unstable, grossly deformed or chronically infected, or when an *arthroplasty would be inadvisable or impossible.

arthrodic joint (gliding joint) a form of *diarthrosis (freely movable joint) in which the bony surfaces slide over each other without angular or rotational movement. Examples are the joints of the carpus and tarsus.

arthrography *n.* an X-ray technique for examining joints. A *contrast medium (either air or a liquid opaque to X-rays) is injected into the joint space, allowing its outline and contents to be traced accurately.

arthropathy *n.* any disease or disorder involving a joint.

arthroplasty *n.* surgical remodelling of a diseased joint. To prevent the ends of the bones fusing after the operation, a large gap may be created between them (*gap arthroplasty*), a barrier of artificial material may be inserted (*interposition arthroplasty*), or one or both bone ends may be replaced by a *prosthesis of metal or plastic (*replacement arthroplasty*).

arthropod *n.* any member of a large group of animals that possess a hard external skeleton and jointed legs and other appendages. Many arthropods are of medical importance, including the *mites, *ticks, and *insects.

arthroscope *n.* an instrument for insertion into the cavity of a joint in order to inspect the contents, before *biopsy or operation on the joint.

arthrotomy *n.* surgical incision of a joint capsule in order to inspect the contents and drain pus (if it is present).

articulation *n.* (in anatomy) the point or type of contact between two bones. *See* joint.

articulator *n.* (in dentistry) an apparatus for relating the upper and lower models of a patient's dentition in a fixed position, usually with maximum tooth contact. Some articulators can reproduce jaw movements. They are used in the construction of crowns, bridges, and dentures.

artifact (artefact) *n.* (in microscopy) a structure seen in a tissue under a microscope that is not present in the living tissue. Artifacts, which are produced by faulty *fixation or staining of the tissue, may give a false impression that disease or abnormality is present in the tissue when it is not.

artificial insemination instrumental introduction of semen into the vagina in order that the woman may conceive. Insemination is timed to coincide with the day on which the woman is expected to ovulate (*see* menstrual cycle). The semen specimen may be provided by the husband (*AIH – artificial insemination husband*) in cases of *impotence or by an anonymous donor (*AID – artificial insemination donor*) in cases where the husband is sterile.

artificial kidney (dialyser) *see* haemodialysis.

artificial lung *see* respirator.

artificial respiration an emergency procedure for maintaining a flow of air into and out of a patient's lungs when the natural breathing reflexes are absent or insufficient. This may occur after drowning, poisoning, etc., or during a surgical operation on the thorax or abdomen when muscle-relaxing drugs are administered. The simplest and most efficient method is the mouth-to-mouth technique (the '*kiss of life*'). In hospital the breathing cycle is maintained by means of a *respirator.

arytenoid cartilage either of the two pyramid-shaped cartilages that lie at the back of the *larynx next to the upper edges of the cricoid cartilage.

asbestosis *n.* a lung disease – a form of *pneumoconiosis – caused by fibres of asbestos inhaled by those who are exposed to large amounts of the mineral. The incidence of lung cancer is high in such patients, particularly if they smoke cigarettes. *See also* mesothelioma.

ascariasis *n.* a disease caused by an infestation with the parasitic worm *Ascaris lumbricoides*. Adult worms in the intestine can cause abdominal pain, vomiting, constipation, diarrhoea, appendicitis, and peritonitis; in large numbers they may cause obstruction of the intestine. The presence of the migrating larvae in the lungs can provoke pneumonia. Ascariasis occurs principally in areas of poor sanitation; it is treated with *piperazine.

Ascaris *n.* a genus of parasitic nematode worms. *A. lumbricoides*, widely distributed throughout the world, is the largest of the human intestinal nematodes – an adult female measures up to 35 cm in length. Eggs, passed out in the stools, may be transmitted to a new host in contaminated food or drink. Larvae

hatch out in the intestine and then undergo a complicated migration, via the hepatic portal vein, liver, heart, lungs, windpipe, and pharynx, before returning to the intestine where they later develop into adult worms (*see also* ascariasis).

ascites (hydroperitoneum) *n.* the accumulation of fluid in the peritoneal cavity, causing abdominal swelling. Causes include infections (such as tuberculosis), heart failure, *portal hypertension, *cirrhosis, and various cancers (particularly of the ovary and liver). *See also* oedema.

ascorbic acid *see* vitamin C.

-ase *suffix denoting* an enzyme. Examples: *lactase*; *dehydrogenase*.

asepsis *n.* the complete absence of bacteria, fungi, viruses, or other microorganisms that could cause disease. Asepsis is the ideal state for the performance of surgical operations and is achieved by using *sterilization techniques. —**aseptic** *adj.*

asparaginase *n.* an enzyme that inhibits the growth of certain tumours and is used in the treatment of acute lymphoblastic leukaemia. It may cause allergic reactions and *anaphylaxis.

asparagine *n. see* amino acid.

aspartic acid (aspartate) *see* amino acid.

aspergillosis *n.* a rare disease in which the fungus *Aspergillus fumigatus* grows freely in pre-existing lesions in the lungs and bronchioles. Occasionally the fungus attacks the mucous membranes of the eyes, nose, or urethra or such internal organs as the lungs, liver, and kidneys.

Aspergillus *n.* a genus of fungi, including many common moulds, some of which cause infections of the respiratory system in man. The species *A. fumigatus* causes *aspergillosis. *A. niger* is commonly found in the external ear and can become pathogenic.

aspermia *n.* strictly, a lack or failure of formation of semen. More usually, however, the term is used to mean the total absence of sperm from the semen (*see* azoospermia).

asphyxia *n.* suffocation: a life-threatening condition in which oxygen is prevented from reaching the tissues by obstruction of or damage to any part of the respiratory system. Drowning, choking, and breathing poisonous gas all lead to asphyxia. Unless the condition is remedied by removing the obstruction (when present) and by artificial respiration if necessary, there is progressive *cyanosis leading to death. Brain cells cannot live for more than about four minutes without oxygen.

aspiration *n.* the withdrawal of fluid from the body by means of suction using an instrument called an *aspirator*. There are various types of aspirator: some employ hollow needles for removing fluid from cysts, inflamed joint cavities, etc.; another kind is used to suck debris and water from the patient's mouth during dental treatment.

aspirin (acetylsalicylic acid) *n.* a widely used drug that relieves pain and also reduces inflammation and fever. It is taken by mouth – alone or in combination with caffeine, phenacetin, or codeine – for the relief of the less severe types of pain, such as headache, toothache, neuralgias, and the pain of rheumatoid arthritis. It is also taken to reduce fever in influenza and the common cold. Aspirin may irritate the lining of the stomach, causing nausea, vomiting, pain, and bleeding. Tablets should not be held on the gum adjacent to a painful tooth as ulceration may occur. High doses cause dizziness, disturbed hearing, mental confusion, and overbreathing. *See also* analgesic.

assay *n.* a test or trial to determine the strength of a solution, the proportion of a compound in a mixture, the potency of a drug, or the purity of a preparation. *See also* bioassay.

assimilation *n.* the process by which food substances are taken into the cells of the body after they have been digested and absorbed.

association area an area of *cerebral cortex that lies away from the main areas that are concerned with the reception of sensory impulses and the start of motor impulses but is linked to them by many neurones known as *association fibres*. The areas of association are thought to be responsible for the elaboration of the information received by the primary sensory areas and its correlation with the information fed in from memory and from other brain areas. They are thus responsible for the maintenance of many higher mental activities. *See also* body image.

association of ideas (in psychology) linkage of one idea to another in a regular way according to their meaning. In *free association* the linkage of ideas arising in dreams or fantasy may be used to discover the underlying motives of the individual. In *word association tests* stimulus words are produced to which the subject has to respond as quickly as possible.

astasia *n.* an inability to stand for which no physical cause can be found. *Astasia-abasia* is an inability to stand or walk in the absence of any recognizable physical illness. The patient's attempts are bizarre and careful examination reveals contradictory features. It is most commonly an expression of *hysteria.

aster *n.* a star-shaped object in a cell that surrounds the *centrosome during mitosis and meiosis and is concerned with the formation of the *spindle.

astereognosis *n.* *see* agnosia.

asthenia *n.* weakness or loss of strength.

asthenic *adj.* describing a personality disorder characterized by low energy, susceptibility to physical and emotional stress, and a diminished capacity for pleasure.

asthenopia *n. see* eyestrain.

asthma *n.* a condition characterized by paroxysmal attacks of *bronchospasm, causing difficulty in breathing. *Bronchial asthma* may be precipitated by exposure to one or more of a large range of stimuli, including *allergens (including some drugs, such as aspirin), exertion, emotions, and infections. The first attacks can occur at any age but are normally in early life, when – in allergic people – they may be associated with other manifestations of hypersensitivity, such as eczema and hay fever. Powerful drugs, including corticosteroids, are now available to control asthmatic attacks, which may be very serious and prolonged (*see* status asthmaticus). Avoidance of known allergens, and *desensitization to them, may help to reduce the frequency of attacks. *Cardiac asthma* occurs in left ventricular heart failure and must be distinguished from bronchial asthma, for which the treatment is different. —**asthmatic** *adj.*

astigmatism *n.* a defect of vision in which the image of an object is distorted, usually in either the vertical or the horizontal axis, because not all the light from it comes to a focus on the retina. Some parts of the object may be in focus but light from other parts may be focused in front of or behind the retina. This is usually due to abnormal curvature of the cornea and/or lens (*see* refraction), whose surface resembles part of the surface of an egg (rather than a sphere). The defect can be corrected by wearing *cylindrical lenses*, which produce exactly the opposite degree of distortion and thus cancel out the distortion caused by the eye itself. —**astigmatic** *adj.*

astragalus *n. see* talus.

astringent *n.* a drug that causes cells to shrink by precipitating proteins from their surfaces. Astringents are used in lotions to harden and protect the skin and to reduce bleeding from minor abrasions. They are also used in mouth washes, throat lozenges, eye drops, etc., and in antiperspirants.

astrocyte (astroglial cell) *n.* a type of cell with numerous sheet-like processes extending from its cell body, found throughout the central nervous system. It is one of the several different types of cell that make up the *glia. The cells have been ascribed the function of providing nutrients for neurones and possibly of taking part in information storage processes.

astrocytoma *n.* a brain tumour derived from non-nervous cells (*glia), which – unlike the neurones – retain the ability to reproduce themselves by mitosis. All grades of malignancy occur, from slow-growing tumours whose histological structure resembles normal glial cells, to rapidly growing highly invasive tumours whose cell structure is poorly differentiated (*see* glioblastoma). In adults astrocytomas are usually found in the cerebral hemispheres but in children they also occur in the cerebellum.

asymbolia *n. see* alexia.

asymptomatic *adj.* not showing any symptoms of disease, whether disease is present or not.

asynclitism *n.* the entry of the head of the baby at birth into the vagina at an oblique angle.

asyndesis *n.* a disorder of thought, in which the normal *association of ideas is disrupted so that thought and speech become fragmentary. It is a symptom of schizophrenia, dementia, or confusion.

asynergia *n. see* dyssynergia.

asystole *n.* a condition in which the heart no longer beats, accompanied by the absence of complexes in the electrocardiogram. The clinical features, causes, and treatment are those of *cardiac arrest.

ataraxia *n.* a state of calmness and freedom from anxiety, especially the state produced by tranquillizing drugs.

atavism *n.* the phenomenon in which an individual has a character or disease known to have occurred in a remote ancestor but not in his parents.

ataxia *n.* the shaky movements and unsteady gait that result from the brain's failure to regulate the body's posture and the strength and direction of limb movements. It may be due to disease of the sensory nerves or the *cerebellum. In *cerebellar ataxia* there is clumsiness of willed movements. The patient staggers when walking; he cannot pronounce words properly and has *nystagmus. *Friedreich's ataxia* is an inherited disorder appearing first in adolescence. It has the features of cerebellar ataxia, together with spasticity of the limbs. The unsteady movements of *sensory ataxia* are exaggerated when the patient closes his eyes (*see* Romberg's sign). *See also* tabes dorsalis (locomotor ataxia). —**ataxic** *adj.*

Atebrin *n. see* mepacrine.

atel- (atelo-) *prefix denoting* imperfect or incomplete development. Examples: *atelencephaly* (of the brain); *atelocardia* (of the heart).

atelectasis *n.* failure of part of the lung to expand. This occurs when the cells lining the air sacs (alveoli) are too immature, as in premature babies, or too damaged by inhaled substances or secretions to produce the wetting agent (surfactant) with which the surface tension between the alveolar walls is overcome. The lung can usually be helped to expand by physiotherapy and supportive measures, but prolonged atelectasis becomes irreversible.

ateleiosis *n.* failure of sexual development owing to lack of *pituitary hormones. *See* infantilism, dwarfism.

atheroma *n.* degeneration of the walls of the arteries due to the formation in them of fatty plaques and scar tissue. This limits blood circulation and predisposes to thrombosis. It is common in adults in Western countries. A diet rich in animal fats (*see* cholesterol) and refined sugar, cigarette smoking, obesity, and inactivity are the principal causes. It may be symptomless but often causes complications from arterial obstruction in middle and late life (such as angina pectoris, heart attack, stroke, and gangrene). Treatment is by prevention, but some symptoms may be ameliorated by drug therapy (e.g. angina by glyceryl trinitrate) or by surgical bypass of the arterial obstruction.

atherosclerosis *n.* a disease of the arteries in which fatty plaques develop on their inner walls, with eventual obstruction of blood flow. *See* atheroma.

athetosis *n.* a writhing involuntary movement especially affecting the hands, face, and tongue. It is usually a form of *cerebral palsy. It impairs the child's ability to speak or use his hands; intelligence is often unaffected.

athlete's foot a fungus infection of the skin between the toes: a type of *ringworm. Medical name: **tinea pedis**.

athyreosis *n.* absence of or lack of function of the thyroid gland, causing *cretinism in infancy and *myxoedema in adult life.

atlas *n.* the first *cervical vertebra, by means of which the skull is articulated to the backbone.

atony *n.* a state in which muscles are floppy, lacking their normal elasticity. —**atonic** *adj.*

atopen *n.* any substance responsible for *atopy.

atopy *n.* a form of *allergy in which the hypersensitivity reaction may be distant from the region of contact with the substance (*atopen*) responsible. For example, a substance that is swallowed may give rise to a form of eczema, called *atopic dermatitis*. —**atopic** *adj.*

ATP (adenosine triphosphate) a compound that contains adenine, ribose, and three phosphate groups and occurs in cells. The chemical bonds of the phosphate groups store energy needed by the cell, for muscle contraction; this energy is released when ATP is split into ADP or AMP. ATP is formed from ADP or AMP using energy produced by the breakdown of carbohydrates or other food substances. *See also* mitochondrion.

atresia *n.* **1.** congenital absence or abnormal narrowing of a body opening. *Biliary atresia* (affecting the bile duct) causes obstructive jaundice in infancy and is lethal unless corrected surgically; *tricuspid atresia* obstructs the blood flow within the heart from the right atrium to the right ventricle. **2.** the degenerative process that affects the majority of ovarian follicles. Usually only one Graafian follicle will ovulate in each menstrual cycle. —**atretic** *adj.*

atri- (atrio-) *prefix denoting* an atrium, especially the atrium of the heart. Example: *atrioventricular* (relating to the atria and ventricles of the heart).

atrioventricular bundle (AV bundle, bundle of His) a bundle of modified heart muscle fibres (*Purkinje fibres*) passing from the *atrioventricular (AV) node forward to the septum between the ventricles, where it divides into right and left bundles, one for each ventricle. The fibres transmit contrac-

tion waves from the atria, via the AV node, to the ventricles.

atrioventricular node a mass of modified heart muscle situated in the lower middle part of the right atrium. It receives the impulse to contract from the *sinoatrial node, via the atria, and transmits it through the *atrioventricular bundle to the ventricles.

atrium *n.* (*pl.* **atria**) **1.** either of the two upper chambers of the *heart. Their muscular walls are thinner than those of the ventricles; the left atrium receives oxygenated blood from the lungs via the pulmonary vein; the right atrium receives deoxygenated blood from the venae cavae. *See also* auricle. **2.** any of various anatomical chambers into which one or more cavities open. —**atrial** *adj.*

Atromid-S *n. see* clofibrate.

atrophy *n.* the wasting away of a normally developed organ or tissue due to degeneration of cells. This may occur through undernourishment, disuse, or ageing. Forms of atrophy peculiar to women include the shrinking of the ovary at the menopause and of the *corpus luteum during the menstrual cycle. *Muscular atrophy* is associated with various diseases, such as poliomyelitis.

atropine *n.* a drug extracted from deadly nightshade (*see* belladonna) that inhibits the action of certain nerves of the autonomic nervous system (*see* parasympatholytic). Atropine relaxes smooth muscle and is used to treat biliary colic and renal colic. It also reduces secretions of the bronchial tubes, salivary glands, stomach, and intestines and is used before general *anaesthesia and to relieve peptic ulcers. It is also used to dilate the pupil of the eye. Atropine is administered by mouth, injection, or as eyedrops; common side-effects include dryness of the throat, thirst, and impaired vision.

attachment *n.* (in psychology) the process of developing the first close selective relationship of a child's life, most commonly with the mother. The relationship acts to reduce anxiety in strange settings and forms a base from which children develop further relationships.

attenuation *n.* reduction of the disease-producing ability (virulence) of a bacterium or virus by chemical treatment, heating, drying, by growing under adverse conditions, or by passing through another organism. Treated (*attenuated*) bacteria or viruses are used for many *immunizations.

attrition *n.* (in dentistry) the wearing of tooth surfaces by the action of opposing teeth. A small amount of attrition occurs with age but accelerated wear may occur in *bruxism and with certain diets.

audi- (audio-) *prefix denoting* hearing or sound.

audiogram *n.* the graphic record of a test of hearing carried out on an audiometer.

audiometer *n.* an apparatus for measuring hearing at different sound frequencies, so helping in the diagnosis of deafness. —**audiometry** *n.*

auditory *adj.* relating to the ear or to the sense of hearing.

auditory nerve *see* vestibulocochlear nerve.

Auerbach's plexus (myenteric plexus) a collection of nerve fibres – fine branches of the *vagus nerve – within the walls of the intestine. It supplies the muscle layers and controls the movements of *peristalsis.

aura *n.* the forewarning of an attack. The true *epileptic aura* is felt as a breeze or coldness passing over the body. The *migrainous aura* usually affects the pa-

tient's eyesight with brilliant flickering lights or blurring of vision.

aural *adj.* relating to the ear.

Aureomycin *n. see* chlortetracycline.

auricle *n.* **1.** a small pouch in the wall of each *atrium of the heart: the term is also used incorrectly as a synonym for *atrium.* **2.** *see* pinna.

auriscope (otoscope) *n.* an apparatus for examining the eardrum and the passage leading to it from the ear (external meatus). It consists of a funnel (speculum), a light, and lenses (see illustration).

An auriscope

auscultation *n.* the process of listening, usually with the aid of a *stethoscope, to sounds produced by movement of gas or liquid within the body. Auscultation is an aid to diagnosis of abnormalities of the heart, lungs, intestines, and other organs according to the characteristic changes in sound pattern caused by different disease processes. —**auscultatory** *adj.*

auscultatory gap a silent period in the knocking sounds heard with a stethoscope over an artery, between the systolic and diastolic blood pressures, when the blood pressure is measured with a *sphygmomanometer.

Australia antigen an antigen that has been detected by serological tests in the serum of patients suffering from serum *hepatitis. This disease is thought to be due to a virus.

aut- (auto-) *prefix denoting* self. Example: *autokinesis* (voluntary movement).

autism *n.* **1. (Kanner's syndrome, infantile autism)** a rare and severe psychiatric disorder of childhood, with an onset before the age of 2½ years. It is marked by an inability to communicate by speech or to form abstract concepts; repetitive and limited patterns of behaviour (*see* stereotypy); and obsessive resistance to tiny changes in familiar surroundings. Autistic children are unable to form normal personal relationships but they can become emotionally attached to objects. Most (but not all) are intellectually subnormal (*see* idiot savant). Genetic factors and brain damage are probably important causes. Treatment is not specific, but lengthy specialized education is usually necessary. Behaviour problems and anxiety can be controlled with behaviour therapy and drugs (such as *phenothiazines). **2.** the condition of retreating from realistic thinking to self-centred fantasy thinking: a symptom of personality disorder and schizophrenia. —**autistic** *adj.*

autoagglutination *n.* the clumping together of the body's own red blood cells by antibodies produced against them, which occurs in acquired haemolytic anaemia (an *autoimmune disease).

autoantibody *n.* an antibody formed against one of the body's own components in an *autoimmune disease.

autochthonous *adj.* **1.** remaining at the site of formation. A blood clot that has not been carried in the bloodstream

from its point of origin is described as autochthonous. **2.** originating in an organ without external stimulus, like the beating of the heart.

autoclave 1. *n.* a piece of equipment for sterilizing surgical instruments, dressings, etc. It consists of a chamber, similar to a domestic pressure cooker, in which the articles are placed and treated with steam at high pressure. **2.** *vb.* to sterilize in an autoclave.

autogenous vaccine *see* autovaccine.

autograft *n.* a tissue graft taken from one part of the body and transferred to another part of the same individual. The repair of burns is often done by grafting on strips of skin taken from elsewhere on the body, usually the upper arm or thigh. Unlike *homografts, autografts are not rejected by the body's immunity defences. *See also* skin graft.

autoimmune disease one of the growing number of otherwise unrelated disorders now suspected of being caused by inflammation and destruction of tissues by the body's own antibodies (*autoantibodies*). These disorders include acquired haemolytic anaemia, pernicious anaemia, rheumatic fever, rheumatoid arthritis, glomerulonephritis, and several forms of thyroid dysfunction, including Hashimoto's disease. It is not known why the body should lose the ability to distinguish between substances that are 'self' and those that are 'non-self'.

autoimmunity *n.* a disorder of the body's defence mechanisms in which antibodies (*autoantibodies*) are produced against certain components or products of its own tissues, treating them as foreign material and attacking them. *See* autoimmune disease, immunity.

autoinoculation *n.* the accidental transfer of inoculated material from one site in the body to another. Following vaccination against smallpox, for example, satellite lesions may occur around the site of inoculation. Sometimes the conjunctiva is affected.

autointoxication *n.* poisoning by a toxin formed within the body.

autologous *adj.* denoting a graft that is derived from the recipient of the graft.

autolysis *n.* the destruction of tissues or cells brought about by the actions of their own enzymes. *See* lysosome.

automatism *n.* one of the symptoms of temporal lobe *epilepsy, in which the patient performs well-organized movements. These movements may be simple and repetitive, such as hand clapping, or they may be so complex as to mimic a person's normal conscious activities.

autonomic nervous system the part of the *nervous system responsible for the control of bodily functions that are not consciously directed, including regular beating of the heart, intestinal movements, sweating, salivation, etc. The autonomic system is subdivided into *sympathetic* and *parasympathetic nervous systems*. Sympathetic nerves lead from the middle section of the spinal cord and parasympathetic nerves from the brain and lower spinal cord. The heart, smooth muscles, and most glands receive fibres of both kinds: the interplay of sympathetic and parasympathetic reflex activity (the actions are often antagonistic) governs their working. Sympathetic nerve endings liberate *noradrenaline as a neurotransmitter; parasympathetic nerve endings release *acetylcholine.

autoploidy *n.* the normal condition in cells or individuals, in which each cell has a chromosome set consisting of *homologous pairs, enabling cells to divide normally. —**autoploid** *adj., n.*

autopsy (necropsy, post mortem) *n.* dissection and examination of a body af-

ter death in order to determine the cause of death or the presence of disease processes.

autoradiography (radioautography) *n.* a technique for examining the distribution of a radioactive *tracer in the tissues of an experimental animal. The tracer is injected into the animal, which is killed after a certain period. Thin sections of its organs are placed in close contact with a radiation-sensitive material, such as a photographic emulsion, and observed under a microscope. Blackening of the film indicates a high concentration of radioactive material.

autosome *n.* any chromosome that is not a *sex chromosome and occurs in pairs in diploid cells. —**autosomal** *adj.*

autosuggestion *n.* self-suggestion or self-conditioning that involves repeating ideas to oneself in order to change psychological or physiological states. Autosuggestion is used primarily in *autogenic training*, a technique used to help patients control their anxiety or their habits. *See* suggestion.

autotransfusion *n.* reintroduction into a patient of blood that has been lost from the patient's circulation during surgical operation. The blood is collected by suction during the operation, filtered to remove bubbles and small blood clots, and returned into one of the patient's veins through a drip.

autotrophic (lithotrophic) *adj.* describing organisms (known as *autotrophs*) that synthesize their organic materials from carbon dioxide and nitrates or ammonium compounds, using an external source of energy. *Photoautotrophic* organisms, including green plants and some bacteria, derive their energy from sunlight; *chemoautotrophic* (*chemosynthetic*) organisms obtain energy from inorganic chemical reactions. All autotrophic bacteria are nonparasitic. *Compare* heterotrophic.

autovaccination n. the use of an *autovaccine.

autovaccine (autogenous vaccine) n. a *vaccine prepared by isolating specimens of bacteria from an infected patient, culturing them, and killing them. By injecting this vaccine back into the patient, it was hoped that the body's resistance to the infection would be stimulated. Although such vaccines were once much favoured for the treatment of boils, there is no good evidence that the dead bacteria are any more likely to stimulate immunity than the living and dead bacteria already present in the body.

aux- (auxo-) prefix denoting increase; growth. Example: auxocardia (enlargement of the heart).

auxotroph n. a strain of a microorganism, derived by mutation, that requires one or more specific factors for growth not needed by the parent organism.

avascular adj. lacking blood vessels or having a poor blood supply. The term is usually used with reference to cartilage.

aversion therapy a form of *behaviour therapy that is used to reduce the occurrence of undesirable behaviour, such as sexual deviations or drug addiction. *Conditioning is used, with repeated pairing of some unpleasant stimulus with a stimulus related to the undesirable behaviour. An example is pairing the taste of beer with electric shock in the treatment of alcoholism. See also sensitization.

avitaminosis n. the condition caused by lack of a vitamin. See also deficiency disease.

avulsion (evulsion) n. **1.** the tearing or forcible separation of part of a structure. For example, a tendon may be torn from the bone to which it attaches or the skin of the scalp may be torn from the underlying tissue and bone. **2.** (in dentistry) the knocking out of a tooth by trauma. The tooth may be *reimplanted.

axilla n. (pl. **axillae**) the armpit. —**axillary** adj.

axis n. **1.** a real or imaginary line through the centre of the body or one of its parts or a line about which the body or a part rotates. **2.** the second *cervical vertebra, which articulates with the atlas vertebra above and allows rotational movement of the head.

axolemma n. the fine cell membrane, visible only under the electron microscope, that encloses the protoplasm of an *axon.

axon n. a nerve fibre: a single process extending from the cell body of a *neurone and carrying nerve impulses away from it. An axon may be over a metre in length in certain neurones. In large nerves the axon has a sheath (neurilemma) made of *myelin; this is interrupted at intervals by gaps called nodes of Ranvier, at which branches of the axon leave. An axon ends by dividing into several branches called telodendria, which make contact with other nerves or with muscle or gland membranes.

axoplasm n. the semifluid material of which the *axon of a nerve cell is composed. It flows slowly outwards from the cell body.

azapetine n. a short-acting drug that relieves spasm of small arteries and capillaries and improves the blood flow to the skin. Its effects and uses are similar to those of *tolazoline. Trade name: **Ilidar**.

azathioprine n. an *immunosuppressive drug, used mainly to aid the survival of organ or tissue transplants. It has also been used in the treatment of acute and chronic leukaemias and inflammatory bowel disease (e.g. ulcerative colitis). Azathioprine may damage bone marrow, causing blood disorders. It may also cause muscle wasting and skin rashes. Trade name: **Imuran**.

azo- (azoto-) *prefix denoting* a nitrogenous compound, such as urea. Example: *azothermia* (fever due to nitrogenous substances in the blood).

azoospermia (aspermia) *n.* the complete absence of sperm from the seminal fluid. This is due either to failure of formation of sperm by the seminiferous tubules within the testes or to a blockage in the ducts that conduct sperm from the testes. A biopsy of the testis is necessary to differentiate these two causes of azoospermia; if a blockage is present it may be possible to relieve it surgically.

azotaemia *n.* a former name for *uraemia.

azoturia *n.* the presence in the urine of an abnormally high concentration of nitrogen-containing compounds, especially urea.

azygos vein an unpaired vein that arises from the inferior vena cava and drains into the superior vena cava, returning blood from the thorax and abdominal cavities.

B

Babinski reflex *see* plantar reflex.

bacillaemia *n.* the presence of bacilli in the blood, resulting from infection.

bacille Calmette-Guérin *see* BCG.

bacilluria *n.* the presence of bacilli in the urine, resulting from a bladder or kidney infection. *See* cystitis.

bacillus *n.* (*pl.* **bacilli**) any rod-shaped bacterium. *See also* Bacillus, Lactobacillus, Streptobacillus.

Bacillus *n.* a large genus of Gram-positive spore-bearing rodlike bacteria. They are widely distributed in soil and air (usually as spores). Most feed on dead organic material and are responsible for food spoilage. The species *B. anthracis* which is nonmotile, causes *anthrax, a disease of farm animals transmissible to man. *B. polymyxa*, commonly found in soil, is the source of the *polymyxin group of antibiotics. *B. subtilis* may cause conjunctivitis in man; it also produces the antibiotic *bacitracin.

bacitracin *n.* an antibiotic produced by certain strains of bacteria and effective against a number of microorganisms. It is usually applied externally, to treat infections of the skin, eyes, or nose, but can be given by mouth as an intestinal antiseptic or by injection. The principal toxic effect is on the kidneys.

backbone (spinal column, spine, vertebral column) *n.* a flexible bony column extending from the base of the skull to the small of the back. It encloses and protects the spinal cord, articulates with the skull, ribs, and hip girdle, and provides attachment for the muscles of the back. It is made up of individual bones (*see* vertebra) connected by discs of fibrocartilage (*see* intervertebral disc) and bound together by ligaments. The backbone of a newborn baby contains 33 vertebrae: seven cervical (neck), 12 thoracic (chest), five lumbar (lower back), five sacral (hip), and four coccygeal. In the adult the sacral and coccygeal vertebrae become fused into two single bones (sacrum and coccyx, respectively); the adult vertebral column therefore contains 26 bones (see illustration). Anatomical name: **rachis**.

bacteraemia *n.* the presence of bacteria in the blood: a sign of infection.

bacteri- (bacterio-) *prefix denoting* bacteria. Example: *bacteriolysis* (dissolution of).

bacteria

cervical
vertebrae
(7)

thoracic
vertebrae
(12)

lumbar
vertebrae
(5)

sacrum
(5 fused)

coccyx
(4 fused)

A   B

The backbone, seen from the back (A) and
left side (B)

bacteria *pl. n.* (*sing.* **bacterium**) a
group of microorganisms all of which
lack a distinct nuclear membrane (and
hence are considered more primitive
than animal and plant cells) and have a
cell wall of unique composition (many
antibiotics act by destroying the bacterial cell wall). Most bacteria are
unicellular; the cells may be spherical
(*coccus), rodlike (*bacillus), spiral
(*Spirillum*), comma-shaped (*Vibrio*)
or corkscrew-shaped (*spirochaete).
Generally, they range in size between
0.5 and 5 μm. Motile species bear one or
more fine hairs (flagella) arising from
their surface. Many possess an outer
slimy *capsule, and some have the
ability to produce an encysted or resting form (*endospore). Bacteria reproduce asexually by simple division of
cells; incomplete separation of daughter

cells leads to the formation of *colonies
of different numbers and arrangements
of cells. Some colonies are filamentous
in shape, resembling those of fungi.
Some bacteria may reproduce sexually
by *conjugation.

Bacteria are very widely distributed.
Some live in soil, water, or air; others
are parasites of man, animals, and
plants. Many parasitic bacteria do not
harm their hosts; some cause diseases
by producing poisons (*see* endotoxin,
exotoxin).

bactericidal *adj.* being capable of
killing bacteria. Substances with this
property include antibiotics, antiseptics, and disinfectants; they are known
as *bactericides*. *Compare* bacteriostatic.

bacteriolysin *n. see* lysin.

bacteriology *n.* the science of bacteria.
See also microbiology. —**bacteriological** *adj.* —**bacteriologist** *n.*

bacteriophage (phage) *n.* a virus that
attacks bacteria. In general, a phage
consists of a head, tail, and tail fibres,
all composed of protein molecules, and
a core of DNA. The tail and tail fibres
are responsible for attachment to the
bacterial surface and for injection of
the DNA core into the host cell. The
phage grows and replicates in the bacterial cell, which is eventually destroyed
with the release of new phages. Each
phage acts specifically against a particular species of bacterium. This is
utilized in *phage-typing*, a technique of
identifying bacteria by the action of
known phages on them. *See also* lysogeny.

bacteriostatic *adj.* capable of inhibiting or retarding the growth and multiplication of bacteria. *Compare* bactericidal.

bacterium *n. see* bacteria.

Bacteroides *n.* a genus of Gram-
negative, mostly nonmotile, anaerobic
rodlike bacteria. They are normally

present in the alimentary and urinogenital tracts of mammals and are found in the mouth, particularly in dental plaque associated with periodontal disease. Some species cause infections (*see* Fusobacterium).

Bactrim *n. see* co-trimoxazole.

Baghdad boil *see* oriental sore.

BAL (British Anti-Lewisite) *see* dimercaprol.

balanitis *n.* inflammation of the glans penis, usually associated with tightness of the foreskin (*phimosis). It is more common in childhood than in adult life. An acute attack is associated with redness and swelling of the glans. Treatment is by antibiotics, and further attacks are prevented by *circumcision.

balanoposthitis *n.* inflammation of the foreskin and the surface of the underlying glans penis. It usually occurs as a consequence of *phimosis and represents a more extensive local reaction than simple *balanitis. The affected areas become red and swollen, which further narrows the opening of the foreskin and makes passing urine difficult and painful. Treatment of an acute attack is by administration of antibiotics, and further attacks are prevented by *circumcision.

balantidiasis *n.* an infestation of the large intestine of man with the parasitic protozoan *Balantidium coli. Man usually becomes infected by ingesting food or drink contaminated with cysts from the faeces of a pig. The parasite invades and destroys the intestinal wall, causing ulceration and *necrosis, and the patient may experience diarrhoea and dysentery. Balantidiasis is a rare cause of dysentery, mainly affecting farm workers; it is treated with various antibiotics, carbarsone, and *diiodohydroxyquinoline.

Balantidium *n.* a genus of one of the largest parasitic *protozoans affecting man (70 μm or more in length). The oval body is covered with threadlike cilia (for locomotion). *B. coli*, normally living in the gut of pigs as a harmless *commensal, occasionally infects man (*see* balantidiasis).

baldness *n. see* alopecia.

ball-and-socket joint *see* enarthrosis.

ballistocardiograph *n.* an instrument for recording the displacement of the whole body produced by the ejection of blood with each heart beat. The normal record produced by such an instrument (*ballistocardiogram*) may be altered by disease of the heart or aortic valve (*see* aortic regurgitation, aortic stenosis).

ballottement *n.* the technique of examining a fluid-filled part of the body to detect a floating object. During pregnancy, a sharp tap with the fingers, applied to the womb through the abdominal wall or the vagina, causes the fetus to move away and then return to impart an answering tap to the examiner's hand as it floats back to its original position. This confirms that swelling of the uterus is due to a fetus rather than a tumour or other abnormality.

balneotherapy *n.* the treatment of disease by bathing, usually in the mineral-containing waters of hot springs. The once fashionable 'water cures', taken at spas, certainly had a more psychological than physical effect. Today, specialized remedial treatment in baths, under the supervision of physiotherapists, is used to alleviate pain and improve blood circulation and limb mobility in arthritis and in nerve and muscle disorders.

bamethan *n.* a drug that relaxes smooth muscle and dilates the peripheral blood vessels. It is used in the treatment of vascular disease to relieve spasm of the arteries and improve blood flow to the tissues. Common side-effects include flushing, gooseflesh, and tingling.

bandage *n.* a piece of material, in the form of a pad or strip, applied to a wound or used to bind around an injured or diseased part of the body.

Bandl's ring *see* retraction ring.

Banti's syndrome a disorder in which enlargement and overactivity of the spleen occurs as a result of increased pressure within the splenic vein. The commonest cause is *cirrhosis of the liver.

barbitone (barbital) *n.* a long-acting *barbiturate, used as a hypnotic, as a sedative, for the suppression of convulsions, as an analgesic, and as an anaesthetic. Prolonged use may lead to *dependence and overdosage has serious toxic effects (*see* barbiturism). Trade name: **Veronal**.

barbitone sodium a barbiturate that has properties, uses, and side-effects similar to those of barbitone but acts more rapidly. It can be given by mouth or by injection.

barbiturate *n.* any of a group of drugs, derived from barbituric acid, that depress activity of the central nervous system. Most barbiturates, including *amylobarbitone and *pentobarbitone, are taken as sleeping pills. Very slow-acting barbiturates (such as *phenobarbitone) are used as sedatives and to control epilepsy; those with a rapid and short-lived effect (such as *thiopentone) are injected as anaesthetics. Because they produce *tolerance and psychological and physical *dependence, have serious toxic side-effects (*see* barbiturism), and can be fatal following large overdosage, barbiturates have been largely replaced in clinical use by safer drugs. The use of barbiturates with alcohol should be avoided since these drugs reinforce each other, producing serious effects.

barbiturism *n.* addiction to drugs of the barbiturate group. Signs of intoxication include confusion, slurring of speech, yawning, sleepiness, loss of memory, loss of balance, and reduction in muscular reflexes. Withdrawal of the drugs must be undertaken slowly, over 1–3 weeks, to avoid the withdrawal symptoms of tremors and convulsions, which can prove fatal.

baritosis *n.* a lung disease – a form of *pneumoconiosis – caused by inhaling barium dust. It gives dramatic shadows on chest X-rays but no respiratory disability.

barium sulphate a barium salt, insoluble in water, that is opaque to X-rays and is used as a contrast medium in radiography of the stomach and intestines. *See also* enema.

baroreceptor (baroceptor) *n.* a collection of sensory nerve endings specialized to monitor changes in blood pressure. The main receptors lie in the *carotid sinuses and the *aortic arch; others are found in the walls of other large arteries and veins and some within the walls of the heart. Impulses from the receptors reach centres in the medulla; from here autonomic activity is directed so that the heart rate and resistance of the peripheral blood vessels can be adjusted appropriately.

barotitis *n.* discomfort in the ears due to changing air pressure during air travel.

barotrauma *n.* damage to the middle ear or *Eustachian tube due to changes in atmospheric pressure associated with air travel.

Barr body *see* sex chromatin.

bartholinitis (vulvovaginitis) *n.* inflammation of the mucus-secreting glands alongside the vaginal opening (*Bartholin's glands). In *chronic bartholinitis* cysts may form in the glands. In *acute bartholinitis* the glands are blocked and an abscess develops.

Bartholin's glands (greater vestibular glands) a pair of glands that open at the junction of the vagina and the external genitalia (vulva). Their secretions lubricate the vulva and so assist penetration by the penis during coitus. The *lesser vestibular glands*, around the vaginal opening, perform the same function.

Bartonella *n.* a genus of parasitic rod-shaped or rounded microorganisms, usually regarded as intermediate between the bacteria and rickettsiae. They occur in the red blood cells and cells of the lymphatic system, spleen, liver, and kidneys. *B. bacilliformis* causes *bartonellosis in man.

bartonellosis *n.* an infectious disease, confined to high river valleys in Peru, Ecuador, and Columbia, caused by the parasitic microorganism **Bartonella bacilliformis*. The parasite, present in red blood cells and cells of the lymphatic system, is transmitted to man by sandflies. There are two clinical types of the disease: *Oroya fever* (*Carrion's disease*), whose symptoms include fever, anaemia, and enlargement of the liver, spleen, and lymph nodes; and *verruga peruana*, characterized by wartlike eruptions on the skin that can bleed easily and ulcerate. Oroya fever accounts for nearly all fatalities. Bartonellosis can be treated successfully with penicillin and other antibiotics and blood transfusions may be given to relieve the anaemia.

basal cell carcinoma *see* rodent ulcer.

basal ganglia several large masses of grey matter embedded deep within the white matter of the *cerebrum (see illustration). They include the *caudate* and *lenticular nuclei* (together known as the *corpus striatum*) and the *amygdaloid nucleus*. The lenticular nucleus consists of the *putamen* and *globus pallidus*. The basal ganglia have complex neural connections with both the cerebral cortex and thalamus: they are involved with the regulation of voluntary movements at a subconscious level.

The basal ganglia and neighbouring parts (seen from the front)

basal metabolism the minimum amount of energy expended by the body to maintain vital processes, e.g. respiration, circulation, and digestion. It is expressed in terms of heat production per unit of body surface area per day (*basal metabolic rate – BMR*), and for an average man the BMR is 1.7 Calories (7.115 kilojoules) per day. BMR may be determined by the direct method, in which the subject is placed in a respiratory chamber and the amount of heat evolved is measured, or (more normally) by the indirect method, based on the *respiratory quotient. Measurements are best taken during a period of least activity, i.e. during sleep and 12–18 hours after a meal, under controlled temperature conditions. Various factors, such as age, sex, and particularly thyroid activity, influence the value of the BMR.

basement membrane the thin delicate membrane that lies at the base of an *epithelium. It is composed of mucopolysaccharide and fibres of protein.

base pairing the linking of the two strands of a DNA molecule by means of hydrogen bonds between the bases of the nucleotides. Adenine always pairs with thymine and cytosine with guanine. *See* DNA.

basilar artery an artery in the base of the brain, formed by the union of the two vertebral arteries. It extends from the lower to the upper border of the pons Varolii and then divides to form the two posterior cerebral arteries.

basilar membrane a membrane in the *cochlea of the ear that separates the two of the three channels (scalae) that run the length of the spiral cochlea. The organ of Corti is situated on the basilar membrane, inside the scala media.

basilic vein a large vein in the arm, extending from the hand along the back of the forearm, then passing forward to the inner side of the arm at the elbow.

basion *n.* the midpoint of the anterior border of the large hole (foramen magnum) at the base of the *skull.

basophil *n.* a variety of white blood cell distinguished by the presence in its cytoplasm of coarse granules that stain purple-black with *Romanowsky stains. The function of basophils is poorly understood, but they are capable of ingesting foreign particles and contain *histamine and *heparin. There are normally $0.03–0.15 \times 10^9$ basophils per litre of blood.

basophilia *n.* **1.** a property of a microscopic structure whereby it shows an affinity for basic dyes. **2.** an increase in the number of certain white blood cells (*basophils) in the blood, which may occur in a variety of blood diseases.

basophilic *adj.* readily stainable by basic dyes: showing *basophilia.

bathyaesthesia *n.* sensation experienced in the deeper parts of the body, such as the joints and muscles.

battered baby syndrome injuries inflicted on babies or young children by their parents, who are often emotionally disturbed or have themselves suffered from physical abuse in infancy or early childhood. The highest incidence of battering occurs in the first six months of life; it commonly takes the form of facial bruises, cigarette burns, bites, head injuries (often with brain damage), and fractured bones. Child abuse may be triggered by such crises as an unwanted pregnancy, unemployment, and debts; frequently, signs of older bruises, fractures, etc., are revealed when the child is brought for treatment. 60% of battered children suffer from further injury if discharged from hospital without the intensive support of a social worker and surveillance of family doctor and health visitor; a care order is often necessary to safeguard a child from further abuse.

Bazin's disease a disease of young women in which tender nodules develop under the skin in the calves. The nodules may break down and ulcerate though they may clear up spontaneously. The cause is unknown but the disease may be associated with tuberculosis or, more commonly, *perniosis. Medical name: **erythema induratum**.

BCG (bacille Calmette-Guérin) a strain of tubercle bacillus that has lost the power to cause tuberculosis but retains its antigenic activity; it is therefore used to prepare a vaccine against the disease.

beclamide *n.* an *anticonvulsant drug used in the treatment of epilepsy. It is administered by mouth and often given together with phenobarbitone. Side-effects may include stomach upsets, dizziness, and nervousness. Trade name: **Nydrane**.

beclomethasone *n.* a *corticosteroid drug that reduces inflammation and is applied externally in the treatment of various skin disorders. High dosage may cause retention of sodium and water and delayed wound healing. Trade name: **Propaderm**.

becquerel *n.* the *SI unit of activity of a radioactive source, being the activity of a radionuclide decaying at a rate of one spontaneous nuclear transition per second. It has replaced the curie. Symbol: Bq.

bed bug a bloodsucking insect of the genus *Cimex*. *C. hemipterus* of the tropics and *C. lectularius* of temperate regions have reddish flattened bodies and vestigial wings. They live and lay their eggs in the crevices of walls and furniture and emerge at night to suck blood; although bed bugs are not known vectors of disease their bites leave a route for bacterial infection. Premises can be disinfested with *DDT.

bed occupancy the number of hospital beds occupied by patients expressed as a percentage of the total beds available in the ward, specialty, hospital, area, or region. It may be recorded in relation to a defined point in time or more usefully for a period, when the calculation is based on bed-days. It is used with other indices (such as *discharge rate) to assess the demands for hospital beds in relation to diseases, specialties, or populations and hence to gauge an appropriate balance between health needs and residential (hospital) resources.

bedsore (decubitus ulcer, pressure sore) *n.* an ulcerated area of skin caused by irritation and continuous pressure on part of the body: a hazard to be guarded against in all bedridden (especially unconscious) patients. Healing is hindered by the reduced blood supply to the area, and careful nursing is necessary to prevent local gangrene. The patient's position should be changed frequently, and the buttocks, heels, elbows, and other regions at risk kept dry and clean.

bedwetting *n. see* enuresis.

behaviourism *n.* an approach to psychology postulating that only observable behaviour need be studied, thus denying any importance to unconscious processes. Behaviourists are concerned with the laws regulating the occurrence of behaviour (*see* conditioning). —**behaviourist** *n.*

behaviour modification the use of the methods of behaviourist psychology (*see* behaviourism) – especially operant *conditioning – to alter people's behaviour. Behaviour modification has wider applications than *behaviour therapy, since it is also used in situations in which the client is not ill; for example, in education. *See also* chaining, prompting.

behaviour therapy treatment based on the belief that psychological problems are the products of faulty learning and not the symptoms of an underlying disease. Treatment is directed at the problem or target behaviour and is designed for the particular patient, not for the particular diagnostic label that has been attached to him. *See also* aversion therapy, conditioning, desensitization.

bejel (endemic syphilis) *n.* a long-lasting nonvenereal form of *syphilis that occurs in the Balkans, Turkey, eastern Mediterranean countries, and the dry savannah regions of North Africa; it is particularly prevalent where standards of personal hygiene are low. The disease is spread among children and adults by direct body contact. Early skin lesions are obvious in the moist areas of the body (mouth, armpits, and groin) and later there may be considerable destruction of the tissues of the skin, nasopharynx, and long bones. Wartlike eruptions in the anal and genital regions are common. Bejel, which is rarely fatal, is treated with penicillin.

bel

bel *n. see* decibel.

belladonna *n.* **1.** deadly nightshade (*Atropa belladonna*): a plant from which the drugs atropine and hyoscyamine are obtained. **2.** the poisonous alkaloid derived from deadly nightshade, from which atropine and hyoscyamine are extracted.

bell and pad a psychological method of treating bed-wetting. When the child starts to pass urine it is detected by a pad (or by sheets of metallic mesh) and this sets off a bell (or loud buzzer), which wakens the child. He then empties his bladder fully. A process of conditioning leads to his learning to be dry. It is effective in about 80% of cases.

Bell's palsy paralysis of the *facial nerve causing weakness of the muscles of one side of the face and an inability to close the eye. In some patients hearing may be affected so that sounds seem abnormally loud, and a loss of taste sensation may occur. The cause of this condition is unknown and recovery normally occurs spontaneously.

belly *n.* **1.** the *abdomen or abdominal cavity. **2.** the central fleshy portion of a muscle.

Bence-Jones protein (Bence-Jones albumose) a protein of low molecular weight found in the urine of patients with multiple *myeloma, *lymphoma, *leukaemia, and *Hodgkin's disease.

bendrofluazide (bendroflumethazide) *n.* a potent diuretic used in the treatment of conditions involving retention of fluid, such as congestive heart failure, hypertension, *oedema, and obesity. Its actions and side-effects are similar to those of *chlorothiazide.

bends *n. see* compressed air illness.

Benedict's test a test for the presence of sugar in urine or other liquids. A few drops of the test solution are added to *Benedict's solution*, prepared from sodium or potassium citrate, sodium car-

bonate, and copper sulphate. The mixture is boiled and shaken for about two minutes, then left to cool. The presence of up to 2% glucose is indicated by the formation of a reddish, yellowish, or greenish precipitate, the highest levels corresponding to the red coloration, the lowest (about 0.05%) to the green.

benethamine penicillin an antibiotic effective against most Gram-positive bacteria (streptococci, staphylococci, and pneumococci). A derivative of benzylpenicillin, it can be administered by mouth but is usually given as an intramuscular injection, from which it liberates benzylpenicillin slowly. Patients hypersensitive to penicillins may suffer allergic reactions. *See also* penicillin.

benign *adj.* **1.** describing a tumour that does not invade and destroy the tissue in which it originates or spread to distant sites in the body, i.e. a tumour that is not cancerous. **2.** describing any disorder or condition that does not produce harmful effects. *Compare* malignant.

benign intracranial hypertension (pseudotumour cerebri) a syndrome of raised pressure within the skull caused by impaired reabsorption of cerebrospinal fluid. The symptoms include headache, vomiting, double vision, and *papilloedema. It normally subsides spontaneously but treatment may be required to protect the patient's vision.

benorylate *n.* a drug, derived from *paracetamol, that relieves pain, inflammation, and fever. It is an alternative to aspirin, particularly in the treatment of rheumatoid arthritis. Side-effects may include drowsiness, noises in the ears, and skin rashes. Trade name: **Benoral**.

benzalkonium *n.* a detergent disinfectant with the same uses and effects as *cetrimide.

benzathine penicillin a long-acting antibiotic, given by mouth or intramuscular injection, that is slowly absorbed and effective against most Gram-positive bacteria (streptococci, staphylococci, and pneumococci). Patients hypersensitive to the penicillins suffer allergic reactions. Trade names: **Bicillin**, **Penidural**. *See also* penicillin.

benzethonium *n.* a detergent disinfectant with uses similar to those of *cetrimide.

benzhexol *n.* a drug that has actions and side-effects similar to those of *atropine. Taken by mouth, it is used mainly to reduce muscle spasm in parkinsonism. Trade names: **Artane**, **Pipanol**.

benzocaine *n.* a local anaesthetic used in the form of an ointment, suppository, or aerosol to relieve painful conditions of the skin and mucous membranes. Virtually non-toxic, it can also be given by mouth to treat such conditions as lacerations of the mouth or tongue and gastric ulcers.

benzodiazepines *n.* a group of pharmacologically active compounds used as minor *tranquillizers and hypnotics. The group includes *chlordiazepoxide, *diazepam, and *oxazepam.

benzoic acid an antiseptic, active against fungi and bacteria, used as a preservative in foods and pharmaceutical preparations, as well as for the treatment of fungal infections of the skin.

benzphetamine *n.* a drug with actions and side-effects similar to those of *amphetamine. It is given by mouth in the treatment of obesity. Trade name: **Didrex**.

benzthiazide *n.* a *diuretic used in the treatment of conditions involving fluid retention, such as congestive heart failure, *oedema, hypertension, and obesity. Trade name: **Exna**.

benztropine *n.* a drug similar to *atropine, but that also acts as an antihistamine, local anaesthetic, and sedative. Given by mouth it is used mainly in the treatment of parkinsonism to reduce rigidity and muscle cramps. It is well tolerated, but produces drowsiness and confusion.

benzyl benzoate an oily aromatic liquid that is applied to the body – in the form of a lotion – for the treatment of scabies. It is also useful in treating pediculosis.

benzylpenicillin *n. see* penicillin.

beriberi *n.* a nutritional disorder due to deficiency of vitamin B$_1$ (thiamin). It is widespread in rice-eating communities in which the diet is based on polished rice, from which the thiamin-rich seed coat has been removed. Beriberi takes two forms: *wet beriberi*, in which there is an accumulation of tissue fluid (*oedema), and *dry beriberi*, in which there is extreme emaciation. There is nervous degeneration in both forms of the disease and death from heart failure is often the outcome.

berylliosis *n.* poisoning by inhalation of beryllium or its compounds. This may be acute and sometimes fatal, but is more often chronic with the development of *fibrosis affecting all parts of the lungs. In Britain some workers with fluorescent light tubes were affected but this use was abolished in 1948.

beta blocker a drug that prevents stimulation of the beta-adrenergic receptors of the nerves of the sympathetic nervous system and therefore decreases the activity of the heart. Beta blockers include *oxprenolol and *propranolol, which are used to control abnormal heart rhythms, to treat angina, and to reduce high blood pressure. Blockade

betamethasone

of beta receptors may cause constriction of air passages in the lungs and care has to be taken with the use of beta blockers in patients with any bronchial conditions. *See also* sympatholytic.

betamethasone *n.* a synthetic corticosteroid drug with effects and uses similar to those of *prednisolone. The side-effects are those of *cortisone. Trade names: **Betnelan, Betnesol, Betnovate**.

betatron *n.* a device used to accelerate a stream of electrons (*beta particles*) into a beam of radiation that can be used in *radiotherapy.

bethanidine *n.* a drug that lowers blood pressure. It is given by mouth and acts by blocking the sympathetic nerves that supply the blood vessels. Common side-effects include dizziness, fainting, oedema, and breathlessness. Trade names: **Bethamid, Esbatal**.

bezoar *n.* a mass of swallowed foreign material within the stomach. The material, which is usually swallowed by psychiatrically disturbed patients, accumulates and ultimately causes gastric obstruction. Its removal often requires a surgical operation. *See also* trichobezoar.

bi- *prefix denoting* two; double. Examples: *biciliate* (having two cilia); *binucleate* (having two nuclei).

biceps *n.* a muscle with two heads. The *biceps brachii* extends from the shoulder joint to the elbow (see illustration). It flexes the arm and forearm and supinates the forearm and hand. The *biceps femoris* is situated at the back of the thigh and is responsible for flexing the knee, extending the thigh, and rotating the leg outwards.

biconcave *adj.* having a hollowed surface on both sides. Biconcave lenses are

The biceps muscle of the arm

used to correct short-sightedness. *Compare* biconvex.

biconvex *adj.* having a surface on each side that curves outwards. Biconvex lenses are used to correct long-sightedness. *Compare* biconcave.

bicornuate *adj.* having two hornlike processes or projections. The term is applied to an abnormal uterus that is divided into two separate halves at the upper end.

bicuspid 1. *adj.* having two *cusps, as in the premolar teeth and the mitral valve of the heart. **2.** *n.* (in the USA) a premolar tooth.

bicuspid valve *see* mitral valve.

bifid *adj.* split or cleft into two parts.

bifocal lenses glasses in which the upper part of the lens is shaped to give a sharp image of distant objects and the lower part is for use in near vision, such as reading. *See also* trifocal lenses, multifocal lenses.

bifurcation *n.* (in anatomy) the point at which division into two branches occurs; for example in blood vessels or in the trachea.

bigeminal body one of the two swellings that develop in the roof of the midbrain during its development in the embryo.

bigeminy *n.* the condition in which alternate *ectopic beats of the heart are transmitted to the pulse and felt as a double pulse beat (*pulsus bigeminus*). It is a common manifestation of digitalis poisoning.

bilateral *adj.* (in anatomy) relating to or affecting both sides of the body or of a tissue or organ or both of a pair of organs (e.g. the eyes, breasts, or ovaries).

bile *n.* a thick alkaline fluid that is secreted by the *liver and stored in the *gall bladder, from which it is ejected intermittently into the duodenum via the common *bile duct. Bile may be yellow, green, or brown, according to the proportions of the *bile pigments (excretory products) present; other constituents are lecithin, cholesterol, and *bile salts. The bile salts help to emulsify fats in the duodenum so that they can be more easily digested by pancreatic *lipase into fatty acids and glycerol. Bile salts also form compounds with fatty acids, which can then be transported into the *lacteals. Bile also helps to stimulate *peristalsis in the duodenum.

bile acids the organic acids in bile; mostly occurring as bile salts (sodium glycocholate and sodium taurocholate). They are cholic acid, deoxycholic acid, glycocholic acid, and taurocholic acid.

bile duct any of the ducts that convey bile from the liver. Bile is drained from the liver cells by many small ducts that unite to form the main bile duct of the liver, the *hepatic duct*. This joins the *cystic duct*, which leads from the *gall bladder, to form the *common bile duct*, which drains into the duodenum.

bile pigments coloured compounds – breakdown products of the blood pigment *haemoglobin – that are excreted in *bile. The two most important bile pigments are *bilirubin*, which is orange or yellow, and its oxidized form *biliverdin*, which is green. Mixed with the intestinal contents, they give the brown colour to the faeces (*see* urobilinogen).

bile salts sodium glycocholate and sodium taurocholate – the alkaline salts of *bile – necessary for the emulsification of fats. After they have been absorbed from the intestine they are transported to the liver for reuse.

Bilharzia *n. see* Schistosoma.

bilharziasis *n. see* schistosomiasis.

bili- *prefix denoting* bile.

biliary *adj.* relating to or affecting the bile duct or bile. *See also* fistula.

biliary colic pain resulting from obstruction of the gall bladder or common bile duct, usually by a stone. The pain, which is very severe, is usually felt in the upper abdomen (in the mid-line or to the right). It often occurs about an hour after a meal (particularly if fatty), may last several hours, and is usually steady in severity (unlike other forms of *colic). Vomiting often occurs simultaneously.

bilious *adj.* **1.** containing bile; for example *bilious vomiting* is the vomiting of bile-containing fluid. **2.** a lay term used to describe attacks of nausea or vomiting.

bilirubin *n. see* bile pigments.

bilirubinaemia *n.* an excess of the *bile pigment bilirubin in the blood. Normally there is under 0.8 mg bilirubin per 100 ml blood; when the concentration of bilirubin is above 1–1.5 mg per 100 ml, visible *jaundice occurs.

biliuria (choluria) *n.* the presence of bile in the urine: a feature of certain forms of jaundice.

biliverdin *n. see* bile pigments.

bimanual *adj.* using two hands to perform an activity, such as a gynaecological examination.

binaural *adj.* relating to or involving the use of both ears.

binder *n.* a bandage that is wound around a part of the body, usually the abdomen, to apply pressure or to give support or protection.

binocular *adj.* relating to or involving the use of both eyes.

binocular vision the ability to focus both eyes on an object at the same time, so that a person sees one image of the object he is looking at. It is not inborn, but acquired during the first few months of life. Binocular vision enables judgment of distance and perception of depth. *See also* stereoscopic vision.

bio- *prefix denoting* life or living organisms. Example: *biosynthesis* (formation of a compound within a living organism).

bioassay *n.* estimation of the activity or potency of a drug or other substance by comparing its effects on living organisms with effects of a preparation of known strength. Bioassay is used to determine the strength of preparations of hormones or other material of biological origin when other physical or chemical methods are not available.

biochemistry *n.* the study of the chemical processes and substances occurring in living things. —**biochemical** *adj.* —**biochemist** *n.*

biofeedback *n.* the giving of immediate information to a subject about his bodily processes (such as heart rate), which are usually unconscious. These processes can then be subject to operant *conditioning. This is an experimental treatment for disturbances of bodily regulation, such as hypertension.

biology *n.* the study of living organisms – plants, animals, and microorganisms – including their structure and working and their relationships with one another and with the inanimate world. —**biological** *adj.*

biometry *n.* the measurement of living things and the processes associated with life, including the application of mathematics, particularly statistics, to problems in biology.

bionics *n.* the science of mechanical or electronic systems that function in the same way as, or have characteristics of, living systems. *Compare* cybernetics. —**bionic** *adj.*

bionomics *n. see* ecology.

biopsy *n.* the removal of a small piece of living tissue from an organ or part of the body for microscopic examination. Biopsy is an important means of diagnosing cancer from examination of a fragment of tumour. It is often carried out with a special hollow needle, inserted into the liver, kidney, or other organ, with relatively little discomfort to the patient.

biostatistics *n.* statistical information and techniques used with special reference to studies of health and social problems. It embraces, overlaps, and is to some extent synonymous with the fields of *vital statistics* (e.g. *fertility and *mortality rates) and *demography.

biotin *n.* a vitamin of the B complex that is essential for the metabolism of fat, being involved in fatty acid synthesis and *gluconeogenesis. A biotin deficiency is extremely rare in man; it can be induced by eating large quantities of raw egg white, which contains a protein – avidin – that combines with biotin, making it unavailable to the body. Rich sources of the vitamin are egg yolk and liver.

bipara *n.* a woman who has been pregnant twice and has given birth to a living child at the end of each pregnancy.

biparous *adj.* giving birth to two children at the end of a pregnancy.

biperiden *n.* a drug with effects similar to those of atropine, used in the treatment of parkinsonism, certain forms of spasticity, and to control the muscular incoordination that may result from the use of some tranquillizers. It is given by mouth; side-effects are those of *atropine. Trade name: **Akineton**.

bipolar *adj.* (in neurology) describing a neurone (nerve cell) that has two processes extending in different directions from its cell body.

birefringence *n.* the property possessed by some naturally occurring substances (such as cell membranes) of doubly refracting a beam of light, i.e. of bending it in two different directions. —**birefringent** *adj.*

birth *n.* (in obstetrics) *see* labour.

birth control the use of *contraception or *sterilization (male or female) to prevent unwanted pregnancies.

birthmark *n.* a skin blemish or mark present at birth. The cause is unknown but most birthmarks grow before the baby is born. *See* naevus.

birth rate *see* fertility rate.

bisacodyl *n.* a *laxative that acts on the large intestine to cause reflex movement and bowel evacuation. It is administered by mouth or in a suppository. The commonest side-effect is the development of abdominal cramps. Trade name: **Dulcolax**.

bisexual *adj.* **1.** describing an individual who is sexually attracted to both men and women. **2.** describing an individual who possesses the qualities of both sexes.

Bismarck brown a basic aniline dye used for staining and counterstaining histological and bacterial specimens.

bistoury *n.* a narrow surgical knife, with a straight or curved blade (see illustration).

Types of bistoury

bite-raiser *n.* an appliance to prevent normal closure of the teeth in the treatment of the *temporomandibular joint syndrome.

bite-wing *n.* a dental X-ray film that provides a view of the crowns of the teeth in part of both upper and lower jaws. This view is used in the diagnosis of caries and periodontal disease.

bivalent *n.* (in genetics) a structure consisting of homologous chromosomes attached to each other by *chiasmata during the first division of *meiosis. —**bivalent** *adj.*

blackdamp (chokedamp) *n.* (in mining) the poisonous gas containing carbon dioxide, carbon monoxide, or other suffocating material, sometimes found in pockets in underground workings. *Compare* firedamp.

Black Death *see* plague.

black eye bruising of the eyelids.

black fly a small widely distributed bloodsucking insect of the genus *Simulium*. Black flies are also known as buffalo gnats from their humpbacked appearance. Female flies can inflict painful bites and constitute a serious pest to man at certain times of the year. *S. damnosum* in Africa and *S. ochraceum* in Central America and Vene-

blackhead

zuela transmit the parasites causing *onchocerciasis.

blackhead *n.* a plug formed of fatty material (sebum and keratin) in the outlet of a *sebaceous gland in the skin. Oxidation of the keratin in the blackhead is the cause of the black coloration. *See also* acne. Medical name: **comedo**.

blackwater fever a rare and serious complication of malignant tertian (falciparum) *malaria in which there is massive destruction of the red blood cells, leading to the presence of the blood pigment haemoglobin in the urine. The condition is probably brought on by inadequate treatment with *quinine; it is marked by fever, bloody urine, jaundice, vomiting, enlarged liver and spleen, anaemia, exhaustion, and – in fatal cases – a reduced flow of urine resulting from a blockage of the kidney tubules. Treatment involves rest, administration of alkaline fluids and intravenous glucose, and blood transfusions.

bladder *n.* **1. (urinary bladder)** a sac-shaped organ that has a wall of smooth muscle and stores the urine produced by the kidneys. Urine passes into the bladder through the *ureters; the release of urine from the bladder is controlled by a sphincter at its junction with the *urethra. **2.** any of several other hollow organs containing fluid, such as the *gall bladder.

bladderworm *n. see* cysticercus.

-blast *suffix denoting* a formative cell. Example: *osteoblast* (formative bone cell).

blastema *n.* any zone of embryonic tissue that is still differentiating and growing into a particular organ. The term is usually applied to the tissue that develops into the kidneys and gonads.

blasto- *prefix denoting* a germ cell or embryo. Example: *blastogenesis* (early development of an embryo).

blastocoele *n.* the fluid-filled cavity that develops within the *blastocyst. The cavity increases the surface area of the embryo and thus improves its ability to absorb nutrients and oxygen.

blastocyst *n.* an early stage of embryonic development that consists of a hollow ball of cells with a localized thickening (the *inner cell mass*) that will develop into the actual embryo; the remainder of the blastocyst is composed of *trophoblast (see illustration). At first the blastocyst is unattached, but it soon implants in the wall of the womb (uterus). *See also* implantation.

Section through a blastocyst

blastomere *n.* any of the cells produced by *cleavage of the zygote, comprising the earliest stages of embryonic development until the formation of the *blastocyst. Blastomeres divide repeatedly without growth and so decrease in size.

blastomycosis *n.* any disease caused by parasitic fungi of the genus *Blastomyces*, which may affect the skin (forming wartlike ulcers and tumours on the face, neck, hands, arms, feet, and legs) or involve various internal tissues, such as the lungs, bones, liver, spleen, and lymphatics. There are two principal forms of the disease: *North American blastomycosis* (*Gilchrist's disease*), caused by *B. dermatitidis*; and *South American blastomycosis*, caused by *B. brasiliensis*. Both diseases are treated with antibiotics (such as amphotericin).

blastopore *n.* the opening that forms as a result of invagination of the surface layer of the early embryo (*gastrula). It is very much reduced in man, in which it gives rise to the archenteric canal (*see* archenteron).

blastula *n.* an early stage of the embryonic development of many animals. The equivalent stage in mammals (including man) is the *blastocyst.

bleeding *n. see* haemorrhage.

blenn- (blenno-) *prefix denoting* mucus. Example: *blennorrhagia* (excessive production of).

blennophthalmia *n. Obsolete.* *conjunctivitis in which there is a sticky yellow discharge from the eye.

blennorrhagia *n.* a copious discharge of mucus, particularly from the urethra. This usually accompanies *urethritis and sometimes acute *prostatitis. Treatment is directed to clearing the underlying causative organism by antibiotic administration.

blennorrhoea *n.* a profuse watery discharge from the urethra. This, like *blennorrhagia, is associated with either prostatitis or urethritis, and is cleared by the usual measures undertaken in the treatment of these conditions.

bleomycin *n.* an antibiotic with action against cancer cells, used in the treatment of Hodgkin's disease and other lymphomas and in squamous-cell carcinoma. It is administered by injection and can cause toxic side-effects in the skin and lungs; it should not be used in patients with impaired kidney function or lung disease.

blephar- (blepharo-) *prefix denoting* the eyelid. Example: *blepharotomy* (incision into).

blepharitis *n.* inflammation of the eyelids. In *squamous blepharitis*, often associated with dandruff of the scalp, white scales accumulate among the lashes. *Chronic ulcerative blepharitis* is characterized by yellow crusts overlying ulcers of the lid margins. The lashes become matted together and tend to fall out or become distorted. *Allergic blepharitis* may occur in response to drugs or cosmetics put in the eye or on the eyelids.

blepharon *n. see* eyelid.

blepharophimosis *n.* narrowing of the aperture between the eyelids. It may be congenital but can be acquired if the skin contracts at the outer corner of the eye as a result of chronic inflammation.

blepharoplasty (tarsoplasty) *n.* any operation to repair or reconstruct the eyelid. It involves either rearrangement of the tissues of the lid or the use of tissue from other sites (e.g. skin or mucous membrane).

blepharospasm *n.* involuntary tight contraction of the eyelids, usually in response to painful conditions of the eye.

blindness *n.* the inability to see. Lack of all light perception constitutes total blindness but there are degrees of visual impairment far less severe than this that may be classed as blindness for administrative or statutory purposes. For example, marked reduction in the *visual field is classified as blindness, even if objects are still seen sharply. The commonest causes of blindness are *trachoma, *onchocerciasis, and vitamin A deficiency (*see* night blindness) but there is wide geographic variation. In Great Britain the commonest causes are diabetes mellitus, myopic degeneration, and *glaucoma.

blind register (in Britain) a list of persons who are technically blind due to reduced visual acuity (inability to read a car number plate from a distance of three metres) or who have severely restricted fields of vision (*see* blindness). Such people are entitled to special education and to financial and other social benefits. *See also* partially sighted register.

blind spot the small area of the *retina of the eye where the nerve fibres from the light-sensitive cells (*see* cone, rod) lead into the optic nerve. There are no rods or cones in this area and hence it does not register light. Anatomical name: **punctum caecum**.

blind trial *see* intervention study.

blinking *n.* the action of closing and opening the eyelids, which wipes the front of the eyeball and helps to spread the *tears. Reflex blinking may be caused by suddenly bringing an object near to the eye: the eyelids close involuntarily in order to protect the eye.

blister *n.* a swelling containing watery fluid (serum) and sometimes also blood (*blood blister*) or pus, within or just beneath the skin. Blisters commonly develop as a result of unaccustomed friction on the hands or feet or at the site of a burn. Blisters may be treated with antiseptics and dressings. An unduly painful blister may be punctured with a sterile needle so that the fluid is released.

block *n.* any interruption of physiological or mental function, brought about intentionally (as part of a therapeutic procedure) or by disease. *See also* heart block, nerve block.

blocking *n.* (in psychiatry) **1.** a sudden halting of the flow of thought or speech. Blocking of thought, accompanied by the sensation of thoughts being removed from the mind, is a symptom of *schizophrenia. Blocking of speech may be a consequence of thought block or a result of a mechanical impediment in speech, such as *stammering. **2.** failure to recall a specific event, or to explore a specific train of thought, because of its unpleasant associations.

blood *n.* a fluid tissue that circulates throughout the body, via the arteries and veins, providing a vehicle by which an immense variety of different substances are transported between the various organs and tissues. It is composed of *blood cells, which are suspended in a liquid medium, the *plasma. An average individual has approximately 70 ml of blood per kilogram body weight (about 5 litres in an average adult male).

blood bank a department within a hospital or blood transfusion centre in which blood collected from donors is stored prior to transfusion. Blood must be kept at a temperature of 4°C and may be used up to three weeks after collection.

blood-brain barrier the mechanism whereby the circulating blood is kept separate from the tissue fluids surrounding the brain cells. It is a semipermeable membrane allowing solutions to pass through it but excluding solid particles and large molecules.

blood cell (blood corpuscle) any of the cells that are present in the blood in health or disease. The cells may be subclassified into two major categories, namely red cells (*erythrocytes), and white cells (*leucocytes), which include granulocytes, lymphocytes, and monocytes (see illustration). Blood cells and *platelets account for approximately 40% of the total volume of the blood in health; red cells comprise the vast majority.

small lymphocyte

erythrocyte

large lymphocyte

neutrophil

monocyte

eosinophil

granulocytes

platelets

basophil

Types of blood cells

blood clot a solid mass formed as the result of *blood coagulation, either within the blood vessels and heart or elsewhere (*compare* thrombus). A blood clot consists of a meshwork of the protein *fibrin in which various blood cells are trapped.

blood clotting *see* blood coagulation.

blood coagulation (blood clotting) the process whereby blood is converted from a liquid to a solid state. The process may be initiated by contact of blood with a foreign surface (*intrinsic system*) or with damaged tissue (*extrinsic system*). These systems involve the interaction of a variety of substances (*coagulation factors) and lead to the production of the enzyme thromboplas-

tin, which converts the soluble blood protein *fibrinogen to the insoluble protein *fibrin. Blood coagulation is an essential mechanism for the arrest of bleeding (*haemostasis).

blood corpuscle *see* blood cell.

blood count the numbers of different blood cells in a known volume of blood, usually expressed as the number of cells per litre. A sample of blood at known dilution is examined in a special counting chamber. Blood-count investigations are important in the diagnosis of blood diseases. *See also* differential leucocyte count.

blood donor a person who gives blood for storage in a *blood bank. The blood can then be used for *transfusion into another patient. In Britain collection is organized by the National Blood Transfusion Services, but the armed forces have their own services. *See also* blood group.

blood group any one of the many types into which a person's blood may be classified, based on the presence or absence of certain inherited antigens on the surface of the red blood cells. Blood of one group contains antibodies in the serum that react against the cells of other groups.

There are more than 30 blood group systems, one of the most important of which is the *ABO system*. This system is based on the presence or absence of antigens A and B: blood of groups A and B contains antigens A and B, respectively; group AB contains both antigens and group O neither. Blood of group A contains antibodies to antigen B; group B blood contains anti-A antibodies; group AB has neither antibody and group O has both. A person whose blood contains either (or both) of these antibodies cannot receive a transfusion of blood containing the corresponding antigens. The table illustrates which blood groups can be used in transfusion for each of the four groups.

blood plasma

Donor's blood group	Blood group of people donor can receive blood from	Blood group of people donor can give blood to
A	A, O	A, AB
B	B, O	B, AB
AB	A, B, AB, O	AB
O	O	A, B, AB, O

blood plasma *see* plasma.

blood poisoning the presence of either bacterial toxins or large numbers of bacteria in the bloodstream causing serious illness. *See* pyaemia, septicaemia, toxaemia.

blood pressure the pressure of blood against the walls of the main arteries. Pressure is highest during *systole, when the ventricles are contracting (*systolic pressure*), and lowest during *diastole, when the ventricles are relaxing and refilling (*diastolic pressure*). Blood pressure is measured – in millimetres of mercury – by means of a *sphygmomanometer at the brachial artery of the arm, where the pressure is most similar to that of blood leaving the heart. The normal range varies with age, but a young adult would be expected to have a systolic pressure of around 120 mm and a diastolic pressure of 80 mm. These are recorded as 120/80.
Individual variations are common. Muscular exertion and emotional factors, such as fear, stress, and excitement, all raise systolic blood pressure (*see* hypertension). Systolic blood pressure is normally at its lowest during sleep. Severe shock may lead to an abnormally low blood pressure and possible circulatory failure (*see* hypotension). Blood pressure is adjusted to its normal level by the *sympathetic nervous system and hormonal controls.

blood serum *see* serum.

blood sugar the concentration of glucose in the blood, normally expressed in millimoles per litre. The normal range is 3.5–5.5 mmol/l. Blood-sugar estimation is an important investigation in a variety of diseases, most notably in diabetes mellitus. *See also* hyperglycaemia, hypoglycaemia.

blood test any test designed to discover abnormalities in a sample of a person's blood, such as the presence of alcohol, drugs, or bacteria, or to determine the *blood group.

blood transfusion *see* transfusion.

blood vessel a tube carrying blood away from or towards the heart. Blood vessels are the means by which blood circulates throughout the body. *See* artery, arteriole, vein, venule, capillary.

blue baby an infant suffering from congenital malformation of the heart as a result of which some or all of the blue (deoxygenated) blood is pumped around the body instead of passing through the lungs to be oxygenated. The skin and lips have a purple colour. Advances in cardiac surgery have enabled remedial operations or even total correction to be performed, usually in the first few days or weeks of life. Those that cannot be corrected or improved may survive for months or years with persistent *cyanosis.

body *n.* 1. an entire animal organism. 2. the trunk of an individual, excluding the limbs. 3. the main or largest part of an organ (such as the stomach or uterus). **4.** a solid discrete mass of tissue; e.g. the carotid body. *See also* corpus.

body image (body schema) the individual's concept of the disposition of his limbs and the identity of the different parts of his body. It is a function of the *association areas of the brain. *See also* Gerstmann's syndrome.

body temperature the intensity of heat of the body, as measured by a thermometer. Body temperature is accurately controlled by a small area at the base of the brain (the *hypothalamus); in normal individuals it is maintained at about 37°C (98.4°F). Heat production by the body arises as the result of vital activities (e.g. respiration, heart beat, circulation, secretion) and from the muscular effort of exercise and shivering. A rise in body temperature occurs in fever.

body type (somatotype) the characteristic anatomical appearance of an individual, based on the predominance of the structures derived from the three germ layers (ectoderm, mesoderm, endoderm). The three types are described as *ectomorphic, *mesomorphic, and *endomorphic.

boil *n.* a tender inflamed area of the skin containing pus. The infection is usually caused by the bacterium *Staphylococcus aureus* entering through a hair follicle or a break in the skin, and local injury or lowered constitutional resistance may encourage the development of boils. Boils usually heal when the pus is released or with antibiotic treatment, though occasionally they may cause more widespread infection. Medical name: **furuncle**.

bolus *n.* a soft mass of chewed food that is ready to be swallowed.

bonding *n.* **1.** (in psychology) the development of a close and selective relationship, such as that of *attachment. *Mother-child bonding* is the supposed process in which physical contact between mother and child in the child's first hours of life promotes the mother's loving and caring for her baby. **2.** (in dentistry) the attachment of dental restorations, sealants, and appliances to teeth. Bonding may be mechanical (*see* acid-etch technique) or chemical, by the use of adhesive *cements.

bone *n.* the hard extremely dense connective tissue that forms the skeleton of the body. It is composed of a matrix of collagen fibres impregnated with bone salts (chiefly calcium carbonate and calcium phosphate). *Compact* (or *cortical*) *bone* forms the outer shell of bones; it consists of a hard virtually solid mass made up of bony tissue arranged in concentric layers (*Haversian systems*). *Spongy* (or *cancellous*) *bone*, found beneath compact bone, consists of a meshwork of bony bars (*trabeculae*) with many interconnecting spaces containing marrow. (See illustration.)

Individual bones may be classed as long, short, flat, or irregular. The outer layer of a bone is called the *periosteum. The *medullary cavity* is lined with *endosteum and contains the marrow. Bones not only form the skeleton but also act as stores for mineral salts and play an important part in the formation of blood cells.

bone marrow (marrow) the tissue contained within the internal cavities of the bones. At birth, these cavities are filled entirely with blood-forming *myeloid tissue* (*red marrow*) but in later life the marrow in the limb bones is replaced by fat (*yellow marrow*). Samples of bone marrow may be obtained for examination by *aspiration through a stout needle or by *trephine biopsy. *See also* haemopoiesis.

bony labyrinth *see* labyrinth.

borax *n.* a mild astringent with a weak antiseptic action, applied externally to skin and mucous membranes. Borax

spongy bone
periosteum
Haversian systems
compact bone

lymphatic vessel

canaliculi
Volkmann canal

two lamellae of matrix

vein
Haversian canal
artery

lacunae containing bone cells

Section of the shaft of a long bone (above) with detail of a single Haversian system (below)

and boric acid are used in mouth and nasal washes, gargles, eye lotions and contact-lens solutions, and in dusting powder. Side-effects from external application are rare; most reported cases of poisoning are in infants.

borborygmus *n.* (*pl.* **borborygmi**) an abdominal gurgle due to movement of fluid and gas in the intestine. Excessive borborygmi occur when intestinal movement is increased, for example in the *irritable bowel syndrome and in intestinal obstruction, or when there is more intestinal gas than normal.

Bordetella *n.* a genus of tiny Gram-negative aerobic bacteria. *B. pertussis* causes *whooping cough, and all the other species are able to break down red blood cells and cause diseases resembling whooping cough.

boric acid *see* borax.

Bornholm disease (devil's grip, epidemic myalgia, epidemic pleurodynia) a disease caused by *Coxsackie viruses. It is spread by contact and epidemics usually occur during warm weather in temperate regions and at any time in the tropics. Symptoms include fever, headache, and attacks of severe pain in the lower chest. The illness lasts about a week and is rarely fatal. There is no specific treatment.

Borrelia *n.* a genus of large parasitic *spirochaete bacteria. The species *B. duttonii*, *B. novyi*, and *B. recurrentis* cause *relapsing fever in W Africa, North America, and Europe, respectively. *B. vincentii* is found in close association with the bacillus *Fusobacterium fusiformis* in *ulcerative gingivitis.

botulism *n.* a serious form of *food poisoning from foods containing the toxin produced by the bacterium *Clostridium botulinum*. The toxin selectively affects the central nervous system; in fatal cases, death is often caused by heart and lung failure resulting from a malfunction of the cardiac and respiratory centres of the brain. The bacterium thrives in improperly preserved foods, typically canned raw meats. The toxin, being rather unstable to heat, is invariably destroyed in cooking.

bougie *n.* a hollow or solid cylindrical instrument, usually flexible, that is inserted into tubular passages, such as the oesophagus (gullet), rectum, or urethra. Bougies are used in diagnosis and treatment, particularly by enlarging *strictures (for example, in the urethra).

bowel *n.* *see* intestine.

Bowen's disease a type of carcinoma of the squamous epidermal cells of the skin that does not spread to the basal layers.

bow-legs *pl. n.* abnormal out-curving of the legs, resulting in a gap between the knees on standing. A certain degree of bowing is normal in small children, but persistence into adult life, or later development of this deformity, results from abnormal growth of the *epiphysis (as in *Still's disease) or arthritis. The condition can be corrected by *osteotomy or interposition *arthroplasty. Medical name: **genu varum**.

Bowman's capsule the cup-shaped end of a *nephron, which encloses a knot of blood capillaries (*glomerulus*). It is the site of primary filtration of the blood into the kidney tubule.

brachi- (brachio-) *prefix denoting* the arm. Example: *brachialgia* (pain in).

brachial *adj.* relating to or affecting the arm.

brachial artery an artery that extends from the axillary artery, at the armpit, down the side and inner surface of the upper arm to the elbow, where it divides into the radial and ulnar arteries.

brachialis *n.* a muscle that is situated at the front of the upper arm and contracts to flex the forearm (see illustration). It works against the triceps brachii.

Brachialis and triceps muscles

brachial plexus a network of nerves, arising from the spine at the base of the neck, from which arise the nerves supplying the arm, forearm and hand, and parts of the shoulder girdle (see illustration). *See also* radial nerve.

The brachial plexus

brachiocephalic artery *see* innominate artery.

brachium

brachium *n.* (*pl.* **brachia**) the arm, especially the part of the arm between the shoulder and the elbow.

brachy- *prefix denoting* shortness. Example: *brachydactylia* (shortness of the fingers or toes).

brachycephaly *n.* shortness of the skull, with a *cephalic index of about 80. —**brachycephalic** *adj.*

brady- *prefix denoting* slowness. Example: *bradylalia* (abnormally slow speech).

bradycardia *n.* slowing of the heart rate to less than 50 beats per minute. *Sinus bradycardia* is often found in healthy individuals, especially athletes, but it is also seen in some patients with reduced thyroid activity, jaundice, hypothermia, or *vasovagal attacks. Bradycardia may also result from *arrhythmias, especially complete *heart block, when the slowing is often extreme and often causes loss of consciousness.

bradykinesia *n.* a symptom of *parkinsonism comprising a difficulty in initiating movements, slowness in executing movements, and an inability to make adjustments to the posture of the body.

bradykinin *n.* a naturally occurring polypeptide consisting of nine amino acids. Bradykinin is a very powerful vasodilator and causes contraction of smooth muscle; it is formed in the blood under certain conditions and is thought to play an important role as a mediator of inflammation. *See* kinin.

braille *n.* an alphabet, developed by Louis Braille (1809–1852) in 1837, in which each letter is represented by a pattern of raised dots, which are read by feeling with the finger tips. It is the main method of reading used by the blind today.

brain *n.* the enlarged and highly developed mass of nervous tissue that forms the upper end of the *central nervous system (see illustration). The average adult human brain weighs about 1400 g (approximately 2% of total body weight) and is continuous below with the spinal cord. It is invested by three connective tissue membranes, the *meninges, and floats in *cerebrospinal fluid within the rigid casing formed by the bones of the skull. The brain is divided into the hindbrain (rhombencephalon), consisting of the *medulla oblongata, *pons Varolii, and *cerebellum; the *midbrain (mesencephalon); and the forebrain (prosencephalon), subdivided into the *cerebrum and the *diencephalon (including the *thalamus and *hypothalamus). Anatomical name: **encephalon**.

brain death *see* death.

brainstem *n.* the enlarged extension upwards within the skull of the spinal cord, consisting of the medulla oblongata, the pons, and the midbrain. The pons and medulla are together known as the *bulb*, or *bulbar area*. Attached to the midbrain are the two cerebral hemispheres. *See* brain.

brain tumour *see* cerebral tumour.

branchial arch *see* pharyngeal arch.

branchial cleft *see* pharyngeal cleft.

branchial cyst a cyst that arises at the site of one of the embryonic *pharyngeal pouches due to a developmental anomaly.

branchial pouch *see* pharyngeal pouch.

breakbone fever *see* dengue.

breast *n.* **1.** the mammary gland of a woman: one of two compound glands that produce milk. Each breast consists of glandular lobules – the milk-secreting areas – embedded in fatty tissue (see illustration). The milk passes from the lobules into ducts, which join up to form 15–20 *lactiferous ducts*. Near the

central sulcus

choroid plexus of
third ventricle

corpus callosum

thalamus

hypothalamus

optic chiasma

infundibulum

pituitary body

mamillary body

pons Varolii

medulla oblongata

pineal body

cerebral aqueduct

fourth ventricle

vermis

white matter of
cerebellum

The brain (midsagittal section)

front of the breast the lactiferous ducts
are dilated into *ampullae*, which act as
reservoirs for the milk. Each lactiferous
duct discharges through a separate orifice in the nipple. The dark area around
the nipple is called the *areola*. *See also*
lactation. Anatomical name: **mamma. 2.**
the front part of the chest (thorax).

breastbone *n. see* sternum.

breast cancer a malignant tumour of
the breast, usually a *carcinoma but
sometimes a *sarcoma. It is rare in men
but is the commonest form of cancer in
women, in some cases involving both
breasts. The cause is not known but it
tends to run in families, and in countries such as Japan, where prolonged
breast feeding is the rule, the incidence
of breast cancer is very low.
The classic sign is a lump in the breast,
which is often noticed after minor local
injury; bleeding or discharge from the
nipple may occur infrequently. Sometimes the first thing to be noticed is a
lump in the armpit, which is due to
spread of the cancer to the drainage
lymph nodes. The tumour may also

clavicle

fatty stroma

milk (lactiferous)
duct

ampulla

nipple

areola

glandular tissue

ribs

Longitudinal section through a breast

spread to the bones, lungs, and liver.
Current treatment of a localized tumour is usually by surgery, with or

breathing

without radiotherapy; cytotoxic drugs and hormone therapy are used for widespread disease.

breathing *n.* the alternation of active *inhalation* (or *inspiration*) of air into the lungs through the mouth or nose with the passive *exhalation* (or *expiration*) of the air. During inhalation the *diaphragm and *intercostal muscles contract, which enlarges the chest cavity and draws air into the lungs. Relaxation of these muscles forces air out of the lungs at exhalation. (See illustration.) Breathing is part of *respiration and is sometimes called external respiration. There are many types of breathing in which the rhythm, rate, or character is abnormal. *See also* apnoea, bronchospasm, Cheyne-Stokes respiration, dyspnoea, stridor.

breathlessness *n. see* dyspnoea.

breath sounds the sounds heard through a stethoscope placed over the lungs during breathing. Normal breath sounds are soft and called *vesicular* – they may be increased or decreased in disease states. The sounds heard over the larger bronchi are louder and harsher. Breath sounds transmitted through consolidated lungs in pneumonia are louder and harsher; they are similar to the sounds heard normally over the larger bronchi and are termed *bronchial breath sounds*. *Crepitations and *rhonchi are sounds added to the breath sounds in abnormal states of the lung. *Amphoric* or *cavernous* sounds have a hollow quality and are heard over cavities in the lung; the amphoric quality may also be heard in voice sounds and on percussion.

breech presentation the position of a baby in the womb such that it is delivered buttocks first (instead of the normal head-first position). Since this can result in a difficult birth, the baby is often turned head first before labour; if this is not possible, the delivery can be facilitated by careful manipulation of the baby during labour.

bregma *n.* the point on the top of the skull at which the coronal and sagittal *sutures meet. In a young infant this is an opening, the anterior *fontanelle.

bridge *n.* (in dentistry) a fixed replacement for missing teeth. The artificial

Position of the diaphragm (from the side) during breathing

tooth is attached to one or more natural teeth, usually by a crown.

Bright's disease *see* nephritis.

British Anti-Lewisite (BAL) *see* dimercaprol.

British thermal unit a unit of heat equal to the quantity of heat required to raise the temperature of 1 pound of water by 1° Fahrenheit. 1 British thermal unit = 1055 joules. Abbrev.: Btu.

Broca's area the area of cerebral motor cortex responsible for the initiation of speech. It is situated in the left frontal lobe in most (but not all) right-handed people, in the region of *Brodmann areas 44 and 45.

Brodie's abscess an abscess of bone: a form of chronic bacterial *osteomyelitis, not due to tuberculosis or syphilis. Treatment is by surgical drainage and antibiotics.

Brodmann areas the numbered areas (1–47) into which a map of the *cerebral cortex may conveniently be divided for descriptive purposes, based upon the arrangement of neurones seen in stained sections under the microscope. On the map area 4, for example, corresponds to primary motor cortex, while the primary visual cortex comes into area 17.

bromhexine *n.* an *expectorant that acts by increasing the volume and reducing the viscosity of bronchial secretions. It is used in the treatment of bronchitis and may cause nausea. Trade name: **Bisolvon**.

bromides *pl. n.* salts of bromine, including potassium bromide, once widely used as sedatives because of their depressant action on the central nervous system. *See also* bromism.

bromidrosis *n.* bacterial breakdown of sweat, usually in the armpit or on the feet, which causes an unpleasant smell.

bromism *n.* a group of symptoms caused by excessive intake of *bromides. Overuse for long periods leads to mental dullness, weakness, drowsiness, loss of sensation, slurred speech, and sometimes coma. A form of acne may also develop. Treatment is by immediate withdrawal.

bromodiphenhydramine *n.* an *antihistamine given by mouth to relieve the symptoms of allergic reactions, especially hay fever and rhinitis. It is also used to prevent travel sickness. Common side-effects include drowsiness, dizziness, dryness of the throat, and digestive upsets. Trade name: **Ambodryl**.

brompheniramine *n.* an antihistamine that has the same uses and side-effects as *bromodiphenhydramine. Trade name: **Dimetane**.

bromsulphthalein *n.* a blue dye used in tests of liver function. A small quantity of the dye is injected into the bloodstream, and its concentration in the blood is measured after 5 and then 45 minutes. The presence of more than 10% of the dose in the circulation after 45 minutes indicates that the liver is not functioning normally.

bronch- (broncho-) *prefix denoting* the bronchial tree. Examples: *broncho-pulmonary* (relating to the bronchi and lungs); *bronchotomy* (incision into).

bronchial tree a branching system of tubes conducting air from the trachea (windpipe) to the lungs: includes the bronchi (*see* bronchus) and their subdivisions and the *bronchioles.

bronchiectasis *n.* widening of the bronchi or their branches. It may be congenital or it may result from infection (especially whooping cough or measles in childhood) or from obstruction, either by an inhaled foreign body or by a growth (including cancer). Pus may form in the widened bronchus so that the patient coughs up purulent sputum, which may contain blood. Diagnosis is on the clinical symptoms and by X-ray. Treatment consists of antibiotic drugs to control the infection and physiotherapy to drain the sputum. Surgery may be used if only a few segments of the bronchi are affected.

bronchiole *n.* a subdivision of the bronchial tree that does not contain cartilage or mucous glands in its wall. Bronchioles open from the fifth or sixth generation of bronchi and extend for up to 20 more generations before reaching the *terminal bronchioles*. Each terminal bronchiole divides into a number of *respiratory bronchioles*, from which the *alveoli open. Each terminal bronchiole conducts air to an acinus in the *lung. —**bronchiolar** *adj.*

bronchiolitis *n.* inflammation of the bronchioles, due to infection by bacteria or viruses. These very small tubes easily become blocked with mucopus, which prevents air from reaching the alveoli of the lungs. The patient becomes short of oxygen (*see* cyanosis); in infants the breathing appears difficult and ineffectual. The condition is treated with oxygen, which is paramount, and antibiotics.

bronchitis *n.* inflammation of the bronchi (*see* bronchus). *Acute bronchitis* is caused by viruses or bacteria and is characterized by coughing, the production of mucopurulent sputum, and narrowing of the bronchi due to spasmodic contraction (*see* bronchospasm). In *chronic bronchitis* the patient coughs up excessive mucus secreted by enlarged bronchial mucous glands; the bronchospasm cannot be relieved by bronchodilator drugs. It is not primarily an inflammatory condition, although it is frequently complicated by acute infections. The disease is particularly prevalent in Britain in association with cigarette smoking, air pollution, and *emphysema.

bronchoconstrictor *n.* a drug that causes narrowing of the air passages by producing spasm of bronchial smooth muscle.

bronchodilator *n.* an agent that causes widening of the air passages by relaxing bronchial smooth muscle. *Sympathomimetic drugs that stimulate beta-receptors, e.g. *ephedrine, *isoprenaline, and *salbutamol, are potent bronchodilators and are used for relief of bronchial asthma and chronic bronchitis. These drugs are often administered as aerosols, giving rapid relief, but at high doses they may stimulate the heart.

bronchography *n.* X-ray examination of the bronchial tree after it has been made visible by the injection of *radio-opaque dye or the inhalation of radio-opaque particles, such as tantalum. It is used particularly in the diagnosis of *bronchiectasis.

bronchophony *n. see* vocal resonance.

bronchopneumonia *n. see* pneumonia.

bronchoscope *n.* an instrument used to look into the trachea and bronchi. In addition to the rigid tubular metal type, used for many years, there is now a narrower flexible *fibre-optic instrument with which previously inaccessible bronchi can be inspected. With either instrument the bronchial tree can be washed out, and samples of tissue and foreign bodies can be removed with long forceps. —**bronchoscopy** *n.*

bronchospasm *n.* narrowing of bronchi by muscular contraction in response to some stimulus, as in *asthma and *bronchitis. The patient can usually inhale air into the lungs, but exhalation may require visible muscular effort and is accompanied by expiratory noises that are clearly audible (*see* wheeze) or detectable with a stethoscope. The condition in which bronchospasm can be relieved by bronchodilator drugs is known as *reversible obstructive airways disease* and includes asthma; that in which bronchodilator drugs have no effect is *irreversible obstructive airways disease* and includes chronic bronchitis.

bronchospirometry *n.* a technique used to assess the efficiency of ventilation of a lung or of a segment of the lung. A catheter with an inflatable cuff is passed into the appropriate airway, through a *bronchoscope, and the volume and rate of gas exchange is estimated.

bronchus *n.* (*pl.* **bronchi**) any of the air passages beyond the *trachea (windpipe) that has cartilage and mucous glands in its wall (see illustration). The trachea divides into two main bronchi, which divide successively into five *lobar bronchi*, 20 *segmental bronchi*, and two or three more divisions. *See also* bronchiole. —**bronchial** *adj.*

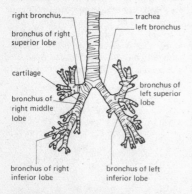

right bronchus
trachea
left bronchus
bronchus of right superior lobe
cartilage
bronchus of left superior lobe
bronchus of right middle lobe
bronchus of right inferior lobe
bronchus of left inferior lobe

The bronchi and their principal (lobar) branches

brown fat a form of fat in adipose tissue that is a rich source of energy and can be converted rapidly to heat. There is speculation that a rapid turnover of brown fat occurs to balance excessive intake of food and unnecessary production of white fat (making up the bulk of adipose tissue). Some forms of obesity may be linked to lack of – or inability to synthesize – brown fat.

Brown-Séquard syndrome the neurological condition resulting when the spinal cord has been partly cut through. In those parts of the body supplied by the damaged segment there is a flaccid weakness and loss of feeling in the skin. Below the lesion there is a spastic paralysis on the same side and a loss of pain and temperature sensation on the opposite side.

Brucella *n.* a genus of Gram-negative aerobic spherical or rodlike parasitic bacteria responsible for *brucellosis (undulant fever) in man and contagious abortion in cattle, pigs, sheep, and goats. The principal species are *B. abortus* and *B. melitensis*. *Brucella ring test* is a diagnostic test for brucellosis involving the clumping together of a standard *Brucella* strain by antibodies in an infected person's serum.

brucellosis (Malta fever, Mediterranean fever, undulant fever) *n.* a chronic disease of farm animals caused by bacteria of the genus *Brucella*, which can be transmitted to man either by contact with an infected animal or by drinking nonpasteurized contaminated milk. Symptoms include headache, sickness, loss of appetite, and weakness, progressing to chronic fever and the swelling of lymph nodes. Untreated the disease may last for years but prolonged administration of antibiotics and sulphonamides is effective.

Brufen *n. see* ibuprofen.

Brugia *n.* a genus of threadlike parasitic worms (*see* filaria). *B. malayi* infects man throughout southeast Asia, causing *filariasis and *elephantiasis (especially of the feet and legs). *B. pahangi*, a parasite of wild cats and domestic animals, produces an allergic condition in man, with coughing, breathing difficulty, and an increase in the number of *eosinophils in the blood. *Brugia* undergoes part of its development in mosquitoes of the genera *Anopheles* and *Mansonia*, which transmit the parasite from host to host.

bruise (contusion) *n.* an area of skin discoloration caused by the escape of blood from ruptured underlying vessels following injury. Initially red or pink, a bruise gradually becomes bluish, and then greenish yellow, as the haemoglobin in the tissues breaks down chemically and is absorbed. It may be necessary to draw off blood from very severe bruises through a needle, to aid healing.

bruit *n. see* murmur.

Brunner's glands compound glands of the small intestine, found in the duodenum and the upper part of the jejunum. They are embedded in the submucosa and secrete mucus.

brush border *see* microvillus.

bruxism *n.* a habit in which an individual grinds his teeth, which leads to excessive wear.

bubo *n.* a swollen inflamed lymph node in the armpit or groin, commonly developing in venereal disease, bubonic plague, and leishmaniasis.

bubonic plague *see* plague.

buccal *adj.* **1.** relating to the mouth or the hollow part of the cheek. **2.** describing the surface of a tooth adjacent to the cheek.

buccal cavity the cavity of the mouth, which contains the tongue and teeth and leads to the pharynx. Here food is tasted, chewed, and mixed with saliva, which begins the process of digestion.

buccal glands small glands in the mucous membrane lining the mouth. They secrete material that mixes with saliva.

buccinator *n.* a muscle of the cheek that has its origin in the maxilla and mandible (jaw bones). It is responsible for compressing the cheek and is important in mastication.

buclizine *n.* an *antihistamine with marked sedative properties. Given by mouth, it is used to treat mild anxiety states and tension, as well as for allergic conditions and vertigo. Side-effects include drowsiness, dizziness, dryness of the throat, and gastro-intestinal upsets. Occasionally teratogenic effects may occur. Trade names: **Softran, Vibazine**.

Budd-Chiari syndrome a rare condition that follows obstruction of the hepatic vein by a blood clot or tumour. It is characterized by ascites and cirrhosis of the liver.

Buerger's disease an inflammatory condition affecting the arteries, especially in the legs, of young male Jews who smoke cigarettes. Intermittent *claudication (pain due to reduced blood supply) and gangrene of the limbs may develop. Coronary thrombosis may occur and venous thrombosis is common. The treatment is similar to that of *atheroma but cessation of smoking is essential to prevent progression of the disease. Medical name: **thromboangiitis obliterans**.

buffer *n.* a solution whose hydrogen ion concentration (pH) remains virtually unchanged by dilution or by the addition of acid or alkali. The chief buffer of the blood and extracellular body fluids is the bicarbonate (H_2CO_3/HCO_3) system. *See also* acid-base balance.

bulb *n.* (in anatomy) any rounded structure or a rounded expansion at the end of an organ or part.

bulbar *adj.* **1.** relating to or affecting the medulla oblongata. **2.** relating to a bulb. **3.** relating to the eyeball.

bulbourethral glands *see* Cowper's glands.

bulimia *n.* insatiable over-eating. This symptom may be psychogenic, occurring, for example, as a phase of *anorexia nervosa (*bulimia nervosa*); or it may be due to neurological causes, such as a lesion of the *hypothalamus.

bulla *n.* (*pl.* **bullae**) **1.** a large blister, containing serous fluid. **2.** (in anatomy) a rounded bony prominence. **3.** a thin-walled air-filled space within the lung, arising congenitally or in *emphysema. It may cause trouble by rupturing into the pleural space (*see* pneumothorax), by adding to the air that does not contribute to gas exchange, and/or by compressing the surrounding lung and making it inefficient. —**bullous** *adj.*

bundle *n.* a group of nerve fibres situated close together and running in the same direction; e.g. the *atrioventricular bundle.

bundle branch block a defect in the specialized conducting tissue of the heart (*see* arrhythmia) that is recognised as an electrocardiographic abnormality. Left or right bundle branch blocks, affecting the respective ventricles, may be seen. Occasionally both left and right bundle branch blocks occur simultaneously and the patient develops complete *heart block. The causes are similar to those of complete heart block.

bundle of His *see* atrioventricular bundle.

bunion *n.* a swelling of the joint between the great toe and the first metatarsal bone. A *bursa often develops over the site and the great toe becomes displaced towards the others. Bunions are usually caused by ill-fitting shoes and may require surgical treatment.

buphenine *n.* a drug whose main action is to dilate blood vessels, particularly those in skeletal muscles. Taken by mouth, it is used to increase the blood flow to muscle, especially in vascular disease due to spasm of the arteries. It may cause palpitations and

stimulate gastric secretion. Trade names: **Arlidin**, **Perdilatal**.

buphthalmos (hydrophthalmos) *n.* infantile or congenital glaucoma: increased pressure within the eye due to a defect in the development of the tissues through which fluid drains from the eye. Since the outer coat (sclera) of the eyeball of children is distensible, the eye enlarges as the inflow of fluid continues. It affects both eyes and may accompany congenital malformations in other parts of the body. Treatment is by surgical operation, e.g. *goniotomy, to improve drainage of fluid from the eye. Spontaneous arrest of buphthalmos may occur before vision is completely lost.

bupivacaine *n.* a potent local anaesthetic, used mainly for regional *nerve block. It is significantly longer-acting than many other local anaesthetics. It has been used in childbirth, but may cause slowing of the baby's heart, with a risk of death. Trade name: **Marcain**.

bur (burr) *n.* a cutting drill that fits in a dentist's handpiece. Burs are mainly used for cutting cavities in teeth.

Burkitt's tumour (Burkitt's lymphoma) a malignant tumour of the lymphatic system, most commonly affecting children and largely confined to tropical Africa in a zone 15° north and south of the equator. It can arise at various sites, most commonly the facial structures, such as the jaw, and in the abdomen. Complications affecting the nervous system occur in up to 50% of cases. Viruses may possibly play a role in the origin and growth of the tumour, which has been shown to be very sensitive to *cytotoxic drug therapy.

burn *n.* tissue damage caused by such agents as heat, chemicals, electricity, sunlight, or nuclear radiation. A *first-degree burn* affects only the outer layer (epidermis) of the skin. In a *second-degree burn* both the epidermis and the underlying dermis are damaged. A *third-degree burn* involves damage or destruction of the skin to its full depth and damage to the tissues beneath. Burns cause swelling and blistering, due to loss of plasma from damaged blood vessels. In serious burns, affecting 15% or more of the body surface in adults (10% or more in children), this loss of plasma results in severe *shock and requires immediate transfusion of blood or saline solution. Burns may also lead to bacterial infection, which can be prevented by administration of antibiotics. Third-degree burns may require skin grafting.

burr *n. see* bur.

bursa *n.* (*pl.* **bursae**) a small sac of fibrous tissue that is lined with *synovial membrane and filled with fluid (synovia). Bursae occur where parts move over one another; they help to reduce friction. They are normally formed round joints and in places where ligaments and tendons pass over bones. However, they may be formed in other places in response to unusual pressure or friction.

bursitis *n.* inflammation of a *bursa, resulting from injury, infection, or rheumatoid *synovitis. It produces pain and tenderness and sometimes restricts movement at a nearby joint; for example, at the shoulder. Treatment of bursitis not due to infection is by rest and corticosteroid injection. *See also* housemaid's knee.

busulphan *n.* a drug that destroys cancer cells by acting on the bone marrow. It is administered by mouth, mainly in the treatment of chronic myeloid leukaemia. It may cause blood disorders producing bleeding. Trade name: **Myleran**.

butacaine *n.* a local anaesthetic used to produce surface anaesthesia, mainly in eye, ear, nose, and throat surgery. Trade name: **Butyn**.

butobarbitone (butobarbital) *n.* an intermediate-acting *barbiturate, used for the treatment of insomnia and for sedation. It produces sleep within 30 minutes when given by mouth and its sedative effect lasts for about six hours. Prolonged administration may lead to *dependence and its use with alcohol should be avoided; overdosage has serious effects (*see* barbiturism). Trade name: **Soneryl**.

byssinosis *n.* an industrial disease of the lungs caused by inhalation of dusts of cotton, flax, or hemp. The patient characteristically has chest tightness and *wheeze after the weekend break, which wears off during the working week. The causal agent has not been identified.

C

cac- (caco-) *prefix denoting* disease or deformity. Example: *cacosmia* (unpleasant odour).

cachet *n.* a flat capsule containing a drug that has an unpleasant taste. The cachet is swallowed intact by the patient.

cachexia *n.* a condition of abnormally low weight, weakness, and general bodily decline associated with chronic disease. It occurs in such conditions as cancer, pulmonary tuberculosis, and malaria.

cacosmia *n.* a disorder of the sense of smell in which scents that are inoffensive to most people are objectionable to the sufferer or in which a bad smell seems to be perpetually present. The disorder is usually due to damage to pathways within the brain rather than in the nose or olfactory nerve.

cadmium *n.* a silvery metallic element that can cause serious lung irritation if the fumes of the molten metal are inhaled. Long-term exposure may also cause kidney damage. Symbol: Cd.

caecostomy *n.* an operation in which the caecum is brought through the abdominal wall and opened in order to drain or decompress the intestine, usually when the colon is obstructed or injured.

caecum *n.* a blind-ended pouch at the junction of the small and large intestines, situated below the *ileocaecal valve. The upper end is continuous with the colon and the lower end bears the vermiform appendix. *See* alimentary canal.

caeruloplasmin *n.* a copper-containing protein present in blood plasma. Congenital deficiency of caeruloplasmin leads to abnormalities of the brain and liver (*see* Wilson's disease).

Caesarean section a surgical operation for delivering a baby through the abdominal wall: it should not be performed before the 28th week of gestation. It is carried out when there are risks to the baby from natural childbirth; for example if it is too large to pass through the birth canal or shows signs of lack of oxygen (anoxia); in a breech presentation that cannot be turned; or if the placenta obstructs the outlet of the womb and may cause dangerous bleeding. It is also performed for the safety of the mother, for example in acute *toxaemia of pregnancy, failure to induce labour, or prolonged ineffectual labour.

caesium-137 *n.* an artificial radioactive isotope of the metallic element caesium. The radiation given off by caesium-137 is employed in the technique of *radiotherapy. Symbol: Cs^{137}. *See also* telecurietherapy.

caffeine *n.* an alkaloid drug, obtained from coffee and tea, that has a stimulant action, particularly on the central nervous system. It is used to promote wakefulness and increase mental activity; it also possesses diuretic properties and will help relieve certain forms of headache. It is often administered with aspirin, codeine, or phenacetin as an analgesic preparation.

caisson disease *see* compressed air illness.

calamine *n.* a preparation of zinc carbonate used as a mild astringent on the skin in the form of a lotion, cream, or ointment.

calc- (calci-, calco-) *prefix denoting* calcium or calcium salts.

calcaneus (heel bone) *n.* the large bone in the *tarsus of the foot that forms the projection of the heel behind the foot. It articulates with the cuboid bone in front and with the talus above.

calcar *n.* a spurlike projection. The *calcar avis* is the projection in the medial wall of the lateral ventricle of the brain.

calcicosis *n.* *pneumoconiosis in marble cutters. The term is not in current use.

calciferol *n. see* vitamin D.

calcification *n.* the deposition of calcium salts in tissue. This occurs as part of the normal process of bone formation (*see* ossification).

calcinosis *n.* the abnormal deposition of calcium salts in the tissues. This may occur only in the fat layer beneath the skin or it may be more widespread.

calcitonin *n. see* thyrocalcitonin.

calcium *n.* a metallic element essential for the normal development and functioning of the body. Calcium is an important constituent of bones and teeth: the matrix of *bone, consisting principally of calcium phosphate, accounts for about 99% of the body's calcium. It is present in the blood at a concentration of about 10 mg/100 ml,

calculosis

being maintained at this level by hormones (see thyrocalcitonin, parathyroid hormone). It is essential for many metabolic processes, including nerve function, muscle contraction, and blood clotting.

The normal dietary requirement of calcium is about 1 g per day: dairy products (milk and cheese) are the principal sources. Its uptake by the body is facilitated by *vitamin D; a deficiency of this vitamin may therefore result in such conditions as *rickets, *osteoporosis, and *osteomalacia. A deficiency of calcium in the blood may lead to *tetany. Excess calcium may be deposited in the body as *calculi (stones), especially in the gall bladder and kidney. Symbol: Ca.

calculosis *n.* the presence of multiple calculi (stones) in the body. *See* calculus.

calculus *n.* (*pl.* **calculi**) **1.** a stone: a hard pebble-like mass formed within the body, particularly in the gall bladder (see gallstone) or anywhere in the urinary tract (see cystolithiasis, nephrolithiasis). Calculi in the urinary tract are commonly composed of calcium oxalate and are usually visible on X-ray examination. Most of these stones cause pain, whether sited in the kidney, ureter, or bladder; stones passing down a duct (such as the ureter) cause severe colicky pain. Such stones are usually removed surgically to prevent or cure urinary obstruction and infection. **2.** a calcified deposit that forms on the surfaces of teeth. *Supragingival calculus* forms above the *gingivae (gums), principally in relation to the openings of the salivary gland ducts. *Subgingival calculus* forms beneath the crest of the gingivae. Calculus hinders the cleaning of teeth.

calibrator *n.* **1.** an instrument used for measuring the size of a tube or opening. **2.** an instrument used for dilating a tubular part, such as the gullet.

calliper (caliper) *n.* **1.** an instrument with two prongs or jaws, used for measuring diameters: used particularly in obstetrics for measuring the diameter of the pelvis. **2.** (also called **calliper splint**) a leg splint that consists of metal rods attached to a padded ring at the top of the leg, taking the weight of the body at the pelvis. Calliper splints can be used to exert *traction on a deformed or paralysed leg as part of orthopaedic treatment.

callosity (callus) *n.* a hard thick area of skin occurring in parts of the body subject to pressure or friction. The soles of the feet and palms of the hands are common sites, and if much hard dead skin develops a callosity can become painful. A *corn is a type of callosity.

callus *n.* **1.** a mass of blood and *granulation tissue, containing bone-forming cells, that forms around the bone ends following a fracture. Callus formation is an essential part of the process of healthy union in a fractured bone. The callus, which is visible on X-ray as a slightly opaque area, eventually becomes calcified and modelled. **2.** see callosity.

calor *n.* heat: one of the classical signs of inflammation in a tissue, the other three being *rubor (redness), *dolor (pain), and *tumor (swelling). An inflamed region has a higher temperature than normal because of the distended blood vessels, which allow an increased flow of blood.

calorie *n.* a unit of heat equal to the amount of heat required to raise the temperature of 1 gram of water from 14.5°C to 15.5°C (the 15° calorie). One Calorie (also known as the *kilocalorie* or *kilogram calorie*) is equal to 1000 calories; this unit is used to indicate the energy value of foods. Except in this context, the calorie has largely been replaced by the *joule (1 calorie = 4.1855 joules).

calorimeter *n.* any apparatus used to measure the heat lost or gained during various chemical and physical changes. For example, calorimeters may be used to determine the total energy values of different foods in terms of calories. —**calorimetry** *n.*

calvaria *n.* the vault of the *skull.

calyx *n.* (*pl.* **calyces**) a cup-shaped part, especially any of the divisions of the pelvis of the *kidney. Each calyx receives urine from the urine-collecting tubes in one sector of the kidney.

camphor *n.* a crystalline substance obtained from the tree *Cinnamomum camphora* that has been used to treat flatulence. It is used in the form of *camphorated oil* (camphor in cottonseed oil) in liniments as a counterirritant.

campimetry *n.* a method of assessing the central part of the *visual field. The patient looks steadily with one eye at a target in the centre of a black screen two metres away. A small object on the end of a black rod is moved onto the screen and the patient tells the examiner when he sees it. This is repeated many times from different directions until a map is built up of the area in front of the eye in which such an object can be seen. Campimetry allows examination only of that part of the field of vision within 30° in all directions from the centre.

camptodactylia *n.* congenital inward bending of a finger, most commonly the little finger.

canal *n.* a tubular channel or passage; e.g. the *alimentary canal and the auditory canal of the ear.

canaliculus *n.* (*pl.* **canaliculi**) a small channel or canal. Canaliculi occur, for example, in compact bone, linking lacunae containing bone cells. *Bile canaliculi* are minute channels within the liver that transport bile to the bile duct.

cancellous *adj.* lattice-like: applied to the bony tissue laid down by *osteoblasts during development of bone and in the *consolidation stage of fracture repair.

cancer *n.* any *malignant tumour, including *carcinoma and *sarcoma. It arises from the abnormal and uncontrolled division of cells that then invade and destroy the surrounding tissues. Spread of cancer cells (*metastasis) may occur via the bloodstream or the lymphatic channels or across body cavities such as the pleural and peritoneal spaces, thus setting up secondary tumours at sites distant from the original tumour. Each individual primary tumour has its own pattern of local behaviour and metastasis; for example, bone metastasis is very common in breast cancer but very rare in cancer of the ovary.
There are probably many causative factors, some of which are known; for example, cigarette smoking is associated with lung cancer, radiation with some bone sarcomas and leukaemia. Some tumours, such as retinoblastoma, are inherited. Treatment of cancer depends on the type of tumour, the site of the primary tumour, and the extent of spread.

cancrum (canker) *n.* ulceration, mainly of the lips and mouth (*cancrum oris*).

candela *n.* the *SI unit of luminous intensity, equal to the intensity in a horizontal direction of a surface of 1/600,000 square metre of a black body at a temperature of 2040 kelvins and a pressure of 101,325 pascals. Symbol: cd.

candicidin *n.* a fungicide, produced by the bacterium *Streptomyces griseus* and used to treat candidiasis, particularly of the vagina.

Candida *n.* a genus of yeastlike fungi (formerly called *Monilia*) that inhabit the vagina and alimentary tract and can

– under certain conditions – cause *candidiasis. The species *C. albicans*, a small oval budding fungus, is primarily responsible for candidiasis of the mouth, lungs, intestine, vagina, skin, and nails.

candidiasis *n.* infection with a yeast-like fungus of the genus *Candida, usually the species *C. albicans*. The infection – formerly called *moniliasis* – is usually superficial, occurring in moist areas of the body, such as the skin folds, mouth, respiratory tract, and vagina (candidiasis of the mouth and vagina is popularly known as *thrush*). Rarely, candidiasis infection may spread throughout the body. Candidiasis of the mouth appears as white patches on the tongue or inside the cheeks. Candidiasis sometimes develops in patients receiving broad-spectrum antibiotics. It is treated with antibiotics – especially *nystatin – applied locally, inhaled, or taken by mouth.

canine *n.* the third tooth from the midline of each jaw. There are thus four canines, two in each jaw, in both the permanent and deciduous (milk) *dentitions. It is known colloquially as the *eye tooth*.

canities *n.* loss of pigment in the hair, which causes greying or whitening. It is usually part of the ageing process, when it starts at the temples. White patches may occur as a result of *alopecia areata or *vitiligo.

canker *n. see* cancrum.

cannabis *n.* a drug prepared from the Indian hemp plant (*Cannabis sativa*), also known as *pot, marihuana, hashish*, and *bhang*. Smoked or swallowed, it produces euphoria and hallucinations and affects perception and awareness, particularly of time. Cannabis has no therapeutic value and its use is illegal: there is evidence that prolonged use may cause brain damage and lead the user onto 'hard' drugs, such as heroin. *See also* dependence.

cannula *n.* a hollow tube designed for insertion into a body cavity, such as the bladder, or a blood vessel. The tube contains a sharp pointed solid core (*trocar*), which facilitates its insertion and is withdrawn when the cannula is in place.

cantharidin *n.* the active principle of *cantharides*, or *Spanish fly* (the dried bodies of a blister beetle, *Lytta vesicatoria*). A toxic and irritant chemical, cantharidin causes blistering of the skin and was formerly used in veterinary medicine as a counterirritant and vesicant. If swallowed it causes nausea, vomiting, and inflammation of the urinary tract, the latter giving rise to its reputation as an aphrodisiac. It is very dangerous and may cause death.

canthus *n.* either corner of the eye; the angle at which the upper and lower eyelids meet. —**canthal** *adj.*

cap *n.* a covering or a cover-like part. The *duodenal cap* is the superior part of the duodenum as seen on X-ray after a barium meal.

Capgras' syndrome (illusion of doubles) the delusion that a person closely involved with the patient has been replaced by an identical-looking impostor. It is often, but not necessarily, a form of paranoid *schizophrenia.

capillary *n.* an extremely narrow blood vessel, approximately 5–20 μm in diameter. Capillaries form networks in most tissues; they are supplied with blood by arterioles and drained by venules. The vessel wall is only one cell thick, which enables exchange of oxygen, carbon dioxide, water, salts, etc., between the blood and the tissues (see illustrations).

A network of capillaries (above); a single capillary (below)

capitate *adj.* head-shaped; having a rounded extremity.

capitate bone a bone of the wrist (*see* carpus). It articulates with the scaphoid and lunate bones behind and with the third metacarpal bone in front.

capitellum *n. see* capitulum.

capitulum *n.* the small rounded end of a bone that articulates with another bone. For example, the *capitulum humeri* (or *capitellum*) is the round prominence at the elbow end of the humerus that articulates with the radius.

capping *n.* (in dentistry) **1.** crowning: the technique of fitting a tooth with an *artificial crown. **2.** the technique of protecting tooth pulp that has been

exposed by caries, by means of a small metal or celluloid cover.

capreomycin *n.* an antibiotic, derived from the bacterium *Streptomyces capreolus*, that is used in the treatment of tuberculosis. It is given with other antituberculosis drugs to reduce the development of resistance by the infective bacteria. Capreomycin is poorly absorbed from the gastro-intestinal tract and therefore must be administered by intramuscular injection. The more serious side-effects include ear and kidney damage.

capsule *n.* **1.** a membrane, sheath, or other structure that encloses a tissue or organ. For example, the kidney, adrenal gland, and lens of the eye are enclosed within capsules. A *joint capsule* is the fibrous tissue, including the synovial membrane, that surrounds a freely movable joint. **2.** a soluble case, usually made of gelatin, in which certain drugs are administered. **3.** the slimy substance that forms a protective layer around certain bacteria. It is usually made of *polysaccharide.

capsulitis *n.* inflammation of the capsule surrounding a joint.

capsulotomy *n.* an incision into the capsule of the lens. In some operations for cataract the lens capsule is not removed and tends to become opaque. A tiny knife (*cystitome*) is inserted into the eye and a hole cut in the centre of the capsule, thus providing a clear path for light rays to reach the retina.

caput succedaneum a temporary swelling of the soft parts of the head of a newly born infant that occurs during birth, due to compression by the muscles of the neck of the womb.

carbachol *n.* a *parasympathomimetic drug used to relieve pressure within the eye in glaucoma. It is also used after surgical operations to restore the function of inactive bowels or bladder. Side-effects may include sweating, nausea, and faintness. Trade name: **Carcholin**.

carbamazepine n. an *anticonvulsant drug used in the treatment of epilepsy and to relieve the pain of trigeminal neuralgia. Common side-effects include drowsiness, dizziness, and muscular incoordination; abnormalities of liver and bone marrow may occur with long-term treatment. Trade name: **Tegretol**.

carbenicillin n. a synthetic penicillin: an antibiotic that is effective against a wide range of bacterial infections. It is poorly absorbed from the gastrointestinal tract and must be given by intramuscular injection. Allergic reactions are common side-effects. Trade name: **Pyopen**.

carbenoxolone n. a drug that reduces inflammation, used mainly to promote healing in the treatment of gastric ulcers or ulcers of the mouth. It is given by mouth; side-effects include the retention of salt and water (see oedema), weight gain, and raised blood pressure. Trade names: **Biogastrone, Bioral**.

carbimazole n. a drug used to reduce the production of thyroid hormone in cases of overactivity of the gland (thyrotoxicosis). It is administered by mouth; some allergic reactions may occur and high dosage may cause enlargement of the thyroid gland, which may obstruct the windpipe. Trade names: **Bimazol, Neo-Merca-zole**.

carbinoxamine n. a short-acting antihistamine, given by mouth in the treatment of allergic conditions, particularly hay fever and rhinitis, and to prevent travel sickness. Trade name: **Clistin**.

carbohydrate n. any one of a large group of compounds, including the *sugars and *starch, that contain carbon, hydrogen, and oxygen and have the general formula $C_x(H_2O)_y$. Carbohydrates are important as a source of energy: they are manufactured by plants and obtained by animals and man from the diet, being one of the three main constituents of food (see also fat, protein). All carbohydrates are eventually broken down in the body to the simple sugar *glucose, which can then take part in energy-producing metabolic processes. Excess carbohydrate, not immediately required by the body, is stored in the liver and muscles in the form of *glycogen. In plants carbohydrates are important structural materials (e.g. cellulose) and storage products (commonly in the form of starch). See also disaccharide, monosaccharide, polysaccharide.

carbol fuchsin a red stain for bacteria and fungi, consisting of carbolic acid and *fuchsin dissolved in alcohol and water.

carbolic acid see phenol.

carbon dioxide a colourless gas formed in the tissues during metabolism and carried in the blood to the lungs, where it is exhaled (an increase in the concentration of this gas in the blood stimulates respiration). Carbon dioxide occurs in small amounts in the atmosphere; it is used by plants in the process of *photosynthesis. It forms a solid (dry ice) at $-75°C$ (at atmospheric pressure) and in this form is used as a refrigerant. Formula: CO_2.

carbon monoxide a colourless almost odourless gas that is very poisonous. When breathed in it combines with haemoglobin in the red blood cells to form *carboxyhaemoglobin, which is bright red in colour. This compound is chemically stable and thus the haemoglobin can no longer combine with oxygen. Carbon monoxide is present in coal gas and motor exhaust fumes. Formula: CO.

carbon tetrachloride a pungent volatile fluid used as a dry-cleaner. When inhaled or swallowed it may severely damage the heart, liver, and kidneys, causing cirrhosis and nephrosis, and it can also affect the optic nerve and other nerves. Treatment is by administration of oxygen.

carboxyhaemoglobin *n.* a substance formed when carbon monoxide combines with the pigment *haemoglobin in the blood. Carboxyhaemoglobin is incapable of transporting oxygen to the tissues and this is the cause of death in carbon monoxide poisoning. Large quantities of carboxyhaemoglobin are formed in carbon monoxide poisoning, and low levels are always present in the blood of smokers and city dwellers.

carboxylase *n.* an enzyme that catalyses the addition of carbon dioxide to a substance.

carbromal *n.* a weak sedative and hypnotic, given by mouth and used in the treatment of mild insomnia. Its action lasts for a few hours but prolonged use may lead to *dependence.

carbuncle *n.* a collection of *boils with multiple drainage channels. The infection is usually caused by *Staphylococcus aureus* and normally results in an extensive slough of skin. Treatment is with antibiotics and sometimes also by surgery.

carcin- (carcino-) *prefix denoting* cancer or carcinoma. Example: *carcinogenesis* (development of).

carcinogen *n.* any substance that, when exposed to living tissue, may cause the production of a *carcinoma. Such substances are known to exist in cigarette smoke and may cause lung cancer. The chemical benzidine, once used in medical laboratories, is also known to be a carcinogen. Many chemicals known to produce cancer in laboratory animals have yet to be proved to do so in man. —**carcinogenic** *adj.*

carcinoid *n. see* argentaffinoma.

carcino-embryonic antigen (CEA) a protein produced in the fetus but not in normal adult life. It may be produced by carcinomas, particularly of the colon, and is a rather insensitive marker of malignancy.

carcinoma *n.* any *cancer that arises in epithelium, the tissue that lines the skin and internal organs of the body. It may occur in any tissue containing epithelial cells. In many cases the site of origin of the tumour may be identified by the nature of the cells it contains. Organs may exhibit more than one type of carcinoma; for example, an adenocarcinoma and a squamous carcinoma may be found in the cervix (but not usually concurrently). Treatment depends on the nature of the primary tumour, different types responding to different drug combinations. —**carcinomatous** *adj.*

carcinomatosis *n.* carcinoma that has spread widely throughout the body. Spread of the cancer cells occurs via the lymphatic channels and bloodstream and across body cavities, for example the peritoneal cavity.

carcinosarcoma *n.* a malignant tumour of the cervix, uterus, or vagina containing a mixture of *adenocarcinoma, sarcoma cells, and stroma. It is often bulky and polypoid, with grapelike fronds (*sarcoma botryoides*). Tissues of mesodermal origin, such as bone, cartilage, or striated muscle, may also be present.

cardi- (cardio-) *prefix denoting* the heart. Examples: *cardiomegaly* (enlargement of); *cardiopathy* (disease of).

cardia *n.* **1.** the opening at the upper end of the *stomach that connects with the oesophagus (gullet). **2.** the heart.

cardiac *adj.* **1.** of, relating to, or affecting the heart. **2.** of or relating to the upper part of the stomach (*see* cardia).

cardiac arrest the cessation of effective pumping action of the heart, which most commonly occurs when the muscle fibres of the ventricles start to beat rapidly without pumping any blood (ventricular *fibrillation) or when the heart stops beating completely (*asystole). There is abrupt loss of consciousness, absence of the pulse, and breathing stops. The most common cause is *myocardial infarction. Unless treated promptly, irreversible brain damage and death follow within minutes. Some patients may be resuscitated by massage of the heart, artificial respiration, and *defibrillation.

cardiac cycle the sequence of events between one heart beat and the next, normally occupying less than a second. The atria contract simultaneously and force blood into the relaxed ventricles. The ventricles then contract very strongly and pump blood out through the aorta and pulmonary artery. During ventricular contraction, the atria relax and fill up again with blood. *See* diastole, systole.

cardiac muscle the specialized muscle of which the walls of the *heart are composed. It is composed of a network of branching elongated cells (fibres) whose junctions with neighbouring cells are marked by irregular transverse bands known as *intercalated discs*.

cardiac reflex reflex control of the heart rate. Sensory fibres in the walls of the heart are stimulated when the heart rate increases above normal. Impulses are sent to the cardiac centre in the brain, stimulating the vagus nerve and leading to slowing of the heart rate.

cardinal veins two pairs of veins in the embryo that carry blood from the head (*anterior cardinal veins*) and trunk (*posterior cardinal veins*); they unite to form the *common cardinal vein*, which drains into the sinus venosus of the heart.

cardiology *n.* the science concerned with the study of the structure, function, and diseases of the heart. *See also* nuclear cardiology. —**cardiologist** *n.*

cardiomyopathy *n.* any chronic disorder affecting the muscle of the heart. It may be inherited but can be caused by various conditions, including virus infections, alcoholism, beriberi (vitamin B deficiency), and amyloidosis. The cause is often unknown. It may result in enlargement of the heart, *heart failure, *arrhythmias, and embolism. There is often no specific treatment but patients improve following the control of heart failure and arrhythmias.

cardiomyotomy *n. see* achalasia.

cardioplegia *n.* a technique for extending the life of a heart in the absence of a blood supply by injecting it with a solution of salts. This has enabled complex cardiac surgery and transplants to be performed safely.

cardiopulmonary bypass a method by which the circulation to the body is maintained while the heart is deliberately stopped during heart surgery. The function of the heart and lungs is carried out by a pump-oxygenator (*heart-lung machine) until the natural circulation is restored.

cardiospasm *n. see* achalasia.

cardiotomy syndrome (postcardiotomy syndrome) a condition that may develop weeks or months after surgery to the heart and the membrane surrounding it (pericardium) and is characterized by fever and *pericarditis. Pneumonia and pleurisy may form part of the syndrome. It is thought to be an *autoimmune condition and may be recurrent. A similar syndrome (*Dressler's syndrome*) may follow myocardial infarction. It may respond to anti-inflammatory drugs.

cardiovascular system (circulatory system) the heart together with two networks of blood vessels – the *systemic circulation and the *pulmonary circulation (see illustration). The cardiovascular system effects the circulation of blood around the body, which brings about transport of nutrients and oxygen to the tissues and the removal of waste products.

cardioversion (countershock) *n.* a method of restoring the normal rhythm of the heart in patients with increased heart rate due to arrhythmia. A controlled direct-current shock, synchronized with the R wave of the electrocardiograph, is given through electrodes placed on the chest wall of the anaesthetized patient. The apparatus is called a *cardiovertor* and is a modified defibrillator (*see* defibrillation).

caries *n.* decay and crumbling of the substance of a tooth (*see* dental caries) or a bone. —**carious** *adj.*

carina *n.* a keel-like structure, such as the keel-shaped cartilage at the bifurcation of the trachea into the two main bronchi.

cariogenic *adj.* causing caries, particularly dental caries.

carisoprodol *n.* a drug with muscle-relaxant, analgesic, and tranquillizing

Diagram of the cardiovascular system

action. It is used in the treatment of spastic conditions, such as parkinsonism, and for back pain, sprains, and other injuries. It is administered by mouth; there are few side-effects, but drowsiness or dizziness may occur. Trade names: **Carisoma**, **Rela**, **Soma**.

carminative *n.* a drug that relieves flatulence, used to treat gastric discomfort and colic.

carneous mole a fleshy mass that develops from blood clots, membranes, or pieces of placenta left in the womb after abortion.

carotenaemia *n. see* xanthaemia.

carotene *n.* a yellow or orange plant pigment – one of the carotenoids – that occurs in three forms: alpha (α), beta (β), and gamma (γ). The most important form is β-carotene, which can be converted in the body to retinol (vitamin A). Foods containing β-carotene (milk and some vegetables) are therefore a source of the vitamin.

carotenoid *n.* any one of a group of about 100 naturally occurring yellow to red pigments found mostly in plants. The group includes the *carotenes.

carotid artery either of the two main arteries in the neck whose branches supply the head and neck. The *common carotid artery* arises on the left side directly from the aortic arch and on the right from the innominate artery. They ascend the neck on either side as far as the thyroid cartilage (Adam's apple), where they each divide into two branches, the *internal carotid*, supplying the cerebrum, forehead, nose, eye, and middle ear, and the *external carotid*, sending branches to the face, scalp, and neck.

carotid body a small mass of tissue in the carotid sinus containing *chemore-

ceptors that monitor levels of oxygen, carbon dioxide, and hydrogen ions in the blood. If the oxygen level falls, the chemoreceptors send impulses to the cardiac and respiratory centres in the brain, which promote increases in heart and respiration rates.

carotid sinus a pocket in the wall of the carotid artery, at its division in the neck, containing receptors that monitor blood pressure (*see* baroreceptor). When blood pressure is raised, impulses travel from the receptors to the vasomotor centre in the brain, which initiates a reflex *vasodilatation and slowing of heart rate to lower the blood pressure to normal.

carp- (carpo-) *prefix denoting* the wrist (carpus).

carpal 1. *adj.* relating to the wrist. **2.** *n.* any of the bones forming the carpus.

carpal tunnel the space between the carpal bones of the wrist and the connective tissue (retinaculum) over the flexor tendons. It contains the flexor tendons and the median nerve.

carpal tunnel syndrome compression of the median nerve as it enters the palm of the hand (*see* carpal tunnel). This causes pain and numbness in the index and middle fingers and weakness of the abductor muscle of the thumb.

carphology (floccillation) *n.* plucking at the bedclothes by a delirious patient. This is often a sign of extreme exhaustion and may be the prelude to death.

carpopedal spasm *see* spasm.

carpus *n.* the eight bones of the wrist (see illustration). The carpus articulates with the metacarpals distally and with the humerus and radius proximally.

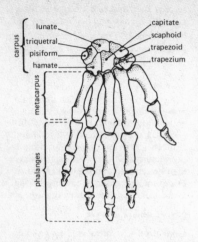

Bones of the left wrist and hand (from the front)

carrier *n.* **1.** a person who harbours the microorganisms causing a particular disease without experiencing signs or symptoms of infection and who can transmit the disease to others. **2.** (in genetics) a person who bears a gene for an abnormal trait without showing signs of the disorder; the carrier is usually *heterozygous for the gene concerned, which is *recessive. **3.** an animal, usually an insect, that passively transmits infectious organisms from one animal to another or from an animal to man. *See also* vector.

cartilage *n.* a dense connective tissue composed of a matrix produced by cells called *chondroblasts*, which become embedded in the matrix as *chondrocytes*. It is a semiopaque grey or white substance, consisting chiefly of *chondroitin sulphate, that is capable of withstanding considerable pressure. There are three types: *hyaline cartilage*, *elastic cartilage*, and *fibrocartilage* (see illustration). In the fetus and infant cartilage occurs in many parts of the body, but most of this cartilage disap-

pears during development. In the adult hyaline cartilage is found in the costal cartilages, larynx, trachea, bronchi, nose, and at the joints of movable bones. Elastic cartilage occurs in the external ear, and fibrocartilage in the intervertebral discs and tendons.

Hyaline cartilage

Elastic cartilage

Fibrocartilage

Types of cartilage

caruncle *n.* a small red fleshy swelling. The *lacrimal caruncle* is the red prominence at the inner angle of the eye.

Hymenal caruncles occur around the mucous membrane lining the vaginal opening.

caseation *n.* the breakdown of diseased tissue into a dry cheeselike mass: a type of degeneration associated with tubercular lesions.

case control study comparison of a group of people who have a disease with another group free from that disease, in terms of *variables in their backgrounds (e.g. cigarette smoking in those who have died from lung cancer and in those dying from other causes). In the more precise *matched pair study* every individual with the disease is paired with a control matched on the basis of (say) age, sex, or occupation in order to place greater emphasis on a factor for which the pairs have not been matched. *Compare* cohort study, cross-sectional study.

case fatality ratio the number of fatalities from a specified disease in a given period per 100 episodes of the disease arising in the same period. Unless all such deaths occur rapidly after the onset of the disease (e.g. cholera) they are likely to be the outcome of episodes that started in an earlier period (hence the term *ratio* rather than *rate*). Comparison of the annual number of admissions and fatalities in a given hospital in respect of a specific disease is known as the *hospital fatality ratio*.

casein *n.* a milk protein. Casein is precipitated out of milk in acid conditions or by the action of rennin: it is the principal protein of cheese. Casein is very easily prepared and is useful as a protein supplement, particularly in the treatment of malnutrition.

case work *see* social services.

cassette *n.* (in radiography) a thin light-proof box in which a piece of X-ray film is placed during the taking of an X-ray. It usually contains special screens that fluoresce under the influence of X-rays and so intensify the image that is formed on the film.

cast *n.* **1.** a rigid casing for a limb, made with open-woven bandage impregnated with plaster of Paris and applied while wet. A plaster cast is designed to protect a broken bone and prevent movement of the aligned bone ends until healing has progressed sufficiently. **2.** a mass of dead cellular, fatty, and other material that forms within a body cavity and takes its shape. It may then be released and appear elsewhere. For example, *granular casts appearing in the urine indicate kidney disease.

castor oil *see* laxative.

castration *n.* removal of the sex glands (the testes or the ovaries). Castration in childhood causes failure of sexual development but when done in adult life (usually as part of hormonal treatment for cancer) it produces less marked physical changes in both sexes. Castration inevitably causes sterility but it need not cause impotence or loss of sexual desire.

cata- *prefix denoting* downward or against.

catabolism *n.* the chemical decomposition of complex substances by the body to form simpler ones, accompanied by the release of energy. The substances broken down include nutrients in food (carbohydrates, proteins, etc.) as well as the body's storage products (such as glycogen). *See also* metabolism. —**catabolic** *adj.*

catalase *n.* an enzyme, present in many cells (including red blood cells and liver cells), that catalyses the breakdown of hydrogen peroxide.

catalepsy *n.* the abnormal maintenance of postures or physical attitudes, occurring in *catatonia. These may have arisen spontaneously or they may be induced by the examiner. There is no resistance to passive movements, which distinguishes it from *flexibilitas cerea.

catalyst *n.* a substance that alters the rate of a chemical reaction but is itself unchanged at the end of the reaction. The catalysts of biochemical reactions are the *enzymes.

catamenia *n. see* menstruation.

cataphoresis *n.* the introduction into the tissues of positively charged ionized substances (cations) by the use of a direct electric current. *See* iontophoresis.

cataplasia *n.* degeneration of tissues to an earlier developmental form.

cataplexy *n.* a recurrent condition in which the patient suddenly collapses to the ground without loss of consciousness. Laughter or any strong emotion can provoke an attack. It is usually associated with *narcolepsy.

cataract *n.* any opacity in the lens of the eye, resulting in blurred vision. The commonest type is *senile cataract*, seen frequently in the elderly, but some cataracts are congenital, while others are due to metabolic disease, such as *diabetes, *galactosaemia, and *hypocalcaemia. Cataracts may also result from direct or indirect injury to the lens and prolonged exposure of the eye to infrared rays (e.g. *glass-blowers' cataract*) or ionising radiation. Minor degrees of cataract do not necessarily impair vision seriously.
Cataract is treated by surgical removal of the affected lens (*cataract extraction*). The lens is usually removed intact (*intracapsular extraction*), but there are several techniques in which the capsule of the lens is left behind (*extracapsular extraction*).

catarrh *n.* the excessive secretion of thick phlegm or mucus by the mucous membrane of the nose, nasal sinuses, nasopharynx, or air passages. The term is not used in any precise or scientific sense.

catatonia *n.* a syndrome of motor abnormalities associated with an abnormal mental state. The symptoms may be *excited*: *stereotypy, stilted overactivity, and purposeless violence; or *inhibited*: stupor, *catalepsy, *flexibilitas cerea, and *negativism. Commonly they are features of catatonic *schizophrenia but they are also seen in other conditions, including encephalitis and hysteria. The syndrome can often be modified by *suggestion. The symptoms usually respond transiently to intravenous *barbiturates. The major *tranquillizers are effective therapy, and *electroconvulsive therapy is sometimes used. —**catatonic** *adj.*

catchment area the geographic area from which a hospital can expect to receive patients and on which in Britain the designated population of the hospital is based. There is no statutory requirement forcing patients to use the hospital(s) of their area, but a code of zoning practice exists for some specialties (e.g. geriatrics, mental illness). A hospital may have a smaller catchment area (e.g. a National Health Service District) for common specialties than for rarer ones, which may be shared between several districts or regions.

catecholamines *pl. n.* a group of physiologically important substances, including *adrenaline, *noradrenaline, and *dopamine, having various different roles (mainly as *neurotransmitters) in the functioning of the sympathetic and central nervous systems. Chemically, all contain a benzene ring with adjacent hydroxyl groups (catechol) and an amine group on a side chain.

catgut *n.* a fibrous material prepared from the tissues of animals, usually from the walls of sheep intestines, twisted into strands of different thicknesses and used to sew up wounds (*see* suture) and tie off blood vessels during surgery. The catgut gradually dissolves and is absorbed by the tissues, so that the stitches do not have to be removed later. This also minimizes the possibility of long-term irritation at the site of operation. Some catgut is treated with chromic acid for different periods during manufacture. This gives catguts of various 'lives', lasting for different lengths of time before absorption is complete.

catharsis *n.* purging or cleansing out of the bowels by giving the patient a *laxative (cathartic) to stimulate intestinal activity.

cathartic *n. see* laxative.

cathepsin *n.* one of a group of enzymes found in animal tissues, particularly the spleen, that digest proteins.

catheter *n.* a tube for insertion into a narrow opening so that fluids may be introduced or removed. *Urinary catheters* are passed into the bladder through the urethra to allow drainage of urine in certain disorders and to empty the bladder before abdominal operations.

catheterization *n.* the introduction of a *catheter into a hollow organ. This is most often performed as *urethral catheterization*, when a catheter is introduced into the bladder to relieve obstruction to the outflow of urine. *Cardiac catheterization* entails the introduction of special catheters into the arteries and veins of the arms or legs through which their tips are manipulated into the various chambers of the heart. Cardiac catheterization provides data on pressures and blood flow within the various chambers of the heart. It permits *angiocardiography.

cation-exchange resins complex insoluble chemical compounds that may be administered with the diet to alter the *electrolyte balance of the body in the treatment of heart, kidney, and metabolic disorders. For example, in patients on a strict low-sodium diet such resins combine with sodium in the food so that it cannot be absorbed and passes out in the faeces.

CAT scanner *see* computerized axial tomography.

cat-scratch fever an infectious virus disease transmitted to man following injury to the skin by a cat scratch, splinter, or thorn. Mild fever and glandular swelling develop about a week after infection. In some cases serious abscess formation occurs, but generally recovery is complete.

cauda *n.* a tail-like structure. The *cauda equina* is a bundle of nerve roots from the lumbar, sacral, and coccygeal spinal nerves that descend nearly vertically from the spinal cord until they reach their respective openings in the vertebral column.

caudal *adj.* relating to the lower part or tail end of the body.

caul *n.* **1.** (in obstetrics) a membrane that may cover an infant's head at birth. This membrane is part of the sac (*amnion) that encloses the fetus during pregnancy. **2.** (in anatomy) *see* omentum.

causal agent a factor associated with the definitive onset of an illness (or other response, including an accident). Examples of causal agents are bacteria, trauma, and noxious agents. The relationship is more direct than in the case of a *risk factor.

causalgia *n.* an intensely unpleasant burning pain felt in a limb where there has been partial damage to the sympathetic and somatic sensory nerves. The blood supply to the limb and the growth of the skin and nails may also be abnormal.

caustic *n.* an agent, such as silver nitrate, that causes irritation and burning and destroys tissue. Caustic agents may be used to remove dead skin, warts, etc., but care must be taken not to damage the surrounding area.

caustic soda *see* sodium hydroxide.

cauterize *vb.* to destroy tissues by direct application of a heated instrument (known as a *cautery*): used for the removal of small warts or other growths. —**cautery** *n.*

cavernitis *n.* inflammation of the corpora cavernosa of the *penis or the corpus cavernosum of the clitoris.

cavernous breathing *see* breath sounds.

cavernous sinus one of the paired cavities within the *sphenoid bone, at the base of the skull behind the eye sockets, into which blood drains from the brain, eye, nose, and upper cheek before leaving the skull through connections with the internal jugular and facial veins. Through the sinus, in its walls, pass the internal carotid artery and the abducens, oculomotor, trochlear, ophthalmic, and maxillary nerves.

cavity *n.* **1.** (in anatomy) a hollow enclosed area; for example, the abdominal cavity or the buccal cavity (mouth). **2.** (in dentistry) **a.** the hole in a tooth caused by *caries or abrasion. **b.** the hole shaped in a tooth by a dentist to retain a filling.

cavity varnish (in dentistry) a solution of natural or synthetic resin in an organic solvent. It is used as a sealer for amalgam fillings or as a coating over newly inserted cement fillings.

CBW (Chemical and Biological Warfare) the use of poison gases and other chemicals, bacteria, viruses, and toxins during war.

-cele (-coele) *suffix denoting* swelling, hernia, or tumour. Example: *gastrocele* (hernia of the stomach).

cell *n.* the basic unit of all living organisms, which can reproduce itself

exactly (*see* mitosis). Each cell is bounded by a *cell membrane* of lipids and protein, which controls the passage of substances into and out of the cell. Cells contain *cytoplasm, in which are suspended a *nucleus and other structures (*organelles) specialized to carry out particular activities in the cell (see illustration).

Complex organisms such as man are built up of millions of cells that are specially adapted to carry out particular functions. The process of cell differentiation begins early in the development of the embryo and cells of a particular type (e.g. blood cells, liver cells) always give rise to cells of the same type. Each cell has a particular number of *chromosomes in its nucleus. The sex cells (sperm and ova) always contain half the number of chromosomes of all the other cells of the body (*see* meiosis); at fertilization a sperm and ovum combine to form a cell with a complete set of chromosomes that will develop into the embryo.

cell body (perikaryon) the enlarged portion of a *neurone (nerve cell), containing the nucleus. It is concerned more with the nutrition of the cell than with propagation of nerve impulses.

cell division reproduction of cells by division first of the chromosomes (karyokinesis) and then of the cytoplasm (cytokinesis). Cell division to produce more body (somatic) cells is by *mitosis; cell division during the formation of gametes is by *meiosis.

cellulitis *n.* inflammation of the connective tissue between adjacent tissues and organs. This is commonly due to bacterial infection and usually requires antibiotic treatment to prevent its spread to the bloodstream.

cellulose *n.* a carbohydrate consisting of linked glucose units. It is an important constituent of plant cell walls. Cellulose cannot be digested by man

plasma membrane

cytoplasm

centrosome

nucleus

nucleolus

fibrils

nucleoplasm

pores in nuclear membrane

rough endoplasmic reticulum

ribosomes

glycogen granules

Golgi apparatus

centrioles

lysosomes

nuclear membrane

chromatin

smooth endoplasmic reticulum

fat droplets

mitochondria

An animal cell (microscopical structure)

and is a component of *dietary fibre (roughage).

Celsius temperature (centigrade temperature) temperature expressed on a scale in which the melting point of ice is assigned a temperature of 0° and the boiling point of water a temperature of 100°. For many medical purposes this scale has superseded the Fahrenheit scale (*see* Fahrenheit temperature). The formula for converting from Celsius (C) to Fahrenheit (F) is: $F = \frac{9}{5}(C + 32)$.

cement *n.* **1.** any of a group of materials used in dentistry either as fillings or as *lutes for crowns. Glass ionomer cements are used for filling, and zinc phosphate, zinc polycarboxylate, and glass ionomer cements are used for luting. Zinc oxide–eugenol cements are widely used as temporary fillings. **2.** *see* cementum.

cementocyte *n.* a cell found in cementum.

cementoma *n.* a benign overgrowth of cementum.

cementum (cement) *n.* a thin layer of hard tissue on the surface of the root of a *tooth. It attaches the fibres of the periodontal membrane to the tooth.

censor *n.* (in psychology) the mechanism, postulated by Freud, that suppresses or modifies desires that are inappropriate or feared. The censor is usually regarded as being located in the *superego but was also described by Freud as being in the *ego itself.

-centesis *suffix denoting* puncture or perforation. Example: *amniocentesis* (surgical puncture of the amnion).

centi- *prefix denoting* one hundredth or a hundred.

centigrade temperature *see* Celsius temperature.

Central Manpower Committee *see* manpower committee.

central nervous system (CNS) the *brain and the *spinal cord, as opposed to the cranial and spinal nerves and the *autonomic nervous system, which together form the *peripheral nervous sys-*

tem. The CNS is responsible for the *integration of all nervous activities.

centre *n*. (in neurology) a collection of neurones (nerve cells) whose activities control a particular function. The *respiratory* and *cardiovascular centres*, for example, are regions in the lower brainstem that control the movements of respiration and the functioning of the circulatory system, respectively.

centrencephalic *adj*. (in electroencephalography) describing discharges that can be recorded synchronously from all parts of the brain. The source of this activity is in the *reticular formation of the midbrain. *Centrencephalic epilepsy* is associated with a congenital predisposition to fits.

centri- *prefix denoting* centre. Example: *centrilobular* (in the centre of a lobule (especially of the liver)).

centrifugal *adj*. moving away from a centre, as from the brain to the peripheral tissues.

centrifuge *n*. a device for separating components of different densities in a liquid, using centrifugal force. The liquid is placed in special containers that are spun at high speed around a central axis.

centriole *n*. a small particle found in the cytoplasm of cells, near the nucleus. Centrioles are involved in the formation of the *spindle and aster during cell division. During interphase there are usually two centrioles in the *centrosome; when cell division occurs these separate and move to opposite sides of the nucleus, and the spindle is formed between them.

centripetal *adj*. moving towards a centre, as from the peripheral tissues to the brain.

centromere (kinetochore) *n*. the part of a chromosome that joins the two *chromatids to each other and becomes attached to the spindle during *mitosis

and *meiosis. When chromosome division takes place the centromeres split longitudinally.

centrosome (centrosphere) *n*. an area of clear cytoplasm, found next to the nucleus in nondividing cells, that contains the *centrioles.

centrosphere *n*. **1.** an area of clear cytoplasm seen in dividing cells around the poles of the spindle. **2.** *see* centrosome.

centrum *n*. (*pl*. **centra**) the solid rod-shaped central portion of a *vertebra.

cephal- (cephalo-) *prefix denoting* the head. Example: *cephalalgia* (pain in).

cephalad *adj*. towards the head.

cephalexin *n*. a semisynthetic antibiotic, administered by mouth, used in the treatment of a variety of infections. *See* cephalosporin. Trade names: **Ceporex**, **Keflex**.

cephalhaematoma *n*. an egg-sized swelling on the head caused by a collection of bloody fluid between one of the skull bones (usually the *parietal bone) and its covering membrane (periosteum). It is most commonly seen in newborn infants delivered with the aid of forceps or subjected to pressures during passage through the birth canal. No treatment is necessary and the swelling disappears in a few weeks. A cephalhaematoma in an older baby or child is evidence of some recent injury to the head; occasionally an unsuspected fracture is revealed on X-ray.

cephalic *adj*. of or relating to the head.

cephalic index a measure of the shape of a skull, commonly used in *craniometry: the ratio of the greatest breadth, multiplied by 100, to the greatest length of the skull. *See also* brachycephaly, dolichocephaly.

cephalic version a procedure for turning a fetus that is lying in a breech or transverse position so that its head will enter the birth passage first. It cannot be performed after labour is well advanced.

cephalin *n.* one of a group of *phospholipids that are constituents of cell membranes and are particularly abundant in the brain.

cephalocele *n. see* neural tube defects.

cephaloglycin *n.* a semisynthetic antibiotic, given by mouth for the treatment of urinary tract infections. The main side-effects are gastrointestinal irritation and allergy. Cross-sensitivity with the penicillins may occur and cephaloglycin should be used with caution in patients known to be sensitive to these drugs. *See* cephalosporin.

cephalogram *n.* a special standardized X-ray picture that can be used to measure alterations in the growth of skull bones.

cephalometry *n.* the study of facial growth by examination of standardized lateral radiographs of the head. It is used mainly for diagnosis in *orthodontics.

cephaloridine *n.* a semisynthetic antibiotic, given by intravenous or intramuscular injection. It is used in the treatment of a variety of severe infections, including those of bones, joints, the bloodstream, and the urinary and respiratory tracts. *See* cephalosporin. Trade name: **Loridine**.

cephalosporin *n.* any one of a group of semisynthetic antibiotics, derived from the mould *Cephalosporium*, which are effective against a wide range of microorganisms and are therefore used in a variety of infections (*see* cephalexin, cephaloglycin, cephaloridine, cephalothin sodium). Cross-sensitivity with penicillin may occur and the principal side-effects are allergic reactions and irritation of the digestive tract.

cephalothin sodium a semisynthetic antibiotic, given by intramuscular or intravenous injection in the treatment of a number of infections. *See* cephalosporin. Trade name: **Keflin**.

cercaria *n.* (*pl.* **cercariae**) the final larval stage of any parasitic trematode (*see* fluke). The cercariae, which have tails but otherwise resemble the adults, are released into water from the snail host in which the parasite undergoes part of its development. Several thousand cercariae may emerge from a single snail in a day.

cerebellum *n.* the largest part of the hindbrain, bulging back behind the pons and the medulla oblongata and overhung by the occipital lobes of the cerebrum. Like the cerebrum, it has an outer grey cortex and a core of white matter. Three broad bands of nerve fibres – the inferior, middle, and superior cerebellar peduncles – connect it to the medulla, the pons, and the midbrain respectively. It has two hemispheres, one on each side of the central region (the *vermis*), and its surface is thrown into thin folds called *folia* (see illustration). Within lie four pairs of nuclei.

The cerebellum (anterior view)

The cerebellum is essential for the maintenance of muscle tone, balance, and the synchronization of activity in groups of muscles under voluntary control, converting muscular contractions into smooth coordinated movement. It does not, however, initiate movement and plays no part in the perception of conscious sensations or in intelligence. —**cerebellar** *adj.*

cerebr- (cerebri-, cerebro-) *prefix denoting* the cerebrum or brain.

cerebral aqueduct (aqueduct of Sylvius) the narrow channel, containing cerebrospinal fluid, that connects the third and fourth *ventricles of the brain.

cerebral cortex the intricately folded outer layer of the *cerebrum, making up some 40% of the brain by weight and composed of an estimated 15 thousand million neurones (*see* grey matter). This is the part of the brain most directly responsible for consciousness, with essential roles in perception, memory, thought, mental ability, and intellect, and it is responsible for initiating voluntary activity. It has connections, direct or indirect, with all parts of the body. The folding of the cortex provides a large surface area, the greater part lying in the clefts (*sulci*), which divide the upraised convolutions (*gyri*). On the basis of its microscopic appearance in section, the cortex is mapped into *Brodmann's areas; it is also divided into functional regions; including *motor cortex, *sensory cortex, and *association areas. Within, and continuous with it, lies the *white matter, through which connection is made with the rest of the nervous system.

cerebral haemorrhage bleeding from a cerebral artery into the tissue of the brain. It is usually caused by degenerative disease of the blood vessels and high blood pressure. The extent and severity of the symptoms depend upon the site and volume of the haemorrhage; they vary from a transient weakness or numbness to profound coma

and death. *See also* atheroma, hypertension, stroke.

cerebral hemisphere one of the two paired halves of the *cerebrum.

cerebral palsy a developmental abnormality of the brain resulting in weakness and incoordination of the limbs. The brain damage may be caused by injury during birth, haemorrhage, lack of oxygen before birth, meningitis, viral infection, or faulty development. The most common disability is a *spastic paralysis (an affected child is called a *spastic*), which may slowly increase from contractures to cause fixed deformities of the limbs. Defective sensory perception, including lack of balance, is always present in some degree, and intelligence is often impaired. Posture and speech may be severely affected. Other disabilities that may occur include involuntary writhing movements (*athetosis) and epilepsy. Management of cerebral palsy is aimed at improving movement (by physiotherapy and other means), combined with prevention or surgical amelioration of fixed deformities due to muscle imbalance and the judicious use of appliances or locomotor aids. Speech therapy may also be required.

cerebral tumour an abnormal multiplication of brain cells. This forms a swelling that compresses or destroys the healthy brain cells and – because of the rigid nature of the skull – increases the pressure on the brain tissue. Malignant tumours grow rapidly, spreading through the otherwise normal brain tissue and causing progressive neurological disability. Benign tumours grow slowly and compress the brain tissue, sometimes causing epileptic fits.

cerebration *n.* **1.** the functioning of the brain as a whole. **2.** the unconscious activities of the brain.

cerebroside *n.* one of a group of compounds occurring in the *myelin sheaths of nerve fibres. They are *gly-colipids, containing *sphingosine, a fatty acid, and a sugar (usually galactose or glucose).

cerebrospinal fever (spotted fever) a type of *meningitis caused by the bacterium *Neisseria meningitidis*. Bacteria are transmitted by coughing and sneezing: outbreaks occur most commonly in overcrowded conditions, and children are more susceptible than adults. After an incubation period of 3–5 days, symptoms appear suddenly, including severe headache, fever, stiffness of the neck muscles, and a rash of small red spots on the trunk. Occasionally the disease enters a chronic state in which deafness, blindness, and serious mental deterioration may occur. Without treatment death can occur within a week, but administration of penicillin or sulphonamide drugs is usually effective.

cerebrospinal fluid (CSF) the clear watery fluid that surrounds the brain and spinal cord. It is contained in the *subarachnoid space and circulates in the *ventricles of the brain and in the central canal of the spinal cord. The brain floats in the fluid (its weight so being reduced from about 1400 g to less than 100 g) and is cushioned by it from contact with the skull when the head is moved vigorously. The CSF is secreted by the *choroid plexuses in the ventricles, circulates through them to reach the subarachnoid space, and is eventually absorbed into the bloodstream through the *arachnoid villi. Its normal contents are glucose, salts, enzymes, and a few white cells, but no red blood cells.

cerebrovascular disease any disorder of the blood vessels of the brain and its covering membranes (meninges). Most cases are due to atheroma and/or hypertension, clinical effects being caused by rupture of diseased blood vessels (*cerebral or *subarach-noid haemorrhage) or inadequacy of the blood supply to the brain (ischaemia), due to cerebral thrombosis or embolism. The term *cerebrovascular accident* is sometimes given to the clinical syndrome accompanying a sudden and severe attack, which leads to a *stroke.

cerebrum (telencephalon) *n.* the largest and most highly developed part of the brain, composed of the two *cerebral hemispheres*, separated from each other by the *longitudinal fissure* in the midline (see illustration). Each hemisphere has an outer layer of grey matter, the *cerebral cortex, below which lies white matter containing the *basal ganglia. Connecting the two hemispheres at the bottom of the longitudinal fissure is the *corpus callosum*, a massive bundle of nerve fibres. Within each hemisphere is a crescent-shaped fluid-filled cavity (lateral *ventricle), connected to the central third ventricle in the *diencephalon. The cerebrum is responsible for the initiation and coordination of all voluntary activity in the body and for governing the functioning of lower parts of the nervous system. The cortex is the seat of all intelligent behaviour. —**cerebral** *adj.*

cerumen (earwax) *n.* the waxy material that is secreted by the sebaceous glands in the external auditory meatus of the outer ear. Its function is to protect the delicate skin that lines the inside of the meatus.

cervic- (cervico-) *prefix denoting* 1. the neck. Example: *cervicodynia* (pain in). 2. the cervix, especially of the uterus. Example: *cervicectomy* (surgical removal of).

cervical *adj.* 1. of or relating to the neck. 2. of, relating to, or affecting the cervix (neck region) of an organ, especially the cervix of the womb.

cervical cancer cancer in the neck (cervix) of the womb. The growth can

parieto-occipital fissure
parietal lobe
central sulcus
frontal lobe
lateral sulcus
temporal lobe
occipital lobe

Lobes of the cerebrum (from the right side)

be detected at an early stage by periodic microscopical examination of cells released from the affected region (*see* cervical smear), and it can then be eradicated before it has been able to spread. Vaginal discharge, especially with blood, may be a symptom.

cervical smear a specimen of cellular material scraped from the neck (cervix) of the womb and examined under a microscope in order to determine whether cancer is present.

cervical vertebrae the seven bones making up the neck region of the *backbone. The first cervical vertebra – the *atlas* – consists basically of a ring of bone that supports the skull by articulating with the occipital condyles (*see* occipital bone). The second vertebra – the *axis* – has an upward-pointing process (the *odontoid process* or *dens*) that forms a pivot on which the atlas can rotate, enabling the head to be turned. *See also* vertebra.

cervicitis *n.* inflammation of the neck (cervix) of the womb.

cervix *n.* a necklike part, especially the *cervix uteri*, the narrow passage at the lower end of the uterus (womb), which

connects with the vagina. Its cavity is normally filled with mucus, the viscosity of which changes throughout the menstrual cycle. The cervix is capable of very wide dilation during childbirth.

cestode *n. see* tapeworm.

cetrimide *n.* a detergent disinfectant, used for cleansing skin surfaces and wounds, sterilizing surgical instruments and babies' napkins, and in shampoos. There are few adverse reactions from external application; most toxic effects are due to poisoning from ingestion. Trade name: **Cetavlon**.

cetylpyridinium *n.* a detergent disinfectant, used for the disinfection of skin, wounds, and burns and as a mouthwash.

Chagas' disease a disease caused by the protozoan parasite *Trypanosoma cruzi*. It is transmitted to man when the trypanosomes, present in the faeces of nocturnal bloodsucking *reduviid bugs, come into contact with wounds and scratches on the skin or the delicate internal tissues of the nose and mouth. The presence of the parasite in the heart muscles and central nervous system results in serious inflammation and lesions, which can prove fatal. The disease, limited to poor rural areas of South and Central America, is especially prevalent in children and young adults. There is no effective treatment. *See also* trypanosomiasis.

chaining *n.* a technique of *behaviour modification in which a complex skill is taught by being broken down into its separate components, which are gradually built up into the full sequence. Usually the last component in the sequence is taught first, as it is this component that is followed by *reinforcement: this is termed *backwards chaining*.

chalazion (meibomian cyst) *n.* a swollen sebaceous gland in the eyelid, caused by chronic inflammation following blockage of the gland's duct. The gland becomes converted into a jelly-like mass, producing disfigurement of the lid. It may become secondarily infected, when it will be painful and may discharge. Treatment is by application of antibiotic ointments or surgical incision and curettage of the gland.

chalicosis *n.* pneumoconiosis occurring in stone cutters: a variety of *silicosis. The term is not in current use.

chancre *n.* a painless ulcer that develops on the lips, penis, urethra, or eyelid as the primary symptom of such infections as sleeping sickness and syphilis.

chancroid *n. see* soft sore.

Charcot-Leyden crystals fine colourless sharp-pointed crystals seen in the sputum of asthmatics.

Charcot-Marie-Tooth disease (peroneal muscular atrophy) an inherited disease of the peripheral nerves causing a gradually progressive weakness and wasting of the muscles of the legs and the lower part of the thighs. The hands and arms are eventually affected.

Charcot's joint a damaged, swollen, and deformed joint, often the knee, resulting from repeated minor injuries of which the patient is unaware because the nerves that normally register pain are not functioning. The condition may occur in syphilis, diabetes mellitus, and syringomyelia.

Charnley clamps parallel metal rods driven through the ends of two bones that are to be joined to form an *arthrodesis. The rods are connected on each side of the joint by bolts bearing wing nuts; tightening of the screw arrangements forces the surfaces of the bones together. When the two bones have joined, by growth and reshaping, the clamps can be removed.

cheil- (cheilo-) *prefix denoting* the lip(s). Example: *cheiloplasty* (plastic surgery of).

cheilitis *n.* inflammation of the lips.

cheiloplasty *n. see* labioplasty.

cheiloschisis *n. see* harelip.

cheilosis *n.* swollen cracked bright-red lips. This is a common symptom of many nutritional disorders, including ariboflavinosis (vitamin B_2 deficiency).

cheir- (cheiro-) *prefix denoting* the hand(s). Examples: *cheiralgia* (pain in); *cheiroplasty* (plastic surgery of).

cheiropompholyx *n.* a type of eczema affecting the sides and fronts of the palms and fingers, with a similar distribution on the feet. The thickness of the skin in these areas prevents the eczema vesicles from breaking and eventually the skin peels after a period of intense itching. Attacks start suddenly, often in the summer, and last up to six weeks. Secondary infection is common.

chelating agent a chemical compound that forms complexes by binding metal ions. Some chelating agents, including *desferrioxamine and *penicillamine, are drugs used to treat metal poisoning: the metal is bound to the drug and excreted safely. Chelating agents often form the active centres of enzymes.

cheloid *n. see* keloid.

chem- (chemo-) *prefix denoting* chemical or chemistry.

chemoreceptor *n.* a cell or group of cells that responds to the presence of specific chemical compounds by initiating an impulse in a sensory nerve. Chemoreceptors are found in the taste buds and in the mucous membranes of the nose. *See also* receptor.

chemosis *n.* swelling (oedema) of the *conjunctiva. It is usually due to inflammation but may occur if the drainage of blood and lymph from around the eye is obstructed.

chemotaxis *n.* movement of a cell or organism in response to the stimulus of a gradient of chemical concentration.

chemotherapy *n.* the prevention or treatment of disease by the use of chemical substances. The term is sometimes restricted to the treatment of infectious diseases with antibiotics and other drugs or to the control of cancer with antimetabolites and similar drugs (in contrast to *radiotherapy).

chest *n. see* thorax.

Cheyne-Stokes respiration a striking form of breathing in which there is a cyclical variation in the rate, which becomes slower until breathing stops for several seconds before speeding up to a peak and then slowing again. It occurs when the sensitivity of the respiratory centres in the brain is impaired, particularly in states of coma.

chiasma *n.* (*pl.* **chiasmata**) **1.** (in genetics) the point at which homologous chromosomes remain in contact after they have started to separate in the first division of *meiosis. Chiasmata occur from the end of prophase to anaphase and represent the point at which mutual exchange of genetic material takes place (*see* crossing over). **2.** *see* optic chiasma.

chickenpox *n.* a mild highly infectious disease caused by a *herpesvirus that is transmitted by airborne droplets. After an incubation period of 11–18 days a mild fever develops, followed within 24 hours by an itchy rash of dark red pimples. The pimples spread from the trunk to the face, scalp, and limbs; they develop into blisters and then scabs, which drop off after about 12 days. The only treatment is bed rest and the application of calamine lotion to the spots to discourage scratching. Scarring is unusual. The patient is infectious from the onset of symptoms until all the spots have gone. Since an attack in childhood generally confers life-long immunity, chickenpox is rare among adults. Medical name: **varicella**.

chiclero's ulcer a form of *leishmaniasis of the skin caused by the parasite *Leishmania tropica mexicana*. The disease, occurring in Panama, Honduras, and the Amazon, primarily affects men who visit the forests to collect chicle (gum) and takes the form of an ulcerating lesion on the ear lobe. The sore usually heals spontaneously within six months.

Chief Administrative Medical Officer a physician at Area level under the NHS (Scotland) Act. *See* National Health Service.

chigger *n. see* Trombicula.

chigoe *n. see* Tunga.

Chikungunya fever a disease, occurring in Africa and Asia, caused by an *arbovirus and transmitted to man by mosquitoes of the genus *Aëdes*. The disease is similar to *dengue and symptoms include fever, headache, generalized body pain, and an irritating rash. The patient is given drugs to relieve the pain and reduce the fever.

chilblain *n.* a red round itchy swelling of the skin, occurring generally on the fingers or toes in cold weather. Chilblains form part of a group of related conditions (*see* perniosis). Treatment is by keeping the limbs warm, though vasodilator drugs may help. Medical name: **pernio**.

childbed *n. see* puerperium.

childbirth *n. see* labour.

child health clinic (CHC) (in Britain) a special clinic for the routine care of infants and preschool children, formerly known as a *child welfare centre*. Sometimes these clinics are staffed by doctors, *health visitors, and clinic nurses employed by District Health

Authorities; the children attending them are drawn from the district around the clinic. Alternatively general practitioners may run their own CHC, say once a week, with health visitors and other staff in attendance; it is unusual for children not registered with the practice to attend such clinics. The service provides screening tests for congenital dislocation of hips, suppressed squint (*see* cover test), and impaired speech and/or hearing. The *Guthrie test may also be performed if this has not been done before the baby leaves hospital. The staff of CHCs also educate mothers (especially those having their first child) in feeding techniques and hygiene and see that children receive the recommended immunizations against infectious diseases. They also ensure that the families of handicapped children receive maximum support from health and social services and that such children achieve their maximum potential in the preschool period.

chir- (chiro-) *prefix denoting* the hand(s). *See also* cheir-.

chiropody (podiatry) *n.* the study and care of the foot, including its normal structure, its diseases, and their treatment. —**chiropodist** *n.*

chiropractic *n.* a system of treating diseases by manipulation, mainly of the vertebrae of the backbone. It is based on the theory that nearly all disorders can be traced to the incorrect alignment of bones, with consequent malfunctioning of nerves and muscle throughout the body.

Chlamydia *n.* a genus of virus-like microorganisms that cause disease in man and birds. Some *Chlamydia* infections of birds can be transmitted to man (*see* ornithosis, parrot disease). *Chlamydia trachomatis* is the causative agent of the eye disease *trachoma. The organisms appear to resemble bacteria but are of similar size to viruses and all are obligate parasites.

chloasma (melasma) *n.* the appearance of brown patches, up to several centimetres in diameter, mainly on the forehead, temples, and cheeks. It is due to a localized increase in the dark pigment *melanin and occurs sometimes in pregnancy (when the nipples also turn brown), as well as during the menopause. Women taking the contraceptive pill may also develop chloasma.

chlor- (chloro-) *prefix denoting* **1.** chlorine or chlorides. **2.** green.

chloracne *n.* an occupational acne-like skin disorder that occurs after regular contact with chlorinated hydrocarbons. These chemicals are derived from oil and tar products; 'cutting oils' used in engineering also cause the disease. The skin develops blackheads, papules, and pustules, mainly on hairy parts (such as the forearm). Warts and skin cancer may develop after many years of exposure to these chemicals.

chloral hydrate a sedative and hypnotic drug used, mainly in children and the elderly, to induce sleep or as a daytime sedative. It is rapidly absorbed from the alimentary canal and is usually given by mouth as a syrup, although it can be administered rectally. Toxic effects are usually only seen with overdosage. Prolonged use may lead to *dependence. Trade names: **Noctec, Somnos.**

chlorambucil *n.* a drug that destroys cancer cells. It is given by mouth and used mainly in the treatment of chronic leukaemias. Prolonged large doses may cause damage to the bone marrow. Trade name: **Leukeran.**

chloramphenicol *n.* an antibiotic, derived from the bacterium *Streptomyces venezuelae* and also produced synthetically, that is effective against a wide variety of microorganisms. However, due to its serious side-effects, especially damage to the bone marrow, it is usually reserved for serious infections (such as typhoid fever) when less toxic drugs are ineffective. Trade names: **Chloromycetin, Mycinol**, etc.

chlorbutol *n.* an antibacterial and antifungal agent used as a preservative in injection solutions, in eye and nose drops, in powder form for topical use in irritational skin conditions, and occasionally by mouth as a mild sedative in travel sickness.

chlorcyclizine *n.* an *antihistamine drug that is slow-acting but produces long-lasting effects. Given by mouth, it is used mainly to relieve the symptoms of allergic reactions and to prevent travel sickness. Principal side-effects are drowsiness, dizziness, and dryness of the mouth and throat. Trade names: **Di-paralene, Histantine**.

chlordantoin *n.* an antifungal drug, used mainly for the treatment of fungus infections (candidiasis) of the vagina. It is applied in the form of a cream or pessaries, and local skin reactions occasionally occur.

chlordiazepoxide *n.* a sedative and tranquillizing drug with *muscle relaxant properties, used to relieve tension, fears and anxiety and in the treatment of alcoholism. It is administered by mouth or injection. Common side-effects are nausea, skin reactions, and muscular incoordination. Trade names: **Librium, Diapox, Elenium**. *See also* tranquillizer.

chlorhexadol *n.* a sedative and hypnotic drug with uses similar to those of *chloral hydrate. Trade name: **Medodorm**.

chlorhexidine *n.* an antiseptic used as a general disinfectant for skin and mucous membranes or as a preservative (for example, in eye drops). Chlorhexidine is used in solution, creams, gels, and lozenges and in some preparations is combined with *cetrimide. In very dilute solutions it can be used as an effective mouthwash for the control of infections of the mouth. Skin sensitivity to chlorhexidine occurs rarely. Trade name: **Hibitane**.

chlorination *n.* the addition of noninjurious traces of chlorine (often one part per million) to water supplies before human consumption to ensure that disease-causing organisms are destroyed.

chlorine *n.* an extremely pungent gaseous element with antiseptic and bleaching properties. It is widely used to sterilize drinking water and purify swimming baths. In high concentrations it is toxic; it was used in World War I as a poison gas in the trenches. Symbol: Cl.

chlormadinone *n.* a synthetic sex hormone (*see* progestogen) that was formerly used in oral contraceptives as a sequential and progestogen-only pill. Chlormadinone produces variations in the length of the menstrual cycle and abnormal bleeding; nausea, vomiting, and weight gain may also occur.

chlormethiazole *n.* a *sedative and hypnotic drug used to treat insomnia in the elderly (when associated with confusion, agitation, and restlessness) and drug withdrawal symptoms (especially in alcoholism). It is administered by mouth or injection and the most common side-effects are tingling sensations in the nose and sneezing. Trade name: **Heminevrin**.

chlormezanone *n.* a tranquillizing drug used in the treatment of mild anxiety and tension, including premenstrual tension. It is also used to relieve pain and muscle spasm. Chlormezanone is administered by mouth; the most common side-effects are drowsiness and dizziness. Trade name: **Trancopal**.

chlorocresol *n.* an antiseptic derived from phenol, used as a general disinfectant and, at low concentrations, as a preservative in injections, creams, and lotions and also in eye drops. Strong solutions applied to the skin may cause sensitivity reactions.

chloroform *n.* a volatile liquid formerly widely used as a general anaesthetic. Because its use as such causes liver damage and affects heart rhythm, chloroform is now used only in low concentrations as a flavouring agent and preservative, in the treatment of flatulence, and in liniments as a *rubefacient.

chloroma *n.* a tumour that arises in association with *myeloid leukaemia and consists essentially of a mass of leukaemic cells. A freshly cut specimen of the tumour appears green, but the colour rapidly disappears on exposure to air. It shows red fluorescence with ultraviolet light and responds to specific antileukaemic treatment.

chlorophenothane *n. see* DDT.

chlorophyll *n.* one of a group of green pigments, found in all green plants and some bacteria, that absorb light to provide energy for the synthesis of carbohydrates from carbon dioxide and water (photosynthesis). The two major chlorophylls, a and b, consist of a porphyrin/magnesium complex.

chloropsia *n.* green vision: a rare symptom of digitalis poisoning.

chloropyrilene *n.* an *antihistamine administered by mouth to treat allergies and other reactions involving release of histamine.

chloroquine *n.* a drug used principally in the treatment and prevention of malaria but also used in rheumatoid arthritis, certain liver infections and skin conditions, and lupus erythematosus. It is administered by mouth or injection; a side-effect of prolonged use in large doses is eye damage. Trade names: **Avloclor, Nivaquine**.

chlorosis *n.* a severe form of *anaemia produced by gross deficiency of iron, so

called because of the greenish skin pallor that it produces.

chlorothiazide *n.* a *diuretic used to treat fluid retention (oedema) and high blood pressure (hypertension). It is administered by mouth and may cause skin sensitivity reactions, stomach pains, nausea, and reduced blood potassium levels. Trade name: **Saluric**.

chlorotrianisene *n.* a synthetic *oestrogen administered by mouth to treat symptoms of the menopause, to suppress lactation in mothers not breast feeding, and to relieve symptoms in cancer of the prostate gland. Trade name: **Tace**.

chloroxylenol *n.* an *antiseptic, derived from *phenol but less toxic and more selective in bactericidal activity, used mainly in solution as a skin disinfectant. Trade name: **Dettol**.

chlorphenesin *n.* a compound, active against bacteria and fungi, that is applied to the skin as a cream or dusting powder to treat fungal infections, such as athlete's foot. Trade name: **Mycil**.

chlorpheniramine *n.* a potent *antihistamine used to treat such allergies as hay fever, rhinitis, and urticaria. It is administered by mouth or, to relieve severe conditions, by injection. Trade name: **Piriton**.

chlorphenoxamine *n.* a drug with atropine-like and *antihistamine action, administered by mouth to treat muscle stiffness in parkinsonism; it does not affect tremor. Trade name: **Clorevan**.

chlorphentermine *n.* a drug used to suppress appetite in the treatment of obesity. It has a similar action to *amphetamine but is less potent. It is administered by mouth and may cause dizziness, insomnia, or drowsiness.

chlorproguanil *n.* a drug administered by mouth to prevent and treat malaria. Side-effects are rare, but large doses may cause stomach discomfort and vomiting.

chlorpromazine *n.* a major *tranquillizer and antipsychotic drug. It is used in the treatment of *schizophrenia and *mania; to control severe anxiety and agitation; and to control nausea and vomiting. It also enhances the effects of *analgesics and is used in terminal illness and preparation for anaesthesia. Chlorpromazine is administered by mouth or injection or as a rectal suppository; common side-effects are drowsiness and dry mouth. It also causes abnormalities of movement, especially *dystonias, *dyskinesia, and *parkinsonism. Trade names: **Chloractil, Largactil**.

chlorpropamide *n.* a drug that reduces blood sugar levels and is used to treat diabetes in adults. It is administered by mouth and can cause such side-effects as skin sensitivity reactions and digestive upsets. Trade names: **Diabinese, Melitase**. *See also* sulphonylurea.

chlorprothixene *n.* a major *tranquillizer and sedative used to treat agitation, anxiety, insomnia, delusions, and hallucinations. It is administered by mouth; common side-effects are dry mouth and drowsiness. Trade name: **Taractan**.

chlortetracycline *n.* an *antibiotic active against many bacteria and fungi. It is administered by mouth or injection or as ointment or cream (for skin and eye infections); side-effects are those of the other *tetracyclines. Trade names: **Aureomycin, Chlortetrin, Deteclo**.

chlorthalidone *n.* a *diuretic used to treat fluid retention (oedema) and high blood pressure (hypertension). It is administered by mouth and may cause skin sensitivity reactions, stomach pains, nausea, and reduced blood potassium levels. Trade name: **Hygroton**.

choana *n.* (*pl.* **choanae**) a funnel-shaped opening, particularly either of the two openings between the nasal cavity and the pharynx.

chokedamp *n.* *see* blackdamp.

chol- (chole-, cholo-) *prefix denoting* bile. Example: *cholemesis* (vomiting of).

cholagogue *n.* a drug that stimulates the flow of bile from the gall bladder and bile ducts into the duodenum.

cholangiography *n.* X-ray examination of the bile ducts, used to demonstrate the site and nature of any obstruction to the ducts or to show the presence of stones within them. A medium that is opaque to X-rays is introduced into the ducts either by injection into the bloodstream (*intravenous cholangiography*); direct injection into the liver (*percutaneous transhepatic cholangiography*); direct injection into the bile ducts at operation (*operative cholangiography*); or by injection into the duodenal opening of the ducts through a *duodenoscope (*endoscopic retrograde cholangiopancreatography*; see* ERCP).

cholangiolitis *n.* inflammation of the smallest bile ducts (*cholangioles*). *See* cholangitis.

cholangioma *n.* a rare tumour originating from the bile duct.

cholangitis *n.* inflammation of the bile ducts. It usually occurs when the ducts are obstructed, especially by stones, or after operations on the bile ducts. Symptoms include intermittent fever, usually with *rigors, and intermittent jaundice. Initial treatment is by antibiotics, but removal of the obstruction is essential for permanent cure. Liver abscess is a possible complication, and recurrent episodes of cholangitis lead to secondary biliary *cirrhosis.

cholecalciferol *n.* *see* vitamin D.

cholecyst- *prefix denoting* the gall bladder. Example: *cholecystotomy* (incision of).

cholecystectomy *n.* surgical removal of the gall bladder, usually for *cholecystitis or gallstones.

cholecystenterostomy *n.* a surgical procedure in which the gall bladder is joined to the small intestine. It is performed in order to allow bile to pass from the liver to the intestine when the common bile duct is obstructed by an irremovable cause.

cholecystitis *n.* inflammation of the gall bladder. *Acute cholecystitis* is due to bacterial infection, causing fever and acute pain over the gall bladder. It is usually treated by rest and antibiotics. *Chronic cholecystitis* is often associated with *gallstones and causes recurrent episodes of upper abdominal pain. Recurrent bacterial infection may be the cause, but the physical processes leading to gallstone formation may also be important. It may require treatment by *cholecystectomy. *See also* cholesterosis.

cholecystoduodenostomy *n.* a form of *cholecystenterostomy in which the gall bladder is joined to the duodenum.

cholecystogastrostomy *n.* a form of *cholecystenterostomy in which the gall bladder is joined to the stomach. It is rarely performed.

cholecystography *n.* X-ray examination of the gall bladder. A compound containing iodine and therefore opaque to X-rays is taken by mouth, absorbed by the intestine, and excreted by the liver into the bile, which is concentrated in the gall bladder. An X-ray photograph (*cholecystogram*) of the gall bladder indicates whether or not it is functioning, and gallstones may be seen as contrasting (nonopaque) areas within it. A fatty meal is usually also given, to demonstrate the ability of the gall bladder to contract.

cholecystokinin-pancreozymin *n.* a hormone from the small intestine (duodenum) that causes contraction of the gall bladder and expulsion of bile into the intestine and stimulates the production of digestive enzymes by the pancreas. *See also* pancreatic juice.

cholecystotomy *n.* a surgical operation in which the gall bladder is opened, usually to remove gallstones. It is performed only when *cholecystectomy would be impracticable or dangerous.

choledoch- (choledocho-) *prefix denoting* the common bile duct. Example: *choledochoplasty* (plastic surgery of).

choledocholithiasis *n.* stones within the common bile duct. The stones usually form in the gall bladder and pass into the bile duct, but they may develop within the duct after *cholecystectomy.

choledochotomy *n.* a surgical operation in which the common bile duct is opened, to search for or to remove stones within it. It may be performed at the same time as *cholecystectomy or if stones occur in the bile duct after cholecystectomy.

cholelithiasis *n.* the formation of stones in the gall bladder (*see* gallstone).

cholelithotomy *n.* removal of gallstones by *cholecystotomy.

cholera *n.* an acute infection of the small intestine by the bacterium *Vibrio cholerae*, which causes severe vomiting and diarrhoea (known as *ricewater stools*) leading to dehydration. The disease is contracted from food or drinking water contaminated by faeces from a patient. Cholera often occurs in epidemics; outbreaks are rare in good sanitary conditions. After an incubation period of 1–5 days symptoms commence suddenly; the resulting dehydration and imbalance in the concentration of body fluids can cause death within 24 hours. Treatment involves intravenous infusion of salt solution; antibiotics only hasten recovery. The mortality rate in untreated cases is over 50%. Vaccination against cholera is effective for only 6–9 months.

choleresis *n.* the production of bile by the liver.

choleretic *n.* an agent that stimulates the secretion of bile by the liver thereby increasing the flow of bile.

cholestasis *n.* failure of normal amounts of bile to reach the intestine, resulting in obstructive *jaundice. The cause may be a mechanical block in the bile ducts, such as a stone (*extrahepatic biliary obstruction*), or liver disease, such as that caused by the drug *chlorpromazine in some hypersensitive individuals (*intrahepatic cholestasis*). The symptoms are jaundice with dark urine, pale faeces, and usually itching (pruritus).

cholesteatoma *n.* a mass consisting mainly of cellular debris in which cholesterol crystals may be demonstrated. Cholesteatomas occur mainly in the middle ear and, by pressure, cause destruction of surrounding structures. They may also occur in other parts of the skull and nervous system.

cholesterol *n.* a fatlike material (a *sterol) present in the blood and most tissues, especially nervous tissue. Cholesterol and its esters are important constituents of cell membranes and are precursors of many steroid hormones and bile salts. Western dietary intake is approximately 500–1000 mg/day. Cholesterol is synthesized in the body from acetate, mainly in the liver, and blood concentration is normally 140–300 mg/100 ml (3.6–7.8 mmol/l). Elevated blood concentration is often associated with *atheroma, of which cholesterol is a major component. Cholesterol is also a constituent of *gallstones.

cholesterosis *n.* a form of chronic *cholecystitis in which small crystals of cholesterol are deposited on the inter-

nal wall of the gall bladder, like the pips of a strawberry: hence its descriptive term *strawberry gall bladder*. The crystals may enlarge to become *gallstones.

cholestyramine *n.* a drug that binds with bile salts so that they are excreted. It is administered by mouth to relieve conditions due to irritant effects of bile salts – such as the itching that occurs in obstructive jaundice – and also to lower the blood levels of cholesterol and other fats. Common side-effects include constipation, diarrhoea, heartburn, and nausea. Trade names: **Cuemid, Questran.**

cholic acid (cholalic acid) *see* bile acids.

choline *n.* a basic compound important in the synthesis of phosphatidylcholine (lecithin) and other *phospholipids and of *acetylcholine. It is also involved in the transport of fat in the body. Choline is sometimes classed as a vitamin but, although it is essential for life, it can be synthesized in the body.

cholinergic *adj.* describing nerve fibres that release *acetylcholine as a neurotransmitter. *Compare* adrenergic.

choline salicylate an analgesic, related to *aspirin, that is applied locally to relieve earache, mouth ulcers, and other painful conditions. Trade names: **Audax, Bonjela, Teejel.**

cholinesterase *n.* an enzyme that breaks down a choline ester into its choline and acid components. The term usually refers to *acetylcholinesterase*, which breaks down the neurotransmitter *acetylcholine into choline and acetic acid. It is found in all *cholinergic nerve junctions, where it rapidly destroys the acetylcholine released during the transmission of a nerve impulse so that subsequent impulses may pass. Other cholinesterases are found in the blood and other tissues.

choline theophyllinate a drug used to dilate the air passages in asthma and chronic bronchitis. It is administered by mouth and can cause digestive upsets and nausea. Trade name: **Choledyl.**

choluria *n.* bile in the urine, which occurs when the level of bile in the blood is raised, especially in obstructive *jaundice. The urine becomes dark brown or orange, and bile pigments and bile salts may be detected in it.

chondr- (chondro-) *prefix denoting* cartilage. Example: *chondrogenesis* (formation of).

chondrin *n.* a material that resembles gelatin, produced when cartilage is boiled.

chondriosome *n. see* mitochondrion.

chondroblast *n.* a cell that produces the matrix of *cartilage.

chondroblastoma *n.* a tumour derived from *chondroblasts, having the appearance of a mass of well-differentiated cartilage.

chondrocalcinosis *n.* the presence of calcium phosphate crystals in joint cartilage, as seen by X-ray in *pseudogout.

chondroclast *n.* a cell that is concerned with the absorption of cartilage.

chondrocranium *n.* the embryonic skull, which is composed entirely of cartilage and is later replaced by bone. *See also* meninx.

chondrocyte *n.* a *cartilage cell, found embedded in the matrix.

chondrodysplasia (chondro-osteodystrophy, chondrodystrophy, Morquio-Brailsford disease) *n.* a hereditary disorder of cartilage formation, due to a defect in mucopolysaccharide metabolism. It results in deformities in the weight-bearing bones, which leads to dwarfism. *Osteoporosis is marked, and the cornea and heart may also develop abnormally. The condition is diagnosed by X-rays, which show characteristic malformation of the growing ends (epiphyses) of the bones, and examination of the urine.

chondrodystrophy *n. see* chondrodysplasia.

chondroitin sulphate a mucopolysaccharide that forms an important constituent of cartilage, bone, and other connective tissues. It is composed of glucuronic acid and N-acetyl-D-galactosamine units.

chondroma *n.* a benign tumour of cartilage-forming cells, which may occur at the growing end of any bone but is found most commonly in the bones of the feet and hands. *See also* dyschondroplasia, enchondroma, ecchondroma.

chondromalacia *n.* degeneration of cartilage at a joint. *Chondromalacia patellae* is a roughening of the inner surface of the kneecap, resulting in a pain, a grating sensation, and a feeling of instability on movement.

chondro-osteodystrophy *n. see* chondrodysplasia.

chondrosarcoma *n.* a malignant tumour of cartilage cells, occurring in a bone. Treatment is by surgical removal, which may necessitate amputation of a limb, and radiotherapy.

chord- (chordo-) *prefix denoting* 1. a cord. Example: *chordotomy* (surgical incision of the spinal cord). 2. the notochord.

chorda *n.* (*pl.* **chordae**) a cord, tendon, or nerve fibre. The *chordae tendineae* are stringlike processes in the heart that attach the margins of the mitral and tricuspid valve leaflets to projections of the wall of the ventricle (*papillary muscles*). Rupture of the chordae, through injury, endocarditis, or degenerative changes, results in *mitral incompetence.

chordee *n.* acute angulation of the penis. In *Peyronie's disease, this is due to a localized fibrous plaque in the penis, which fails to engorge on erection. As a result, the penis angulates at this point making intercourse impossible. In a child, downward chordee is an associated deformity in *hypospadias and the more severe forms are corrected surgically.

chorditis *n.* inflammation of a vocal cord. *See* laryngitis.

chordoma *n.* a tumour arising from remnants of the embryologic *notochord. The classical sites are the base of skull and the region of the sacrum.

chorea *n.* a jerky involuntary movement particularly affecting the shoulders, hips, and face. Each movement is sudden but the resulting posture may be prolonged for a few seconds. The symptoms are due to disease of the *basal ganglia. In *Huntington's chorea* the involuntary movements are accompanied by a progressive *dementia: there is widespread neuronal degeneration throughout the brain. It is inherited as a *dominant characteristic, appearing in half of the children of the patients with this condition. *Senile chorea* occurs sporadically in elderly people and there is no dementia. *Sydenham's chorea* affects children and is associated with rheumatic fever. It responds to mild sedatives.

chorion *n.* the embryonic membrane that totally surrounds the embryo from the time of implantation. It is formed from *trophoblast lined with mesoderm and becomes closely associated with the *allantois. The blood vessels (supplied by the allantois) are concentrated in the region of the chorion that is attached to the wall of the womb and forms the *placenta. *See also* villus. —**chorionic** *adj.*

chorionepithelioma (choriocarcinoma) *n.* a rare form of cancer originating in the outermost of the membranes (chorion) surrounding the fetus and affecting the womb or the site of a pregnancy outside the womb, e.g. a Fallopian tube (*see* ectopic pregnancy). Chorionepithelioma, which rapidly invades and causes secondary deposits, is highly malignant; it may occur after *hydatidiform mole, pregnancy, or abortion.

chorionic gonadotrophin (human chorionic gonadotrophin, HCG) a hormone, similar to the pituitary *gonadotrophins, produced by the placenta during pregnancy. Large amounts are excreted in the urine, and this is used as the basis for most *pregnancy tests. HCG maintains the secretion of *progesterone by the corpus luteum of the ovary, the secretion of pituitary gonadotrophins being blocked during pregnancy. HCG is given by injection to treat delayed puberty, undescended testes, premenstrual tension, and (with *follicle-stimulating hormone) sterility due to lack of ovulation.

choroid *n.* the layer of the eyeball between the retina and the sclera. It contains blood vessels and a pigment that absorbs excess light and so prevents blurring of vision. *See* eye.

choroiditis *n.* inflammation of the choroid layer of the eye. It may be inflamed together with the iris and ciliary body, but often is involved alone and in patches (*focal* or *multifocal choroiditis*). Vision becomes blurred but the eye is usually painless. *See* uveitis.

choroid plexus a rich network of blood vessels, derived from those of the pia mater, in each of the brain's ventricles. It is responsible for the production of *cerebrospinal fluid.

Christmas disease a disorder that is identical in its effects to *haemophilia, but is due to a deficiency of a different blood coagulation factor, the *Christmas factor* (Factor IX).

chrom- (chromo-) *prefix denoting* colour or pigment.

chromaffin *n.* tissue in the medulla of the *adrenal gland consisting of modified neural cells containing granules that are stained brown by chromates. Adrenaline and noradrenaline are released from the granules when the adrenal gland is stimulated by its sympathetic nerve supply. *See also* neurohormone.

-chromasia *suffix denoting* staining or pigmentation.

chromat- (chromato-) *prefix denoting* colour or pigmentation.

chromatid *n.* one of the two threadlike strands formed by longitudinal division of a chromosome during *mitosis and *meiosis. They remain attached at the *centromere. Chromatids can be seen between early prophase and metaphase in mitosis and between diplotene and the second metaphase of meiosis, after which they divide at the centromere to form daughter chromosomes.

chromatin *n.* the material of a cell nucleus that stains with basic dyes and consists of DNA and protein: the substance of which the chromosomes are made. *See* euchromatin, heterochromatin.

chromatography *n.* any of several techniques for separating the components of a mixture by selective absorption. Two such techniques are quite widely used in medicine, for example to separate mixtures of amino acids. In one of these, *paper chromatography*, a sample of the mixture is placed at the edge of a sheet of filter paper. As the solvent soaks along the paper, the components are absorbed to different extents and thus move along the paper at different rates. In *column chromatography* the components separate out

along a column of a powdered absorbent, such as silica or aluminium oxide.

chromatolysis *n.* the dispersal or disintegration of the microscopic structures within the nerve cells that normally produce proteins. It is part of the cell's response to injury.

chromatophore *n.* a cell containing pigment. In man chromatophores containing *melanin are found in the skin, hair, and eyes.

chromatopsia *n.* abnormal coloured vision: a rare symptom of various conditions. Sometimes everything looks reddish to patients after removal of their cataracts; patients suffering from digitalis poisoning may see things in green or yellow. Similar disturbances of colour may be experienced by people recovering from inflammation of the optic nerve.

chromoblastomycosis (chromomycosis) *n.* a chronic fungal infection of the skin usually caused by injury; for example, a wound from a wood splinter. It produces pigmented wartlike lumps – mainly on the feet and legs – that sometimes ulcerate. The disease is often found in rural communities.

chromosome *n.* one of the threadlike structures in a cell nucleus that carry the genetic information in the form of *genes. It is composed of a long double filament of *DNA coiled into a helix together with associated proteins, with the genes arranged in a linear manner along its length. It stains deeply with basic dyes during cell division (*see* meiosis, mitosis). The nucleus of each human somatic cell contains 46 chromosomes, 23 being of maternal and 23 of paternal origin (see illustration). Each chromosome can duplicate an exact copy of itself between each cell division (*see* interphase) so that each new cell formed receives a full set of chromosomes. *See also* chromatid, centromere, sex chromosome. —**chromosomal** *adj.*

Human male chromosomes, arranged in numbered pairs according to a standard classification. The female set differs only in the sex chromosomes (XX instead of XY).

chron- (chrono-) *prefix denoting* time. Example: *chronophobia* (abnormal fear of).

chronaxie *n.* a measurement of the electrical excitability of a nerve or muscle, formerly used in the detection of damage to the motor nerves. Its use has largely been superseded by *electromyography, the direct recording of electrical activity in the muscles.

chronic *adj.* describing a disease of long duration involving very slow changes. Such disease is often of gra-

dual onset. The term does not imply anything about the severity of a disease. *Compare* acute.

Chronic Sick and Disabled Persons Act (1970) (in Britain) an Act providing for the identification and care of those suffering from a chronic or degenerative disease for which there is no cure and which can be only partially alleviated by treatment. Such patients are usually distinguished from the elderly who may also suffer from chronic diseases. It is the responsibility of local authorities to identify those with such problems and to ensure that services are available to meet their needs and that the people concerned are aware of the available services. Identification can be difficult unless doctors and health visitors notify the appropriate Social Service Departments, but there is no compulsion to make such notifications.

chrys- (chryso-) *prefix denoting* gold or gold salts.

Chrysops *n.* a genus of bloodsucking flies, commonly called deer flies. Female flies, found in shady wooded areas, bite man during the day. Certain species in Africa may transmit the tropical disease *loiasis to man. In the USA *C. discalis* is a vector of *tularaemia.

chrysotherapy *n.* the treatment of disease by the administration of gold or its compounds. The injection of gold salts is claimed by some authorities to be extremely effective in the treatment of arthritis. However, many patients develop severe side-effects, including blood disorders, dermatitis, and upsets of liver and kidney function.

chyle *n.* an alkaline milky liquid found within the *lacteals after a period of absorption. It consists of lymph with a suspension of minute droplets of digested fats, which have been absorbed from the small intestine. It is transported in the lymphatic system to the

chylomicron

thoracic duct, which drains into the subclavian vein.

chylomicron *n.* a microscopic particle of fat present in the blood after fat has been digested and absorbed from the small intestine.

chyluria *n.* the presence of *chyle in the urine.

chyme *n.* the semiliquid acid mass that is the form in which food passes from the stomach to the small intestine. It is produced by the action of *gastric juice and the churning movements of the stomach.

chymotrypsin *n.* a protein-digesting enzyme (*see* peptidase). It is secreted by the pancreas in an inactive form, *chymotrypsinogen*, that is converted into chymotrypsin in the duodenum by the action of *trypsin.

chymotrypsinogen *n. see* chymotrypsin.

cicatrix *n.* a scar: any mark left after the healing of a wound, where the damaged tissues fail to repair themselves completely and are replaced by connective tissue.

-cide *suffix denoting* killer or killing. Examples: *bactericide* (of bacteria); *infanticide* (of children).

ciliary body the part of the *eye that connects the choroid with the iris. It consists of three zones: the *ciliary ring*, which adjoins the choroid; the *ciliary processes*, a series of about 70 radial ridges behind the iris to which the suspensory ligament of the lens is attached; and the *ciliary muscle*, contraction of which alters the curvature of the lens (*see* accommodation).

cilium *n.* (*pl.* **cilia**) **1.** a hairlike process, large numbers of which are found on certain epithelial cells and on certain (ciliate) protozoa. Cilia are particularly characteristic of the epithelium that lines the upper respiratory tract, where their beating serves to remove particles of dust and other foreign material. **2.** an eyelash or eyelid. —**ciliary** *adj.*

cimetidine *n.* a drug that reduces secretion of acid in the stomach and is used to treat stomach and duodenal ulcers, inflammation of the oesophagus, and other digestive disorders. It is administered by mouth or injection and the most common side-effects are dizziness, diarrhoea, muscular pains, and rash. Trade name: **Tagamet**.

Cimex *n. see* bed bug.

cinchocaine *n.* a local anaesthetic used in dental and other operations and to relieve pain. It is applied directly to the skin or mucous membranes or injected at the site where anaesthesia is required or into the spine. Side-effects such as yawning, restlessness, excitement, nausea, vomiting, and allergic reactions sometimes occur.

cinchona *n.* the dried bark of *Cinchona* trees, formerly used in medicine to stimulate the appetite and to prevent haemorrhage and diarrhoea. Taken over prolonged periods, it may cause *cinchonism. Cinchona is the source of *quinine.

cinchonism *n.* poisoning caused by an overdose of cinchona or the alkaloids quinine, quinidine, or cinchonine derived from it. The symptoms are commonly ringing noises in the ears, dizziness, blurring of vision (and sometimes complete blindness), rashes, fever, and low blood pressure. Treatment with *diuretics increases the rate of excretion of the toxic compounds from the body.

cineangiocardiography *n.* a form of *angiocardiography in which the X-ray pictures are recorded on cine film. This allows the dynamic movements of the heart to be studied when the film is projected.

cinefluorography *n.* the technique of taking a rapid succession of photo-

118

graphs of the fluorescent screen of a *fluoroscope, so that the recorded events may be later analysed.

cineradiography *n.* the technique of taking a rapid succession of X-ray photographs, to capture on film events that occur rapidly during a particular radiographic investigation.

cingulectomy *n.* surgical excision of the cingulum. The procedure is sometimes carried out as *psychosurgery for intractable mental illness.

cingulum *n.* (*pl.* **cingula**) **1.** a curved bundle of nerve fibres in each cerebral hemisphere, nearly encircling its connection with the corpus callosum. *See* cerebrum. **2.** a small protuberance on the lingual surface of the crowns of incisor and canine teeth.

circle of Willis a circle on the undersurface of the brain formed by linked branches of the arteries that supply the brain (see illustration). This helps to maintain the blood supply in the event of a feeding vessel being blocked. Most cerebral *aneurysms occur on or near the circle of Willis.

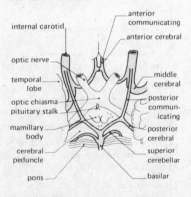

Arterial branches forming the circle of Willis
(from below)

circulatory system *see* cardiovascular system.

circum- *prefix denoting* around; surrounding. Example: *circumanal* (around the anus).

circumcision *n.* surgical removal of the foreskin of the penis. This operation is usually performed for religious and ethnic reasons but is sometimes required for medical conditions, mainly *phimosis and *paraphimosis.

circumduction *n.* a circular movement, such as that made by a limb.

circumflex nerve a mixed sensory and motor nerve of the upper arm. It arises from the fifth and sixth cervical segments of the spinal cord and is distributed to the deltoid muscle of the shoulder and the overlying skin.

circumoral *adj.* situated around the mouth.

circumstantiality *n.* a disorder of thought in which thinking and speech proceed slowly and with many unnecessary trivial details. It is sometimes seen in organic *psychosis, in *schizophrenia, and in people of pedantic and obsessional personality.

cirrhosis *n.* a condition in which the liver responds to injury or death of some of its cells by producing interlacing strands of fibrous tissue between which are nodules of regenerating cells. The liver becomes tawny and characteristically knobbly (due to the nodules). Causes include *alcoholism (*alcoholic cirrhosis*), viral *hepatitis (*postnecrotic cirrhosis*), chronic obstruction of the common bile duct (*secondary biliary cirrhosis*), autoimmune diseases (*chronic aggressive hepatitis*, *primary biliary cirrhosis*), and chronic heart failure (*cardiac cirrhosis*). In at least half the cases of cirrhosis no cause is found (*cryptogenic cirrhosis*). Complications include *portal hypertension, *ascites, *hepatic encephalopathy, and *hepatoma. Cirrhosis cannot be cured but its progress may be stopped if the cause can be removed. This particularly applies in alcoholism (when all alcohol must be prohibited); in hepatitis (in which corticosteroid treatment may reduce inflammation); in secondary biliary cirrhosis (in which surgery may relieve obstruction); and in cardiac failure that can be treated. —**cirrhotic** *adj.*

cirs- (cirso-) *prefix denoting* a varicose vein. Example: *cirsectomy* (excision of).

cirsoid *adj.* describing the distended knotted appearance of a varicose vein. The term is used for a type of tumour of the scalp (*cirsoid aneurysm*), which is an arteriovenous aneurysm.

cisplatinum *n.* a heavy-metal compound: a *cytotoxic drug that impedes cell division by damaging DNA. Administered intravenously, it is important in the treatment of testicular and ovarian tumours. It is highly toxic; side-effects include nausea, vomiting, kidney damage, peripheral neuropathy, and hearing loss. Trade name: **Neoplatin.**

cisterna *n.* (*pl.* **cisternae**) **1.** one of the enlarged spaces beneath the *arachnoid that act as reservoirs for cerebrospinal fluid. The largest (*cisterna magna*) lies beneath the cerebellum and behind the medulla oblongata. **2.** a dilatation at the lower end of the thoracic duct, into which the great lymph ducts of the lower limbs drain.

cistron *n.* the section of a DNA or RNA chain that controls the amino-acid sequence of a single polypeptide chain in protein synthesis. A cistron can be regarded as the functional equivalent of a *gene.

citric acid an organic acid found naturally in citrus fruits. Citric acid is formed in the first stage of the *Krebs cycle, the important energy-producing cycle in the body.

citric acid cycle *see* Krebs cycle.

citrullinaemia *n.* an inborn lack of one of the enzymes concerned with the chemical breakdown of proteins to urea: in consequence both the amino acid citrulline and ammonia accumulate in the blood. Affected children fail to thrive, and show signs of mental retardation.

citrulline *n.* an *amino acid produced by the liver as a by-product during the conversion of ammonia to *urea.

clamp *n.* a surgical instrument designed to compress a structure, such as a blood vessel or a cut end of the intestine (see illustration). A variety of clamps have been designed for specific surgical procedures. Blood-vessel clamps are used to stop bleeding from the cut vessels. Intestinal clamps prevent the intestinal contents from leaking into the abdominal cavity during operations on the intestines and are designed not to damage the intestinal wall.

noncrushing clamp

twin gastrointestinal clamp

Intestinal clamps

clasmocyte *n. see* macrophage.

clasp *n.* (in dentistry) the part of a *denture that keeps it in place. It is made of flexible metal.

claudication *n.* limping. *Intermittent claudication* is a cramping pain, induced by exercise and relieved by rest, that is caused by an inadequate supply of blood to the affected muscles. It is most often seen in the calf and leg muscles as a result of *atheroma of the leg arteries. The leg pulses are often absent and the feet may be cold. The treatment is that of atheroma.

claustrophobia *n*. a morbid fear of enclosed places. *See also* phobia.

claustrum *n*. a thin vertical layer of grey matter in each cerebral hemisphere, between the surface of the *insula and the lenticular nucleus (*see* basal ganglia).

clavicle *n*. the collar bone: a long slender curved bone, a pair of which form the front part of the shoulder girdle. Each clavicle articulates laterally with the *scapula and medially with the manubrium of the sternum (breastbone). —**clavicular** *adj.*

clavus *n*. **1.** *see* corn. **2.** a sharp pain in the head, as if a nail were being driven in.

claw-foot *n*. an excessively arched foot, giving an unnaturally high instep. In most cases the cause is unknown, but the deformity may sometimes be due to an imbalance between the muscles flexing the toes and the shorter muscles that extend them; this type is found in some neuromuscular diseases, such as Friedreich's *ataxia. Surgical treatment is effective in childhood but less so in adult life. Medical name: **pes cavus**.

claw-hand *n*. flexion and contraction of the fingers with extension at the joints between the fingers and the hand, giving a claw-like appearance. Any kind of damage to the nerves or muscles may lead to claw-hand; causes include injuries, *syringomyelia, and leprosy. *See also* Dupuytren's contracture.

clearance (renal clearance) *n*. a quantitative measure of the rate at which waste products are removed from the blood by the kidneys. It is expressed in terms of the volume of blood that could be completely cleared of a particular substance in one minute.

clearing *n*. (in microscopy) the process of removing the cloudiness from microscopical specimens after *dehydration by means of a *clearing agent*. This increases the transparency of the specimens. Xylene, cedar oil, methyl benzoate plus benzol, and methyl salicylate plus benzol are commonly used as clearing agents.

cleavage *n*. (in embryology) the process of repeated cell division of the fertilized egg to form a ball of cells that becomes the *blastocyst. The cells (*blastomeres*) do not grow between divisions and so they decrease in size.

cleft palate a fissure in the midline of the palate due to failure of the two sides to fuse in embryonic development. Only part of the palate may be affected, or the cleft may extend the full length with bilateral clefts at the front of the maxilla; it may be accompanied by a *harelip and disturbance of tooth formation. Cleft palates can be corrected by surgery.

cleid- (cleido-, clid-, clido-) *prefix denoting* the clavicle (collar bone). Example: *cleidocranial* (of the clavicle and cranium).

cleidocranial dysostosis a congenital defect of bone formation in which the skull bones ossify imperfectly and the collar bones (clavicles) are absent.

clemizole *n*. an *antihistamine used to treat such allergies as hay fever and urticaria. It is administered by mouth or injection or applied to the skin as a cream.

client-centred therapy (Rogerian therapy) a method of psychotherapy in which the therapist refrains from directing his client in what he should do and instead concentrates on communicating understanding and acceptance. Frequently he reflects the client's own words or feelings back to him. The aim is to enable the client to solve his own problems.

climacteric

climacteric *n.* **1.** *see* menopause. **2.** declining sexual drive and fertility in men, usually occurring in middle age.

clindamycin *n.* an *antibiotic used to treat serious bacterial infections. It is administered by mouth; possible side-effects are nausea, vomiting, diarrhoea, and occasional hypersensitivity reactions.

clinic *n.* **1.** an establishment or department of a hospital devoted to the treatment of particular diseases or the medical care of out-patients. **2.** a gathering of instructors, students, and patients, usually in a hospital ward, for the examination and treatment of the patients.

clinical medicine the branch of medicine dealing with the study of patients in bed and the diagnosis and treatment of disease at the bedside, as opposed to the study of disease by *pathology or other laboratory work.

clioquinol *n.* an iodine-containing antiseptic active against amoebae and other microorganisms. It is used to treat bowel infections, such as dysentery, and skin infections and is administered by mouth, as suppositories, or in ointments, creams, or lotions.

clitoris *n.* the female counterpart of the penis, which contains erectile tissue (*see* corpus cavernosum) but is unconnected with the urethra. Like the penis it becomes erect under conditions of sexual stimulation, to which it is very sensitive.

clivus *n.* (in anatomy) a surface that slopes, such as occurs in part of the sphenoid bone.

cloaca *n.* the most posterior part of the embryonic *hindgut. It becomes divided into the rectum and the urinogenital sinus, which receives the bladder together with the urinary and genital ducts.

clofibrate *n.* a drug that reduces the levels of blood lipids, including cholesterol, and is used to treat atherosclerosis and angina. It is administered by mouth; side-effects can include stomach discomfort, nausea, and diarrhoea. Trade names: **Atromid-S, Liprinal**.

clomipramine *n.* a drug used to treat various depressive states (*see* antidepressant). It is administered by mouth or injection; common side-effects are dry mouth and blurred vision. Trade name: **Anafranil**.

clomocycline *n.* an *antibiotic used to treat infections caused by a variety of microorganisms and also used for long-term treatment of acne. It is administered by mouth and may cause digestive upsets and allergic reactions. Trade name: **Megaclor**.

clonazepam *n.* a drug with *anticonvulsant properties, used to treat epilepsy and other conditions involving seizures. It is administered by mouth or injection; drowsiness is a common side-effect. Trade name: **Rivotril**.

clone 1. *n.* a group of cells (usually bacteria) descended from a single cell by asexual reproduction and therefore genetically identical to each other and to the parent cell. **2.** *vb.* to form a clone.

clonic *adj.* of, relating to, or resembling clonus. The term is most commonly used to describe the rhythmical limb movements in convulsive epilepsy (*see* grand mal).

clonidine *n.* a drug used to treat high blood pressure (hypertension) and migraine. It is administered by mouth or injection and commonly causes drowsiness and dry mouth. Trade name: **Catapres**.

clonorchiasis *n.* a condition caused by the presence of the fluke *Clonorchis sinensis* in the bile ducts. The infection, common in the Far East, is acquired through eating undercooked, salted, or pickled freshwater fish harbouring the larval stage of the parasite. Symptoms include fever, abdominal pain, diarrhoea, liver enlargement, loss of appetite, emaciation and – in advanced cases – cirrhosis and jaundice. Treatment is unsatisfactory although *chloroquine diphosphate has proved beneficial in some cases.

Clonorchis *n.* a genus of liver flukes, common parasites of man and other fish-eating mammals in the Far East. The adults of *C. sinensis* cause clonorchiasis. Eggs are passed out in the stools and the larvae undergo their development in two other hosts, a snail and a fish.

clonus *n.* rhythmical contraction of a muscle in response to a suddenly applied and then sustained stretch stimulus. It is most readily obtained at the ankle when the examiner bends the foot sharply upwards and then maintains an upward pressure on the sole. It is caused by an exaggeration of the stretch reflexes and is usually a sign of disease in the brain or spinal cord.

clopamide *n.* a *diuretic used to treat fluid retention (oedema) and high blood pressure (hypertension). It is administered by mouth and side-effects are uncommon. Trade name: **Brinaldix**.

clorazepate potassium a tranquillizing drug used to relieve anxiety, tension, and agitation. It is administered by mouth; side-effects can include dizziness, digestive upsets, blurred vision, and, occasionally, drowsiness. Trade name: **Tranxene**.

clorexolone *n.* a *diuretic with prolonged action, used to treat fluid retention (oedema) and high blood pressure (hypertension). It is administered by mouth; common side-effects are nausea and loss of appetite, and reduced blood potassium levels may develop. Trade name: **Nefrolan**.

clorindione *n.* an *anticoagulant used to prevent further blood clotting in coronary and other thromboses. It is administered by mouth and side-effects can include nausea, diarrhoea, hair loss, itching, and skin damage.

Clostridium *n.* a genus of mostly Gram-positive anaerobic spore-forming rodlike bacteria commonly found in soil and in the intestinal tract of man and animals. Many species cause disease in man and animals and produce extremely potent *exotoxins. *C. botulinum* grows freely in badly preserved canned foods, producing a toxin causing serious food poisoning (*botulism). *C. histolyticum*, *C. oedematiens*, and *C. septicum* all cause *gas gangrene when they infect wounds. *C. tetani* lives as a harmless *commensal in the intestine of animals and man but causes *tetanus on contamination of wounds (with manured soil). The species *C. welchii* (*C. perfringens*) – Welch's bacillus – causes blood poisoning, *food poisoning, and gas gangrene.

clotrimazole *n.* an antiseptic used to treat all types of fungal skin infections, including ringworm and infections of the genital organs. It is applied to the infected part as cream or solution or as vaginal pessaries and occasionally causes mild burning or irritation. Trade name: **Canesten**.

clotting factors *see* coagulation factors.

clotting time *see* coagulation time.

cloxacillin sodium an antibiotic, derived from penicillin, used to treat many bacterial infections. It is administered by mouth or injection; diarrhoea sometimes occurs and hypersensitivity reactions occur in penicillin-sensitive patients. Trade name: **Orbenin**.

clubbing *n.* thickening of the tissues at the bases of the finger and toe nails so that the normal angle between the nail and the digit is filled in. The nail becomes convex in all directions and in extreme cases the digit end becomes bulbous like a club or drumstick. Clubbing is seen in pulmonary tuberculosis, bronchiectasis, empyema, infective endocarditis, cyanotic congenital heart disease, and lung cancer and as a harmless congenital abnormality.

club-foot (talipes) *n.* a deformity of one or both feet in which the patient cannot stand with the sole of the foot flat on the ground. In the most common variety (*talipes equinovarus*) the foot is twisted downwards and inwards so that the patient walks on the outer edge of the upper surface of his foot. Other varieties are *talipes varus*, in which the sole of the foot is turned inwards, and *talipes valgus*, in which it is twisted outwards. The defect is present at birth and can be corrected by orthopaedic splinting in the early months of infancy. It may also occur as a complication of muscular paralysis due to poliomyelitis.

clumping *n. see* agglutination.

Clutton's joint a swollen joint, usually the knee, caused by inflammation of the synovial membranes due to congenital syphilis.

clyster *n.* an old-fashioned term for an *enema.

CNS *see* central nervous system.

coagulant *n.* any substance capable of converting blood from a liquid to a solid state. *See* blood coagulation.

coagulase *n.* an enzyme, formed by disease-producing varieties of certain bacteria of the genus *Staphylococcus*, that causes blood plasma to coagulate. Staphylococci that are positive when tested for coagulase production are classified as belonging to the species *Staphylococcus aureus*.

coagulation *n.* the process by which a colloidal liquid changes to a jellylike mass. *See* blood coagulation.

coagulation factors (clotting factors) a group of substances present in blood plasma that, under certain circumstances, undergo a series of chemical reactions leading to the conversion of blood from a liquid to a solid state (*see* blood coagulation). Although they have specific names, most coagulation factors are referred to by an agreed set of Roman numerals. Lack of any of these factors in the blood results in the inability of the blood to clot. *See also* haemophilia.

coagulation time (clotting time) the time taken for blood or blood plasma to coagulate (*see* blood coagulation). When measured under controlled conditions and using appropriate techniques, coagulation times may be used to test the function of the various stages of the blood coagulation process.

coagulum *n.* a mass of coagulated matter, such as that formed when blood clots.

coalesce *vb.* to grow together or unite. —**coalescence** *n.*

coarctation *n.* (of the aorta) a congenital narrowing of a short segment of the aorta. The most common site of coarctation is just beyond the origin of the left subclavian artery from the aorta. This results in high blood pressure (*hypertension) in the upper part of the body and arms and low blood pressure in the legs. The defect is corrected surgically.

cobalamin *n. see* vitamin B_{12}.

cobalt *n.* a metallic element. The artificial radioisotope *cobalt-60*, or *radiocobalt*, is a powerful emitter of gamma radiation and is used in the radiation treatment of cancer (*see* radiotherapy, telecurietherapy). Cobalt itself forms part of the *vitamin B_{12} molecule. Symbol: Co.

cobalt-chromium *n.* a silver-coloured nonprecious alloy of cobalt and chromium used for the metal frame of partial *dentures.

cocaine *n.* an alkaloid, derived from the leaves of the coca plant (*Erythroxylon coca*) or prepared synthetically, sometimes used as a local anaesthetic in eye, ear, nose, and throat surgery. It constricts the small blood vessels at the site of application and therefore need not be given with *adrenaline. Since it causes feelings of exhilaration and may lead to psychological *dependence, cocaine has largely been replaced by safer anaesthetics.

cocainism *n.* **1.** the habitual use of, or addiction to, *cocaine in order to experience its intoxicating effects. **2.** the mental and physical deterioration resulting from addiction to cocaine.

cocarcinogen *n.* a substance that enhances the effect of a *carcinogen.

coccidioidomycosis *n.* an infection caused by inhaling the spores of the fungus *Coccidioides immitis*. In the primary form there is an influenza-like illness that usually resolves within about eight weeks. In a few patients the disease becomes progressive and resembles tuberculosis. Severe or progressive infections are treated with intravenous injections of amphotericin-B. The disease is endemic only in the southwestern US, Mexico, and Venezuela.

coccobacillus *n.* a rod-shaped bacterium (bacillus) that is so small that it resembles a spherical bacterium (coccus). Examples of such bacteria are *Bacteroides* and *Brucella*.

coccus *n.* (*pl.* **cocci**) any spherical bacterium. *See also* gonococcus, meningococcus, Micrococcus, pneumococcus, Staphylococcus, Streptococcus.

coccy- (coccyg-, coccygo-) *prefix denoting* the coccyx. Example: *coccygectomy* (excision of).

coccydynia *n.* pain in the lowermost segment of the spine (coccyx) and the neighbouring area.

coccyx *n.* (*pl.* **coccyges** or **coccyxes**) the lowermost element of the *backbone: the vestigial human tail. It consists of four rudimentary *coccygeal vertebrae* fused to form a triangular bone that articulates with the sacrum. *See also* vertebra. —**coccygeal** *adj.*

cochlea *n.* the spiral organ of the *labyrinth of the ear, which is concerned with the reception and analysis of sound. As vibrations pass from the middle ear through the cochlea, different frequencies cause particular regions of the basilar membrane to vibrate: high notes cause vibration in the region nearest the middle ear; low notes cause vibration in the region nearest the tip of the spiral. The *organ of Corti*, which lies within a central triangular membrane-bound canal (*scala media* or *cochlear duct*), contains sensory hair cells attached to an overlying *tectorial membrane* (see illustration). When the basilar membrane vibrates the sensory cells become distorted and send nerve impulses to the brain via the *cochlear nerve. —**cochlear** *adj.*

cochlear duct (scala media) *see* cochlea.

cochlear nerve the nerve connecting the cochlea to the brain and therefore responsible for the nerve impulses relating to hearing. It forms part of the *vestibulocochlear nerve (cranial nerve VIII).

codeine *n.* an *analgesic derived from morphine but less potent as a pain killer and sedative and less toxic. It is administered by mouth or injection to relieve pain and also to suppress coughs. Common side-effects include constipation, nausea, vomiting, dizziness, and drowsiness, but *dependence is uncommon.

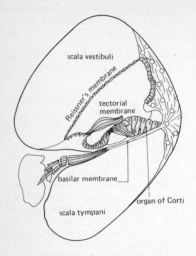

scala vestibuli

Reissner's membrane

tectorial membrane

basilar membrane

organ of Corti

scala tympani

Section through a turn of the cochlea

codon *n.* the unit of the *genetic code that determines the synthesis of one particular amino acid. Each codon consists of a section of the DNA molecule, and the order of the codons along the molecule determines the order of amino acids in each protein made in the cell.

-coele *suffix denoting* **1.** a body cavity. Example: *blastocoele* (cavity of blastocyst). **2.** *see* -cele.

coeli- (coelio-) *prefix denoting* the abdomen or belly. Example: *coeliectasia* (abnormal distention of).

coeliac *adj.* of or relating to the abdominal region. The *coeliac trunk* is a branch of the abdominal *aorta supplying the stomach, spleen, liver, and gall bladder.

coeliac disease a condition in which the small intestine fails to digest and absorb food. It affects 0.1–0.2% of the population and is due to sensitivity of the intestinal lining to the protein gliadin, which is contained in *gluten in the germ of wheat and rye and causes atrophy of the digestive and absorptive cells of the intestine. Symptoms include stunted growth, distended abdomen, and pale frothy foul-smelling stools; the disease can be diagnosed by *biopsy of the jejunum and is treated successfully by a strict and lifelong gluten-free diet. Medical name: **gluten enteropathy**.

coelioscopy *n.* the technique of introducing an *endoscope through an incision in the abdominal wall to examine the intestines and other organs within the abdominal cavity.

coelom *n.* the cavity in an embryo between the two layers of mesoderm. It develops into the body cavity.

coenzyme *n.* a nonprotein organic compound that, in the presence of an *enzyme, plays an essential role in the reaction that is catalysed by the enzyme. Coenzymes, which frequently contain the B vitamins in their molecular structure, include *coenzyme A, *FAD, and *NAD.

coenzyme A a *nucleotide containing pantothenic acid, which is an important coenzyme in the Krebs cycle and in the metabolism of fatty acids.

cofactor *n.* a nonprotein substance that must be present in suitable amounts before certain *enzymes can act. Cofactors include *coenzymes and metal ions (e.g. sodium and potassium ions).

Cogwheel division *see* medical committee (hospital).

cohort study (longitudinal study, prospective study) a systematic follow-up of a group of people for a defined period of time or until the occurrence of a specified event (e.g. retirement or death) in order to observe their pattern of disease and/or cause of death. On the basis of factors prevailing at the outset of the study or arising during the period of follow-up, two or more separate cohorts may be identified and compared in relation to outcome.

coitus (sexual intercourse, copulation) *n.* sexual contact between a man and a woman during which the erect penis enters the vagina and is moved within it by pelvic thrusts until *ejaculation occurs. *See also* orgasm. —**coital** *adj.*

coitus interruptus a contraceptive method in which the penis is removed from the vagina before ejaculation of semen (orgasm). The method is unreliable (10–20 pregnancies per 100 woman-years) and it may lead to sexual disharmony and anxiety in one or both partners.

col- (coli-, colo-) *prefix denoting* the colon. Example: *coloptosis* (prolapse of).

colchicine *n.* a drug obtained from the meadow saffron (*Colchicum autumnale*), used to relieve pain in attacks of gout. It is administered by mouth; common side-effects are nausea, vomiting, diarrhoea, and stomach pains.

cold (common cold) *n.* a widespread infectious virus disease causing inflammation of the mucous membranes of the nose, throat, and bronchial tubes. The disease is transmitted by coughing and sneezing. Symptoms commence 1–2 days after infection and include a sore throat, stuffy or runny nose, headache, cough, and general malaise. The disease is mild and lasts only about a week but it can prove serious to young babies and to patients with a pre-existing respiratory complaint.

cold sore (herpes simplex) *see* herpes.

colectomy *n.* surgical removal of the colon. *Total colectomy* is removal of the whole colon, usually for extensive *colitis; *partial colectomy* is removal of a segment of the colon. *See also* hemicolectomy, proctocolectomy.

colic *n.* severe abdominal pain, usually of fluctuating severity, with waves of pain seconds or a few minutes apart. *Infantile colic* is common among babies, due to wind in the intestine associated with feeding difficulties. *Intestinal colic* is due to partial or complete obstruction of the intestine or to constipation. Colic arising from the small intestine is felt in the upper abdomen; colic from the colon is felt in the lower abdomen. Medical names: **enteralgia, tormina**. *See also* biliary colic.

coliform bacteria a group of Gram-negative rodlike bacteria that are normally found in the gastrointestinal tract and have the ability to ferment the sugar lactose. It includes the genera *Enterobacter*, *Escherichia*, and *Klebsiella*.

colistin *n.* an *antibiotic administered by mouth to treat gastroenteritis and other bacterial infections. Colistin is a mixture of antimicrobial substances produced by a strain of the bacterium *Bacillus polymyxa*. Trade name: **Colomycin**.

colitis *n.* inflammation of the colon. The usual symptoms are diarrhoea, sometimes with blood and mucus, and lower abdominal pain. It is diagnosed by demonstrating inflammation of the colon's lining (mucosa) by *sigmoidoscopy or barium *enema X-ray. Colitis may be due to infection by *Entamoeba histolytica* (*amoebic colitis*) or by bacteria (*infective colitis*); it may also occur in *Crohn's disease (*Crohn's colitis*). *Ulcerative colitis* (*idiopathic proctocolitis*) almost always involves the rectum (*see* proctitis) as well as a varying amount of the colon, which become inflamed and ulcerated. Its cause is unknown. It varies in severity from month to month, relapses being treated by drugs, including corticosteroids and sulphasalazine (as tablets, injections, or enemas), and bed rest. Severe, continu-

collagen

ous, or extensive colitis may be treated by surgery (*see* colectomy, proctocolectomy). Diarrhoea or pain where inflammation is absent is often due to *mucous colitis* (*see* irritable bowel syndrome).

collagen *n.* a protein that is the principal constituent of white fibrous connective tissue (as occurs in tendons). Collagen is also found in skin, bone, cartilage, and ligaments. It is relatively inelastic but has a high tensile strength.

collagen disease (connective-tissue disease) any one of a group of diseases that are characterized by degenerative changes in collagen – the principal component of connective tissue. Collagen diseases, which affect any part of the body in which collagen is found, include *dermatomyositis, *lupus erythematosus, and *polyarteritis nodosa.

collar bone *see* clavicle.

collateral 1. *adj.* accessory or secondary. 2. *n.* a branch (e.g. of a nerve fibre) that is at right angles to the main part.

collateral circulation 1. an alternative route provided for the blood by secondary vessels when a primary vessel becomes blocked. 2. the channels of communication between the blood vessels supplying the heart. At the apex of the heart, where the coronary arteries form *anastomoses, these are very complex.

Colles' fracture fracture of the wrist, across the lower end of the *radius, usually caused by a fall on the outstretched hand. The hand and wrist below the fracture are displaced backwards. The bone is restored to its normal position under anaesthesia, and a plaster slab is applied. The fracture usually unites within six weeks. *Malunion is a common complication, resulting in deformity.

colliculus *n.* (*pl.* **colliculi**) a small protuberance or swelling. Two pairs of colliculi, the *superior* and *inferior colliculi*, protrude from the roof of the midbrain (*see* tectum).

collimation *n.* the production of a thin parallel-sided beam of radiation by means of adjustable slits placed at strategic points along the beam. A collimated beam of radiation is necessary in the technique of scintigraphy, when an organ is scanned for radioactivity (*see* scintigram).

collodion *n.* a syrupy solution of nitrocellulose in a mixture of alcohol and ether. When applied to the surface of the body it evaporates to leave a thin clear transparent skin, useful for the protection of minor wounds. Flexible collodion also contains camphor and castor oil, which allow the skin to stretch a little more.

collyrium *n.* a medicated solution used to bathe the eyes.

coloboma *n.* a defect in the development of the eye causing abnormalities ranging in severity from a notch in the lower part of the iris, making it pear-shaped, to defects in the lower part of the retina and choroid (the inner layers of the eyeball). Vision is usually poor in the severer cases. A coloboma of the eyelid is a congenital notch in the lid margin.

colon *n.* the main part of the large intestine, which consists of four sections – the *ascending, transverse, descending,* and *sigmoid colons* (see illustration). The colon has no digestive function but it absorbs large amounts of water and electrolytes from the undigested food passed on from the small intestine. At intervals strong peristaltic movements move the dehydrated contents (faeces) towards the rectum. —**colonic** *adj.*

splenic flexure
descending colon
transverse colon
ileum
hepatic flexure

haustra

sigmoid colon
rectum
appendix
ascending colon
caecum

The colon

colonic irrigation washing out the contents of the large bowel by means of copious enemas, using either water, with or without soap, or other medication.

colonoscopy *n.* a procedure for examining the interior of the entire colon and rectum using a flexible illuminated *fibreoptic instrument (*colonoscope*) introduced through the anus and guided up the colon by a combination of visual and X-ray control. It is possible to obtain specimens for microscopic examination using flexible forceps passed through the colonoscope and to remove polyps using a *diathermy snare.

colony *n.* a discrete population or mass of microorganisms, usually bacteria, all of which are considered to have developed from a single parent cell. Bacterial colonies that grow on agar plates differ in shape, size, colour, elevation, translucency, and surface texture, depending on the species. This is used as a

means of identification. *See also* culture.

colorimeter *n.* an instrument for determining the concentration of a particular compound in a preparation by comparing the intensity of colour in it with that in a standard preparation of known concentration. The instrument is used particularly for measuring the amount of haemoglobin in the blood.

colostomy *n.* a surgical operation in which a part of the colon is brought through the abdominal wall and opened in order to drain or decompress the intestine. The part of the colon chosen depends on the site of obstruction. An *iliac colostomy* opens onto the left lower abdomen; a *transverse colostomy* on the upper abdomen. The colostomy may be temporary, eventually being closed after weeks or months to restore continuity; or permanent, usually when the rectum or lower colon has been removed. An appliance is usually worn over the colostomy opening (*stoma) to prevent soiling the clothes.

colostrum *n.* the first secretion from the breast, occurring shortly after, or sometimes before, birth. It contains serum, white blood cells, and protective antibodies.

colour blindness any of various conditions in which certain colours are confused with one another. True lack of colour appreciation is extremely rare (*see* monochromat), but some defect of colour discrimination is present in about 8% of Caucasian males, and 0.4% of Caucasian females. The most common type of colour blindness is *Daltonism* (*protanopia*) – red-blindness – in which the person cannot distinguish between reds and greens. Occasional cases are due to acquired disease of the retina but in the vast majority it is inherited. The defect is thought to be in the functioning of the light-sensitive cells in the retina responsible for colour

colp-

perception (*see* cone). *See also* deuteranopia, trichromatic.

colp- (colpo-) *prefix denoting* the vagina. Example: *colpoplasty* (plastic surgery of).

colpocele (vaginocele) *n.* **1.** a hernia protruding into the vagina. **2.** *see* colpoptosis.

colpoperineorrhaphy (colpoperineoplasty) *n.* a tissue grafting operation for repairing tears in the vagina and the area surrounding its opening (perineum).

colpopexy *n.* the stitching of a displaced vagina to the abdominal wall. Loss of the normal position of the vagina may be caused by the action of gravity if the supporting tissues are weak.

colpoptosis (colpocele) *n.* the dropping of the vagina from its normal position, which may happen under the action of gravity if the supporting tissues are weak. The condition can be corrected by *colpopexy.

colporrhaphy *n.* stitching of the vagina (by 'pleating') in order to reduce its laxity in cases of prolapse of the bladder (*anterior colporrhaphy*) or rectum (*posterior colporrhaphy*).

colposcope (vaginoscope) *n.* an instrument that is inserted into the vagina and permits visual examination of the neck of the womb and the upper part of the vagina in which it lies. **—colposcopy** *n.*

colpotomy *n.* an incision made into the wall of the vagina.

columella *n.* (in anatomy) a part resembling a small column. For example, the *columella cochleae* (*modiolus*) is the central pillar of the cochlea, around which the spiral cochlear canal winds. The *columella nasi* is the anterior part of the nasal septum.

column *n.* (in anatomy) any pillar-shaped structure, especially any of the tracts of grey matter found in the spinal cord.

coma *n.* a state of unrousable unconsciousness. Its severity is sometimes graded according to the presence or absence of withdrawal responses to painful stimuli and pupillary and corneal reflexes.

comedo *n.* (*pl.* **comedones**) *see* blackhead.

commando operation a major operation performed to remove a malignant tumour from the head and neck. Extensive dissection, often involving the face, is followed by reconstruction to restore function and cosmetic acceptability.

commensal *n.* an organism that lives in close association with another of a different species without either harming or benefiting it. For example, some microorganisms living in the gut obtain both food and a suitable habitat but neither harm nor benefit man. *Compare* symbiosis. **—commensalism** *n.*

comminuted fracture a fracture in which the bone is broken into more than two pieces. A crushing force is usually responsible and there is often extensive injury to surrounding soft tissues.

commissure *n.* **1.** a bundle of nerve fibres that crosses the midline of the central nervous system, often connecting similar structures on each side. **2.** any other tissue connecting two similar structures.

communicable disease (contagious disease, infectious disease) any disease that can be transmitted from one person to another. This may occur by direct physical contact, by common handling of an object that has picked up infective microorganisms (*see* fomes), through a disease *carrier, or by spread of infected droplets coughed or exhaled into the air. The most dangerous communicable diseases are on the list of *notifiable diseases.

communicans *adj.* communicating or connecting. The term is applied particularly to blood vessels or nerve fibres connecting two similar structures.

community dentistry the branch of NHS dentistry under the control of the health authorities. It is principally concerned with the treatment of children. Its staff are all salaried.

Community Health Council (CHC) (in Britain) a group of local residents (usually one per district) appointed to voice the views of patients in relation to the *National Health Service. Serviced by a salaried secretary, these Councils have no executive power but their views must be sought by District Health Authorities (DHA) on all matters that affect the provision of health services in the district. The DHA must also receive and consider the annual report of each CHC within its district. Members of a CHC may pay site visits to hospitals or other health service property but not to the private premises of general practitioners. Patients who are dissatisfied with treatment may be advised by the CHC as to how to submit complaints to the DHA; indeed a letter from the secretary of the CHC showing an interest in such a complaint will usually ensure serious consideration even though the CHC lack the authority of the *health service commissioner to investigate complaints.

community medicine the branch of medicine concerned with assessing needs and trends in health and disease of populations as distinct from individuals. Formerly known as *social medicine*, it includes *epidemiology, public health, *preventive medicine, health care planning, and evaluation of services.

community nurses (in Britain) a generic term for *health visitors, *domiciliary midwives, and *home nurses. *See also* domiciliary services.

community physician (in Britain) a doctor of consultant status with special postgraduate training in community medicine. Community physicians undertake executive functions at each tier of the *National Health Service, as *Regional Medical Officer* (*RMO*) or *District Medical Officer* (*DMO*). In most appointments the DMO also acts as *Proper Officer* to the appropriate local authority, giving epidemiological and other medical advice to the *Environmental Health Officer. Other *Specialists in Community Medicine* (*SCM*) have responsibility for advising on and coordinating appropriate services (e.g. child health, social service, information and planning, and manpower).

community services *see* domiciliary services.

comparative mortality figure *see* occupational mortality.

compatibility *n.* the degree to which the body's defence systems will tolerate the presence of intruding foreign material, such as blood when transfused or a kidney when transplanted. Complete compatibility exists between identical twins: a blood transfusion between identical twins will evoke no *antibody formation in the recipient. In severe *incompatibility*, for example between completely unrelated people, there are likely to be swift immune reactions as antibodies attack and destroy any offending antigenic material. *See also* histocompatibility, immunity. —**compatible** *adj.*

compensation *n.* the act of making up for a functional or structural deficiency. For example, compensation for the loss of a diseased kidney is brought about by an increase in size of the remaining kidney, so restoring the urine-producing capacity.

complement *n.* a substance in the blood, consisting of a group of nine different fractions, that aids the body's defences when antibodies combine with invading antigens. Complement is involved with the breaking up (*lysis), *agglutination, and *opsonization of foreign cells. Following antibody-antigen reaction it may also attract scavenging cells (*phagocytes) to the area of conflict. *See also* immunity.

complement fixation the binding of *complement to the complex that is formed when an antibody reacts with a specific antigen. Because complement is taken up from the serum only when such a reaction has occurred, testing for the presence of complement after mixing a suspension of a known organism with a patient's serum can give confirmation of infection with a suspected organism. The *Wasserman reaction for diagnosis of syphilis is a complement-fixation test.

complex *n.* (in psychoanalysis) an emotionally charged and repressed group of ideas and beliefs that is capable of influencing an individual's behaviour. The term in this sense was originally used by Jung, but it is now widely used in a looser sense to denote an unconscious motive.

complication *n.* a disease or condition arising during the course of or as a consequence of another disease.

composite resin a tooth-coloured filling material for anterior teeth. It is composed of two different materials: an inorganic filler held in an organic resin.

compress *n.* a pad of material soaked in hot or cold water and applied to an injured part of the body to relieve the pain of inflammation.

compressed air illness (caisson disease) a syndrome occurring in people working under high pressure in diving bells or at great depths with breathing apparatus. On return to normal atmospheric pressure nitrogen dissolved in the bloodstream expands to form bubbles, causing pain (the *bends*) and blocking the circulation in small blood vessels in the brain and elsewhere (*decompression sickness*). Pain, paralysis, and other features may be eliminated by returning the victim to a higher atmospheric pressure and reducing this gradually, so causing the bubbles to redissolve. Chronic compressed air illness may cause damage to the bones (*avascular necrosis*), heart, and lungs.

compulsion *n.* an *obsession that takes the form of a motor act, such as repetitive washing based on a fear of contamination.

compulsory admission (in Britain) the entry and detention of a person within an institution (hospital or Part III Accommodation) without his consent, either because of mental illness (*see* Mental Health Act) or severe social deprivation (*see* National Assistance Act). Application by a *mental welfare officer or *social worker supported by a general practitioner and/or a suitably qualified specialist must be approved by a court of law except in emergencies relating to mental illness, in which the patient must either agree to stay as a voluntary admission or the emergency order is ratified by a court within seven days. When a patient has committed a dangerous act the court may order compulsory admission to a hospital with special security arrangements (e.g. Broadmoor). *Compare* voluntary admission.

computerized axial tomography (CAT) a development of diagnostic radiology for the examination of the soft tissues of the body. For example, within the skull it can be used to reveal the normal anatomy of the brain, the ventricles, and other structures and to distinguish pathological conditions, such as tumours, abscesses, and haematomas. The technique involves the recording of 'slices' of the body with an X-ray scanner (*CAT scanner*); these records are then integrated by computer to give a cross-sectional image. This investigation is without risk to the patient. *See also* tomography. *Compare* positron emission tomography (PET).

conation *n.* the group of mental activities (including drives, will, and *instincts) that leads to purposeful action.

conception *n.* **1.** (in gynaecology) the start of pregnancy, when a male germ cell (sperm) fertilizes a female germ cell (ovum) in the *Fallopian tube. **2.** (in psychology) an idea or mental impression.

conceptus *n.* the products of conception: the developing infant and its enclosing membrane at all stages in the womb.

concha *n.* (*pl.* **conchae**) (in anatomy) any part resembling a shell. For example, the *concha auriculae* is a depression on the outer surface of the pinna (auricle), which leads to the external auditory meatus of the outer ear. *See also* nasal concha.

concordance *n.* similarity of any physical characteristic that is found in both of a pair of twins.

concretion *n.* a stony mass formed within such an organ as the kidney, especially the coating of an internal organ (or a foreign body, such as a urinary catheter) with calcium salts. *See also* calculus.

concussion *n.* a limited period of unconsciousness caused by injury to the head. It may last for a few seconds or a few hours. There is no recognizable structural damage to the brain, although repeated concussion eventually causes symptoms suggesting brain damage. *See also* punch drunk syndrome.

condenser *n.* (in microscopy) an arrangement of lenses beneath the stage of a microscope. It can be adjusted to provide correct focusing of light on the microscope slide.

conditioned reflex a reflex in which the response occurs not to the sensory stimulus that normally causes it but to a separate stimulus, which has been learnt to be associated with it. In Pavlov's classic experiments, dogs learned to associate the sound of a bell with feeding time and would salivate at the bell's sound whether food was then presented to them or not.

conditioning *n.* the establishment of new behaviour by modifying the stimulus/response associations. In *classical conditioning* a stimulus not normally associated with a particular response is presented together with the stimulus that evokes the response automatically. This is repeated until the first stimulus evokes the response by itself (*see* conditioned reflex). In *operant conditioning* a response is rewarded (or punished) each time it occurs, so that in time it comes to occur more (or less) frequently (*see* reinforcement).

condom (French letter, rubber) *n.* a sheath made of latex rubber, plastic, or silk that is fitted over the penis during sexual intercourse. Use of a condom protects both partners against the transmission of venereal diseases and, carefully used, it is a reasonably reliable contraceptive (between 2 and 10 pregnancies per 100 woman-years).

condylarthrosis (condyloid joint) *n.* a form of *diarthrosis (freely movable joint) in which an ovoid head fits into an elliptical cavity. Examples are the knee joint and the joint between the mandible (lower jaw) and the temporal bone of the skull.

condyle *n.* a rounded protuberance that occurs at the ends of some bones, e.g. the *occipital bone, and forms an articulation with another bone.

condyloma *n.* a raised wartlike growth. The commonest type, *condyloma acuminatum*, is found on the vulva, under the foreskin, or on the skin of the anal region. Condylomas are infectious and are probably transmitted during sexual contact. *Condyloma latum* is an infectious warty lesion of the secondary stage of syphilis, occurring around the vulva or anus.

cone *n.* one of the two types of light-sensitive cells in the *retina of the eye (*compare* rod). The human retina contains 6–7 million cones; they function best in bright light and are essential for acute vision (receiving a sharp accurate image). The area of the retina called the *fovea contains the greatest concentration of cones. Cones can also distinguish colours. It is thought that there are three types of cone, each sensitive to the wavelength of a different primary colour – red, green, or blue. Other colours are seen as combinations of these three primary colours.

confabulation *n.* the invention of circumstantial but fictitious detail about events supposed to have occurred in the past. Usually this is to disguise an inability to remember past events. It may be a symptom of any form of loss of memory, but typically occurs in *Korsakoff's syndrome.

confection *n.* (in pharmacy) a sweet substance that is combined with a medicinal preparation to make it suitable for administration.

conflict *n.* (in psychology) the state produced when a stimulus produces two opposing reactions. The basic types of conflict situation are *approach–approach*, in which the individual is drawn towards two attractive – but mutually incompatible – goals; *ap-*proach–avoidance*, where the stimulus evokes reactions both to approach and to avoid; and *avoidance–avoidance*, in which the avoidance reaction to one stimulus would bring the individual closer to an equally unpleasant stimulus. Conflict has been used to explain the development of neurotic disorders, and the resolution of conflict remains an important part of psychoanalysis. *See also* conversion.

confluence *n.* a point of coalescence. The *confluence of the sinuses* is the meeting point of the superior sagittal, transverse, straight, and occipital venous sinuses in the dura mater in the occipital region of the skull.

congenital *adj.* describing a condition that is recognized at birth or that is believed to have been present since birth. Congenital malformations include all disorders present at birth whether they are inherited or caused by an environmental factor.

congestion *n.* an accumulation of blood within an organ, which is the result of back pressure within its veins (for example congestion of the lungs and liver occurs in heart failure). Congestion may be associated with *oedema (accumulation of fluid in the tissues). It is relieved by treatment of the cause.

Congo red a dark-red or reddish-brown pigment that becomes blue in acidic conditions. It is used as a histological *stain. *Amyloidosis is indicated if over 60% of the dye disappears from the blood within one hour of injection.

coniine *n.* an extremely poisonous alkaloid, found in hemlock (*Conium maculatum*), that paralyses the nerves, mainly the motor nerves. Coniine has been included in drug preparations for the treatment of asthma and whooping cough.

conization *n.* surgical removal of a cone of tissue. The technique is commonly used in excising a portion of the cervix (neck) of the womb.

conjugate (conjugate diameter, true conjugate) *n.* the distance between the front and rear of the pelvis measured from the most prominent part of the sacrum to the back of the pubic symphysis. Since the true conjugate cannot normally be measured during life it is estimated by subtracting 1.3–1.9 cm from the *diagonal conjugate*, the distance between the lower edge of the symphysis and the sacrum (usually about 12.7 cm). If the true conjugate is less than about 10.2 cm, delivery of an infant through the natural passages may be difficult or impossible, and *Caesarean section may have to be performed.

conjugation *n.* the union of two microorganisms in which genetic material (DNA) passes from one organism to the other. In some bacteria a minute projection on the donor 'male' cell (a *pilus*) forms a bridge with the recipient 'female' cell through which the DNA is transferred. Conjugation is comparable to sexual reproduction in higher organisms.

conjunctiva *n.* the delicate mucous membrane that covers the front of the eye and lines the inside of the eyelids. The conjunctiva lining the eyelids contains many blood vessels but that over the eyeball contains few and is transparent. —**conjunctival** *adj.*

conjunctivitis (pink eye) *n.* inflammation of the conjunctiva, which becomes red and swollen and produces a watery or pus-containing discharge. It causes discomfort rather than pain and does not usually affect vision. Conjunctivitis is caused by infection (in which case it usually spreads rapidly to the other eye), allergy, or physical or chemical irritation. The patient usually recovers with no after-effects in one to three weeks; bacterial infections respond to antibiotic eye drops. *See also* trachoma, ophthalmia neonatorum.

connective tissue the tissue that supports, binds, or separates more specialized tissues and organs or functions as a packing tissue of the body. It consists of an amorphous *ground substance* of mucopolysaccharides in which may be embedded white (collagenous), yellow (elastic), and reticular fibres, fat cells, *fibroblasts, *mast cells, and *macrophages (see illustration). Variations in chemical composition of the ground substance and in the proportions and quantities of cells and fibres give rise to tissues of widely differing characteristics, including bone, cartilage, tendons, and ligaments as well as *adipose, *areolar, and *elastic tissues.

Loose (areolar) connective tissue

connective-tissue disease *see* collagen disease.

consanguinity *n.* relationship by blood; the sharing of a common ancestor within a few generations.

conservative treatment treatment aimed at preventing a condition from becoming worse, in the expectation that either natural healing will occur or progress of the disease will be so slow that no drastic treatment will be justified. *Compare* radical treatment.

consolidation *n.* 1. the state of the lung in which the alveoli (air sacs) are filled with fluid produced by inflamed tissue, as in *pneumonia. It is diagnosed from its dullness to *percussion, bronchial breathing (*see* breath sounds) in the patient, and from the distribution of shadows on the chest X-ray. 2. the stage of repair of a broken bone following *callus formation, during which the callus is transformed by *osteoblasts into mature bone.

constipation *n.* a condition in which bowel evacuations occur infrequently, or in which the faeces are hard and small, or where passage of faeces causes difficulty or pain. The frequency of bowel evacuation varies considerably from person to person and the normal cannot be precisely defined. Constipation developing in a person of previously regular bowel habit may be a symptom of intestinal disease. Recurrent or longstanding constipation is treated by increasing *dietary fibre (roughage), *laxatives, or *enemas.

constrictor *n.* any muscle that compresses an organ or causes a hollow organ or part to contract.

consultant *n.* a fully trained specialist in a branch of medicine who accepts total responsibility for patient care. In Britain consultants are usually responsible for the care of patients in hospital wards but they are allowed to opt for some sessions in private practice in addition to any National Health Service commitments. After registration, doctors continuing in hospital service are appointed successively *senior house officer*, *registrar*, and *senior registrar* (all full-time training grades with increasing responsibilities). While in the training grades specialist examinations are taken and consultant appointment is based on a combination of qualifications by examination and practical experience in post. *See also* doctor.

consumption *n.* any disease causing wasting of tissues, especially (formerly) pulmonary tuberculosis. —**consumptive** *adj.*

contact *n.* transmission of an infectious disease by touching or handling an infected person or animal (*direct contact*) or by *indirect contact* with airborne droplets, faeces, etc., containing the infective microorganism.

contact lenses glass or plastic lenses worn directly against the eye, separated from it only by a film of tear fluid. *Corneal microlenses* cover only the cornea, while *haptic lenses* cover some of the surrounding sclera as well. Contact lenses are used mainly in place of glasses to correct long and short sightedness and other errors of refraction, but they may be used in a protective capacity in some types of corneal disease.

contact therapy a form of *radiotherapy in which a radioactive substance is brought into close contact with the part of the body being heated. Needles or capsules of the isotope may be implanted in or around a tumour so that the radiation they emit will destroy it. *Compare* telecurietherapy.

contagious disease originally, a disease transmitted only by direct physical contact: now usually taken to mean any *communicable disease.

contra- *prefix denoting* against or opposite. Example: *contraversion* (turning away from).

contraception *n.* the prevention of unwanted pregnancy. Fertilization may be prevented by mechanical methods, including *coitus interruptus, the *condom, or the *diaphragm; by fitting the woman with an intrauterine contraceptive device (*IUD); by *sterilization; or by altering the woman's hormonal balance by regular doses of an *oral contraceptive (the Pill) or by long-acting injections of a hormonal drug (a *progestogen). Couples whose religious beliefs forbid the use of mechanical or hormonal contraceptives may use the *rhythm method, in which intercourse is limited to those days in the menstrual cycle when conception is least likely.

contraction *n.* the shortening of a muscle in response to a motor nerve impulse. This generates tension in the muscle, usually causing movement.

contracture *n.* *fibrosis of muscle tissue producing shrinkage and shortening of the muscle without generating any strength. It is usually a consequence of pain in or disuse of a muscle or limb. *See also* Dupuytren's contracture.

contraindication *n.* any factor in a patient's condition that makes it unwise to pursue a certain line of treatment. For example, an attack of pneumonia in a patient would be a strong contraindication against the use of a general anaesthetic.

contralateral *adj.* on or affecting the opposite side of the body: applied particularly to paralysis (or other symptoms) occurring on the opposite side of the body from the brain lesion that caused them.

contrast medium any substance that is used to improve the visibility of structures during radiography. Barium, given orally or as an enema to show up the alimentary tract on X-ray, is an example of a contrast medium. Air is occasionally useful as a contrast me-

dium; it may be used to displace the cerebrospinal fluid during X-ray examination of the ventricles of the brain. *See also* radio-opaque.

contrecoup *n.* injury of a part resulting from a blow on its opposite side. This may happen, for example, if a blow on the back of the head causes the front of the brain to be pushed against the inner surface of the skull.

contusion *n. see* bruise.

conus arteriosus the front upper portion of the right ventricle adjoining the pulmonary arteries.

conus medullaris the conical end of the spinal cord, at the level of the lower end of the first lumbar vertebra.

convergence *n.* (in neurology) the formation of nerve tracts by fibres coming together into one pathway from different regions of the brain.

conversion *n.* (in psychiatry) the expression of *conflict as physical symptoms. Psychiatrists believe that the repressed instinctual drive is manifested as motor or sensory loss, such as paralysis, rather than as speech or action. This is thought to be one of the ways in which *hysteria is produced.

convolution *n.* a folding or twisting, such as one of the many that cause the fissures, sulci, and gyri of the surface of the *cerebrum.

convulsion *n.* an involuntary contraction of the muscles producing contortion of the body and limbs. Rhythmic convulsions of the limbs are part of *grand mal epilepsy. *Febrile convulsions* are provoked by fever in otherwise healthy infants and young children. An afebrile *infantile convulsion* is likely to be due to birth injury or a developmental defect of the brain.

Cooley's anaemia *see* thalassaemia.

Coomb's test a means of detecting antibodies on the surface of red blood cells that can precipitate simple proteins (globulins) in the blood serum. The test is used in the diagnosis of haemolytic *anaemia (resulting from the destruction of red blood cells).

copr- (copro-) *prefix denoting* faeces. Example: *coprophobia* (abnormal fear of).

coprolalia *n.* the repetitive speaking of obscene words. It can be involuntary, as part of the *Gilles de la Tourette syndrome.

coprolith *n.* a mass of hard faeces within the colon or rectum, due to chronic constipation. It may become calcified.

coproporphyrin *n.* a *porphyrin compound that is formed during the synthesis of protoporphyrin IX, a precursor of *haem. Coproporphyrin is excreted in the faeces during the process of red blood cell formation.

copulation *n.* *see* coitus.

cor *n.* the heart.

coracoid process a beaklike process that curves upwards and forwards from the top of the *scapula, over the shoulder joint.

cord *n.* any long flexible structure, which may be solid or tubular. Examples include the spermatic cord, spinal cord, umbilical cord, and vocal cord.

cordectomy *n.* surgical removal of a vocal cord.

cordotomy *n.* a surgical procedure for the relief of severe and persistent pain in the pelvis or lower limbs. The nerve fibres transmitting the sensation of pain to consciousness pass up the spinal cord in special tracts (the *spinothalamic tracts*). In cordotomy the spinothalamic tracts are severed in the cervical (neck) region.

Cordylobia *n.* *see* tumbu fly.

core-and-cluster *n.* a form of housing for handicapped or subnormal people. Institutional organizations are replaced by small self-contained living units associated with a central facility providing more intensive resources.

corectopia *n.* displacement of the pupil towards one side from its normal position in the centre of the iris. When present from birth, the displacement is usually inwards towards the nose. Scarring of the iris from inflammation may also draw the pupil out of position.

corium *n.* *see* dermis.

corn *n.* an area of hard thickened skin on or between the toes: a type of *callosity produced by ill-fitting shoes. The horny skin layers form an inverted pyramid that presses down into the deeper skin layers, causing pain. A corn may be treated by soaking in hot water or applying softening agents. Medical name: **clavus.**

cornea *n.* the transparent circular part of the front of the eyeball. It refracts the light entering the eye onto the lens, which then focuses it onto the retina. The cornea contains no blood vessels and it is extremely sensitive to pain. —**corneal** *adj.*

corneal graft *see* keratoplasty.

cornification *n.* *see* keratinization.

cornu *n.* (*pl.* **cornua**) (in anatomy) a horn-shaped structure, such as the horn-shaped processes of the hyoid bone and thyroid cartilage. *See also* horn.

corona *n.* a crown or crownlike structure. The *corona capitis* is the crown of the head.

coronal *adj.* relating to the crown of the head or of a tooth. The *coronal plane* divides the body into dorsal and ventral parts.

coronal suture *see* suture (def. 1).

corona radiata 1. a series of radiating fibres between the cerebral cortex and the internal capsule of the brain. **2.** a layer of follicle cells that surrounds a freshly ovulated ovum. The cells are elongated radially to the ovum when seen in section.

coronary angioplasty a procedure, not requiring *thoracotomy, in which a segment of coronary artery narrowed by atheroma is stretched by the inflation of a balloon introduced into it by means of cardiac *catheterization under X-ray screening. The site of the obstruction is identified by prior *angiocardiography. Not all narrowed segments can be improved by angioplasty. *See also* coronary bypass grafting.

coronary arteries the arteries supplying blood to the heart. The *right* and *left coronary arteries* arise from the aorta, just above the aortic valve, and form branches that encircle the heart. *See* coronary angioplasty, coronary bypass grafting.

coronary bypass grafting coronary revascularization in which a segment of a coronary artery narrowed by atheroma is bypassed by an autologous section of healthy saphenous vein or internal mammary artery at *thoracotomy. The improved blood flow resulting from one or more such grafts relieves *angina pectoris and reduces the risk of *myocardial infarction.

coronary revascularization a surgical method of improving the blood flow through coronary arteries narrowed by atheroma. *See* coronary bypass grafting.

coronary thrombosis the formation of a blood clot (thrombus) in the coronary artery, which obstructs the flow of blood to the heart. This is usually due to *atheroma and results in the death (infarction) of part of the heart muscle. For symptoms and treatment *see* myocardial infarction.

coroner *n.* the official who presides at an *inquest. He must be either a medical practitioner or a lawyer of at least five years standing.

coronoid process 1. a process on the upper end of the *ulna. It forms part of the notch that articulates with the humerus. **2.** the process on the ramus of the *mandible to which the temporalis muscle is attached.

cor pulmonale enlargement of the right ventricle of the heart that results from diseases of the lungs or the pulmonary arteries. Such diseases include those affecting the structure of the lungs (e.g. emphysema) or their function (e.g. obesity) except when these changes result from congenital heart disease or diseases primarily affecting the left side of the heart.

corpus *n.* (*pl.* **corpora**) any mass of tissue that can be distinguished from its surroundings.

corpus albicans the residual body of scar tissue that remains in the ovary at the point where a *corpus luteum has regressed after its secretory activity has ceased.

corpus callosum the broad band of nervous tissue that connects the two cerebral hemispheres, containing an estimated 300 million fibres. *See* cerebrum.

corpus cavernosum either of a pair of cylindrical blood sinuses that form the erectile tissue of the *penis and clitoris. In the penis a third sinus, the corpus spongiosum, encloses the urethra and extends into the glans. All these sinuses have a spongelike structure that allows them to expand when filled with blood.

corpuscle *n.* any small particle, cell, or mass of tissue.

corpus luteum the glandular tissue in the ovary that forms at the site of a ruptured *Graafian follicle after ovulation. It secretes the hormone *progesterone, which prepares the womb for implantation. If implantation fails the corpus luteum becomes inactive and degenerates. If an embryo becomes implanted the corpus luteum continues to secrete progesterone until the fourth month of pregnancy, by which time the placenta has taken over this function.

corpus spongiosum the blood sinus that surrounds the urethra of the male. Together with the corpora cavernosa, it forms the erectile tissue of the *penis. It is expanded at the base of the penis to form the urethral bulb and at the tip to form the glans penis.

corpus striatum the part of the *basal ganglia in the cerebral hemispheres of the brain consisting of the caudate nucleus and the lentiform nucleus.

correlation *n.* (in statistics) the extent to which one of a pair of characteristics affects the other in a series of individuals. Such pairs of observations can be plotted as a series of points on a graph. If all the points on the resulting *scatter diagram* are in a straight line (which is neither horizontal nor vertical), the *correlation coefficient* of 0 indicates no dependence of the one characteristic on the other of a straight line type. The *regression coefficient* is the average extent to which a unit increase of one characteristic influences the increase/decrease of the other. Where several factors appear to correlate with the onset of disease the relative importance of each may be calculated by the statistical technique known as *multivariate analysis*.

cortex *n.* (*pl.* **cortices**) the outer part of an organ, situated immediately beneath its capsule or outer membrane; for example, the *adrenal cortex* (*see* adrenal glands), *renal cortex* (*see* kidney), or *cerebral cortex. —**cortical** *adj.*

corticosteroid (corticoid) *n.* any steroid hormone synthesized by the adrenal cortex. There are two main groups of corticosteroids. The *glucocorticoids* (e.g. *hydrocortisone (cortisol), *cortisone, and corticosterone) are essential for the utilization of carbohydrate, fat, and protein by the body and for a normal response to stress. Naturally occurring and synthetic glucocorticoids have very powerful anti-inflammatory effects and are used to treat conditions involving inflammation. The *mineralocorticoids* (e.g. *aldosterone) are necessary for the regulation of salt and water balance.

corticosterone *n.* a steroid hormone (*see* corticosteroid) synthesized and released in small amounts by the adrenal cortex.

corticotrophin *n. see* ACTH.

cortisol *n. see* hydrocortisone.

cortisone *n.* a naturally occurring *corticosteroid that is used mainly to treat deficiency of corticosteroid hormones in *Addison's disease and following surgical removal of the adrenal glands. It is administered by mouth or injection and may cause serious side-effects such as stomach ulcers and bleeding, nervous and hormone disturbances, muscle and bone damage, and eye changes.

cor triloculare a rare congenital condition in which there are three instead of four chambers of the heart due to the presence of a single common ventricle. *Cyanosis (blueness) is common. Most patients die in infancy.

Corynebacterium *n.* a genus of Gram-positive, mostly aerobic, nonmotile rodlike bacteria that frequently bear club-shaped swellings. Many species cause disease in man, domestic animals, birds, and plants; some are found in dairy products. The species *C. diphtheriae* (*Klebs-Loeffler bacillus*) is the causative organism of *diphtheria, producing a powerful *exotoxin that is harmful to heart and nerve tissue. It occurs in one of three forms: *gravis*, *intermedius*, and *mitis*.

coryza (cold in the head) *n.* a catarrhal inflammation of the mucous membrane in the nose due to either a *cold or *hay fever. *See also* catarrh.

cost- (costo-) *prefix denoting* the rib(s). Example: *costectomy* (excision of).

costal *adj.* of or relating to the ribs.

costal cartilage a cartilage that connects a *rib to the breastbone (*sternum). The first seven ribs (true ribs) are directly connected to the sternum by individual costal cartilages. The next three ribs are indirectly connected to the sternum by three costal cartilages, each of which is connected to the one immediately above it.

costalgia *n.* pain localized to the ribs. This term is now rarely used.

costive *adj.* constipated.

costochondritis *n. see* Tietze's syndrome.

cot death the death of a baby, usually occurring overnight while it is in its cot, from an unidentifiable cause. Some 20% of infant deaths in the UK occur in this way. The causes may include virus infections or allergic reactions, but evidence is growing that cot deaths are less likely in breast-fed babies and more likely in households with very low income levels.

co-trimoxazole *n.* an antibacterial drug consisting of *sulphamethoxazole and *trimethoprim. Since both these drugs are well absorbed and rapidly excreted – and each potentiates the action of the other – co-trimoxazole is taken by mouth and is particularly useful for treating urinary-tract infections (such as cystitis). Side-effects are those of the *sulphonamides. Trade names: **Bactrim**, **Septrin**.

cotyledon *n.* any of the major convex subdivisions of the mature *placenta. Each cotyledon contains a major branch of the umbilical blood vessels, which branch further into the numerous villi that make up the surface of the cotyledon.

cotyloid cavity *see* acetabulum.

couching *n.* an operation for cataract in which the lens is pushed out of the pupil downwards and backwards into the jelly-like vitreous humour by a small knife inserted through the edge of the cornea. It was widely employed in ancient Hindu civilizations and has been practised ever since. Its sole advantage is speed of performance, but modern developments in surgery and anaesthesia leave little place for it today. The complication rate is very high.

coughing *n.* a form of violent exhalation by which irritant particles in the airways can be expelled. Stimulation of the cough reflexes results in the glottis being kept closed until a high expiratory pressure has built up, which is then suddenly released. Medical name: **tussis**.

coulomb *n.* the *SI unit of electric charge, equal to the quantity of electricity transferred by 1 ampere in 1 second. Symbol: C.

counselling *n.* a method of approaching psychological difficulties in adjustment that aims to help the client work out his own problems. The counsellor listens sympathetically, attempting to identify with the client, tries to clarify current problems, and sometimes gives advice. It involves less emphasis on insight and interpretation than does psychotherapy or psychoanalytic therapy. *See also* client-centred therapy.

counterextension *n.* an orthopaedic procedure consisting of *traction on one part of a limb, while the remainder of the limb is held steady: used particularly in the treatment of a fractured femur (thigh bone).

counterirritant *n.* an agent, such as methyl salicylate, that causes irritation when applied to the skin and is used in order to relieve more deep-seated pain or discomfort. —**counterirritation** *n.*

countertraction *n.* the use of a balancing opposing force during *traction, when a strong continuous pull is applied to a limb so that broken bones can be kept in alignment during healing. To arrange that traction on a limb by weights and pulleys does not pull the patient out of bed, countertraction is often produced by applying tension to metal pins temporarily inserted into the opposite end of the bone.

couvade *n.* **1.** a custom in some tribes whereby a father takes to his bed during or after the birth of his child. **2.** a symptom of abdominal pain experienced by a man in relation to his wife's giving birth. It may be due to hysteria, anxiety, or sympathy.

cover-slip *n.* an extremely thin square or circle of glass used to protect the upper surface of a preparation on a microscope slide.

cover test a test used to detect a suppressed *strabismus (squint) in children. The child is asked to look fixedly at an object with one eye while the other is kept open but covered by the hand of the observer. The hand is then withdrawn: if the eye that had been covered is seen to move towards the nose to adjust to the focus of the uncovered eye the child is assumed to have a divergent squint; movement of the eye away from the nose implies a convergent squint.

Cowper's glands (bulbourethral glands) a pair of small glands that open into the urethra at the base of the penis. Their secretion contributes to the seminal fluid, but less than that of the prostate gland or seminal vesicles.

cowpox *n.* a virus infection of cows' udders, transmitted to man by direct contact, causing very mild symptoms similar to *smallpox. An attack confers immunity to smallpox. Medical name: **vaccinia**.

cox- (coxo-) *prefix denoting* the hip. Example: *coxalgia* (pain in).

coxa *n.* (*pl.* **coxae**) **1.** the hip bone. **2.** the hip joint.

Coxiella *n.* a genus of rickettsia-like microorganisms that cause disease in animals and man. They are smaller than *rickettsiae, are transmitted by air-borne droplets rather than by insects, and they produce diseases characterized by inflammation of the lungs, without a rash (*compare* typhus). The species *C. burnettii* causes *Q fever.

Coxsackie virus one of a group of RNA-containing viruses that are able to multiply in the gastrointestinal tract (*see* enterovirus). About 30 different types exist. *Type A Coxsackie viruses* generally cause less severe and less well-defined diseases, although some cause meningitis and severe throat infections (*see* herpangina). *Type B Coxsackie viruses* cause inflammation or degeneration of brain, skeletal muscle, or heart tissue (*see* Bornholm disease).

crab louse *see* Phthirus.

cradle *n.* a framework of metal strips or other material that forms a cage over an injured part of the body of a patient lying in bed, to protect it from the pressure of the bedclothes.

cramp *n.* prolonged painful contraction of a muscle. It is sometimes caused by an imbalance of the salts in the body, but is more often a result of fatigue, imperfect posture, or stress. Spasm in the muscles making it impossible to perform a specific task but allowing the use of these muscles for any other movement is called *occupational cramp*. It most often affects the hand muscles for writing (*writer's cramp*).

crani- (cranio-) *prefix denoting* the skull. Example: *cranioplasty* (plastic surgery of).

cranial nerves the 12 pairs of nerves that arise directly from the brain and leave the skull through separate apertures; they are conventionally given Roman numbers, as follows: I *olfactory; II *optic; III *oculomotor; IV *trochlear; V *trigeminal; VI *abducens; VII *facial; VIII *vestibulocochlear; IX *glossopharyngeal; X *vagus; XI *accessory; XII *hypoglossal. *Compare* spinal nerves.

cranioclasm (cranioclasis, cranioclasty) *n.* the crushing of the head of the fetus in the womb by means of a special instrument (*cranioclast*). This may be done in difficult childbirth.

craniopagus (dicephalus) *n.* *Siamese twins united by their heads.

craniopharyngioma *n.* a brain tumour derived from remnants of *Rathke's pouch*, an embryologic structure from which the pituitary gland is partly formed. The patient may show raised intracranial pressure and *diabetes insipidus due to reduced secretion of the hormone *vasopressin. An X-ray of the skull typically shows calcification within the tumour and loss of the normal skull structure around the pituitary gland.

craniostenosis *n.* premature closing of the *sutures between the cranial bones during development, resulting in deformities of the skull.

craniotomy *n.* **1.** surgical removal of a portion of the skull, performed to expose the brain and *meninges for inspection or biopsy or to relieve excessive intracranial pressure (as in a subdural *haematoma). **2.** surgical perforation of the skull of a dead fetus during difficult labour, so that delivery may continue.

For both operations the instrument used is called a *craniotome*.

cranium *n.* the part of the skeleton that encloses the brain. It consists of eight bones connected together by immovable joints (*see* skull). —**cranial** *adj.*

creatinase (creatine kinase) *n.* an enzyme involved in the metabolic breakdown of creatine to creatinine.

creatine *n.* a product of protein metabolism found in muscle. Its phosphate, *creatine phosphate* (*phosphocreatine, phosphagen*), acts as a store of high-energy phosphate in muscle and serves to maintain adequate amounts of *ATP (the source of energy for muscular contraction).

creatinine *n.* a substance derived from creatine and creatine phosphate in muscle. Creatinine is excreted in the urine.

creatinuria *n.* an excess of the nitrogenous compound creatine in the urine.

creatorrhoea *n.* the passage of excessive nitrogen in the faeces due to failure of digestion or absorption in the small intestine. It is found particularly in pancreatic failure. *See* cystic fibrosis, pancreatitis.

Credé's method 1. a technique for expelling the placenta from the womb. Downward pressure is applied to the womb through the abdominal wall in the direction of the birth canal. **2.** the application of 1% silver nitrate solution to the eyes of a newborn baby whose mother has gonorrhoea. The treatment aims to prevent the development of *ophthalmia neonatorum in the infant.

creeping eruption (larva migrans) a skin disease caused either by larvae of certain nematode worms (e.g. *Ancylos-*

crenation

toma braziliense) normally parasitic in dogs and cats or by the maggots of certain flies (*see* Hypoderma, Gasterophilus). The larvae burrow within the skin tissues, their movements marked by long thin red lines that cause the patient intense irritation. The nematode infections are treated with diethylcarbamazine or thiabendazole; maggots can be surgically removed.

crenation *n.* an abnormal appearance of red blood cells seen under a microscope, in which the normally smooth cell margins appear crinkly or irregular. Crenation may be a feature of certain blood disorders, but most commonly occurs as a result of prolonged storage of a blood specimen prior to preparation of a blood film.

crepitation (rale) *n.* a soft fine crackling sound heard in the lungs through the stethoscope. Crepitations are made either by air passages and alveoli (air sacs) opening up during inspiration or by air bubbling through fluid. They are not normally heard in healthy lungs but their interpretation is somewhat controversial.

crepitus *n.* **1.** a crackling sound or grating feeling produced by bone rubbing on bone or roughened cartilage, detected on movement of an arthritic joint. Crepitus in the kneejoint is a common sign of *chondromalacia patellae in the young and *osteoarthritis in the elderly. **2.** a similar sound heard with a stethoscope over an inflamed lung when the patient breathes in.

cresol *n.* a strong antiseptic effective against many microorganisms and used mostly in soap solutions as a general disinfectant. It is sometimes used in low concentrations as a preservative in injections. Cresol solutions irritate the skin and if taken by mouth are corrosive and cause pain, nausea, and vomiting.

crest *n.* a ridge or linear protuberance, particularly on a bone. Examples in-

clude the crest of fibula and the iliac crest (of the ilium).

cretinism *n.* a syndrome of *dwarfism, mental retardation, and coarseness of the skin and facial features due to lack of thyroid hormone from birth (congenital *hypothyroidism).

cribriform plate *see* ethmoid bone.

cricoid cartilage the cartilage, shaped like a signet ring, that forms part of the anterior and lateral walls and most of the posterior wall of the *larynx.

crisis *n.* **1.** the turning point of a disease, after which the patient either improves or deteriorates. Since the advent of antibiotics, infections seldom reach the point of crisis. **2.** the occurrence of sudden severe pain in certain diseases. *See also* Dietl's crisis.

crista *n.* (*pl.* **cristae**) **1.** the sensory structure within the ampulla of a *semicircular canal within the inner ear (see illustration). The cristae respond to changes in the rate of movement of the head, being activated by pressure from the fluid in the semicircular canals. **2.** one of the infoldings of the inner membrane of a *mitochondrion. **3.** any anatomical structure resembling a crest.

Crohn's disease a condition in which segments of the alimentary tract become inflamed, thickened, and ulcerated. It usually affects the terminal part of the ileum; its acute form (*acute ileitis*) may mimic *appendicitis. Chronic disease often causes partial obstruction of the intestine, leading to pain, diarrhoea, and *malabsorption. *Fistulae around the anus, between adjacent loops of intestine, or from intestine to skin, bladder, etc., are characteristic complications. The cause is unknown. Treatment includes rest, corticosteroids, immunosuppressive drugs, antibiotics, or (in some cases) surgical removal of the affected part of the intestine. Alternacupula

gelatinous matrix

processes of hair cell

supporting cells

hair cells

fibres of vestibular nerve

A crista in the ampulla of a semicircular canal

tive names: **regional enteritis, regional ileitis**.

cromolyn sodium a drug used to prevent and treat asthma and allergic bronchitis. It is administered by inhalation and may cause throat irritation. Trade name: **Intal**.

crossbite *n.* a condition in which some or all of the lower teeth close outside the upper teeth when the mandible is as far back as it will go.

crossing over (in genetics) the exchange of sections of chromatids between pairs of homologous chromosomes, which results in the recombination of genetic material. It occurs during *meiosis at a *chiasma.

cross-over trial *see* intervention study.

cross-sectional study the collection and analysis of information relating to persons in a population or group at a defined point in time, with particular reference to their individual characteristics and exposure to factors thought likely to predispose to disease.

crotamiton *n.* a drug that destroys mites and is used to treat scabies and similar skin infections and also to relieve itching. It is applied to the skin as a lotion or ointment and sometimes causes reddening and hypersensitivity reactions. Trade name: **Eurax**.

croup *n.* inflammation and obstruction of the larynx in young children (usually aged between six months and two years). In the past diphtheria was the most common cause, but now croup generally results from a viral infection of the respiratory tract (*see* laryngotracheobronchitis). The symptoms are those of *laryngitis, accompanied by signs of obstruction – harsh difficult breathing (*see* stridor), a rising pulse rate, restlessness, and *cyanosis. Treatment by humidification and mild sedation usually reverses the alarming symptoms. In severe cases the obstruction may require treatment by *tracheostomy or nasotracheal *intubation. *See also* epiglottitis.

crown *n.* **1.** the part of a tooth normally visible in the mouth and usually covered by enamel. **2.** a dental *restoration that covers most or all of the natural crown. It may be made of porcelain, gold, a combination of these, or less commonly other materials. Most crowns are like thimbles and are custom made to fit over a trimmed-down tooth. A *post crown* is used to restore a tooth when insufficient of the natural crown remains. A post is inserted into the root and the missing centre of the tooth is built up; over it is fitted a thimble-like crown to restore the natural shape of the tooth. *Root treatment is required before such a crown can be made.

crowning *n.* **1.** the stage of labour when the upper part of the infant's head is tightly encircled by the margins of the vaginal opening. Only the top of the head is visible at this stage. **2.** the fitting of an artificial *crown to a tooth.

crude rate the total number of events (e.g. cases of lung cancer) expressed as a percentage (or rate per 1000, etc.) of the whole population. When factors such as age structure or sex of populations may seriously affect their rates (as in *mortality or *morbidity rates) it is more meaningful to compare age/sex specific rates using one or more age groups of a designated sex (e.g. lung cancer in males aged 55–64 years). More complex calculations, which take account of the age bias of a population as a whole, can produce *standardized rates* or – as currently used for deciding resource allocation in the British National Health Service – *standardized mortality ratios* (SMR). In these the ratios of subgroups are expressed as percentages of that for a designated or standard population (e.g. England and Wales), particularly applied to the age bracket 15–64 years.

crural *adj.* **1.** relating to the thigh or leg. **2.** relating to the crura cerebri (*see* crus).

crus *n.* (*pl.* **crura**) an elongated process or part of a structure. The *crus cerebri* is one of two symmetrical nerve tracts situated between the medulla oblongata and the cerebral hemispheres.

cry- (cryo-) *prefix denoting* cold.

cryaesthesia *n.* **1.** exceptional sensitivity to low temperature. **2.** a sensation of coldness.

cryoglobulin *n.* an abnormal protein – an *immunoglobulin (*see* paraprotein) – that may be present in the blood in certain diseases. Cryoglobulins become insoluble at low temperatures, leading to obstruction of small blood vessels in the fingers and toes in cold weather and producing a characteristic rash. The presence of cryoglobulins (*cryoglobulinaemia*) may be a feature of a variety of diseases, including *macroglobulinaemia, systemic *lupus erythematosus and certain infections.

cryoprecipitate *n.* a precipitate produced by freezing and thawing under controlled conditions. An example of a cryoprecipitate is the residue obtained from fresh frozen blood plasma that has been thawed at 4°C. This residue is extremely rich in a clotting factor, Factor VIII (antihaemophilic factor), and is used in the control of bleeding in *haemophilia.

cryoprobe *n. see* cryosurgery.

cryostat *n.* **1.** a chamber in which frozen tissue is sectioned with a *microtome. **2.** a device for maintaining a specific low temperature.

cryosurgery *n.* the use of extreme cold in a localized part of the body to freeze and destroy unwanted tissues. Cryosurgery is usually undertaken with an instrument called a *cryoprobe*, which has a fine tip cooled by allowing carbon dioxide or nitrous oxide gas to expand within it. Cryosurgery is commonly used for the removal of cataracts and the destruction of certain bone tumours.

cryotherapy *n.* the use of cold in the treatment of disorders. *See* cryosurgery, hypothermia (def. 2). *Compare* thermotherapy.

crypt *n.* a small sac, follicle, or cavity; for example, the crypts of Lieberkuhn (*see* Lieberkuhn's glands), which are intestinal glands.

crypt- (crypto-) *prefix denoting* concealed. Example: *cryptogenic* (of unknown origin).

cryptococcosis (torulosis) *n.* a rare disease occurring in the USA, caused by the fungus *Cryptococcus neoformans*. The fungus attacks the lungs, causing tumour-like lesions (*torulomas*), but it may also spread to the brain, causing meningitis. Treatment with *amphotericin B may be effective.

Cryptococcus *n.* a genus of unicellular yeastlike fungi that cause disease in man. They are found in soil (particularly when enriched with pigeon droppings), and they are common in pigeon roosts and nests. The species *C. neoformans* causes *cryptococcosis.

cryptomenorrhoea *n.* absence of blood flow when the internal symptoms of menstruation are present. The condition may arise because the hymen at the entrance to the vagina lacks an opening or because of some other obstruction.

cryptophthalmos *n.* apparent absence of the eyes due to the skin having grown over the eyeballs during embryonic development.

cryptorchidism (cryptorchism) *n.* the condition in which the testes fail to descend into the scrotum and are retained within the abdomen or inguinal canal. The operation of *orchidopexy is necessary to bring the testes into the scrotum before puberty to allow subsequent normal development; it is thought that the higher temperature in the abdomen interferes with sperm production. —**cryptorchid** *adj., n.*

crystal violet (gentian violet) an antiseptic dye used to treat some skin infections due to bacteria and fungi and also some worm infestations. Crystal violet is administered by mouth, as pessaries, or as ointments, paints, and solutions; side-effects are uncommon but can include nausea, vomiting, and diarrhoea. The dye is also used to stain tissues and microorganisms for microscopical study.

CSF *see* cerebrospinal fluid.

CS gas a powerful incapacitating gas used in warfare and riot control. The sufferer experiences a burning sensation in the eyes, difficulty in breathing, tightness of the chest, nausea, vomiting, and streaming from the eyes and nose. In confined spaces the gas can prove fatal.

cubital *adj.* relating to the elbow or forearm; for example the *cubital fossa* is the depression at the front of the elbow.

cuboid bone the outer bone of the *tarsus, which articulates with the fourth and fifth metatarsal bones in front and with the calcaneus (heel bone) behind.

cuirass *n. see* respirator.

culdoscope *n.* a tubular instrument with lenses and a light source, used for direct observation of the womb, ovaries, and Fallopian tubes (*culdoscopy*). The instrument is passed through the wall of the vagina behind to the neck of the womb. *See also* endoscope.

Culex *n.* a genus of mosquitoes, worldwide in distribution, of which there are some 600 species. Certain species are important as vectors of filariasis (*see also* Wuchereria) and viral encephalitis.

culicide *n.* an agent that destroys mosquitoes or gnats.

culmen *n.* an area of the upper surface of the *cerebellum, anterior to the declive and posterior to the central lobule and separated from them by deep fissures.

culture 1. *n.* a population of microorganisms, usually bacteria, grown in a solid or liquid laboratory medium (*culture medium*), which is usually *agar, broth, or *gelatin. A *pure culture* consists of a single bacterial species. A *stab culture* is a bacterial culture growing in a plug of solid medium within a bottle (or tube); the medium is inoculated by 'stabbing' with a bacteria-coated straight wire. A *stock culture* is a permanent bacterial culture, from which subcultures are made. *See also* tissue culture. 2. *vb.* to grow bacteria or other microorganisms in cultures.

cumulative action the toxic effects of a drug produced by repeated administration of small doses at intervals that are not long enough for it to be either broken down or excreted by the body.

cumulus oophoricus a cluster of follicle cells that surround a freshly ovulated ovum. By increasing the effective size of the ovum they may assist its entrance into the end of the Fallopian tube. They are dispersed at fertilization by the contents of the *acrosome.

cuneiform bones three bones in the *tarsus – the *lateral* (external), *intermediate* (middle), and *medial* (internal) cuneiform bones – that articulate respectively with the first, second, and third metatarsal bones in front. All three bones articulate with the navicular bone behind.

cuneus *n.* a wedge-shaped area of *cerebral cortex that forms the inner surface of the occipital lobe.

Cuniculus *n.* a genus of large forest-dwelling rodents, the pacas or spotted cavies, found in South and Central America. In Brazil these animals are a natural reservoir of the parasite *Leishmania braziliensis*, which causes espundia (*see* leishmaniasis).

cupola *n.* **1.** the small dome at the end of the cochlea. **2.** any of several dome-shaped anatomical structures.

cupping *n.* the former practice of applying a heated cup to the skin and allowing it to cool, which causes swelling of the tissues beneath and an increase in the flow of blood in the area. This was thought to draw out harmful excess blood from diseased organs nearby and so promote healing. In *wet cupping* the skin was previously cut, so that blood would actually flow into the cup and could be removed.

cupula *n.* a small dome-shaped structure consisting of sensory hairs embedded in gelatinous material, forming part of a *crista in the ampullae of the semicircular canals of the ear.

curare *n.* an extract from the bark of South American trees (*Strychnos* and *Chondodendron* species) that relaxes and paralyses voluntary muscle. Used for centuries as an arrow poison by South American Indians, curare was formerly employed to control the muscle spasms of tetanus and, more recently, as a muscle relaxant in surgical operations. It has now been replaced in surgery by *tubocurarine.

curettage (curettement) *n.* the scraping of the internal surface of an organ or body cavity by means of a spoon-shaped instrument (*curette*). Curettage is usually performed to remove diseased tissue or to obtain a specimen for diagnostic purposes. *See also* dilatation and curettage.

curette *n.* a spoon-shaped instrument for scraping tissue from a cavity (*see* curettage).

curie *n.* a former unit for expressing the activity of a radioactive substance. It has been replaced by the *becquerel. Symbol: Ci.

Curschmann's spirals elongated *casts of the smaller bronchi, which are coughed up in bronchial asthma. They unroll to a length of 2 cm or more and have a central core ensheathed in mucus and cell debris.

Cushing's syndrome the condition resulting from excess amounts of *corticosteroid hormones in the body. Symptoms include weight gain, reddening of the face and neck, excess growth of body and facial hair, raised blood pressure, loss of mineral from the bones (osteoporosis), raised blood glucose levels, and sometimes mental disturbances. The syndrome may be due to overstimulation of the adrenal glands by excessive amounts of the hormone ACTH, secreted either by a tumour of the pituitary gland (*Cushing's disease*) or by a malignant tumour in the lung or elsewhere. Other causes include a benign or malignant tumour of the adrenal gland(s) resulting in excess activity of the gland and prolonged therapy with high doses of corticosteroid drugs (such as prednisone).

cusp *n.* **1.** any of the cone-shaped prominences on teeth, especially the molars and premolars. **2.** a pocket or fold of the membrane (endocardium) lining the heart or of the layer of the wall of a vein, several of which form a *valve. When the blood flows backwards the cusps fill up and become distended, so closing the valve.

cutaneous *adj.* relating to the skin.

cuticle *n.* **1.** the *epidermis of the skin. **2.** a layer of solid or semisolid material that is secreted by and covers an *epithelium. **3.** a layer of cells, such as the outer layer of cells in a hair.

cutis *n. see* skin.

cyan- (cyano-) *prefix denoting* blue.

cyanide *n.* any of the notoriously poisonous salts of hydrocyanic acid. Cyanides combine with and render inactive the enzymes of the tissues responsible for cellular respiration, and therefore they kill extremely quickly; unconsciousness is followed by convulsions and death. Hydrogen cyanide vapour is fatal in less than a minute when inhaled. Sodium or potassium cyanide taken by mouth may also kill within minutes. Prompt treatment with amyl nitrite and sodium thiosulphate or cobalt EDTA may save life. Cyanides give off a smell of bitter almonds.

cyanocobalamin *n. see* vitamin B_{12}.

cyanopsia *n.* a condition in which everything looks bluish.

cyanosis *n.* a bluish discoloration of the skin and mucous membranes resulting from an inadequate amount of oxygen in the blood. Cyanosis is associated with heart failure, lung diseases, the breathing of oxygen-deficient atmospheres, and asphyxia. Cyanosis is also seen in *blue babies, because of congenital heart defects. —**cyanotic** *adj.*

cybernetics *n.* the science of communication processes and automatic control systems in both machines and living things: a study linking the working of the brain and nervous system with the functioning of computers and automated feedback devices. *See also* bionics.

cycl- (cyclo-) *prefix denoting* **1.** cycle or cyclic. **2.** the ciliary body. Example: *cyclectomy* (excision of).

cyclamate *n.* either of two compounds, sodium or calcium cyclamate, that are thirty times as sweet as sugar and, unlike saccharin, stable to heat. Cyclamates were used as sweetening agents in the food industry until 1969, when their use was banned because they were suspected of causing cancer.

cyclandelate *n.* a *vasodilator drug used to improve circulation in cerebrovascular disease and other conditions in which blood flow is reduced. It is administered by mouth; side-effects are rare but high doses sometimes cause nausea, digestive upsets, and flushing. Trade name: **Cyclospasmol.**

cyclitis *n.* inflammation of the *ciliary body of the eye (*see* uveitis).

cyclizine *n.* a drug with *antihistamine properties, used to prevent and relieve nausea and vomiting in travel sickness, vertigo, disorders of the inner ear, and postoperative sickness. It is administered by mouth; common side-effects are drowsiness and dizziness. Trade names: **Marzine, Valoid.**

cyclobarbitone *n.* a *barbiturate drug used as a hypnotic and sedative in cases of insomnia and anxiety. It is administered by mouth and prolonged use can cause *dependence. Trade name: **Phanodorm.**

cyclodialysis *n.* an operation for *glaucoma in which part of the *ciliary body is separated from its attachment to the sclera, producing a cleft between the two. The aqueous humour comes into contact with the exposed surface of the ciliary body and some of it is absorbed from this surface. The pressure within the eye will be reduced if this absorption adds significantly to the drainage of fluid from the eye.

cyclomethycaine *n.* a local anaesthetic applied to the skin in solution to relieve discomfort in cuts, abrasions, and minor skin irritations. It sometimes causes skin sensitivity reactions.

cyclopentamine *n.* a drug that constricts small blood vessels and raises blood pressure (*see* sympathomimetic). It is administered by injection to maintain blood pressure during surgery and is also used in nasal decongestants. Large doses sometimes cause giddiness, headache, nausea, and vomiting.

cyclopenthiazide *n.* a *diuretic used to treat fluid retention (oedema), high blood pressure (hypertension), and heart failure. It is administered by mouth and may cause skin sensitivity reactions, nausea, constipation, diarrhoea, and reduced blood potassium levels. Trade name: **Navidrex**.

cyclopentolate *n.* a drug, similar to *atropine, that is used in eye drops to paralyse the ciliary muscles and dilate the pupil for eye examinations and to treat some types of eye inflammation. Trade names: **Mydrilate, Cyclopentolate Hydrochloride Minims**.

cyclophoria *n.* a type of squint (*see* strabismus) in which the eye, when covered, tends to rotate slightly clockwise or anticlockwise.

cyclophosphamide *n.* a drug used to treat some cancers, often in combination with other *cytotoxic drugs. It also has *immunosuppressive properties and is used in prolonging the survival of tissue transplants and in other conditions requiring reduced immune response. Cyclophosphamide is administered by mouth or by injection; common side-effects are nausea, vomiting, and – particularly at high doses – hair loss. Trade name: **Endoxana**.

cycloplegia *n.* paralysis of the ciliary muscle of the eye (*see* ciliary body). This causes inability to alter the focus of the eye and is usually accompanied by paralysis of the muscles of the pupil, resulting in fixed dilation of the pupil (*mydriasis*). It is induced by the use of atropine or similar drugs in order to rest the muscle in cases of inflammation of the iris and ciliary body. It may also occur after injuries to the eye.

cyclopropane *n.* a general *anaesthetic, administered by inhalation for all types of surgical operation. It can cause postoperative nausea, vomiting, and headache.

cycloserine *n.* an *antibiotic, active against a wide range of bacteria, used as supporting treatment in tuberculosis and in some infections of the urinary tract. It is administered by mouth; side-effects, which can be severe, include dizziness, drowsiness, convulsions, and mental confusion.

cyclosporin A a drug that suppresses the immune system and is administered to prevent and treat rejection of a transplanted organ or bone marrow.

cyclothymia *n.* the occurrence of marked swings of mood from cheerfulness to misery. These fluctuations are not as great as those of *manic-depressive psychosis. They usually represent a personality disorder, for which *psychotherapy is sometimes helpful.

cyclotron *n.* a machine in which charged particles following a spiral path within a magnetic field are accelerated by an alternating electric field. It produces electromagnetic radiation, which has been used in the treatment of certain cancers.

cyesis *n. see* pregnancy.

cyn- (cyno-) *prefix denoting* a dog or dogs. Example: *cynophobia* (morbid fear of).

cyproheptadine *n.* a potent *antihistamine administered by mouth to treat allergies and itching skin conditions; it is also used to stimulate the appetite. Drowsiness is a common side-effect. Trade name: **Periactin.**

cyproterone *n.* a steroid drug that inhibits the effects of male sex hormones (androgens) and is used to treat various sexual disorders in men. It is administered by mouth and common side-effects include tiredness, loss of strength, inhibition of sperm formation, infertility, and breast enlargement (gynaecomastia).

cyrtometer *n.* a device for measuring the shape of the chest and its movements during breathing.

cyst *n.* **1.** an abnormal sac or closed cavity lined with *epithelium and filled with liquid or semisolid matter. There are many varieties of cysts occurring in different parts of the body. *Retention cysts* arise when the outlet of a glandular duct is blocked, as in *sebaceous cysts. Some cysts are congenital, due to abnormal embryonic development; for example, *dermoid cysts. Others are tumours containing cells that secrete mucus or other substances, and another type of cyst is formed by parasites in the body (*see* hydatid cyst). Cysts may occur in the jaws: a *dental cyst* occurs at the apex of a tooth, a *dentigerous cyst* occurs around the crown of an unerupted tooth, and an *eruption cyst* forms over an erupting tooth. *See also* ovarian cyst. **2.** a dormant stage produced during the life cycle of certain protozoan parasites of the alimentary canal, including *Giardia* and *Entamoeba*. Cysts, passed out in the faeces, have tough outer coats that protect the parasites from unfavourable conditions. The parasites emerge from their cysts when they are eaten by a new host. **3.** a structure formed by and surrounding the larvae of certain parasitic worms.

cyst- (cysto-) *prefix denoting* **1.** a bladder, especially the urinary bladder. Example: *cystoplasty* (plastic surgery of). **2.** a cyst.

cystadenoma *n.* an *adenoma showing a cystic structure.

cystalgia *n.* pain in the urinary bladder. This is common in *cystitis and when there are stones in the bladder and is occasionally present in bladder cancer. Treatment is directed to the underlying cause.

cystectomy *n.* surgical removal of the urinary bladder. This is necessary in the treatment of certain bladder conditions, notably cancer. The ureters draining the urine from the kidneys are reimplanted into the colon (*see* ureterosigmoidostomy) or into an isolated segment of intestine (usually the ileus), which is brought to the skin surface as a spout (*see* ileal conduit).

cysteine *n.* a sulphur-containing *amino acid that is an important constituent of many enzymes. The disulphide (S–S) links between adjacent cysteine molecules in polypeptide chains contribute to the three-dimensional molecular structure of proteins.

cystic *adj.* **1.** of, relating to, or characterized by cysts. **2.** of or relating to the gall bladder or urinary bladder.

cystic duct *see* bile duct.

cysticercosis *n.* a disease caused by the presence of tapeworm larvae (*see* cysticercus) of the species *Taenia soleum* in any of the body tissues. Man becomes infected on ingesting tapeworm eggs in contaminated food or drink. The presence of cysticerci in the muscles causes pain and weakness; in the brain the symptoms are more serious, including mental deterioration, paralysis, giddiness, epileptic attacks, and convulsions, which may be fatal. There is no specific treatment for this cosmopolitan disease although surgical removal of cysticerci may be necessary to relieve pressure on the brain.

cysticercus (bladderworm) *n.* a larval stage of some *tapeworms in which the scolex and neck are invaginated into a large fluid-filled cyst. The cysts develop in the muscles or brain of the host following ingestion of tapeworm eggs. *See* cysticercosis.

cystic fibrosis (fibrocystic disease of the pancreas, mucoviscidosis) a hereditary disease affecting the exocrine glands (including mucus-secreting glands, sweat glands, and others). The abnormality results in the production of thick mucus, which obstructs the intestinal glands (causing meconium *ileus in newborn babies), pancreas (causing deficiency of pancreatic enzymes), and bronchi (causing *bronchiectasis). Respiratory infections, which may be severe, are a common complication. The sweat contains excessive amounts of sodium and chloride, which is an aid to diagnosis. Treatment consists of minimizing the effect of the disease by administration of pancreatic enzymes and bronchial physiotherapy and by preventing and combating secondary infection.

cystine *n.* see amino acid.

cystinosis *n.* an inborn defect in the absorption and metabolism of amino acids, leading to abnormal accumulation of the amino acid cystine in the blood, kidneys, and lymphatic system. Excess excretion of cystine in the urine (*cystinuria*) leads to the formation of cystine stones in the kidneys. *See also* Fanconi syndrome.

cystinuria *n.* see cystinosis.

cystitis *n.* inflammation of the urinary bladder, often caused by infection (most commonly by the bacterium *Escherichia coli*). It is usually accompan-

ied by the desire to pass urine frequently, with a degree of burning. More severe attacks are often associated with the painful passage of blood in the urine, accompanied by a cramplike pain in the lower abdomen persisting after the bladder has been emptied. An acute attack is treated by antibiotic administration and a copious fluid intake.

cystitome *n.* a small knife with a tiny curved or hooked blade, used to cut the lens capsule in the type of operation for cataract in which the capsule is left behind (*extracapsular cataract extraction*). *See also* capsulotomy.

cystocele *n.* prolapse of the base of the bladder in women. It is usually due to weakness of the pelvic floor after childbirth and causes bulging of the anterior wall of the vagina on straining. When accompanied by stress incontinence of urine, surgical repair (anterior *colporrhaphy) is indicated.

cystography *n.* X-ray examination of the urinary bladder after the injection of a contrast medium. The X-ray photographs or films thus obtained are known as *cystograms*. Cystography is most commonly performed to detect reflux of urine from the bladder to the ureters, usually in children (*see* vesicoureteric reflux). If films are taken during voiding then the ureters can also be observed (*see* urethrography).

cystolithiasis *n.* the presence of stones (calculi) in the urinary bladder. The stones are either formed in the bladder, due to obstruction, urinary retention, and infection (*primary calculi*), or pass to the bladder after being formed in the kidneys (*secondary calculi*). They cause pain, the passage of bloody urine, and interruption of the urinary stream and should be removed surgically. *See* calculus.

cystometer *n.* an apparatus for measuring pressure within the bladder.

Modern investigations also include measurement of urine flow, and the resultant bladder pressure/flow study (*urodynamic investigation*) provides useful information regarding bladder function.

cystopexy (vesicofixation) *n.* a surgical operation to fix the urinary bladder (or a portion of it) in a different position. It may be performed as part of the repair or correction of a prolapsed bladder.

cystosarcoma phylloides a malignant tumour of the connective tissue of the breast: it accounts for approximately 1% of all breast cancers. Such tumours may show a wide variation in cell structure. The best treatment for a localized tumour is simple *mastectomy.

cystoscopy *n.* examination of the bladder by means of an instrument (*cystoscope*) inserted via the urethra. The cystoscope consists of a metal sheath surrounding a telescope and light-conducting bundles. Irrigating fluid is conducted via the sheath into the bladder and additional channels are available for the catheters to be inserted into the ureters, diathermy electrodes for removing polyps, etc., or biopsy forceps for taking specimens of tumours or other growths.

cystostomy *n.* the operation of creating an artificial opening between the bladder and the anterior abdominal wall. This provides a temporary or permanent drainage route for urine.

cystotomy *n.* surgical incision into the urinary bladder, usually by cutting through the abdominal wall above the pubic symphysis (*suprapubic cystotomy*). This is necessary for such operations as removing stones or tumours from the bladder and for gaining access to the prostate gland in the operation of transvesical *prostatectomy.

cyt- (cyto-) *prefix denoting* **1.** cell(s). **2.** cytoplasm.

cytarabine *n.* a *cytotoxic drug used to suppress the symptoms of some types of leukaemia. It is administered by injection and can damage the bone marrow, leading to various blood cell disorders. Other side-effects are nausea, vomiting, mouth ulcers, and diarrhoea. Trade name: **Cytosar**.

-cyte *suffix denoting* a cell. Examples: *chondrocyte* (cartilage cell); *osteocyte* (bone cell).

cytidine *n.* a compound containing cytosine and the sugar ribose. *See also* nucleoside.

cytochemistry *n.* the study of chemical compounds and their activities in living cells.

cytochrome *n.* a compound consisting of a protein linked to *haem. Cytochromes act as electron transfer agents in biological oxidation-reduction reactions, particularly those associated with the mitochondria in cellular respiration. *See* electron transport chain.

cytogenetics *n.* a science that links the study of inheritance (genetics) with that of cells (cytology); it is concerned mainly with the study of the *chromosomes, especially their origin, structure, and functions.

cytokinesis *n.* division of the cytoplasm of a cell, which occurs at the end of cell division, after division of the nucleus, to form two daughter cells. *Compare* karyokinesis.

cytology *n.* the study of the structure and function of cells. The examination of cells under a microscope is used in the diagnosis of various diseases, e.g. cancer (*see* cervical smear). *See also* biopsy. —**cytological** *adj.*

cytolysis *n.* the breakdown of cells, particularly by destruction of their outer membranes.

cytomegalovirus (CMV) *n.* a member of the herpes group of viruses (*see* herpesvirus). It commonly occurs in man and normally produces symptoms milder than the common cold. However, in individuals whose immune systems are disturbed (e.g. by cancer) it can cause more severe effects, and it has been found to be the cause of congenital handicap in infants born to women who have contracted the virus during pregnancy.

cytometer *n.* an instrument for determining the number of cells in a given quantity of fluid, such as blood, cerebrospinal fluid, or urine. *See* haemocytometer.

cytomorphosis *n.* the changes undergone by a cell in the course of its life cycle.

cytopenia *n.* a deficiency of one or more of the various types of blood cells. *See* eosinopenia, erythropenia, lymphopenia, neutropenia, pancytopenia, thrombocytopenia.

cytophotometry *n.* the study of chemical compounds in living cells by means of a *cytophotometer*, an instrument that measures light intensity through stained areas of cytoplasm.

cytoplasm *n.* the jelly-like substance that surrounds the nucleus of a cell. *See also* ectoplasm, endoplasm, protoplasm. —**cytoplasmic** *adj.*

cytoplasmic inheritance the inheritance of characters controlled by factors present in the cell cytoplasm rather than by genes on the chromosomes in the cell nucleus. Cytoplasmic inheritance is known to occur in lower animals and in plants but has not so far been found in man.

cytosine *n.* one of the nitrogen-containing bases (*see* pyrimidine) that occurs in the nucleic acid DNA.

cytosome *n.* the part of a cell that is outside the nucleus.

cytotoxic drug a drug that damages or destroys cells and is used to treat various types of cancer, with or without the use of *radiotherapy. Examples are *cyclophosphamide, *cytarabine, and *mustine; they offer successful treatment in some conditions and help reduce symptoms and prolong life in others. Cytotoxic drugs destroy cancer cells by inhibiting cell division (i.e. they are *antimitotic*) but they also affect normal cells, particularly in bone marrow, skin, stomach lining, and fetal tissue, and dosage must be carefully controlled. *See also* antimetabolite.

cytotrophoblast *n.* the part of a *trophoblast that retains its cellular structure and does not invade the maternal tissues. It forms the outer surface of the *chorion.

D

dacry- (dacryo-) *prefix denoting* 1. tears. 2. the lacrimal apparatus.

dacryoadenitis *n.* inflammation of the tear-producing gland (*see* lacrimal apparatus). It usually occurs only in people who are in generally poor health.

dacryocystitis *n.* inflammation of the lacrimal sac (in which tears collect), usually occurring when the duct draining the tears into the nose is blocked (*see* lacrimal apparatus).

dacryocystorhinostomy *n.* an operation to relieve blockage of the nasolacrimal duct (which drains tears into the nose), in which a communication is made between the lacrimal sac and the nose by removing the intervening bone. *See* dacryocystitis, lacrimal apparatus.

dacryops *n. Obsolete.* a watering eye.

dactyl- *prefix denoting* the digits (fingers or toes). Examples: *dactylomegaly* (abnormal size of); *dactylospasm* (painful contraction of).

dactylitis *n.* inflammation of a finger or toe caused by bone infection (as in tuberculous *osteomyelitis) or rheumatic disease.

dactylology *n.* the representation of speech by finger movements: deaf and dumb language.

Daltonism (protanopia) *n.* red-blindness: a defect in colour vision in which a person cannot distinguish between reds and greens. The term has been used to refer to *colour blindness in general.

damp *n.* (in mining) any gas encountered underground other than air. *See* blackdamp, firedamp.

D and C *see* dilatation and curettage.

dandruff (scurf) *n.* a common condition in which the scalp is covered with small flakes of dead skin. The flakes, which come away when the hair is brushed or combed, represent an increase in the normal loss of the outermost skin layer. Some types of dandruff are accompanied by inflammation of the scalp to give a type of seborrhoeic dermatitis (*see.* eczema). If too little sebum is produced the hair becomes dry and brittle, with the formation of white skin flakes; too much sebum gives greasy hair and yellow flakes. Treatment is by regular washing with a detergent shampoo. Medical name: **pityriasis capitis**.

dangerous drugs *see* Misuse of Drugs Act (1971).

danthron *n.* a *laxative administered by mouth; it sometimes colours the urine pink or red.

dapsone *n.* a drug (*see* sulphone) used to treat leprosy and some types of dermatitis. It is administered by mouth or injection; the commonest side-effects are allergic skin reactions.

dark adaptation the changes that take place in the retina and pupil of the eye enabling vision in very dim light. Dark adaptation involves activation of the *rods – the cells of the retina that function best in dim light – and the reflex enlargement of the pupil (*see* pupillary reflex). *Compare* light adaptation.

day blindness comparatively good vision in poor light but poor vision in good illumination. The condition is usually congenital and associated with poor *visual acuity and defective colour vision. Acquired cases occur when the *cones (light-sensitive cells) at the back of the retina are selectively destroyed by disease. Medical name: **hemeralopia**. *Compare* night blindness.

day hospital a hospital in which patients spend a substantial part of the day under medical supervision but do not stay overnight. Day hospitals are mainly used for the treatment of elderly patients and those with mental disorders.

DDT (chlorophenothane, dicophane) *n.* a powerful insecticide that has been in wide use for many years against lice, fleas, flies, bed bugs, cockroaches, and other disease-carrying and destructive insects. It is a relatively stable compound that is stored in animal fats, and the quantities now present in the environment – in the form of stores accumulated in animal tissues – raise the question of possible harmful effects on the body. Acute poisoning, from swallowing more than 20 g, produces nervous irritability, muscle twitching, convulsions, and coma, but only a few fatalities have been reported.

de- *prefix denoting* **1.** removal or loss. Examples: *demineralization* (of minerals from bones or teeth); *devascularization* (of blood supply). **2.** reversal.

deafness *n.* partial or total loss of hearing in one or both ears. *Conductive* *deafness* is due to a defect in the conduction of sound from the external ear to the internal ear, most commonly an infection affecting the small bones in the middle ear (*otitis media) but also caused by an abnormal condition of the inner ear (*see* otosclerosis) that affects the conduction of sound. *Perceptive deafness* is due to a lesion of the *cochlea in the inner ear, the auditory nerve, or the auditory centres in the brain. It may be present from birth (for example if the mother was affected with German measles during pregnancy). In adults it may be brought on by injury, disease (e.g. *Ménière's disease), or prolonged exposure to loud noises; progressive perceptive deafness (*presbyacusis*) is common with advancing age. The type of deafness can be diagnosed by various hearing tests (*see* Rinne's test, Weber's test), and the treatment depends on the cause. *See also* hearing aid.

deamination *n.* a process, occurring in the liver, that occurs during the metabolism of amino acids. The amino group ($-NH_2$) is removed from an amino acid and converted to ammonia, which is ultimately converted to *urea and excreted.

death *n.* absence of vital functions. Medically, death used to be defined as permanent cessation of the heart beat. More recently emphasis has switched to *brain death*, defined as permanent functional death of the centres in the brainstem that control the breathing, pupillary, and other vital reflexes. Usually two independent medical opinions are required before brain death is agreed, but organs such as kidneys may then legally be removed for transplantation surgery before the heart has stopped.

death certificate a medical certificate stating the cause of a person's death, usually also stating the deceased's marital status, occupation, and age. A doc-tor's diagnosis of the main cause of death, and any contributory causes of death, and his signature are registered in Great Britain at Somerset House. Death certificates are required by law in the majority of countries throughout the world.

debridement *n.* the process of cleaning an open wound by removal of foreign material and dead tissue, so that healing may occur without hindrance.

debrisoquine *n.* a potent drug used to treat high blood pressure (hypertension). It is administered by mouth; common side-effects are nausea, headache, sweating, and general malaise. Trade name: **Declinax**.

dec- (deca-) *prefix denoting* ten.

Decadron *n. see* dexamethasone.

decalcification *n.* loss or removal of calcium salts from a bone or tooth.

decapitation *n.* removal of the head, usually the head of a dead fetus to enable delivery to take place. This procedure is very rare nowadays, being undertaken only in dire circumstances when the fetal head is too large to pass through the birth canal, the mother's life is endangered, and Caesarean section impossible.

decapsulation *n.* the surgical removal of a *capsule from an organ; for example, the stripping of the membrane that envelops the kidney.

decay *n.* (in bacteriology) the decomposition of organic matter due to microbial action.

decerebration *n.* the removal of the higher centres of the brain or cutting across the brain below the cerebrum so that cerebral functions are eliminated. This procedure is carried out on experimental animals, but certain injuries to the brain in man may cause the same severe neurological signs as occur in an animal that has been decerebrated.

deci- *prefix denoting* a tenth.

decibel (db) *n.* one tenth of a bel: a unit for comparing levels of power (especially sound) on a logarithmic scale. A power source of intensity P has a power level of $10 \log_{10} P/P_0$ decibels, where P_0 is the intensity of a reference source. The decibel is much more widely used than the bel. Silence is 0 db; a whisper has an intensity of 20 db, normal speech 50 db, heavy traffic 80 db, and a jet aircraft 120 db.

decidua *n.* the modified mucous membrane that lines the wall of the uterus (womb) during pregnancy and is shed with the afterbirth at parturition (*see* endometrium). There are three regions: the *decidua capsularis*, a thin layer that covers the embryo; the *decidua basalis*, where the embryo is attached; and the *decidua parietalis*, which is not in contact with the embryo. —**decidual** *adj.*

deciduoma *n.* a mass of tissue within the womb derived from remnants of *decidua. See also* chorionepithelioma (malignant deciduoma).

deciduous teeth the primary teeth, which are shed just before eruption of their permanent successors. In the absence of permanent successors they can remain functional for many years. *See* dentition.

decigravida *n.* a woman who has been pregnant ten times.

decipara *n.* a woman who has been pregnant at least ten times and has given birth to a child capable of survival after each of ten pregnancies.

declive *n.* an area of the upper surface of the *cerebellum, posterior to the culmen and anterior to the folium of the middle lobe.

decomposition *n.* the gradual disintegration of dead organic matter, usually foodstuffs or tissues, by the chemical action of bacteria and/or fungi.

decompression *n.* **1.** the reduction of pressure on an organ or part of the body by surgical intervention. Surgical decompression can be effected at many sites: the pressure of tissues on a nerve may be relieved by incision; raised pressure in the fluid of the brain can be lowered by cutting into the *dura mater; and cardiac compression – the abnormal presence of blood or fluid round the heart – can be cured by cutting the sac (pericardium) enclosing the heart. **2.** the gradual reduction of atmospheric pressure for deep-sea divers, who work at artificially high pressures. *See* compressed air illness.

decompression sickness *see* compressed air illness.

decongestant *n.* an agent that reduces or relieves nasal congestion. Most nasal decongestants are *sympathomimetic drugs, applied either locally, in the form of nasal sprays or drops, or taken by mouth.

decortication *n.* **1.** the removal of the outside layer (cortex) from an organ or structure, such as the kidney. **2.** an operation for removing the blood clot and scar tissue that forms after bleeding into the chest cavity (haemothorax).

decubitus *n.* the recumbent position.

decubitus ulcer *see* bedsore.

decussation *n.* a point at which two or more structures of the body cross to the opposite side. The term is used particularly for the point at which nerve fibres cross over in the central nervous system.

deer fly *see* Chrysops.

defence mechanism the means whereby an undesirable impulse can be avoided or controlled (*see* censor). Many defence mechanisms have been described, including *repression, *projection, and *reaction formation. They may be partly responsible for such

deferent

problems as tics, stammering, and phobias.

deferent *adj.* **1.** carrying away from or
down from. **2.** relating to the vas
deferens.

defervescence *n.* the disappearance of
a fever, a process that may occur
rapidly or take several days, depending
upon the cause and treatment given.

defibrillation *n.* administration of a
controlled electric shock to restore normal heart rhythm in cases of cardiac
arrest due to ventricular *fibrillation.
The apparatus (*defibrillator*) administers the shock either through electrodes
placed on the chest wall over the heart
or directly to the heart after the chest
has been opened surgically.

defibrination *n.* the removal of *fibrin,
one of the plasma proteins that causes
coagulation, from a sample of blood. It
is normally done by whisking the blood
with a bundle of fine wires, to which the
strands of fibrin that form in the blood
adhere.

deficiency *n.* (in genetics) *see* deletion.

deficiency disease any disease caused
by the lack of an essential nutrient in
the diet. Such nutrients include *vitamins, *essential amino acids, and *essential fatty acids.

deflorescence *n.* a disappearance of a
rash in those diseases in which a rash is
a characteristic part of the illness.

degeneration *n.* the deterioration and
loss of specialized function of the cells
of a tissue or organ. The changes may
be caused by a defective blood supply
or by disease. Degeneration may involve the deposition of calcium salts, fat
(*see* fatty degeneration), or fibrous tissue in the affected organ or tissue. *See
also* infiltration.

deglutition *n.* *see* swallowing.

dehiscence *n.* a splitting open, as of a
surgical wound.

dehydration *n.* **1.** loss or deficiency of
water in body tissues. The condition
may result from inadequate water intake and/or from excessive removal of
water from the body; for example, by
sweating, vomiting, or diarrhoea.
Symptoms include great thirst, nausea,
and exhaustion. The condition is
treated by drinking plenty of water;
severe cases require intravenous administration of water and salts (which have
been lost with the water). **2.** the removal
of water from tissue during its preparation for microscopical study, by placing
it successively in stronger solutions of
ethyl alcohol. Dehydration follows *fixation and precedes *clearing.

dehydrogenase *n.* *see* oxidoreductase.

déjà vu a vivid psychic experience in
which immediately contemporary
events seem to be a repetition of previous happenings. It is a symptom of
temporal lobe *epilepsy. *See also* jamais vu.

deletion (deficiency) *n.* (in genetics) a
type of chromosome mutation in which
a part of the chromosome, and therefore the genes carried on that part, is
lost.

Delhi boil *see* oriental sore.

delirium *n.* an acute disorder of the
mental processes accompanying organic brain disease. It may be manifested by illusions, disorientation, hallucinations, or extreme excitement and
occurs in metabolic disorders, intoxication, deficiency diseases, and infections.

delirium tremens a psychosis caused
by *alcoholism, usually seen as a withdrawal syndrome in chronic alcoholics.
Typically it is precipitated by a head
injury or an acute infection causing
abstinence from alcohol. Features include anxiety, tremor, sweating, and
vivid and terrifying visual and sensory
hallucinations, often of animals and
insects. Severe cases may end fatally.

158

deltoid *n.* a thick triangular muscle that covers the shoulder joint (see illustration). It is responsible for raising the arm away from the side of the body.

The deltoid muscle

delusion *n.* an irrationally held belief that cannot be altered by rational argument. In mental illness it is often a false belief that the individual is persecuted by others, is very powerful, is controlled by others, or is a victim of physical disease (*see* paranoia). It may be a symptom of schizophrenia, *manic-depressive psychosis, or an organic psychosis.

dementia *n.* a chronic or persistent disorder of the mental processes due to organic brain disease. It is marked by memory disorders, changes in personality, deterioration in personal care, impaired reasoning ability, and disorientation. *Presenile dementia* occurs in young or middle-aged people. The term is sometimes reserved for Alzheimer's disease and Pick's disease, but it is important to distinguish these conditions from those brain diseases for which curative treatment may be available.

demethylchlortetracycline *n.* an antibiotic that is active against a wide range of bacteria and is used to treat various infections. It is administered by mouth; common side-effects are nausea, diarrhoea, and symptoms resulting from the growth of organisms not sensitive to the drug. Trade name: **Ledermycin**.

demi- *prefix denoting* half.

Demodex *n.* a genus of harmless parasitic mites, the follicle mites, found in the hair follicles and associated sebaceous glands of the face. They resemble tiny worms, about 0.4 mm in length, and their presence may give rise to dermatitis.

demography *n.* the study of the populations of the world, their racial make-up, movements, birth rates, death rates, and other factors affecting the quality of life within them. *See also* biostatistics.

demulcent *n.* a soothing agent that protects the mucous membranes and relieves irritation. Demulcents form a protective film and are used in mouth washes, gargles, etc., to soothe irritation or inflammation in the mouth.

demyelination *n.* a disease process selectively damaging the *myelin sheaths in the central or peripheral nervous system. This in turn affects the function of the nerve fibres, which the myelin normally supports. Demyelination may be the primary disorder, as in *multiple sclerosis, or it may occur after head injury or strokes.

denaturation *n.* the changes in the physical and physiological properties of a protein that are brought about by heat, X-rays, or chemicals. These changes include loss of activity (in the case of enzymes) and loss (or alteration) of antigenicity (in the case of *antigens).

dendrite *n.* one of the shorter branching processes of the cell body of a *neurone, which makes contact with other neurones at synapses and carries nerve impulses from them into the cell body.

dendritic ulcer a branching ulcer of the surface of the cornea caused by herpes simplex virus. A similar appearance may be produced by a healing corneal abrasion. Dendritic ulcers tend to recur because the virus lies dormant in the tissues; years may elapse between attacks.

denervation *n.* interruption of the nerve supply to the muscles and skin. The muscle is paralysed and its normal tone (elasticity) is lost. The muscle fibres shrink and are replaced by fat. A denervated area of skin loses all forms of sensation and its subsequent ability to heal and renew its tissues is impaired.

dengue (breakbone fever) *n.* a viral disease transmitted to man principally by the mosquito *Aëdes aegypti.* Symptoms, which last for a few days, include severe pains in the joints and muscles, headache, sore throat, fever, running of the eyes, and an irritating rash. These symptoms recur in a usually milder form after an interval of two or three days. Death rarely occurs, but the patient is left debilitated and requires considerable convalescence. Dengue occurs throughout the tropics and subtropics. Patients are given aspirin and codeine to relieve the pain and calamine lotion is helpful in easing the irritating rash.

dens *n.* a tooth or tooth-shaped structure.

dens invaginatus literally, an infolded tooth: a specific type of tooth malformation that mainly affects upper lateral incisors to varying degrees.

dent- (denti-, dento-) *prefix denoting* the teeth. Example: *dentoalveolar* (relating to the teeth and associated jaw).

dental auxiliary any of several assistants to a dentist. A *dental hygienist* performs scaling and instruction in oral hygiene under the supervision of the dentist. A *dental surgery assistant* helps the dentist at the chairside by preparing materials, passing instruments, and aspirating the mouth. A *dental technician* constructs dentures, crowns, and orthodontic appliances in the laboratory for the dentist. A *dental therapist* performs treatment on children under the direction of a dentist in the community dental services and in hospitals.

dental caries decay and crumbling of the substance of a tooth. Dental caries is caused by the metabolism of the bacteria in *plaque attached to the surface of the tooth. Acid formed by bacterial breakdown of sugar in the diet gradually etches and decomposes the enamel of the tooth. If left unrepaired it spreads in and progressively destroys the tooth completely, first exposing the deeper dentine, causing toothache, and eventually opening the pulp to allow ingress of infection into the bone and abscess formation (*see* apical abscess). Frequent intake of sugar is a major cause, and the disease is more common in young people and has a predilection for specific sites. Repair consists of removing the decayed part of the tooth using a *drill and replacing it with a *filling. The resistance of enamel to dental caries can be increased by the application of *fluoride salts to the tooth surface from toothpastes or mouth rinses. *Fluoridation of water also makes teeth resistant to caries during the period of tooth development.

dental committee (local) *see* medical committee (local).

dental floss fine thread, usually of nylon, used to clean some surfaces of teeth.

dental nerve either of two nerves that supply the teeth. The *inferior dental* *nerve* supplies the lower teeth and for most of its length exists as a single large bundle; thus anaesthesia of it has a widespread effect (*see* inferior dental block). The *superior dental nerve*, which supplies the upper teeth, breaks into separate branches at some distance from the teeth and it is possible to anaesthetize these individually with less widespread effect for the patient.

dental unit a major piece of dental equipment to which are attached the dental drills, aspirator, and compressed air syringes.

dentate *adj.* serrated; having toothlike projections.

dentifrice *n.* a paste or powder for cleaning the teeth. Toothpastes contain a fine abrasive; an essential ingredient is suitable flavouring to make their use pleasant. Most toothpastes contain *fluoride salts, which help to prevent dental caries.

dentine *n.* a hard tissue that forms the bulk of a tooth. The dentine of the crown is covered by enamel and that of the root by cementum. The dentine is permeated by fine tubules, which close to the centre of the tooth contain cellular processes from the pulp. Exposed dentine is sensitive to touch, heat, and cold.

dentinogenesis *n.* the formation of *dentine by *odontoblasts. Although dentine continues to be formed throughout life, very little is formed later than a few years after tooth eruption. *Dentinogenesis imperfecta* is a hereditary condition in which dentine formation is disturbed, resulting in loss of overlying enamel.

dentist *n.* a member of the dental profession, who in the UK must be registered with the General Dental Council unless he holds a medical qualification.

dentistry *n.* the study, management, and treatment of diseases and conditions affecting the mouth, jaws, teeth, and their supporting tissues. *See* endodontics, orthodontics, periodontics, preventive dentistry.

dentition *n.* the arrangement of teeth in the mouth. The *deciduous dentition* comprises the teeth of young children. It consists of 20 teeth, made up of incisors, canines, and molars only. The lower incisor erupts first at about 6 months of age, and all the deciduous teeth have usually erupted by the age of 2–3. The lower incisors are shed first at about 6 years of age, and from this time until about 12 years old both deciduous and permanent teeth are present; i.e. there is a *mixed dentition*. The *permanent dentition* consists of up to 32 teeth, made up of incisors, canines, premolars, and molars. The first tooth to erupt is the first molar (at the age of 6) and most have appeared by the age of 14 years, although the third molars may not erupt until the age of 18–21 years. See illustrations.

denture (prosthesis) *n.* a removable replacement for one or more teeth carried on some type of plate or frame. A *complete denture* replaces all the teeth in one jaw. It is usually made entirely of acrylic resin. A *partial denture* replaces some teeth because others still remain. It is designed to restore function with the least potential damage to the remaining teeth. The framework of the denture base is often made of metal (*cobalt-chromium) because of its strength. *Denture sore mouth* is a form of candidiasis related to inadequately cleaned denture bases. *Denture hyperplasia* is an overgrowth of fibrous tissue covered by mucous membrane, resulting from chronic irritation by a denture.

deodorant *n.* an agent that reduces or removes unpleasant body odours by destroying bacteria that live on the skin

deontology

molars | incisors | molars
canines | canines

Deciduous dentition

R   L

molars premolars | incisors | premolars molars
canines | canines

Permanent dentition

and break down sweat. Deodorant preparations often contain an antiseptic.

deontology *n.* the study of ethics and correct behaviour or duty. In medicine this includes consideration of the proper behaviour of a doctor towards his patient, whether a patient should be told if his condition is fatal or not, and similar problems for which there may be *Hippocratic oath.

deoxycholic acid *see* bile acids.

deoxycorticosterone *n.* a hormone, synthesized and released by the adrenal cortex, that regulates salt and water balance. *See also* corticosteroid.

deoxyribonuclease *n.* an enzyme, located in the *lysosomes of cells, that splits DNA at specific places in the molecule.

deoxyribonucleic acid *see* DNA.

Department of Health and Social Security a department of central government that supports the Secretary of State for Health and Social Services in meeting his obligations, which include the *National Health Service and the prevention and control of infectious diseases. Information is collated, priorities assessed, and resources allocated to Regional and District Health Authorities. Similar assessments and allocations are made to local authorities for *social services. The department is staffed by civil servants, including medical and nursing personnel and those from other health professions. Equivalent departments support the ministers responsible for similar services in Scotland, Wales, and Northern Ireland.

dependence (drug dependence) *n.* the physical and/or psychological effects produced by the habitual taking of certain drugs, characterized by a compulsion to continue taking the drug. In *physical dependence* withdrawal of the drug causes specific symptoms (*withdrawal symptoms*), such as sweating, vomiting, or tremors, that are reversed

162

by further doses. Substances that may induce physical dependence include alcohol and the 'hard' drugs morphine, heroin, and cocaine. Dependence on 'hard' drugs carries a high mortality, partly because overdosage may be fatal and partly because their casual injection intravenously may lead to infections such as *hepatitis. Treatment is difficult and requires specialist skills. Much more common is *psychological dependence*, in which repeated use of a drug induces reliance on it for a state of well-being and contentment, but there are no physical withdrawal symptoms if use of the drug is stopped. Substances that may induce psychological dependence include nicotine in tobacco, cannabis, and many 'soft' drugs, such as barbiturates and amphetamines.

depersonalization *n.* a state in which a person feels himself becoming unreal or strangely altered, or feels that his mind is becoming separated from his body. Minor degrees of this feeling are common in normal people under stress. Severe feelings of depersonalization occur in anxiety neurosis, in states of *dissociation, in depression and schizophrenia, and in epilepsy (particularly temporal-lobe epilepsy). *See also* derealization.

depilatory *n.* an agent applied to the skin to remove hair.

depolarization *n.* the sudden surge of charged particles across the membrane of a nerve or muscle cell that accompanies a physicochemical change in the membrane and cancels out, or reverses, its resting potential to produce an *action potential. The passage of a *nerve impulse is a rapid wave of depolarization along the membrane of a nerve fibre.

depressant *n.* an agent that reduces the normal activity of any body system or function. Drugs such as general *anaesthetics, *barbiturates, and opiates are depressants of the central

nervous system and respiration. *Cytotoxic drugs, such as azathioprine, are depressants of the levels of white blood cells.

depression *n.* a mental state characterized by excessive sadness. Activity can be agitated and restless or slow and retarded. Behaviour is governed by pessimistic or despairing beliefs, and sleep, appetite, and concentration are disturbed. There are several causes. *Manic-depressive psychosis causes severe depressions, in which there may be delusions of being worthless, ill, wicked, or impoverished and hallucinations of accusing voices. Loss and frustration also cause depression, which may be prolonged and disproportionate in depressive *neurosis. Treatment is with *antidepressant drugs and/or *psychotherapy. Severe cases may need *electroconvulsive therapy. *See also* endogenous, reactive.

depressor *n.* **1.** a muscle that causes lowering of part of the body. The *depressor labii inferioris* is a muscle that draws down and everts the lower lip. **2.** a nerve that lowers blood pressure.

dequalinium *n.* an antiseptic, active against some bacteria and fungi, used as lozenges or paint to treat mouth and throat infections.

deradenitis *n.* inflammation of the lymph nodes in the neck.

derealization *n.* a feeling of unreality in which the environment is experienced as unreal and as flat, dull, or strange. The experience is unwelcome and often frightening. It occurs in association with *depersonalization or with the conditions that cause depersonalization.

dereism *n.* undirected fantasy thinking that fails to respect the realities of life. When this becomes markedly dominant it may be a feature of *schizoid personality or of *schizophrenia.

derm- (derma-, dermo-, dermat(o)-)
prefix denoting the skin.

-derm *suffix denoting* **1.** the skin. **2.** a germ layer.

Dermacentor *n.* a genus of hard *ticks, worldwide in distribution, the adults of which are parasites of man and other mammals. The wood tick, *D. andersoni*, transmits Rocky Mountain spotted fever to man in the western USA and the dog tick, *D. variabilis*, is the vector of the milder form of this disease in the east.

dermal *adj.* relating to or affecting the skin, especially the *dermis.

Dermanyssus *n.* a genus of wide-spread parasitic mites. The red poultry mite, *D. gallinae*, is a common parasite of wild birds in temperate regions but can also infest poultry. It occasionally attacks and takes a blood meal from man, causing itching and mild dermatitis.

dermatitis *n.* inflammation of the skin caused by an outside agent: a condition with many causes. The skin is red and itchy and small blisters may develop. In most cases the condition is associated with certain typical changes in the skin that are described as *eczema (*eczematous dermatitis*). Eczematous dermatitis may result from direct irritation of the skin by a substance (such as a chemical) or it may be an allergic reaction to a particular substance that has been in contact with the skin, injected, or taken by mouth. In cases associated with a different reaction the disorder is described as *noneczematous dermatitis*. Industrial substances are a common cause of noneczematous dermatitis, which is sometimes called *occupational dermatitis*. Other types of dermatitis can be caused by soaps or detergents (for example, in nappies) or by sunlight. Treatment of dermatitis depends upon the cause.

Dermatobia *n.* a genus of nonblood-sucking flies inhabiting lowland woods and forests of South and Central America. The parasitic maggots of *D. hominis* can cause a serious disease of the skin in man (*see* myiasis). The maggots burrow into the skin, after emerging from eggs transported by bloodsucking insects (e.g. mosquitoes), and produce painful boil-like swellings. Treatment involves surgical removal of the maggots.

dermatofibrosarcoma protuberans a tumour probably derived from *histiocytes that may occur in any part of the body. It is locally invasive but does not *metastasize. It often recurs locally despite excision.

dermatoglyphics *n.* the study of the patterns of finger, palm, toe, and sole prints. These patterns are formed by skin ridges, the distribution of which is unique to each individual. As well as being of value in criminology, dermatoglyphics is of interest to anthropologists and to doctors studying genetic disorders. *See also* fingerprint.

dermatology *n.* the medical specialty concerned with the diagnosis and treatment of skin disorders. —**dermatological** *adj.* —**dermatologist** *n.*

dermatome *n.* **1.** a surgical instrument used for cutting thin slices of skin in some skin grafting operations. **2.** that part of the segmented mesoderm in the early embryo that forms the deeper layers of the skin (dermis) and associated tissues. *See* somite.

dermatomyositis *n.* an inflammatory disorder of the skin and underlying tissues, including the muscles (where breakdown of the muscle fibres occurs). The condition is one of the *collagen diseases. A bluish-red skin eruption occurs on the face, scalp, neck, shoulders, and hands and is later accompanied by severe swelling. Dermatomyositis is often associated with internal cancer.

Dermatophagoides *n.* a genus of *mites that have been detected in samples of dust taken from houses in various parts of Europe. The mites may occasionally infest the skin of the scalp and cause dermatitis.

dermatophyte *n.* any microscopic fungus that grows on the skin and mucous membranes. There are three main genera: *Microsporum*, *Epidermophyton*, and *Trichophyton*. These do not invade the deeper tissues of the body.

dermatophytosis *n.* any fungus infection of the skin; more specifically, an infection caused by the parasitic fungus *Epidermophyton*.

dermatoplasty *n.* replacement of damaged or destroyed skin by surgery. *See* plastic surgery, skin graft.

dermatosis *n.* any disease of skin, particularly one without inflammation.

dermis (corium) *n.* the true *skin: the thick layer of living tissue that lies beneath the epidermis. It consists mainly of loose connective tissue within which are blood capillaries, lymph vessels, sensory nerve endings, sweat glands and their ducts, hair follicles, sebaceous glands, and smooth muscle fibres. —**dermal** *adj.*

dermographia *n.* a local allergic reaction caused by pressure on the skin. People with such highly sensitive skin can 'write' on it with a finger or blunt instrument, the pressure producing lasting weals.

dermoid 1. *adj.* resembling the skin. **2.** *n. see* dermoid cyst.

dermoid cyst (dermoid) a cyst containing hair, hair follicles, and *sebaceous glands, usually found at sites marking the fusion of developing sections of the body in the embryo. Sometimes a dermoid cyst may develop after an injury. Treatment is by surgical removal.

Descemet's membrane the elastic membrane that lines the inner surface of the cornea of the eye, next to the aqueous humour.

desensitization *n.* **1.** (*or* **hyposensitization**) a method for reducing the effects of a known allergen by injecting, over a period, gradually increasing doses of the allergen, until resistance is built up. *See* allergy. **2.** a technique used in the *behaviour therapy of phobic states. The thing that is feared is very gradually introduced to the patient, first in imagination and then in reality. At the same time the patient is taught relaxation to inhibit the development of anxiety (*see* relaxation therapy). In this way he is able to cope with progressively closer approximations to the feared object or situation.

deserpidine *n.* a drug that reduces blood pressure and is used to treat essential hypertension (*see* sympatholytic). It is administered by mouth; side-effects include stuffiness of the nose, diarrhoea, nausea, headache, lethargy, and depression. Trade name: **Harmonyl**.

desferrioxamine *n.* a drug that combines with iron in body tissues and fluids and is used to treat iron poisoning (including that resulting from prolonged or constant blood transfusion, as for thalassaemia), diseases involving iron storage in parts of the body (*see* haemochromatosis), and for the diagnosis of such diseases. It is administered by mouth, injection, or as eye drops; reactions and pain sometimes occur on injection. Trade name: **Desferal**.

desipramine *n.* a tricyclic *antidepressant drug administered by mouth or injection; common side-effects are dry mouth, blurred vision, insomnia, and unsteadiness in walking. Trade name: **Pertofran**.

desmosome *n.* an area of contact between two adjacent cells, occurring particularly in epithelia. The cell membranes at a desmosome are thickened and fine fibres (*tonofibrils*) extend from the desmosome into the cytoplasm.

desquamation *n.* the process in which the outer layer of the *epidermis of the skin is removed by scaling.

detached retina separation of the retina from the layer of the eyeball (choroid) to which it is attached. It commonly occurs when one or more holes in the retina allow fluid from the vitreous cavity of the eyeball to accumulate between the retina and choroid, which are only delicately attached. Sometimes the detachment is secondary to inflammation or tumour of the choroid or disorder of the vitreous humour. Vision is lost in the affected part of the retina. The condition can be treated surgically by creating patches of scar tissue between the retina and the choroid (by application of extreme heat or cold; *see* photocoagulation), which, combined with *plombage, stick it back into place.

detergent *n.* a synthetic cleansing agent that removes all impurities from a surface by reacting with grease and suspended particles, including bacteria and other microorganisms. Some detergents, e.g. *cetrimide, are used solely for cleansing; others may be used as *antiseptics and *disinfectants.

detoxication (detoxification) *n.* the process whereby toxic substances are removed or toxic effects neutralized. It is one of the functions of the liver.

detrition *n.* the process of wearing away solid bodies (e.g. bones) by friction or use.

Dettol *n. see* chloroxylenol.

detumescence *n.* **1.** the reverse of erection, whereby the erect penis or clitoris becomes flaccid after orgasm. **2.** subsidence of a swelling.

deut- (deuto-, deuter(o)-) *prefix denoting* two, second, or secondary.

deuteranopia *n.* a defect in colour vision in which reds, yellows, and greens are confused. It is thought that the mechanisms for perceiving red light and green light are in some way combined in people with this defect. *Compare* protanopia, tritanopia. *See also* colour blindness.

deutoplasm *n. see* yolk.

deviance *n.* variation from normal behaviour beyond the limits acceptable to the majority of the conforming peer group; particularly (though not exclusively) applied to sexual habits (*see also* perversion).

deviation *n.* (in ophthalmology) any abnormal position of one or both eyes. For example, if the eyes are both looking to one side when the head is facing forwards, they are said to be *deviated* to that side. Such deviations of both eyes may occur in brain disease. Deviations of one eye come into the category of squint (*see* strabismus).

Devic's disease *see* neuromyelitis optica.

devitalization *n.* (in dentistry) removal of the pulp of a tooth. *See* root treatment.

dexamethasone *n.* a *corticosteroid drug used principally to treat severe allergies, skin and eye diseases, rheumatic and other inflammatory conditions, and hormone and blood disorders. It is administered by mouth or injection; side-effects include sodium and fluid retention, muscle weakness, convulsions, vertigo, headache, and hormonal disturbances (including menstrual irregularities). Trade names: **Decadron**, **Oradexon**.

dexamphetamine *n.* a drug with actions and effects similar to those of *amphetamine. Trade names: **Dexamed**, **Dexedrine**.

dextr- (dextro-) *prefix denoting* **1.** the right side. Example: *dextroposition* (displacement to the right). **2.** (in chemistry) dextrorotation.

dextran *n.* a carbohydrate, consisting of branched chains of glucose units, that is a storage product of bacteria and yeasts. Preparations of dextran solution are used in transfusions, to increase the volume of plasma.

dextrin *n.* a carbohydrate formed as an intermediate product in the digestion of starch by the enzyme amylase. Dextrin is used in the preparation of pharmaceutical products (as an *excipient) and surgical dressings.

dextrocardia *n.* a congenital defect in which the position of the heart is a mirror image of its normal position, with the apex of the ventricles pointing to the right. It may be associated with other congenital defects and is often combined with *situs invertus*, in which the appendix and liver lie on the left side of the abdomen and the stomach lies on the right side. Isolated dextrocardia produces no adverse effects.

dextromethorphan *n.* a drug used in lozenges, syrups, and linctuses to suppress coughs (*see* antitussive). It sometimes causes drowsiness, dizziness, and digestive upsets.

dextromoramide *n.* an *analgesic used to relieve moderate or severe pain. It is given by mouth, injection, or as suppositories and sometimes causes dizziness, reduced blood pressure, nausea, vomiting, and sleepiness. Dextromoramide is similar to *morphine and can cause morphine-type dependence. Trade name: **Palfium**.

dextropropoxyphene *n.* an *analgesic used to relieve mild or moderate pain.

It is administered by mouth, often in combination with other analgesics, and sometimes causes dizziness, drowsiness, nausea, and vomiting.

dextrose *n. see* glucose.

dextrothyroxine *n.* a *thyroid hormone used to reduce blood cholesterol levels in patients with normally working thyroid glands and also to treat hypothyroidism. It is administered by mouth and side-effects commonly involve chest pains due to angina.

dhobie itch a skin disease – a type of allergic *dermatitis – caused by clothes laundry-marked with ink used in India by native laundrymen (or women).

di- *prefix denoting* two or double.

dia- *prefix denoting* **1.** through. **2.** throughout or completely. **3.** apart.

diabetes *n.* any disorder of metabolism causing excessive thirst and the production of large volumes of urine. Used alone, the term most commonly refers to *diabetes mellitus. *See also* diabetes insipidus, haemochromatosis (bronze diabetes). —**diabetic** *adj., n.*

diabetes insipidus a rare metabolic disorder in which the patient produces large quantities of dilute urine and is constantly thirsty. It is due to deficiency of the pituitary hormone *vasopressin, which regulates reabsorption of water in the kidneys, and is treated by administration of the hormone.

diabetes mellitus a disorder of carbohydrate metabolism in which sugars in the body are not oxidized to produce energy due to lack of the pancreatic hormone *insulin. The accumulation of sugar leads to its appearance in the blood (*hyperglycaemia*), then in the urine; symptoms include thirst, loss of weight, and the excessive production of urine. The use of fats as an alternative source of energy leads to disturbances of the *acid-base balance, the accumulation of ketones in the bloodstream

diaclasia

(*ketosis), and eventually to convulsions preceding *diabetic coma*. There appears to be an inherited tendency to diabetes; the disorder may be triggered by various factors, including physical stress. Diabetes that starts in childhood or adolescence is usually more severe than that beginning in middle or old age. Treatment is based on a carefully controlled diet, with adequate carbohydrate for the body's needs, together with injections of insulin or drugs (such as *tolbutamide) that are taken by mouth to lower blood-glucose levels. Lack of balance in the diet or in the amount of insulin taken leads to *hypoglycaemia. Long-term complications of diabetes include thickening of the arteries, which can affect the eyes (diabetic *retinopathy).

diaclasia *n.* a fracture made deliberately by a surgeon to correct a deformity in a bone, which has usually resulted from a badly set or untreated fracture.

diaclast *n.* a surgical instrument used for the destruction of the skull of a fetus. This rare procedure enables a dead fetus to be delivered through the birth canal.

diagnosis *n.* the process of determining the nature of a disorder by considering the patient's *signs and *symptoms, medical background, and – when necessary – results of laboratory tests and X-ray examinations. *See also* differential diagnosis, prenatal diagnosis. *Compare* prognosis. —**diagnostic** *adj.*

diakinesis *n.* the final stage in the first prophase of *meiosis, in which homologous chromosomes, between which crossing over has occurred, are ready to separate.

dialyser *n.* a piece of apparatus for separating components of a liquid mixture by *dialysis, especially an artificial kidney (*see* haemodialysis).

dialysis *n.* a method of separating particles of different dimensions in a liquid mixture, using a thin semipermeable membrane whose pores are too small to allow the passage of large particles, such as proteins, but large enough to permit the passage of dissolved crystalline material. A solution of the mixture is separated from distilled water by the membrane; the solutes pass through the membrane into the water while the proteins, etc., are retained. The principle of dialysis is used in the artificial kidney (*see* haemodialysis).

diamorphine *n.* see heroin.

diamthazole *n.* a drug with antifungal activity used to treat skin infections such as athlete's foot and some types of ringworm. It is applied to the infected part as ointment, dusting powder, or tincture and sometimes causes irritation and hypersensitivity reactions.

diapedesis *n.* migration of cells through the walls of blood capillaries into the tissue spaces. Diapedesis is an important part of the reaction of tissues to injury (*see* inflammation).

diaphoresis *n.* the process of sweating, especially excessive sweating. *See* sweat.

diaphoretic (sudorific) *n.* a drug that causes an increase in sweating, such as *pilocarpine, which stimulates the sweat glands directly. *Antipyretic drugs also have diaphoretic activity, which helps reduce the body temperature in fevers.

diaphragm *n.* **1.** (in anatomy) a thin musculomembranous dome-shaped muscle that separates the thoracic and abdominal cavities. The diaphragm is attached to the lower ribs at each side and to the breastbone and the backbone at the front and back. It bulges upwards against the heart and the lungs, arching over the stomach, liver, and spleen. There are openings in the diaphragm through which the oesophagus, blood vessels, and nerves pass. The diaphragm plays an important role in *breathing. It contracts with each inspiration, becoming flattened downwards and increasing the volume of the thoracic cavity. With each expiration it relaxes and is restored to its dome shape. **2.** a hemispherical rubber cap fitted inside the vagina over the neck of the womb as a contraceptive. When combined with the use of a chemical spermicide the diaphragm provides reliable contraception with a failure rate as low as 2–10 pregnancies per 100 woman-years.

diaphysial aclasis a hereditary abnormality of cartilage and bone growth, resulting in many cartilaginous outgrowths (exostoses) from the long bones. Bone growth may also be retarded, causing stunting and deformity.

diaphysis *n.* the shaft (central part) of a long bone. *Compare* epiphysis.

diaphysitis *n.* inflammation of the diaphysis (shaft) of a bone, through infection or rheumatic disease. It may result in impaired growth of the bone and consequent deformity.

diarrhoea *n.* frequent bowel evacuation or the passage of abnormally soft or liquid faeces. It may be caused by intestinal infections, other forms of intestinal inflammation (such as *colitis or *Crohn's disease), *malabsorption, anxiety, and the *irritable bowel syndrome. Severe or prolonged diarrhoea may lead to excess losses of fluid, salts, and nutrients in the faeces.

diarthrosis (synovial joint) *n.* a freely movable joint. The ends of the adjoining bones are covered with a thin cartilaginous sheet, and the bones are linked by a ligament (*capsule*) lined with *synovial membrane, which secretes synovial fluid (see illustration). Such joints are classified according to the type of connection between the

bones and the type of movement allowed. *See* arthrodic joint, condylarthrosis, enarthrosis, ginglymus, saddle joint, trochoid joint.

A synovial joint

diaschisis *n.* a temporary loss of reflex activity in the brainstem or spinal cord following destruction of the cerebral cortex. As time passes this state of suppressed reflex activity is replaced by one of unduly exaggerated reflexes and spasticity of the limbs.

diastase *n.* an enzyme that hydrolyses starch in barley grain to produce maltose during the malting process. It has been used to aid the digestion of starch in some digestive disorders.

diastole *n.* the period between two contractions of the heart, when the muscle of the heart relaxes and allows the chambers to fill with blood. The term usually refers to *ventricular diastole*, which lasts about 0.5 seconds in a normal heart rate of about 70/minute. During exertion this period shortens, so allowing the heart rate to increase. *See also* blood pressure, systole. —**diastolic** *adj.*

diastolic pressure *see* blood pressure.

diathermy *n.* the production of heat in a part of the body by means of a high-frequency electric current passed between two electrodes placed on the patient's skin. The heat generated increases blood flow and can be used in the treatment of deep-seated pain in rheumatic and arthritic conditions. *See also* microwave therapy.

The principle of diathermy is also utilized in various surgical instruments: a *diathermy knife*, for example, is used to coagulate tissues. The knife is itself one electrode, the other being a large moistened pad applied to another part of the patient's body. Because blood is coagulated as the knife is used, and small vessels sealed off, virtually bloodless incisions may be made. *Diathermy snares* and *needles* can be used to destroy unwanted tissue (*see* electrocautery).

diathesis *n.* a higher than average tendency to acquire certain diseases, such as allergies, rheumatic diseases, or gout. Such diseases may run in families, but they are not inherited.

diazepam *n.* a *tranquillizer with *muscle-relaxant and *anticonvulsant properties, used to relieve anxiety and tension and in the treatment of epilepsy and muscular rheumatism. It is administered by mouth or injection; common side-effects are drowsiness and lethargy. Trade name: **Valium**.

diazoxide *n.* a drug used to lower blood pressure in patients with hypertension and also used to treat conditions in which the levels of blood sugar are low (including *insulinoma). It is usually administered (by mouth or (for hypertension) injection) with a diuretic as it causes salt and water retention.

dibenzepin *n.* an *antidepressant drug administered by mouth. Common side-effects include dry mouth, blurred vision, constipation, sweating, drowsiness, and reduced blood pressure. Trade name: **Noveril**.

dicephalus *n. see* craniopagus.

dichloralphenazone *n.* a *sedative used to relieve pain, fever, and restlessness, mainly in children and elderly patients. It is administered by mouth and sometimes causes skin reactions, nausea, vomiting, and headache. It can also cause *dependence of the barbiturate-alcohol type. Trade names: **Paedo-Sed**, **Welldorm**.

dichlorophen *n.* an *anthelmintic drug used to treat human tapeworm infestation. It is administered by mouth and commonly causes abdominal pain and discomfort, diarrhoea, nausea, and vomiting. Trade name: **Anthiphen**.

dichlorphenamide *n.* a *diuretic used to reduce pressure within the eye in the treatment of glaucoma. It is administered by mouth; side-effects include drowsiness, dizziness, digestive upsets, and skin rashes. Trade names: **Daranide**, **Oratrol**.

dichromatic *adj.* describing the state of colour vision of those who can appreciate only two of the three primary colours. People with such vision match any given colour by a mixture of the two they can distinguish. *Compare* trichromatic.

Dick test a test for susceptibility to *scarlet fever. If a small quantity of toxin from the bacteria responsible (haemolytic streptococci) is injected under the skin of a person not immune to the disease, a positive reaction results, causing local reddening of the skin.

dicophane *n. see* DDT.

dicoumarol *n.* an *anticoagulant drug used in the treatment of coronary and venous thrombosis. It is administered by mouth and may cause nausea, vomiting, and diarrhoea. Dicoumarol has now largely been replaced in clinical use by *phenindione or *warfarin because it is slow acting, has unpredictable effects, and may produce bleeding from overdosage.

dicrotism *n.* a condition in which the pulse is felt as a double beat for each contraction of the heart. It may be seen in typhoid fever. —**dicrotic** *adj.*

dictyoma *n.* a tumour of the epithelium lining the *ciliary body of the eye. It may be benign or malignant.

dicyclomine *n.* a drug that reduces spasms of smooth muscle and is used to relieve peptic ulcer, infantile colic, colitis, and related conditions. It is administered by mouth; side-effects include dry mouth, thirst, and dizziness. Trade name: **Merbentyl**.

didym- (didymo-) *prefix denoting* the testis.

dieldrin *n.* an insecticide that attacks the central nervous system of insects and has proved useful in the control of various beetles, flies, and larvae that attack crops. Because of its toxic effects, there has been considerable anxiety over its widespread use in situations where food may be contaminated.

diencephalon *n.* an anatomical division of the forebrain, consisting of the epithalamus, thalamus (dorsal thalamus), hypothalamus, and ventral thalamus (subthalamus). *See* brain.

dienoestrol *n.* a synthetic female sex hormone (*see* oestrogen) administered by mouth to treat symptoms of the menopause, to suppress lactation, and to relieve symptoms in cancer of the breast or prostate. It is also applied as a cream to relieve itching or inflammation of the vagina and in acne. Trade name: **Hormofemin**.

diet *n.* the mixture of foods that a person eats. A *balanced diet* contains adequate quantities of all the *nutrients.

dietary fibre (roughage) the part of food that cannot be digested and absorbed to produce energy. Dietary fibre falls into four groups: *cellulose, hemicelluloses, lignins,* and *pectins.* Highly refined foods, such as sucrose, contain no dietary fibre. Foods with a high fibre content include wholemeal cereals and flour, root vegetables, nuts, and fruit. Dietary fibre is considered by some to be helpful in the prevention of many of the diseases of Western civilization, such as *diverticulosis, constipation, appendicitis, obesity, and diabetes mellitus. Communities consuming high-fibre diets very rarely have any of these diseases.

dietetics *n.* the application of the principles of *nutrition to the selection of food and the feeding of individuals and groups.

diethylcarbamazine *n.* an anthelmintic drug that destroys filariae and is therefore used in the treatment of filariasis, loiasis, and onchocerciasis. It is administered as tablets. Side-effects may include headache, malaise, joint pains, nausea, and vomiting.

diethylpropion *n.* a drug, similar to *amphetamine, that suppresses the appetite and is used in the treatment of obesity. It is administered by mouth and may cause dry mouth, insomnia, depression, headache, constipation, and allergic rashes. Dependence of the amphetamine type can occur. Trade names: **Apesate, Tenuate**.

diethylstilboestrol *n.* a synthetic female sex hormone (*see* oestrogen) used to treat symptoms of the menopause, menstrual disorders, inflammation of the female genital organs, and cancer of the breast and prostate. It is administered by mouth or injection or as creams and pessaries; side-effects include loss of appetite, abdominal pain, and diarrhoea.

Dietl's crisis acute obstruction of a kidney causing severe pain in the loins. The obstruction usually occurs at the junction of the renal pelvis and the ureter, causing the kidney to become distended with accumulated urine (*see* hydronephrosis). Sometimes the pelvis drains spontaneously, with relief of pain, but acute decompression of the kidney may be required with surgical relief of the obstruction (*pyeloplasty).

differential diagnosis *diagnosis of a condition whose signs and/or symptoms are shared by various other conditions. For example, abdominal pain may be due to any of a large number of different disorders, which must be ruled out in arriving at a correct diagnosis.

differential leucocyte count (differential blood count) a determination of the proportions of the different kinds of white cells (leucocytes) present in a sample of blood. Usually 100 white cells are counted and classified under the microscope, so that the results can readily be expressed as percentages of the total number of leucocytes and the absolute numbers per litre of blood. The information often aids diagnosis of disease.

differentiation *n.* the process in embryonic development during which unspecialized cells or tissues become specialized for particular functions.

digestion *n.* the process in which ingested food is broken down in the alimentary canal into a form that can be absorbed and assimilated by the tissues of the body. Digestion includes mechanical processes, such as chewing, churning, and grinding food, as well as the chemical action of digestive enzymes and other substances (bile, acid, etc.). Chemical digestion begins in the mouth with the action of *saliva on food, but most of it takes place in the stomach and small intestine, where the food is subjected to *gastric juice, *pancreatic juice, and *succus entericus.

digitalis *n.* an extract from the dried leaves of foxgloves (*Digitalis* species), which contains various substances, including *digitoxin and *digoxin, that stimulate heart muscle. Used to treat heart failure, it is administered by mouth or, in emergency, by injection. High doses can cause nausea, vomiting, loss of appetite, diarrhoea, abdominal pain, and abnormal heart activity. *See also* digitalization.

digitalization *n.* the administration of the drug digitalis or one of its purified derivatives to a patient with heart failure until the optimum level has been reached in the heart tissues. At this stage the control of heart failure should be adequate and there should be few side-effects. The process of digitalization may take several days.

digitoxin *n.* a drug that increases heart muscle contraction and is used in heart failure. It is slow-acting but the effects are prolonged. Digitoxin is administered by mouth or injection; side-effects are those of *digitalis.

digoxin *n.* a drug that increases heart muscle contraction and is used in heart failure. It is rapidly effective and the effects are short-lived. Digoxin is administered by mouth or injection; side-effects are those of *digitalis.

dihydrallazine *n.* a drug used to lower blood pressure in moderate hypertension. It is administered by mouth, often in combination with reserpine or other hypotensive agents, since side-effects (fast heart rate, headache, loss of appetite, nausea, and vomiting) may be severe.

dihydrocodeine *n.* a drug used to relieve pain and suppress coughs (*see* analgesic, antitussive). It is administered by mouth or injection and sometimes causes nausea, dizziness, and constipation. Dependence of the *morphine type can also occur, but this is rare.

dihydroergotamine *n.* a derivative of *ergotamine used to prevent and relieve migraine attacks. It is administered by mouth or injection; side-effects are rare but nausea sometimes occurs.

diiodohydroxyquinoline *n.* an antiseptic used to treat bowel infections and dysentery. It is administered by mouth or as pessaries and occasionally causes irritation of the digestive system, headache, itching, and boils. Trade name: **Diodoquin**.

diiodotyrosine *n.* an iodine-containing substance produced in the thyroid gland from which the *thyroid hormones are derived.

dilaceration *n.* a condition affecting some teeth after traumatic injury, in which the root and crown are at an abnormal angle to each other. It usually necessitates removal of the tooth.

dilatation *n.* the enlargement or expansion of a hollow organ (such as a blood vessel) or cavity.

dilatation and curettage (D and C) an operation in which the neck of the womb is expanded, using an instrument called a *dilator, and the lining of the womb is peeled off with a curette (*see* curettage). It is performed for a variety of reasons, including the removal of any remaining material left after a miscarriage, removal of cysts or tumours, and examination of the womb lining in the diagnosis of gynaecological disorders.

dilator *n.* **1.** an instrument used to enlarge a body opening or cavity. For example, the male urethra may become narrowed by disease and it can sometimes be restored to its original size by inserting a dilator. Dilators are also used to enlarge the canal in the neck of the womb in the procedure of *dilatation and curettage. **2.** a drug, applied either locally or systemically, that causes expansion of a structure, such as the pupil of the eye or a blood vessel. *See also* vasodilator. **3.** a muscle that, by its action, opens an aperture or orifice in the body.

diloxanide *n.* an antiseptic used to treat bowel infections. It is administered by mouth and occasionally causes vomiting, flatulence, itching, and skin rash.

dimenhydrinate *n.* an *antihistamine used to prevent and treat travel sickness, nausea and vomiting due to other causes, vertigo, and inner ear disturbances. It is administered by mouth or injection and commonly causes drowsiness, dizziness, digestive upsets, dry mouth, and headache. Trade name: **Dramamine**.

dimercaprol *n.* a drug that combines with metals in the body and is used to treat poisoning by antimony, arsenic, bismuth, gold, mercury, and thallium and in Wilson's disease. It is administered by injection and commonly causes nausea, vomiting, and watering of the eyes. Trade name: **British Anti-Lewisite (BAL)**.

dimethisterone *n.* a synthetic female sex hormone (*see* progestogen) used to treat amenorrhoea and disorders of the lining of the womb and formerly used in sequential *oral contraceptives. It is administered by mouth; side-effects are abdominal pains, breast turgidity, nausea, and vertigo.

dimethothiazine *n.* an *antihistamine used to treat allergies such as hay fever. It is administered by mouth; side-effects include drowsiness, dry mouth, nausea, stomach pain, vertigo, diarrhoea, and mild headache. Trade name: **Banistyl**.

dimethyl sulphoxide (DMSO) a chemical used in an ointment to treat skin inflammations or in combination with other topically applied drugs to improve their absorption. It may cause skin irritation.

dimetria (uterus duplex, uterus didelphys) *n.* the condition of having a double womb.

dioctyl sodium sulphosuccinate

dioctyl sodium sulphosuccinate a softening agent that is given by mouth or in suppositories, often together with a laxative, to relieve constipation. It is also used in solution to soften ear wax.

diodone *n.* an iodine-containing compound that is *radio-opaque and therefore useful in radiographic examination of parts of the body. Injected into the bloodstream, it is concentrated by the kidneys as it is excreted and forms a useful medium for showing up the urinary tract and any abnormalities that may be present (*see* pyelography).

dioptre *n.* the unit of measurement of the power of *refraction of a lens. One dioptre is the power of a lens that brings parallel light rays to a focus at a point one metre from the lens, after passing through it. A stronger lens brings light rays to a focus at a point closer to it than a weaker lens and is a higher number of dioptres in power.

dipeptidase *n.* an enzyme, found in digestive juices, that splits certain products of protein digestion (dipeptides) into their constituent amino acids. The latter are then absorbed by the body.

dipeptide *n.* a compound consisting of two amino acids joined together by a peptide bond (e.g. glycylalanine, a combination of the amino acids glycine and alanine). *See* dipeptidase.

diphenhydramine *n.* an *antihistamine used to treat allergic conditions, such as hay fever and rhinitis, and in cough mixtures. It is administered by mouth or injection; side-effects include drowsiness, dry mouth, dizziness, and nausea. Trade name: **Benadryl.**

diphenoxylate *n.* a drug used, often in combination with *atropine, to treat diarrhoea. It is also used after *colostomy or ileostomy to reduce the frequency and fluidity of the stools. It is administered by mouth; side-effects can include nausea, drowsiness, dizziness, skin reactions, and restlessness.

diphtheria *n.* an acute highly contagious infection, caused by the bacterium *Corynebacterium diphtheriae*, generally affecting the throat but occasionally other mucous membranes and the skin. The disease is spread by direct contact with a patient or carrier or by contaminated milk. After an incubation period of 2–6 days a sore throat, weakness, and mild fever develop. Later, a soft grey membrane forms across the throat, constricting the air passages and causing difficulty in breathing and swallowing; a *tracheostomy may be necessary. Bacteria multiply at the site of infection and release a toxin into the bloodstream, which damages heart and nerves. Death from heart failure or general collapse can follow within four days but prompt administration of antitoxin and penicillin arrests the disease; complete recovery requires prolonged bed rest. An effective immunization programme has now made diphtheria rare in most Western countries (*see also* Schick test).

diphtheroid *adj.* resembling diphtheria (especially the membrane formed in diphtheria) or the bacteria that cause it.

diphyllobothriasis *n.* an infestation of the intestine with the broad tapeworm, *Diphyllobothrium latum*, which sometimes causes nausea, malnutrition, diarrhoea, and anaemia resulting from impaired absorption of vitamin B_{12} through the gut. The infestation, common in Baltic countries, is contracted following ingestion of uncooked fish infected with the larval stage of the tapeworm. The tapeworm can be expelled from the gut with the anthelmintic *mepacrine.

Diphyllobothrium *n.* a genus of large tapeworms that can grow to a length of 3–10 m. The adult of *D. latum*, the broad (or fish) tapeworm, infects fish-eating mammals including man, in whom it may cause serious anaemia (*see* diphyllobothriasis). The parasite has two intermediate hosts: a freshwater crustacean and a fish (*see also* plerocercoid).

dipipanone *n.* a potent *analgesic drug used to relieve severe pain. It is administered by mouth or injection and may cause nausea, vomiting, dizziness, and drowsiness.

dipl- (diplo-) *prefix denoting* double.

diplacusis *n.* perception of a single sound as double owing to a defect of the *cochlea in the inner ear.

diplegia *n.* paralysis involving both sides of the body and affecting the legs more severely than the arms. *Cerebral diplegia* is a form of *cerebral palsy in which there is widespread damage, in both cerebral hemispheres, of the brain cells that control the movements of the limbs. —**diplegic** *adj.*

diplococcus *n.* any of a group of nonmotile parasitic spherical bacteria that occur in pairs. The group includes the *pneumococcus.

diploë *n.* the lattice-like tissue that lies between the inner and outer layers of the *skull.

diploid *adj.* describing cells, nuclei, or organisms in which each chromosome except the Y sex chromosome is represented twice. *Compare* haploid, triploid. —**diploid** *n.*

diplopia *n.* double vision: the simultaneous awareness of two images of the one object. It is usually due to a disturbance in the coordinated movements of the muscles that move the eyeball, and covering one eye will abolish it. A very slight degree of doubling, which does not disappear when one eye is covered, may be experienced by introspective people. This is *uniocular diplopia*, and only in the rarest cases is there any abnormality of the eye.

diplotene *n.* the fourth stage in the first prophase of *meiosis, in which *crossing over occurs between the paired chromatids of homologous chromosomes, which then begin to separate.

diprophylline *n.* a drug that relaxes bronchial muscle and stimulates heart muscle. It is used to relieve symptoms in asthma and bronchitis and to treat congestive heart failure. It is administered by mouth, injection, or in suppositories and may cause nausea and vomiting, headache, palpitations, and dizziness, especially following injection. *See also* bronchodilator. Trade names: **Neutraphylline, Silbephylline**.

diprosopus *n.* a fetal monster with a single trunk and normal limbs but with some degree of duplication of the face.

dipsomania *n.* morbid and insatiable craving for alcohol, occurring in paroxysms. Only a small proportion of alcoholics show this symptom. *See* alcoholism.

Diptera *n.* a large group of insects, including *mosquitoes, gnats, midges, house flies and *tsetse flies, that possess a single pair of wings. The mouthparts of many species, e.g. mosquitoes and tsetse flies, are specialized for sucking blood; these forms are important in the transmission of disease (*see* vector). *See also* fly.

Dipylidium *n.* a genus of tapeworms. *D. caninum*, a common parasite of the small intestine of dogs and cats, occasionally infects man but usually produces no obvious symptoms. Fleas are the intermediate hosts, and children in close contact with pets become infected on ingesting fleas harbouring the parasite.

dipyridamole *n.* a drug that dilates the blood vessels of the heart. It is used to treat reduced heart activity and is given by mouth or injection. It may cause headache, stomach upsets, and dizziness.

director *n.* an instrument used to guide the extent and direction of a surgical incision.

dis- *prefix denoting* separation.

disability *n. see* handicap.

Disabled Living Foundation (in Britain) a voluntary agency interested in all aspects of the care of those with *handicaps and in improving their quality of life. It is particularly concerned with aids to daily living, which can be inspected by clients, doctors, and others at a permanent exhibition at the headquarters of the Foundation.

disabled person *see* Employment Service Division.

disaccharide *n.* a carbohydrate consisting of two linked *monosaccharide units. The most common disaccharides are *maltose, *lactose, and *sucrose.

disarticulation *n.* separation of two bones at a joint. This may be the result of an injury or it may be done by the surgeon at operation in the course of amputation; for example of a limb, finger, or toe.

disc *n.* (in anatomy) a rounded flattened structure, such as an *intervertebral disc or the *optic disc.

discharge rate the number of cases of a specified disease discharged from hospitals related to the population of the *catchment area: usually expressed regionally per 10,000.

discission *n.* an operation for cataract in which the front of the lens capsule is cut extensively by a fine knife or needle inserted through the edge of the cornea. Subsequently the lens is absorbed naturally into the surrounding fluid of the eye. It is usually necessary to perform *capsulotomy later.

disease *n.* a disorder with a specific cause and recognizable signs and symptoms; any bodily abnormality or failure to function properly, except that resulting directly from physical injury (the latter, however, may open the way for disease).

disimpaction *n.* the process of separating the broken ends of a bone when they have been forcibly driven together during a fracture. *Traction may be required to keep the bone ends separate but in good alignment.

disinfectant *n.* an agent that destroys or removes bacteria and other microorganisms and is used to cleanse surgical instruments and other objects. Examples are *cresol, *hexachlorophane, and *phenol. Dilute solutions of some disinfectants may be used as *antiseptics or as preservatives in solutions of eye drops or injections.

disinfection *n.* the process of eliminating infective microorganisms from contaminated instruments, clothing, or surroundings by using physical means or chemicals (*disinfectants).

disinfestation *n.* the destruction of insect pests and other animal parasites. This generally involves the use of insecticides applied either topically, as in delousing, or as a spray for eliminating an infestation of fleas or bed bugs in the home.

disintegrative psychosis *see* Heller's syndrome.

disjunction *n.* the separation of pairs of homologous chromosomes during meiosis or of the chromatids of a chromosome during *anaphase of mitosis or meiosis. *Compare* nondisjunction.

dislocation (luxation) *n.* displacement from their normal position of bones meeting at a joint. Dislocation of the shoulder is common in sports injuries, and congenital abnormalities may lead to repeated dislocations of the hip. The bones are restored to their normal positions by manipulation, which may require local or general anaesthesia (*see* reduction). *Compare* subluxation.

dismemberment *n.* the amputation of a leg, arm, or part of a limb.

disoma *n.* a double-bodied fetal monster with a single head.

disopyramide *n.* a *parasympatholytic drug used to treat various heart conditions involving abnormal heart rates. It is administered by mouth; side-effects such as dry mouth, blurred vision, difficulty in urination, and digestive upsets may occur. Trade names: **Norpace**, **Rythmodan**.

disorientation *n.* the state produced by loss of awareness of space, time, or personality. It can be the result of drugs, anxiety, or organic disease (such as dementia or *Korsakoff's syndrome).

dispensary *n.* a place where medicines are made up by a pharmacist according to the doctor's prescription and dispensed to patients. A dispensary is often part of an out-patient department in a hospital.

displacement *n.* (in psychology) the substitution of one type of behaviour for another, usually the substitution of a relatively harmless activity for a harmful one; for example, kicking the cat instead of one's boss.

dissection *n.* the cutting apart and separation of the body tissues along the natural divisions of the organs and different tissues in the course of an operation. Dissection of corpses is carried out for the study of anatomy.

disseminated *adj.* widely distributed in an organ (or organs) or in the whole body. The term may refer to disease organisms or to pathological changes.

disseminated sclerosis *see* multiple sclerosis.

dissociation *n.* (in psychiatry) the process whereby thoughts and ideas can be split off from consciousness and may function independently, thus (for example) allowing conflicting opinions to be held at the same time about the same object. Dissociation may be the main factor in cases of hysterical *fugue and multiple personalities.

distal *adj.* **1.** (in anatomy) situated away from the origin or point of attachment or from the median line of the body. For example, the term is applied to a part of a limb that is furthest from the body; to a blood vessel that is far from the heart; and to a nerve fibre that is far from the central nervous system. *Compare* proximal. **2.** (in dentistry) describing the surface of a tooth away from the midline of the jaw.

distichiasis *n.* a very rare condition in which there is an extra row of eyelashes behind the normal ones. They may rub on the cornea.

District Health Authority *see* National Health Service.

District Management Team *see* National Health Service.

District Medical Committee *see* medical committee.

District Medical Officer (DMO) *see* community physician.

district nurse *see* home nurse.

District Planning Team a multidisciplinary group of doctors, nurses, and others established in a health district to identify gaps in the services and to suggest how they can be improved. Outside agencies (e.g. *social services) are included when appropriate. Some teams are permanent (e.g. those dealing with the elderly and mentally sick); others are established on an *ad hoc* basis.

disulfiram *n.* a drug used in the treatment of chronic alcoholism. It acts as a deterrent by producing unpleasant effects when taken with alcohol, includ-

dithiazanine

ing flushing, breathing difficulties, headache, palpitations, nausea, and vomiting. It is administered by mouth; common side-effects are fatigue, nausea, and constipation. Trade name: **Antabuse**.

dithiazanine *n.* an *anthelmintic drug used to treat certain worm infestations. It is administered by mouth and stains the stools bluish-green. Other side-effects include nausea, vomiting, diarrhoea, fluid retention, and fever.

dithranol *n.* a drug applied to the skin as an ointment or paste to treat ringworm infections, psoriasis, and other skin conditions. It may irritate the skin on application.

diuresis *n.* increased secretion of urine by the kidneys. This normally follows the drinking of more fluid than the body requires, but it can be stimulated by the administration of a *diuretic.

diuretic *n.* a drug that increases the volume of urine produced by promoting the excretion of salts and water from the kidney. Examples are the *thiazide diuretics* (e.g. *chlorothiazide and *chlorthalidone), *frusemide, *spironolactone, and *triamterene. Diuretics are used to reduce the oedema due to salt and water retention in disorders of the heart, kidneys, liver, or lungs. Some mild diuretics, including *acetazolamide, are used to reduce the pressure within the eyeball in glaucoma. Diuretics are also used – in conjunction with other drugs – in the treatment of high blood pressure. Treatment with thiazide diuretics often results in potassium deficiency; this is corrected by simultaneous administration of potassium salts.

divagation *n.* rambling discursive thought and speech. It is not specific to any one psychiatric condition.

divaricator *n.* a scissor-like surgical instrument used to divide portions of

tissue into two separate parts during an operation.

diverticular disease a condition in which there are diverticula (*see* diverticulum) in the colon associated with lower abdominal pain and disturbed bowel habit. The pain is due to spasm of the muscles of the intestine and not to inflammation of the diverticula (*compare* diverticulitis).

diverticulitis *n.* inflammation of a *diverticulum, most commonly of one or more colonic diverticula. This type of diverticulitis is caused by infection and causes lower abdominal pain with diarrhoea or constipation; it may lead to abscess formation, which often requires surgical drainage. A Meckel's diverticulum sometimes becomes inflamed due to infection, causing symptoms similar to *appendicitis. Diverticula elsewhere in the alimentary tract are not subject to diverticulitis. *Compare* diverticular disease.

diverticulosis *n.* a condition in which diverticula exist in a segment of the intestine without evidence of inflammation (*compare* diverticulitis).

diverticulum *n.* (*pl.* **diverticula**) a sac or pouch formed at weak points in the walls of the alimentary tract. They may be caused by increased pressure from within (*pulsion diverticula*) or by pulling from without (*traction diverticula*). A *pharyngeal diverticulum* occurs in the pharynx and may cause difficulty in swallowing. *Oesophageal diverticula* occur in the middle or lower oesophagus (gullet); they may be associated with muscular disorders of the oesophagus but rarely cause symptoms. *Gastric diverticula* affect the stomach (usually the upper part) and cause no symptoms. *Duodenal diverticula* occur on the concave surface of the duodenal loop; they may be associated with *dyspepsia but usually cause few symptoms. *Jeju-*

nal diverticula affect the small intestine, are often multiple, and may give rise to abdominal discomfort and *malabsorption due to growth of bacteria within them. *Meckel's diverticulum* occurs in the ileum, about 35 cm from its termination, as a congenital abnormality. It may become inflamed, mimicking *appendicitis; if it contains embryonic remnants of stomach mucosa it may form a *peptic ulcer, causing pain, bleeding, or perforation. *Colonic diverticula*, affecting the colon (particularly the lowest portion), become commoner with increasing age and often cause no symptoms. However they are sometimes associated with abdominal pain or altered bowel habit (*see* diverticular disease) or they may become inflamed (*see* diverticulitis).

division *n.* the separation of an organ or tissue into parts by surgery.

divulsor *n.* a surgical instrument used to dilate forcibly any canal or cavity, usually the urethra.

dizygotic twins *see* twins.

DNA (deoxyribonucleic acid) the genetic material of nearly all living organisms, which controls heredity and is located in the cell nucleus (*see* chromosome, gene). DNA is a *nucleic acid composed of two strands made up of units called *nucleotides (see illustration). The two strands are wound around each other into a double helix and linked together by hydrogen bonds between the bases of the nucleotides (*see* base pairing). The genetic information of the DNA is contained in the sequence of bases along the molecule (*see* genetic code); changes in the DNA cause *mutations. The DNA molecule can make exact copies of itself by the process of *replication, thereby passing on the genetic information to the daughter cells when the cell divides.

A	adenine	
G	guanine	} bases
T	thymine	
C	cytosine	

H hydrogen
S deoxyribose sugar
P phosphate
---- hydrogen bond

Structure of part of a DNA molecule

Doctor *n.* **1.** the title given to a recipient of a higher university degree than a Master's degree. The degree *Medicinae Doctor* (MD) is awarded by some British universities as a research degree. In the US the degree is awarded on qualification. **2.** a courtesy title given to a qualified medical practitioner, i.e. one who has been registered by the General Medical Council (GMC). Most doctors in the UK obtain bachelors' degrees in medicine and surgery (MB, BS) or the diplomas of the conjoint boards of the Royal College of Physicians and the Royal College of Surgeons (LRCP, MRCS): these degrees or diplomas and one year's hospital experience are required by the GMC before they will register a person as a doctor. Normally it is compulsory to hold two full-time *preregistration appointments* in general subjects at hospitals recognized for this purpose. The doctor has the title *house physician* (or *surgeon*), *resident*, or *intern* and is debarred from independent practice. Surgeons in the UK do not use the title Doctor and are referred to, as a mark of distinction, as Mr. In the US qualified dentists and pharmacists also use the courtesy title Doctor. *See also* consultant.

dolich- (dolicho-) *prefix denoting* long. Example: *dolichocolon* (abnormally long colon).

dolichocephaly *n.* the condition of having a relatively long skull, with a *cephalic index of 75 or less. —**dolichocephalic** *adj.*

dolor *n.* pain: one of the classical signs of inflammation in a tissue, the other three being *calor (heat), *rubor (redness), and *tumor (swelling). The pain in inflammation is thought to be due to the release of chemicals from damaged cells.

dolorimetry *n.* the measurement of pain. *See* algesimeter.

domiciliary midwife (in Britain) a State Registered Nurse with special training in midwifery (both hospital and domiciliary practice). She must be registered with the Central Midwives' Board in order to practise; this requires regular refresher courses to supplement the basic qualification of *State Certified Midwife* (*SCM*). Planned home deliveries are comparatively rare; the work of domiciliary midwives is mainly concerned with antenatal and postnatal care, especially in those discharged 48 hours or less after delivery, and in some cases conducting deliveries in community hospitals.

domiciliary services (in Britain) health and social services that are available in the home and are distinguished from hospital-based services. They include the services of such personnel as community nurses employed by Area Health Authorities (*see* home nurse, domiciliary midwife, health visitor) and social workers, home helps,

and bath attendants employed by social service departments of local authorities. Also included are services such as meals on wheels, loan equipment for home care, and ambulatory aids. The term *community services* is also applied to these services, but strictly speaking, hospitals and other residential institutes should be included under the latter heading.

dominant *adj.* (in genetics) describing a gene (or its corresponding characteristic) whose effect is shown in the individual whether its *allele is the same or different. If the allele is different it is described as *recessive* and its effect is masked. —**dominant** *n.*

domiphen *n.* an *antiseptic administered in the form of lozenges to treat bacterial and fungal infections of the mouth and throat. It is also used in solution for cleansing wounds and burns, for treating fungal infections of the skin, and for general disinfection of skin and mucous membranes.

donor *n.* a person who makes his own tissues or organs available for use by someone else. For example, a donor may provide blood for transfusion (*see* blood donor) or a kidney for transplantation.

dopa *n.* dihydroxyphenylalanine: a physiologically important compound that forms an intermediate stage in the synthesis of catecholamines (dopamine, adrenaline, and noradrenaline) from the essential amino acid tyrosine. It also plays a role itself in the functioning of certain parts of the brain. The form *L-dopa* is administered for the treatment of *parkinsonism, a disease in which there is a deficiency of dopamine in the brain.

dopamine *n.* a *catecholamine derived from dopa that is an intermediate in the synthesis of noradrenaline. It is found in high concentrations in the adrenal medulla and is also in the brain, in the caudate nucleus (*see* basal ganglia), where it may function as a *neurotransmitter.

dopamine hypothesis the theory that schizophrenia is caused in part by abnormalities in the metabolism of *dopamine and can be treated in part by drugs (such as *chlorpromazine) that antagonize its action as a neurotransmitter.

dors- (dorsi-, dorso-) *prefix denoting* 1. the back. Example: *dorsalgia* (pain in). 2. dorsal.

dorsal *adj.* relating to or situated at or close to the back of the body or to the posterior part of an organ.

dorsiflexion *n.* backward flexion of the foot or hand or their digits; i.e. bending towards the upper surface.

dorsoventral *adj.* (in anatomy) extending from the back (dorsal) surface to the front (ventral) surface.

dorsum *n.* 1. the back. 2. the upper or posterior surface of a part of the body; for example, of the hand. *See also* dorsal.

dose *n.* a carefully measured quantity of a drug that is prescribed by a doctor to be given to a patient at any one time. The *median effective dose* (ED_{50}) is the dose of a drug that produces desired effects in 50% of individuals tested. *See also* LD_{50}.

dosimeter *n.* a device to record the amount of radiation received by workers with X-rays or other radiation, usually consisting of a small piece of photographic film in a holder attached to the clothing. At regular intervals the film is examined to discover the amount of radiation it (and therefore the wearer) have received.

dosimetry *n.* the calculation of appropriate doses for given conditions, usually the calculation of correct amounts of radiation for the treatment of cancer

in different parts of the body. *See* radiotherapy.

double-bind *n.* a disordered pattern of family relationships in which one family member gives contradictory instructions to another (as when a mother asks her child verbally for affection but simultaneously, by her gestures, indicates that the child should remain distant). The result is that any action the child makes will be wrong, and furthermore he cannot escape from the situation. This has been supposed, but not proved, to be a factor in causing schizophrenia.

double-blind trial *see* intervention study.

double vision *see* diplopia.

douche *n.* a forceful jet of water used for cleaning any part of the body, most commonly the vagina. A vaginal douche is extremely unreliable as a method of contraception.

Down's syndrome a form of mental subnormality due to a chromosome defect (there are three no. 21 chromosomes instead of the usual two). The main physical features are a slightly oblique slant to the eyes, as in the Mongolian races (hence the former name of this condition – *mongolism*); a round head; flat nasal bridge; fissured tongue; abnormalities of the palms, including single transverse creases and characteristic dermal ridges; small round or knotty ears; and short stature. Many of these features are present at birth, enabling an early diagnosis; the condition can also be diagnosed prenatally, by *amniocentesis. The ultimate mental attainment is about that of a five-year-old child, i.e. an IQ of 50–60. Rare partial forms of Down's syndrome occur with a slightly higher IQ (*see* mosaicism). Medical name: **trisomy 21**.

doxepin *n.* a drug used to relieve depression, especially when associated with anxiety (*see* antidepressant, tranquillizer). It is administered by mouth; side-effects can include drowsiness, dry mouth, blurred vision, and digestive upsets. Trade name: **Sinequan.**

doxorubicin *n.* an *anthracycline antibiotic isolated from *Streptomyces peucetius caesius* and used mainly in the treatment of leukaemia and various other forms of cancer. Doxorubicin acts by interfering with the production of DNA and RNA (*see also* antimetabolite). It is administered by injection or infusion; side-effects include bone marrow depression, baldness, gastrointestinal disturbances, and heart damage. Trade name: **Adriamycin.**

doxycycline *n.* an *antibiotic used to treat infections caused by a wide range of bacteria and other microorganisms. It is administered by mouth and side-effects are those of the other *tetracyclines. Trade name: **Vibramycin.**

DPT vaccine a combined *vaccine against diphtheria, whooping-cough, and tetanus organisms, prepared from their *toxoids and other antigens.

drachm *n.* **1.** a unit of weight used in pharmacy. 1 drachm = 3.883 g (60 grains). **2.** a unit of volume used in pharmacy. 1 fluid drachm = 3.696 ml (1/8 fluid ounce).

dracontiasis *n.* a tropical disease caused by the parasitic nematode *Dracunculus medinensis* (*see* guinea worm) in the tissues beneath the skin. The disease is transmitted to man via contaminated drinking water. The initial symptoms, which appear a year after infection, result from the migration of the worm to the skin surface and include itching, giddiness, difficulty in breathing, vomiting, and diarrhoea. Later a large blister forms on the skin, usually on the legs or arms, which eventually bursts and may ulcerate and become infected. Dracontiasis is common in India and West Africa but also occurs in Arabia, Iran, East Africa, and Afghanistan. Treatment involves killing the adult worms with injections of phenolthiazine.

Dracunculus *n. see* guinea worm.

dragee *n.* a *pill that has been coated with sugar.

drain 1. *n.* a device, usually a tube or wick, used to draw fluid from an internal body cavity to the surface. A drain is sometimes inserted during an operation to ensure that any fluid formed immediately passes to the surface, so preventing an accumulation that may become infected or cause pressure in the operation site. **2.** *vb. see* drainage.

drainage *n.* the drawing off of fluid from a cavity in the body, usually fluid that has accumulated abnormally. For example, serous fluid may be drained from a swollen joint, pus removed from an internal abscess, or urine from an overdistended bladder. *See also* drain.

drastic *n.* any agent causing a major change in a body system or function, e.g. strong laxatives.

draw-sheet *n.* a sheet placed beneath a patient in bed that, when one portion has been soiled or become uncomfortably wrinkled, may be pulled under the patient so that another portion may be used. The bed does not have to be remade, and the patient does not have to leave bed.

drepanocyte (sickle cell) *n. see* sickle-cell disease.

drepanocytosis *n. see* sickle-cell disease.

dressing *n.* material applied to a wound or diseased part of the body, with or without medication, to give protection and assist healing.

drill *n.* (in dentistry) a rotary instrument used to remove tooth substance, particularly in the treatment of caries. It consists of a handpiece that takes variously shaped *burs. Most drilling is done with an air-driven turbine handpiece, but some is performed with a much slower mechanically driven handpiece. Drills usually have a waterspray coolant.

drip (intravenous drip) *n.* apparatus for the continuous injection (*transfusion) of blood, plasma, saline, glucose solution, or other fluid into a vein. The fluid flows under gravity from a suspended bottle through a tube ending in a hollow needle inserted into the patient's vein. The rate of flow can be adjusted according to the rate of drips seen in a transparent section of the tube, which also serves as a trap for bubbles.

drom- (dromo-) *prefix denoting* movement or speed.

dromomania *n.* a pathologically strong impulse to travel, which is said to be present in some vagabonds.

dropsy *n. see* oedema.

Drosophila *n.* a genus of very small flies, commonly called fruit flies, that breed in decaying fruit and vegetables. *D. melanogaster* has been extensively used in genetic research as it has only four pairs of chromosomes and those in its salivary glands are easily recognizable. Adult *D. repleta* sometimes feed on faecal matter and may transmit disease organisms.

drostanolone *n.* a synthetic male sex hormone (*see* androgen) used in the treatment of breast cancer, often in conjunction with other drug treatment or surgery. It is administered by injection and with prolonged use may cause such side-effects as growth of hair and deepening of the voice. Trade name: **Masteril**.

drug *n.* any substance that affects the structure or functioning of a living organism. Drugs are widely used for the prevention, diagnosis, and treatment of disease and for the relief of symptoms. The term *medicine* is sometimes preferred for therapeutic drugs in order to distinguish them from narcotics and other addictive drugs that are used illegally.

drug dependence *see* dependence.

dry socket a painful condition in which the normal healing of a tooth socket has been disturbed. Instead of being filled with a blood clot the socket is empty. The cause is not clear; treatment is palliative and the condition resolves in 10–14 days.

Duchenne dystrophy *see* muscular dystrophy.

duct *n.* a tubelike structure or channel, especially one for carrying glandular secretions.

ductless gland *see* endocrine gland.

ductule *n.* a small duct or channel.

ductus *n.* a duct. The *ductus deferens* is the *vas deferens.

ductus arteriosus a blood vessel in the fetus connecting the pulmonary artery directly to the ascending aorta, so bypassing the pulmonary circulation. It normally closes after birth. Failure of the ductus to close (*patent ductus arteriosus*) produces a continuous *murmur, and the consequences are similar to those of a *septal defect. It may close spontaneously in childhood but often requires surgical closure.

dumbness *n. see* mutism.

Dumdum fever *see* kala-azar.

dumping syndrome a group of symptoms that sometimes occur after stomach operations, particularly *gastrectomy. After a meal, especially one rich in carbohydrate, the patient feels faint and weak and may sweat and become pale. The attack lasts 30 minutes to two hours and is caused by rapid stomach emptying, leading to falls in blood sugar and the drawing of fluid from the blood into the intestine. Avoidance of carbohydrate meals may relieve the syndrome but further surgery is sometimes required.

duo- *prefix denoting* two.

duoden- (duodeno-) *prefix denoting* the duodenum. Example: *duodenectomy* (excision of).

duodenal ulcer an ulcer in the duodenum, caused by the action of acid and pepsin on the duodenal lining (mucosa) of a susceptible individual. It is usually associated with an increased output of stomach acid and affects people with blood group O more commonly than others. Symptoms include pain in the upper abdomen, especially when the stomach is empty, which often disappears completely for weeks or months; vomiting may occur. Complications include bleeding, *perforation, and obstruction due to scarring. Symptoms are relieved by antacid medicines or reduction of stomach acid; surgery is sometimes required for a permanent cure (*see* gastrectomy, vagotomy).

duodenoscope *n.* a *fibrescope for examining the interior of the duodenum. An end-viewing instrument is used for most examinations, but a side-viewing instrument is used for *ERCP.

duodenostomy *n.* an operation in which the duodenum is brought through the abdominal wall and opened, usually in order to introduce food. *See also* gastroduodenostomy.

duodenum *n.* the first of the three parts of the small *intestine. It extends from the pylorus of the stomach to the jejunum. The duodenum receives bile from the gall bladder (via the common bile duct) and pancreatic juice from the pancreas. Its wall contains various glands (including *Brunner's glands*) that

secrete *succus entericus. —**duodenal** *adj.*

Dupuytren's contracture forward curvature of one or more fingers (usually the third and/or fourth) due to fixation of the flexor tendon of the affected finger to the skin of the palm. The condition is treated by surgical *division of the fibrous bands joining tendon and skin.

dura (dura mater, pachymeninx) *n.* the thickest and outermost of the three *meninges surrounding the brain and spinal cord. It consists of two closely adherent layers, the outer of which is identical with the periosteum of the skull. The inner dura extends downwards between the cerebral hemispheres to form the *falx cerebri* and forwards between the cerebrum and cerebellum to form the *tentorium*. A thin film of fluid (not cerebrospinal fluid) separates the inner dura from the arachnoid.

dural *adj.* of, relating to, or affecting the *dura.

dwarfism *n.* abnormally short stature from any cause. The most common type of dwarf is the *achondroplastic dwarf* (*see* achondroplasia). *Pituitary dwarfs* have a deficiency of *growth hormone due to a defect in the pituitary gland; they are well proportioned and show no mental retardation, but may be sexually underdeveloped. *Primordial dwarfs* have a genetic defect in their response to growth hormone. Dwarfism is also associated with thyroid deficiency (*see* cretinism), in which both physical and mental development is retarded; chronic diseases such as rickets; renal failure; and intestinal malabsorption.

dydrogesterone *n.* a synthetic female sex hormone (*see* progestogen) used to treat menstrual abnormalities (such as dysmenorrhoea) and infertility and to prevent miscarriage. It is administered by mouth and may cause mild nausea and breakthrough bleeding. Trade name: **Duphaston**.

dynamometer *n.* a device for recording the force of a muscular contraction. A small hand-held dynamometer may be used to record the strength of a patient's grip. A special optical dynamometer measures the action of the muscles controlling the shape of the lens of the eye.

dyne *n.* a unit of force equal to the force required to impart to a mass of 1 gram an acceleration of 1 centimetre per second per second. 1 dyne $= 10^{-5}$ newton.

-dynia *suffix denoting* pain. Example: *proctodynia* (in the rectum).

dys- *prefix denoting* difficult, abnormal, or impaired. Examples: *dysbasia* (difficulty in walking); *dysgeusia* (impairment of taste).

dysaesthesiae *pl. n.* the abnormal and sometimes unpleasant sensations felt by a patient with partial damage to a peripheral nerve when his skin is touched. *Compare* paraesthesiae.

dysarthria *n.* a speech disorder in which the pronunciation is unclear although the linguistic content and meaning are normal.

dysbarism *n.* any clinical syndrome due to a difference between the atmospheric pressure outside the body and the pressure of air or gas within a body cavity (such as the paranasal sinuses or the middle ear). *See* compressed air illness.

dysbulia *n.* any disturbance of the will or of the mental processes that lead to purposeful action.

dyschezia *n.* a form of constipation resulting from a long period of voluntary suppression of the urge to defecate. The rectum becomes distended with faeces and bowel movements are difficult or painful.

dyschondroplasia *n.* a condition due to faulty ossification of cartilage, resulting in development of many benign cartilaginous tumours (*see* chondroma). The bones involved may become stunted and deformed.

dyscrasia *n.* an abnormal state of the body or part of the body, especially one due to abnormal development or metabolism. In classical medicine the term was used for the imbalance of the four *humours, which was believed to be the basic cause of all diseases.

dysdiadochokinesis (adiadochokinesis) *n.* clumsiness in performing rapidly alternating movements. It is often recognized by asking the patient to tap with his fingers on the back of his other hand. It is a sign of disease of the cerebellum.

dysentery *n.* an infection of the intestinal tract causing severe diarrhoea with blood and mucus. *Amoebic dysentery* (*amoebiasis*) is caused by the protozoan *Entamoeba histolytica* and results in ulceration of the intestines and occasionally in the formation of abscesses in the liver (*see* hepatitis), lungs, testes, or brain. The parasite is spread by food or water contaminated by infected faeces. Symptoms appear days or even years after infection and include diarrhoea, indigestion, loss of weight, and anaemia. Prolonged treatment with drugs, including emetine and tetracyclines, is usually effective in treating the condition. Amoebic dysentery is mainly confined to tropical and subtropical countries.

Bacillary dysentery is caused by bacteria of the genus *Shigella* and is spread by contact with a patient or carrier or through food or water contaminated by their faeces. Epidemics are common in overcrowded insanitary conditions. Symptoms, which develop 1–6 days after infection, include diarrhoea, nausea, cramp, and fever and they persist for about a week. An attack may vary from mild diarrhoea to an acute infection causing serious dehydration and bleeding from the gut. In most cases, provided fluid losses are replaced, recovery occurs within 7–10 days; antibiotics may be given to eliminate the bacteria. *Compare* cholera.

dysgenesis *n.* faulty development; *gonadal dysgenesis* is failure of the ovaries or testes to develop (*see* Turner's syndrome).

dysgerminoma (germinoma, gonocytoma) *n.* a malignant tumour of the ovary, thought to arise from primitive germ cells; it is homologous to the *seminoma of the testis. About 15% of such tumours affect both ovaries; outside the ovary they have been recorded in the anterior mediastinum and near the pineal gland. Dysgerminomas may occur from infancy to old age, but the average age of patients is about 20 years. They are very sensitive to *radiotherapy. Dysgerminomas are also known as *large cell carcinomas* or *alveolar sarcomas of the ovary*.

dysgraphia *n. see* agraphia.

dysidrosis (dyshidrosis) *n.* any abnormality of sweating or the sweat glands other than excessive sweating (*hyperhidrosis*), diminished sweating (*hypohidrosis*), or absence of sweating (*anidrosis*); for example, changes in the colour or smell of sweat.

dyskinesia *n.* a group of involuntary movements that appear to be a fragmentation of the normal smoothly controlled limb and facial movements. They include *chorea, *dystonia, and those involuntary movements occurring as side-effects to the use of L-dopa and the phenothiazines.

dyslalia *n.* a speech disorder in which the patient uses a vocabulary or range of sounds that is peculiar to him. It is a feature of the defective speech acquired

by children who have been aphasic from birth (*see* aphasia).

dyslexia *n.* a developmental disorder selectively affecting a child's ability to learn to read and write. It is an uncommon condition, affecting boys more often than girls, and creates serious educational problems. It is sometimes called *specific dyslexia* or *developmental dyslexia* to distinguish it from acquired difficulties with reading and writing. *Compare* alexia. —**dyslexic** *adj.*

dyslogia *n.* disturbed and incoherent speech. This may be due to *dementia, *aphasia, *subnormality, or mental illness.

dysmenorrhoea *n.* painful or difficult menstruation. The most common type is *primary* (*essential*) *dysmenorrhoea*, which begins with the first period and has no apparent cause. In *secondary dysmenorrhoea* painful menstruation is experienced at some stage following the establishment of normal periods, for reasons including inflammation of the womb lining, the presence of tumours in the muscles of the womb, blockage of the blood flow, and mental disturbance.

dysmnesic syndrome a disorder of memory in which new information is not learned but old material is well remembered. *See* Korsakoff's syndrome.

dysmorphophobia *n.* a fixed distressing belief that one's body is deformed and repulsive, or an excessive fear that it might be so.

dyspareunia *n.* painful or difficult sexual intercourse experienced by a woman. Psychological or physical factors may be responsible (*see* vaginismus).

dyspepsia (indigestion) *n.* disordered digestion: usually applied to pain or discomfort in the lower chest or abdomen after eating and sometimes accompanied by nausea or vomiting. —**dyspeptic** *adj.*

dysphagia *n.* a condition in which the action of swallowing is either difficult to perform, painful (*see* odynophagia), or in which swallowed material seems to be held up in its passage to the stomach. It is caused by painful conditions of the mouth and throat, obstruction of the pharynx or oesophagus by diseases of the wall or pressure from outside, or by abnormalities of muscular activity of the pharynx or oesophagus.

dysphasia *n. see* aphasia.

dysphemia *n. see* stammering.

dysphonia *n.* difficulty in speaking due to a disorder of the larynx, vocal cords, tongue, or mouth. *Compare* dysarthria, aphasia.

dysplasia (alloplasia, heteroplasia) *n.* abnormal development of skin, bone, or other tissues. *See also* fibrous dysplasia.

dyspnoea *n.* laboured or difficult breathing. (The term is often used for a sign of laboured breathing apparent to the doctor, *breathlessness* being used for the subjective feeling of laboured breathing.) Dyspnoea can be due to obstruction to the flow of air into and out of the lungs (as in bronchitis and asthma), various diseases affecting the tissue of the lung (including pneumoconiosis, emphysema, tuberculosis, and cancer), and heart disease.

dyspraxia *n. see* apraxia.

dyssynergia (asynergia) *n.* clumsily uncoordinated movements found in patients with disease of the cerebellum. They include *dysmetria* (the application of inappropriate force for a movement), intention *tremor, *dysdiadochokinesis, and a staggering wide-based gait.

dystocia *n.* difficult birth, caused by abnormalities in the fetus or the mother. The most common causes of *fetal dystocia* are excessive size or *malpresentation of the baby. *Maternal dystocia* may result if the pelvis is abnormally small, the womb muscles fail to contract, or the neck of the womb fails to expand. If the cause of dystocia cannot be eliminated, it may be necessary to deliver the baby by Caesarean section or to operate in such a way that it can be removed with the minimum possible risk to the mother.

dystonia *n.* a postural disorder caused by disease of the *basal ganglia in the brain. There is spasm in the muscles of the shoulders, neck, and trunk. The arm is often held in a rotated position and the head is drawn back and to one side.

dystrophia myotonica a type of *muscular dystrophy in which the muscle weakness and wasting is accompanied by an unnatural prolongation of the muscular contraction after any voluntary effort (*see* myotonia). The muscles of the face, temples, and neck are especially wasted. Baldness, endocrine malfunction, and cataracts also occur. The disease can affect both sexes (it is inherited as an autosomal dominant character) and appears in early middle age.

dystrophy (dystrophia) *n.* a disorder of an organ or tissue, usually muscle, due to impaired nourishment of the affected part. The term is applied to several unrelated conditions; for example, *muscular dystrophy and *dystrophia adiposogenitalis* (*see* Fröhlich's syndrome).

dysuria *n.* difficult or painful urination. This is usually associated with urgency and frequency of urination if due to *cystitis or *urethritis. The pain is burning in nature and is relieved by curing the underlying cause. A high fluid intake usually helps.

E

ear *n.* the sense organ concerned with hearing and balance (see illustration). Sound waves, transmitted from the outside into the external auditory meatus, cause the eardrum (tympanic membrane) to vibrate. The small bones (ossicles) of the middle ear – the malleus, incus, and stapes – transmit the sound vibrations to the fenestra ovalis, which leads to the inner ear (*see* labyrinth). Inside the *cochlea the sound vibrations are converted into nerve impulses. Vibrations emerging from the cochlea could cause pressure to build up inside the ear, but this is released through the *Eustachian tube. The *semicircular canals, *saccule, and *utricle – also in the inner ear – are all concerned with balance.

earache *n. see* otitis, otalgia.

eardrum *n. see* tympanic membrane.

earwax *n. see* cerumen.

eburnation *n.* the wearing down of the cartilage at the articulating surface of a bone, exposing the underlying bone. This is an end result of *osteoarthritis.

ec- *prefix denoting* out of or outside.

ecbolic *n.* an agent, such as *oxytocin, that induces childbirth by stimulating contractions of the womb.

ecchondroma *n.* (*pl.* **ecchondromata**) a benign cartilaginous tumour (*see* chondroma) that protrudes beyond the margins of a bone. *Compare* enchondroma.

ecchymosis *n.* a bruise: an initially bluish-black mark on the skin, resulting from the release of blood into the tissues either through injury or through the spontaneous leaking of blood from the vessels (as in some blood diseases).

eccrine *adj.* **1.** describing sweat glands that are distributed all over the body. Their ducts open directly onto the surface of the skin and they are densest on the soles of the feet and the palms of

Structure of the ear

the hands. *Compare* apocrine. **2.** *see* merocrine.

eccyesis *n.* *see* ectopic pregnancy.

ecdemic *adj.* not occurring normally in the population of a country: applied sometimes to unusual diseases brought in from abroad by immigrants or travellers. *Compare* endemic.

ecdysis *n.* the act of shedding skin; *desquamation.

ECG *n.* *see* electrocardiogram.

echinococciasis (echinococcosis) *n.* *see* hydatid disease.

Echinococcus *n.* a genus of small parasitic tapeworms that reach a maximum length of only 8 mm. Adults are found in the intestines of dogs, wolves, or jackals. If the eggs are swallowed by man, who can act as a secondary host, the resulting larvae penetrate the intestine and settle in the lungs, liver, or brain to form large cysts, usually 5–10 cm in diameter (*see* hydatid disease). Two species causing this condition are *E. granulosus* and *E. multilocularis*.

echoacousia *n.* a false sensation of echoing after normally heard sound.

echocardiography *n.* the use of *ultrasound waves to investigate and display the action of the heart as it beats.

echoencephalography *n.* investigation of structures within the skull by detecting the echoes of ultrasonic pulses. The chief value of the method is in detecting those disorders causing a displacement of the midline structures of the brain.

echography *n.* the technique of using *ultrasound waves to map out and study the internal structure of the body. Ultrasound waves are reflected to different degrees by different structures within the body. The visual recording of these reflected waves is called an *echogram*. *See also* ultrasonics.

echokinesis *n.* *see* echopraxia.

echolalia *n.* pathological repetition of the words spoken by another person. It may be a symptom of language disorders, *autism, *catatonia, or *Gilles de la Tourette syndrome.

echopraxia (echokinesis) *n.* pathological imitation of the actions of another person. It may be a symptom of *catatonia or of *latah.

echotomography *n.* *see* ultrasonotomography.

echovirus *n.* one of a group of about 30 RNA-containing viruses, originally isolated from the human intestinal tract, that were found to produce pathological changes in cells grown in culture, although they were not clearly associated with any specific disease. These viruses – which were accordingly termed *enteric cytopathic human orphan* viruses – are now thought to be the cause of nonspecific meningitis, many gastrointestinal and respiratory tract infections, and of many illnesses producing symptoms of the common cold. *Compare* reovirus.

eclabium *n.* the turning outward of a lip.

eclampsia *n.* a rare and serious condition, affecting women either at the end of pregnancy or shortly after childbirth, in which the whole body is affected by convulsions and the patient eventually passes into a coma. Blood pressure is high, the urine contains proteins, and the ankles and other parts swell because of the accumulation of water in the tissues (oedema). Eclampsia is a threat to the life of both baby and mother. It represents an advanced stage of *toxaemia of pregnancy and can be prevented by regular antenatal examinations.

ecology (bionomics) *n.* the study of the relationships between man, plants and animals, and the environment, including the way in which human activities may affect other animal populations and alter natural surroundings. —**ecological** *adj.* —**ecologist** *n.*

ecraseur *n.* a surgical device, resembling a *snare, that is used to sever the base of a tumour during its surgical removal.

ecstasy *n.* a sense of extreme well-being and bliss. The word applies particularly to *trance states dominated by religious thinking. While not necessarily pathological, it can be caused by epilepsy (especially of the temporal lobe) or by schizophrenia.

ECT *see* electroconvulsive therapy.

ect- (ecto-) *prefix denoting* outer or external.

ectasia (ectasis) *n.* the dilatation of a tube, duct, or hollow organ.

ecthyma *n.* a skin disease – an ulcerative type of *impetigo – in which the infection spreads down to the lower layer of the skin (dermis). Ecthyma heals more slowly than ordinary impetigo and causes scarring.

ectoderm *n.* the outer of the three *germ layers of the early embryo. It gives rise to the nervous system and sense organs, the teeth and lining of the mouth, and the *epidermis and its associated structures (hair, nails, etc.). —**ectodermal** *adj.*

ectomorphic *adj.* describing a *body type that is relatively thin, with a large skin surface in comparison to weight. —**ectomorph** *n.* —**ectomorphy** *n.*

-ectomy *suffix denoting* surgical removal of a segment or all of an organ or part. Examples: *appendicectomy* (of the appendix); *prostatectomy* (of the prostate gland).

ectoparasite *n.* a parasite that lives on the outer surface of its host. Some ectoparasites, such as bed bugs, maintain only periodic contact with their hosts, whereas others, such as the crab louse, have a permanent association. *Compare* endoparasite.

ectopia *n.* **1.** the misplacement, due either to a congenital defect or injury, of a bodily part. **2.** the occurrence of something in an unnatural location (*see* ectopic beat, ectopic pregnancy). —**ectopic** *adj.*

ectopic beat (extrasystole) a heart beat due to an impulse generated somewhere in the heart outside the sinoatrial node. Ectopic beats are generally premature in timing; they are classified as *supraventricular* if they originate in the atria and *ventricular* if they arise from a focus in the ventricles. They may be produced by any heart disease, by nicotine from smoking, or by caffeine from excessive tea or coffee consumption; they are common in normal individuals. The patient may be unaware of their presence or may feel that his heart has 'missed a beat'. Ectopic beats may be suppressed by drugs such as quinidine, propranolol, and lignocaine; avoidance of smoking and reduction in excessive tea or coffee intake may help. *See* arrhythmia.

ectopic pregnancy (extrauterine pregnancy) the development of a fetus at a site other than in the womb. This may happen if the fertilized egg cell remains in the ovary or in the tube leading from near the ovary to the womb (the Fallopian tube) or if it lodges in the free abdominal cavity. The most common type of ectopic pregnancy is a *tubal* (or *oviducal*) *pregnancy*, which occurs in Fallopian tubes that become blocked or inflamed. The growth of the fetus may cause the tube to burst and bleed. In most cases the fetus dies within three months of conception and is absorbed into the woman's body. However, development sometimes continues to a stage at which a live baby can be delivered by Caesarean section. Medical name: **eccyesis**.

ectoplasm *n.* the outer layer of cytoplasm in cells, which is denser than the inner cytoplasm (*endoplasm) and concerned with activities such as cell movement. —**ectoplasmic** *adj.*

ectro- *prefix denoting* congenital absence.

ectrodactyly *n.* congenital absence of all or part of one or more fingers.

ectromelia *n.* congenital absence or gross shortening (aplasia) of the long bones of one or more limbs. *See also* amelia, hemimelia, phocomelia.

ectropion *n.* turning out of the eyelid, away from the eyeball. The commonest type is *senile ectropion*, in which the lower eyelid droops because of loss of the elasticity of its tissues in old age. If the muscle that closes the eye (orbicularis oculi) is paralysed the lower lid also droops. Ectropion may also occur if the lining membrane (conjunctiva) of the lid is very thickened or if scarring causes contraction of the skin.

eczema *n.* a superficial inflammation of the skin, mainly affecting the *epidermis. Eczema causes itching, with a red rash often accompanied by small blisters that weep and become crusted. Subsequent scaling, thickening, or discoloration of the skin may occur. The disorder has several forms, with two major divisions: *eczematous dermatitis*, which results from external factors (*see* dermatitis); and *endogenous* (or *constitutional*) *eczema*, occurring without any obvious external cause. Classification of endogenous eczema is based on its appearance and site. The five types are *atopic*, commonly found in childhood and sometimes associated with a family history of allergy; *discoid*, characterized by small well-defined areas of eczema; *pompholyx, found on the hands and feet; *seborrhoeic*, in which scaly plaques occur in areas of the greatest sebum production (the scalp, face, etc.); and *varicose*, which develops on the legs in association with poor circulation. Treatment of eczema depends on the cause but usually includes the use of locally applied corticosteroids. —**eczematous** *adj.*

edentulous *adj.* lacking teeth: usually applied to people who have lost their teeth.

edrophonium *n.* a drug that stimulates skeletal muscles (*see* parasympathomimetic). It is administered by injection in a test for diagnosis of *myasthenia gravis. Side-effects can include nausea and vomiting, increased saliva flow, diarrhoea, and stomach pains. Trade name: **Tensilon**.

EDTA (**ethylenediamine tetra-acetic acid**) a compound used as a *chelating agent in the treatment of poisoning with several different metals, such as lead and strontium. It is normally administered in the form of its calcium sodium salt, called *calcium sodium edetate*.

EEG (**electroencephalogram**) *see* electroencephalography.

effector *n.* any structure or agent that brings about activity in a muscle or gland, such as a motor nerve that causes muscular contraction or glandular secretion. The term is also used for the muscle or gland itself.

efferent *adj.* **1.** designating nerves or neurones that convey impulses from the brain or spinal cord to muscles, glands, and other effectors; i.e. any motor nerve or neurone. **2.** designating vessels or ducts that drain fluid (such as lymph) from an organ or part. *Compare* afferent.

effleurage *n.* a form of *massage in which the hands are passed continuously and rhythmically over a patient's skin in one direction only, with the aim of increasing blood flow in that direction and aiding the dispersal of any swelling due to *oedema.

effort syndrome a condition of marked anxiety about the condition of one's heart and circulatory system. This is accompanied by a heightened consciousness of heartbeat and respiration, which in turn is worsened by the anxiety it induces. Treatment is commonly with reassurance and *tranquillizers; psychotherapy is only occasionally necessary.

effusion *n.* **1.** the escape of pus, serum, blood, lymph, or other fluid into a body cavity as a result of inflammation or the presence of excess blood or tissue fluid in an organ or tissue. **2.** fluid that has escaped into a body cavity.

egg cell *see* ovum.

ego *n.* (in psychoanalysis) the part of the mind that develops from a person's experience of the outside world and is most in touch with external realities. In Freudian terms the ego is said to reconcile the demands of the *id (the instinctive unconscious mind), the *superego (moral conscience), and reality.

eidetic *adj. see* imagery.

eikonometer *n.* an instrument for measuring the size of images on the retina of the eye.

Eisenmenger reaction a condition in which *pulmonary hypertension is associated with a *septal defect, so that blood flows from the right to the left side of the heart or from the pulmonary artery to the aorta. This allows blue blood, poor in oxygen, to bypass the lungs and enter the general circulation. This reduces the oxygen content of the arterial blood in the aorta and its branches, resulting in a patient with a dusky blue appearance (*cyanosis) and an increased number of red blood cells (*polycythaemia). There is no curative treatment at this stage, but the patient may be helped by the control of heart failure and polycythaemia. The condition may be prevented by appropriate treatment of the septal defect before

irreversible pulmonary hypertension develops.

ejaculation *n.* the discharge of semen from the erect penis at the moment of sexual climax (orgasm) in the male. The constituents of semen are not released simultaneously, but in the following sequence: the secretion of *Cowper's glands followed by that of the *prostate gland and the spermatozoa and finally the secretion of the *seminal vesicles. *See also* premature ejaculation.

elastic cartilage a type of *cartilage in which elastic fibres are distributed in the matrix. It is yellowish in colour and is found in the external ear.

elastic tissue strong extensible flexible *connective tissue rich in yellow *elastic fibres*. These are long, thin, and branching and are composed primarily of an albumin-like protein, *elastin*. Elastic tissue is found in the dermis of the skin, in arterial walls, and in the walls of the alveoli of the lungs.

elastin *n.* protein forming the major constituent of *elastic tissue fibres.

elastosis *n.* degeneration of the yellow fibres in connective tissues and skin (*see* elastic tissue).

elation (exaltation) *n.* a state of cheerful excitement and enthusiasm. Marked elation of mood is a characteristic of *mania or *hypomania.

electroanaesthesia *n.* local or general anaesthesia (usually the latter) brought about by passing an electric current through the tissues.

electrocardiogram (ECG) *n.* a recording of the electrical activity of the heart on a moving paper strip (see illustration). The ECG tracing is recorded by means of an apparatus called an *electrocardiograph* (*see* electrocardiography). It aids in the diagnosis of heart disease, which may produce characteristic changes in the ECG.

Typical electrocardiograms

electrocardiography *n.* a technique for recording the electrical activity of the heart. Electrodes connected to the recording apparatus (*electrocardiograph*) are placed on the skin of the four limbs and chest wall; the record itself is called an *electrocardiogram (ECG). In conventional *scalar electrocardiography* 12 leads (*see* lead[2]) are recorded, but more may be employed in special circumstances (for example, an oesophageal lead, from an electrode within the gullet, may be used in the analysis of arrhythmias).

Vectorcardiography is less commonly used in Britain, but may be employed to obtain a three-dimensional impression of electrical activity of the heart.

electrocardiophonography *n.* a technique for recording heart sounds and murmurs simultaneously with the ECG, which is used as a reference tracing. The sound is picked up by a microphone placed over the heart. The tracing is ·a *phonocardiogram*. It provides a permanent record of heart sounds and murmurs and is useful in their analysis.

electrocautery (galvanocautery) *n.* the destruction of diseased or unwanted tissue by means of a needle or snare that is electrically heated (*see* dia-

thermy). Warts, polyps, and other growths can be burned away by this method; the electricity does not pass through the tissues themselves.

electrocoagulation *n.* the coagulation of tissues by means of a high-frequency electric current concentrated at one point as it passes through them. Electrocoagulation, using a *diathermy knife, permits bloodless incisions to be made during operation.

electroconvulsive therapy (ECT) a treatment for severe depression and occasionally for schizophrenia and mania. A convulsion is produced by passing an electric current through the brain. The convulsion is modified by giving a *muscle relaxant drug and an *anaesthetic, so that in fact only a few muscle twitches are produced. The means by which ECT acts is not yet known. The procedure can also produce confusion, loss of memory, and headache, which almost always pass off within a few hours. These side-effects are reduced by unilateral treatment, in which the current is passed only through the nondominant hemisphere of the brain.

electrodesiccation *n. see* fulguration.

electroencephalogram (EEG) *n. see* electroencephalography.

electroencephalography *n.* the technique for recording the electrical activity from different parts of the brain and converting it into a tracing called an *electroencephalogram (EEG).* The machine that records this activity is known as an *encephalograph.* The pattern of the EEG reflects the state of the patient's brain and his level of consciousness in a characteristic manner. Electroencephalography is used to detect and locate structural disease, such as tumours, in the brain; it is also used in the diagnosis and management of epilepsy.

electrokymography *n.* the technique of recording the movements of an organ, especially the heart, by means of a *fluoroscope and a photoelectric recording system.

electrolyte *n.* a solution that produces ions (an ion is an atom or group of atoms that conduct electricity); for example, sodium chloride solution consists of free sodium and free chloride ions. In medical usage electrolyte usually means the ion itself; thus the term *serum electrolyte level* means the concentration of separate ions (sodium, potassium, chloride, bicarbonate, etc.) in the circulating blood. Concentrations of various electrolyte levels can be altered by many diseases, in which electrolytes are lost from the body (as in vomiting or diarrhoea) or are not excreted and accumulate (as in renal failure). When electrolyte concentrations are severely diminished they can be corrected by administering the appropriate substance by mouth or by intravenous drip. When excess of an electrolyte exists it may be removed by *dialysis or by special resins in the intestine, taken by mouth or by enema.

electromyography *n.* continuous recording of the electrical activity of a muscle by means of electrodes inserted into the muscle fibres. The tracing is displayed on an oscilloscope. The technique is used for diagnosing various nerve and muscle disorders and assessing progress in recovery from some forms of paralysis.

electronarcosis *n.* the induction of sleep by passing weak electrical currents through the brain. It is seldom used in Western psychiatry.

electron microscope a microscope that uses a beam of electrons as a radiation source for viewing the specimen. The resolving power (ability to register fine detail) is a thousand times greater than that of an ordinary light microscope. The specimen must be examined in a vacuum, which necessitates special techniques for preparing it,

and the electrons are usually focused onto a fluorescent screen (for direct viewing) or onto a photographic plate (for a photograph, or *electron micrograph*). A *transmission electron microscope* is used to examine thin sections at high magnification. A *scanning electron microscope* reveals the surfaces of objects at various magnifications; its great depth of focus is advantageous.

electron transport chain a series of enzymes and proteins in living cells through which electrons are transferred, via a series of oxidation-reduction reactions. This ultimately leads to the conversion of chemical energy into a readily usable and storable form. The most important electron transport chain is the *respiratory chain*, present in mitochondria and functioning in cellular respiration.

electrooculography *n.* an electrical method of recording eye movements. Tiny electrodes are attached to the skin at the inner and outer corners of the eye, and as the eye moves an alteration in the potential between these electrodes is recorded. The size of this potential at rest also gives an indication of the health of the retina.

electrophoresis *n.* the technique of separating electrically charged particles, particularly proteins, in a solution by passing an electric current through the solution. The rate of movement of the different components depends upon their charge, so that they gradually separate into bands. Electrophoresis is widely used in the investigation of body chemicals, such as the analysis of the different proteins in blood serum.

electroretinography *n.* a method of recording changes in the electrical potential of the retina when it is stimulated by light. One electrode is placed on the eye in a contact lens and the other is usually attached to the back of the head. In retinal disease the pattern of electrical change is altered. The technique is useful in diagnosing retinal diseases when such things as cataract make it difficult to see the retina or when the disease produces little visible change in the retina.

electrotherapy *n.* the passage of electric currents through the body's tissues to stimulate the functioning of nerves and the muscles that they supply. The technique is used to bring about improvement in the muscles of patients with various forms of paralysis due to nerve disease or muscle disorder. *See also* faradism, galvanism.

electuary *n.* a pharmaceutical preparation in which the drug is made up into a paste with syrup or honey.

elephantiasis *n.* gross enlargement of the skin and underlying connective tissues caused by obstruction of the lymph vessels, which prevents drainage of lymph from the surrounding tissues. Inflammation and thickening of the walls of the vessels and their eventual blocking is commonly caused by the parasitic filarial worms *Wuchereria bancrofti* and *Brugia malayi*. The parts most commonly affected are the legs but the scrotum, breasts, and vulva may also be involved. Elastic bandaging is applied to the affected parts and the limbs are elevated and rested. Larval forms in the blood are killed with diethylcarbamazine. *See also* filariasis.

elevator *n.* **1.** an instrument that is used to raise a depressed broken bone, for example in the skull or cheek. A specialized *periosteal elevator* is used in orthopaedics to strip the fibrous tissue (periosteum) covering bone. **2.** a lever-like instrument used to ease a tooth out of its socket during extraction.

elimination *n.* (in physiology) the entire process of excretion of metabolic waste products from the blood by the kidneys and urinary tract.

elixir *n.* a preparation containing alcohol (ethanol) or glycerine, which is used as the vehicle for bitter or nauseous drugs.

elliptocytosis *n.* the presence of significant numbers of abnormal elliptical red cells (*elliptocytes*) in the blood. Elliptocytosis may occur as a hereditary disorder or be a feature of certain blood diseases, such as *myelofibrosis or iron-deficiency *anaemia.

elutriation *n.* the separation of a fine powder from a coarser powder by mixing them with water and decanting the upper layer while it still contains the finer particles. The heavier coarse particles sink to the bottom more rapidly.

em- *prefix. see* en-.

emaciation *n.* wasting of the body, caused by such conditions as malnutrition, tuberculosis, cancer, or parasitic worms.

emaculation *n.* the removal of spots, freckles, or similar marks from the skin, usually by surgery.

emasculation *n.* strictly, surgical removal of the penis. The term is often used to mean loss of male physical and emotional characteristics, either as a result of removal of the testes (castration) or of emotional stress.

embalming *n.* the preservation of a dead body by the introduction of chemical compounds that delay putrefaction. The ancient Egyptians raised the process to a fine art in the production of their mummies. Today embalming is employed mainly so that a body can be transported long distances and funeral rites can be conducted without undue haste. In the USA embalming is a routine hygienic measure.

embedding *n.* (in microscopy) the fixing of a specimen within a mass of firm material in order to facilitate the cutting of thin sections for microscopi-

embolectomy

cal study. The embedding medium, e.g. paraffin wax for light microscopy or Araldite for electron microscopy, helps to keep the specimen intact.

embolectomy *n.* surgical removal of an *embolus in order to relieve arterial obstruction. The embolus may be removed ·by cutting directly into the affected artery (*arteriotomy*). In some instances it is removed by a balloon *catheter, which is manipulated beyond the embolus from a small arteriotomy in an accessible artery. The catheter is then withdrawn carrying the embolus with it. In some cases of pulmonary embolism, embolectomy may be life saving. It may also prevent gangrene, with loss of a limb, in cases of a limb artery embolus.

embolism *n.* the condition in which an embolus becomes lodged in an artery and obstructs its blood flow. The most common form of embolism is *pulmonary embolism, in which a blood clot is carried in the circulation to lodge in the pulmonary artery. An embolus in any other artery constitutes a *systemic embolism*. In this case a common source of the embolus is a blood clot within the heart in mitral valve disease or following *myocardial infarction. The clinical features depend upon the site at which an embolus lodges (for example, a stroke may result from a cerebral embolism and gangrene from a limb embolism).
Treatment is by *anticoagulant therapy with heparin and warfarin. Major embolism is treated by *embolectomy or *streptokinase to remove or dissolve the embolus. *See also* air embolism.

embolus *n.* (*pl.* **emboli**) material, such as a blood clot, fat, air, amniotic fluid, or a foreign body, that is carried by the blood from one point in the circulation to lodge at another point (*see* embolism).

embrasure *n.* the space formed between adjacent teeth.

embrocation *n.* a lotion that is rubbed onto the body for the treatment of sprains and strains.

embryo *n.* an animal at an early stage of development, before birth. In man the term refers to the products of conception within the womb in the first eight weeks of development, during which time all the main organs are formed (see illustration). *Compare* fetus. —**embryonic** *adj.*

embryology *n.* the study of growth and development of the embryo and fetus from fertilization of the ovum until birth. —**embryological** *adj.*

embryonic disc the early embryo before the formation of *somites. It is a flat disc of tissue bounded dorsally by the amniotic cavity and ventrally by the yolk sac. The formation of the *primitive streak and *archenteron in the embryonic disc determines the orientation of the embryo, which then becomes progressively elongated.

embryotomy *n.* the cutting up of a fetus during difficult birth by means of an instrument called an *embryotome*, in order to aid delivery and reduce the danger to the mother.

emesis *n. see* vomiting.

emetic *n.* an agent that causes vomiting. Strong emetics, such as *apomorphine, are used to induce vomiting following drug overdose. Substances such as common salt, which irritate the stomach nerves if taken in sufficient quantities, also cause vomiting. Some emetics, e.g. *ipecacuanha, are *expectorants at low doses.

emetine *n.* a drug used to treat infections of the liver, bowel, and intestine caused by amoebae, including amoebic dysentery. It is administered by injection, which may be painful, and irritates the stomach lining and other mucous membranes.

A developing embryo

eminence *n.* a projection, often rounded, on an organ or tissue, particularly on a bone. An example is the *iliopubic eminence* on the hip bone.

Emiscan *n.* trade name for *computerized axial tomography.

emissary veins a group of veins within the skull that drain blood from the venous sinuses of the dura mater to veins outside the skull.

emission *n.* the flow of semen from the erect penis, usually occurring while the subject is asleep (*nocturnal emission*).

emmenagogue *n.* an agent that stimulates menstruation.

emmetropia *n.* the state of refraction of the normal eye, in which parallel light rays are brought to a focus on the retina with the accommodation relaxed. Objects further than six metres from the eye are seen clearly without any effort to focus. *Compare* ametropia, hypermetropia, myopia.

emollient *n.* an agent that soothes and softens the skin. Emollients are fats and oils, such as lanolin and liquid paraffin;

they are used chiefly in skin preparations as a base for more active drugs, such as antibiotics.

emotion *n.* a state of arousal that can be experienced as pleasant or unpleasant. Emotions can have three components: *subjective*, *physiological*, and *behavioural*. For example, fear can involve an unpleasant subjective experience, an increase in physiological measures such as heart rate, sweating, etc., and a tendency to flee from the fear-provoking situation.

empathy *n.* the ability to understand the thoughts and emotions of another person. In a psychotherapist empathy is often considered to be one of the necessary qualities enabling successful treatment.

emphysema *n.* air in the tissues. In *pulmonary emphysema* the air sacs (*alveoli) of the lungs are enlarged and damaged, which reduces the surface area for the exchange of oxygen and carbon dioxide. Severe emphysema causes breathlessness, which is made worse by infections. There is no specific treatment, and the patient may become

197

dependent on oxygen. The mechanism by which emphysema develops is not understood, although it is known to be particularly common in men in Britain and is associated with chronic bronchitis, smoking, and advancing age.

In *surgical emphysema* air may escape into the tissues of the chest and neck from leaks in the lungs or oesophagus; occasionally air escapes into other tissues during surgery, and bacteria may form gas in soft tissues. The presence of gas or air gives the affected tissues a characteristic crackling feeling to the touch, and it may be visible on X-rays. It is easily absorbed once the leak or production is stopped.

empirical *adj.* describing a system of treatment based on experience or observation, rather than of logic or reason.

Employment Service Division (ESD) (in Britain) an integral part of the *Manpower Services Commission* (*MSC*) established in 1974 to take over responsibility from the Department of Employment for running public employment services. Along with the *Training Services Division* (*TSD*), it has special responsibility to employ and if necessary train (or retrain) those who are handicapped from any cause. Its *Disablement Resettlement Service* relies on specially trained Officers (*DRO*) who see that those with handicaps find satisfactory employment situations. Recommendations made by DRO include that of registration as *disabled people*, which helps in obtaining and retaining employment. Other ways of assisting include referral to one of 26 *Employment Rehabilitation Centres* for assessment of potential and/or reacclimatization to a working environment for those who have been absent from work through ill-health over a long period. Special training courses may be arranged for handicapped people as part of the *Training Opportunities Scheme* (*TOPS*) of the TSD. These courses, covering a wide range of skilled and semiskilled occupations and lasting about six months, may be held at colleges, *special skill centres*, or at the premises of potential employers. For the blind there are special *Blind Persons Resettlement Officers* (*BPRO*), though *total* blindness is not a prerequisite for registration.

empyema (pyothorax) *n.* pus in the *pleural cavity, usually secondary to infection in the lung or in the space below the diaphragm. It is a life-threatening condition, which can usually only be relieved by surgical drainage of the pus.

emulsion *n.* a preparation in which fine droplets of one liquid (such as oil) are dispersed in another liquid (such as water). In pharmacy medicines are prepared in the form of emulsions to disguise the taste of an oil, which is dispersed in a flavoured liquid.

en- (em-) *prefix denoting* in; inside.

enamel *n.* the extremely hard outer covering of the crown of a *tooth. It is formed before tooth eruption by *ameloblasts.

enanthema *n.* an eruption occurring on a mucus-secreting surface, such as the inside of the mouth or vagina.

enarthrosis *n.* a ball-and-socket joint: a type of *diarthrosis (freely movable joint), e.g. the shoulder joint and the hip joint. Such a joint always involves a long bone, which is thus allowed to move in all planes.

encapsulated *adj.* (of an organ, tumour, etc.) enclosed in a capsule.

encephal- (encephalo-) *prefix denoting* the brain.

encephalin (enkephalin) *n.* either of two peptides occurring naturally in the brain and having effects resembling those of morphine or other opiates. *See also* endorphin.

encephalitis *n.* inflammation of the brain. It may be caused by a viral or bacterial infection or it may be part of an allergic response to a systemic viral illness or vaccination (*see* encephalomyelitis). *Viral encephalitis* is endemic in some parts of the world; it may also occur epidemically or sporadically. One form – *encephalitis lethargica* – reached epidemic proportions shortly after World War I and was marked by headache and drowsiness, progressing to coma (hence its popular name – *sleepy sickness*). Occasional cases still occur as a complication of mumps. It can cause postencephalitic *parkinsonism. Another type of encephalitis that occurs sporadically is due to herpes simplex.

encephalocele *n.* *see* neural tube defects.

encephalography *n.* any of various techniques for recording the structure of the brain or the activity of the brain cells. Examples are *echoencephalography, *electroencephalography, and *pneumoencephalography.

encephaloid *adj.* having the appearance of brain tissue: applied to certain tumours, for example *encephaloid carcinoma of the breast*.

encephalomyelitis *n.* an acute inflammatory disease affecting the brain and spinal cord. It is sometimes part of an overwhelming virus infection but *acute disseminated encephalomyelitis* is a form of delayed tissue hypersensitivity provoked by a mild infection or vaccination 7–10 days earlier. Survival through the acute phase of the illness is often followed by a remarkably complete recovery.

encephalomyelopathy *n.* any condition in which there is widespread disease of the brain and spinal cord. *Necrotizing encephalomyelopathy of childhood* is a progressive illness with extensive destruction of nerve cells throughout the central nervous system. It is thought to be caused by a disorder of metabolism.

encephalon *n.* *see* brain.

encephalopathy *n.* any of various diseases that affect the functioning of the brain. *See* hepatic encephalopathy, Wernicke's encephalopathy.

enchondroma *n.* (*pl.* **enchondromata**) a benign cartilaginous tumour (*see* chondroma) occurring in the growing zone (metaphysis) of a bone and not protruding beyond its margins. Such tumours are often solitary; when multiple the condition is known as *enchondromatosis*. *Compare* ecchondroma.

encopresis *n.* incontinence of faeces. The term is used for faecal soiling associated with psychiatric disturbance.

encounter group a form of group psychotherapy. The emphasis is on encouraging close relationships between group members and on the expression of feelings. To this end, physical contact and confrontations between group members are arranged by the group leader. The stress of the experience can be damaging to maladjusted people.

encysted *adj.* enclosed in a cyst.

end- (endo-) *prefix denoting* within or inner. Example: *endonasal* (within the nose).

endarterectomy *n.* a surgical 're-bore' of an artery that has become obstructed by *atheroma with or without a blood clot (thrombus); the former operation is known as *thromboendarterectomy*. The inner part of the wall is removed together with any clot that is present. This restores patency and arterial blood flow to the tissues beyond the obstruction. The technique is most often applied to obstruction of the carotid arteries or of the arteries that supply the legs.

endarteritis *n.* chronic inflammation of the inner (intimal) portion of the wall of an artery, which most often results from late syphilis. Thickening of the wall produces progressive arterial obstruction and symptoms from inadequate blood supply to the affected part (*ischaemia). The arteries to the brain are often involved, giving rise to meningovascular syphilis. Endarteritis of the aorta may obstruct the mouths of the coronary arteries, supplying the heart. Endarteritis of the arteries to the wall of the aorta (the vasa vasorum) contributes to *aneurysm formation. The syphilitic infection may be eradicated with penicillin.

end artery the terminal branch of an artery, which does not communicate with other branches. The tissue it supplies is therefore probably completely dependent on it for its blood supply.

endemic *adj.* occurring frequently in a particular region or population: applied to diseases that are generally or constantly found among people in a particular area. *Compare* ecdemic, epidemic, pandemic.

endemic syphilis *see* bejel.

endocarditis *n.* inflammation of the lining of the heart cavity (endocardium) and valves. It is most often due to rheumatic fever or results from bacterial infection (*bacterial endocarditis*). Temporary or permanent damage to the heart valves may result. The main features are fever, changing heart murmurs, heart failure, and embolism. Treatment consists of rest and *antibiotics; surgery may be required to repair damaged heart valves.

endocardium *n.* a delicate membrane, formed of flat endothelial cells, that lines the heart and is continuous with the lining of arteries and veins. At the openings of the heart cavities it is folded back on itself to form the cusps of the valves. It presents a smooth slippery surface, which does not impede blood flow. —**endocardial** *adj.*

endocervicitis *n.* inflammation of the membrane lining the neck of the womb, usually resulting from infection. Surface cells (epithelium) may die, resulting in a new growth of healthy epithelium over the affected area. The condition is accompanied by a white or yellow discharge.

endocervix *n.* the mucous membrane (*endometrium) lining the neck (cervix) of the womb.

endochondral *adj.* within the material of a cartilage.

endocrine gland (ductless gland) a gland that manufactures one or more *hormones and secretes them directly into the bloodstream (and not through a duct to the exterior). Endocrine glands include the pituitary, thyroid, parathyroid, and adrenal glands, the ovary and testis, the placenta, and part of the pancreas.

endocrinology *n.* the study of the *endocrine glands and the substances they secrete (*hormones). —**endocrinologist** *n.*

endoderm *n.* the inner of the three *germ layers of the early embryo, which gives rise to the lining of most of the alimentary canal and its associated glands, the liver, gall bladder, and pancreas. It also forms the lining of the bronchi and alveoli of the lung and most of the urinary tract.

endodontics *n.* the study and treatment of diseases of the pulps of teeth and their sequelae. A major part of treatment is *root treatment.

endogenous *adj.* arising within or derived from the body. For example, *endogenous depression* arises from causes inside the body (*see* depression). *Compare* exogenous.

endolymph *n.* the fluid that fills the membranous *labyrinth of the ear.

endolymphatic duct a blind-ended duct that leads from the sacculus and joins a duct from the utriculus of the membranous *labyrinth of the ear.

endometriosis *n.* the presence of membranous material of the kind lining the womb (*see* endometrium) at other sites within the cavity of the pelvis. In *direct* (*internal* or *primary*) *endometriosis*, the endometrium may penetrate the muscular wall of the womb, the ovaries, or the abdominal wall. The fragments of abnormally located tissue pass through the same periodic changes as the womb lining. Since there is no outlet for the bleeding that occurs from them, the patient suffers severe pain for several days each month. This symptom is not experienced during pregnancy or breast-feeding or after the menopause.

endometritis *n.* inflammation of the membrane lining the womb (*endometrium). The condition, sometimes restricted to the neck of the womb, is a reaction to bacterial attack upon the membrane, possibly following physical damage. Ulcers may form and the membrane may be cast off. There may also be excessive menstrual bleeding and pain in the lower regions of the back and abdomen. *Decidual endometritis* occurs during pregnancy; *puerperal endometritis* is an acute form developing immediately after childbirth.

endometrium *n.* the mucous membrane lining the uterus (womb), which becomes progressively thicker and more glandular and has an increased blood supply in the latter part of the menstrual cycle. This prepares the endometrium for implantation of the embryo, but if this does not occur much of the endometrium breaks down and is lost in menstruation. If pregnancy is established the endometrium becomes the *decidua, which is shed after birth.

endomorphic *adj.* describing a *body type that is relatively fat, with highly developed viscera and weak muscular and skeletal development. —**endomorph** *n.* —**endomorphy** *n.*

endomyocarditis *n.* an acute or chronic inflammatory disorder of the muscle and lining membrane of the heart. When the membrane surrounding the heart (pericardium) is also involved the condition is termed *pancarditis*. The principal causes are rheumatic fever and virus infections. There is enlargement of the heart, murmurs, embolism, and frequently arrhythmias. The treatment is that of the cause and complications. *See also* endocarditis.
A chronic condition, *endomyocardial fibrosis*, is seen in African negroes: the cause is unknown.

endomysium *n.* the fine connective tissue sheath that surrounds a single *muscle fibre.

endoneurium *n.* the layer of fibrous tissue that separates individual fibres within a *nerve.

endoparasite *n.* a parasite that lives inside its host, for example in the liver, lungs, gut, or other tissues of the body. *Compare* ectoparasite.

endopeptidase *n.* a digestive enzyme (e.g. *pepsin) that splits a whole protein into small peptide fractions by splitting the linkages between peptides in the interior of the molecule. *Compare* exopeptidase. *See also* peptidase.

endophthalmitis *n.* inflammation confined to the posterior chamber of the eye, i.e. the part behind the lens. *Compare* panophthalmitis.

endoplasm *n.* the inner cytoplasm of cells, which is less dense than the *ectoplasm and contains most of the cell's structures. —**endoplasmic** *adj.*

endoplasmic reticulum (ER) a system of membranes present in the cytoplasm of cells. ER is described as *rough* when it has *ribosomes attached to its surface and *smooth* when ribosomes are absent. It is the site of manufacture of proteins and lipids and is concerned with the transport of these products within the cell (*see also* Golgi apparatus).

end organ a specialized structure at the end of a peripheral nerve, acting as a receptor for a particular sensation. Taste buds, in the tongue, are end organs subserving the sense of taste.

endorphin *n.* one of a group of chemical compounds, similar to the *encephalins, that occur naturally in the brain and have pain-relieving properties similar to those of the opiates. The endorphins are derived from a substance found in the pituitary gland called *beta-lipotropin*; they are thought to be concerned with controlling the activity of the endocrine glands.

endoscope *n.* any instrument used to obtain a view of the interior of the body. Examples of endoscopes include the *auriscope, used for examining the inside of the ear, and the *gastroscope, for examining the inside of the stomach. Essentially, most endoscopes consist of a tube with a light at the end and an optical system for transmitting an image to the examiner's eye. *See also* fibrescope. —**endoscopic** *adj.* —**endoscopy** *n.*

endoscopic retrograde cholangiopancreatography *see* ERCP.

endospore *n.* the resting stage of certain bacteria, particularly species of the genera *Bacillus* and *Clostridium*. In adverse conditions the nucleus and cytoplasm within the normal vegetative stage of the bacterium can become enclosed within a tough protective coat, allowing the cell to survive. On return of favourable conditions the spore changes back to the vegetative form.

endosteum *n.* the membrane that lines the marrow cavity of a bone.

endothelioma *n.* any tumour arising from or resembling endothelium. It may arise from the linings of blood or lymph vessels (*haemangioendothelioma* and *lymphangioendothelioma* respectively); from the linings of the pleural or peritoneal cavities (*see* mesothelioma); or from the meninges (*see* meningioma).

endothelium *n.* the single layer of cells that lines the heart, blood vessels, and lymphatic vessels. It is derived from embryonic mesoderm. *Compare* epithelium.

endothermic *adj.* describing a chemical reaction associated with the absorption of heat. *Compare* exothermic.

endotoxin *n.* a poison generally harmful to all body tissues, contained within a bacterium and released only when the bacterial cell is broken down or dies and disintegrates. *Compare* exotoxin.

end-plate *n.* the area of muscle cell membrane immediately beneath the motor nerve ending at a *neuromuscular junction. Special receptors in this area trigger muscular contraction when the nerve ending releases its *neurotransmitter.

enema *n.* (*pl.* **enemata** or **enemas**) a quantity of fluid infused into the rectum through a tube passed into the anus. An *evacuant enema* (soap or olive oil) is used to remove faeces. A *barium enema* using barium sulphate, which is opaque to X-rays, is given to demonstrate the colon by X-ray. A *therapeutic enema* is used to insert drugs into the rectum, usually corticosteroids in the treatment of *proctocolitis.

enervation *n.* **1.** weakness; loss of strength. **2.** the surgical removal of a nerve.

engram *n.* the supposed physical basis of an individual memory.

enkephalin *n. see* encephalin.

enophthalmos *n.* a condition in which the eye is abnormally sunken into the socket. It may follow fractures of the floor of the orbit that allow the eye to sink downwards and backwards.

ensiform cartilage *see* xiphoid process.

Entamoeba *n.* a genus of widely distributed amoebae, of which some species are parasites of the digestive tract of man. *E. histolytica* invades and destroys the tissues of the intestinal wall, causing *dysentery and ulceration of the gut wall, and the parasite may spread to the liver, where it produces an abscess (*see* amoeboma). *E. coli* is a harmless intestinal parasite; *E. gingivalis*, found within the spaces between the teeth, is associated with periodontal disease and gingivitis.

enter- (entero-) *prefix denoting* the intestine. Example: *enterolith* (calculus in).

enteral *adj.* of or relating to the intestinal tract.

enteralgia *n. see* colic.

enterectomy *n.* surgical removal of part of the intestine.

enteric *adj.* relating to or affecting the intestine.

enteric-coated *adj.* describing tablets that are coated with a substance that enables them to pass through the stomach to the intestine unchanged. Enteric-coated tablets contain drugs that are destroyed by the acid contents of the stomach.

enteric fever *see* paratyphoid fever, typhoid fever.

enteritis *n.* inflammation of the small intestine, usually causing diarrhoea. *Infective enteritis* is caused by viruses or bacteria; *radiation enteritis* is caused by X-rays or radioactive isotopes. *See also* Crohn's disease (regional enteritis), gastroenteritis.

enterobiasis (oxyuriasis) *n.* a disease, common in children throughout the world, caused by the parasitic nematode *Enterobius vermicularis* (*see* pinworm) in the large intestine. The worms do not cause any serious lesions of the gut wall although, rarely, they may provoke appendicitis. The emergence of the female from the anus at night irritates and inflames the surrounding skin, causing the patient to scratch and thereby contaminate fingers and nails with infective eggs. The eggs may reinfect the same child or be spread to other children. Worms may occasionally enter the vulva and cause a discharge from the vagina. Enterobiasis responds well to treatment with *piperazine compounds.

Enterobius (Oxyuris) *n. see* pinworm.

enterocele *n.* a hernia of part of the intestine.

enterocentesis *n.* a surgical procedure in which a hollow needle is pushed through the wall of the stomach or intestines to release an abnormal accumulation of gas or fluid.

enterocolitis *n.* inflammation of the colon and small intestine. *See also* colitis, enteritis.

enterogastrone *n.* a hormone from the small intestine (duodenum) that inhibits the secretion of gastric juice by the stomach. It is released when the stomach contents pass into the small intestine.

enterogenous *adj.* borne by or carried in the intestine.

enterokinase *n.* the former name for *enteropeptidase.

enterolith

enterolith *n.* a stone within the intestine. It usually builds up around a gallstone or a swallowed fruit stone.

enteromegaly *n. Rare.* enlargement (usually increased diameter) of the intestine.

enteropathy *n.* disease of the small intestine. *See also* coeliac disease (gluten-induced enteropathy).

enteropeptidase *n.* an enzyme secreted by the glands of the small intestine that acts on trypsinogen to produce *trypsin. It is part of the *succus entericus.

enteropexy *n.* a surgical operation in which part of the intestine is fixed to the abdominal wall. This was formerly performed for visceroptosis (a condition in which the abdominal organs were thought to have descended to a lower than normal position), but it is no longer carried out.

enteroptosis *n.* a condition in which loops of intestine (especially transverse *colon) are in a low anatomical position. At one time this was thought to cause various abdominal symptoms, and operations were devised to correct it. It is now known that no symptoms result from simple anatomical variations of this sort.

enterorrhaphy *n.* the surgical procedure of stitching an intestine that has either perforated or been divided during an operation.

enterospasm *n.* powerful contraction of the intestine, usually accompanied by pain.

enterostomy *n.* an operation in which the small intestine is brought through the abdominal wall and opened (*see* duodenostomy, jejunostomy, ileostomy) or is joined to the stomach (*gastroenterostomy*) or to another loop of small intestine (*enteroenterostomy*).

enterotomy *n.* surgical incision into the intestine.

enterotoxin *n.* a poisonous substance that has a particularly marked effect upon the gastrointestinal tract, causing vomiting, diarrhoea, and abdominal pain.

enterovirus *n.* any virus that enters the body through the gastrointestinal tract, multiplies there, and then (generally) invades the central nervous system. Enteroviruses include *Coxsackie viruses, *echoviruses, *polioviruses, and *rhinoviruses.

enterozoon *n.* any animal species inhabiting or infecting the gut of another. *See also* endoparasite.

entoptic phenomena visual sensations caused by changes within the eye itself, rather than by the normal light stimulation process. The commonest are tiny floating spots that most people can see occasionally, especially when gazing at a brightly illuminated background (such as a blue sky).

entropion *n.* inturning of the eyelid towards the eyeball. The lashes may rub against the eye and cause irritation (*see* trichiasis). The commonest type is *spastic entropion* of the lower eyelid, due to spasm of the muscle that closes the eye (orbicularis oculi). Entropion may also be caused by scarring of the lining membrane (conjunctiva) of the lid.

enucleation *n.* a surgical operation in which an organ, tumour, or cyst is completely removed. In ophthalmology it is an operation in which the eyeball is removed but the other structures in the socket (e.g. eye muscles) are left in place. Commonly a plastic ball is buried in the socket to provide a firm base on which to fit an artificial eye.

enuresis *n.* the involuntary passing of urine, especially bedwetting at night (*nocturnal enuresis*). This can be caused by underlying disorders of the urinary tract but is usually functional in nature. The condition settles spontaneously as the child grows older, but it may persist into teenage – and rarely adult – life. The condition can be treated successfully by fluid restriction, various drugs, or use of a nocturnal alarm (*see* bell and pad). *See also* incontinence. —**enuretic** *adj.*

environment *n.* any or all aspects of the surroundings of an organism, both internal and external, which influence its growth, development, and behaviour.

Environmental Health Officer (EHO) a person, employed by local authorities, with special training in such aspects of environmental health and pollution as housing, sanitation, food, clean air, and water supplies (formerly known as a *Public Health Inspector*). Though not a registered medical practitioner, the EHO is responsible for the organization of the environmental health department. If medical (epidemiological) advice is required, the appropriate *community physician (Proper Officer) acts in an advisory or consultant capacity.

enzyme *n.* a protein that, in small amounts, speeds up the rate of a biological reaction without itself being used up in the reaction (i.e. it acts as a catalyst). An enzyme acts by binding with the substance involved in the reaction (the *substrate*) and converting it into another substance (the *product* of the reaction). An enzyme is relatively specific in the type of reaction it catalyses; hence there are many different enzymes for the various biochemical reactions. Each enzyme requires certain conditions for optimum activity, particularly correct temperature and pH, the presence of *coenzymes, and the absence of specific inhibitors. Enzymes are unstable and are easily inactivated by heat or certain chemicals. They are produced within living cells and may act either within the cell (as in cellular respiration) or outside it (as in digestion). The names of enzymes usually end in *-ase*; enzymes are named according to the substrate upon which they act (as in *lactase*), or the type of reaction they catalyse (as in *hydrolase*).

Enzymes are essential for the normal functioning and development of the body. Failure in the production or activity of a single enzyme may result in metabolic disorders; such disorders are often inherited and some have serious effects. —**enzymatic** *adj.*

eonism *n.* the adoption of female manners and dress by a man. *See* transsexualism, transvestitism.

eosin *n.* a red acidic dye, produced by the reaction of bromine and fluorescein, used to stain biological specimens for microscopical examination. Eosin may be used in conjunction with a contrasting blue alkaline dye taken up by different parts of the same specimen.

eosinopenia *n.* a decrease in the number of eosinophils in the blood.

eosinophil *n.* a variety of white blood cell distinguished by the presence in its cytoplasm of coarse granules that stain orange-red with *Romanowsky stains. The function of the eosinophil is poorly understood, but it is capable of ingesting foreign particles, is present in large numbers in lining or covering surfaces within the body, and is involved in allergic responses. There are normally $0.04–0.4 \times 10^9$ eosinophils per litre of blood.

eosinophilia *n.* an increase in the number of eosinophils in the blood. Eosinophilia occurs in a variety of diseases, including allergies, parasitic infestations, and certain forms of leukaemia.

eparterial *adj.* situated on or above an artery.

ependyma *n.* the extremely thin membrane, composed of cells of the *glia (*ependymal cells*), that lines the ventricles of the brain and the choroid plexuses. It is responsible for helping to form cerebrospinal fluid. —**ependymal** *adj.*

ependymoma *n.* a cerebral tumour derived from the glial (non-nervous) cells lining the cavities of the ventricles of the brain (*see* ependyma). It may obstruct the flow of cerebrospinal fluid, causing a *hydrocephalus.

ephebiatrics *n.* the branch of medicine concerned with the common disorders of children and adolescents. *Compare* paediatrics.

ephedrine *n.* a drug that causes constriction of blood vessels and widening of the bronchial passages (*see* sympathomimetic). It is used mainly in the treatment of asthma and other allergic conditions and chronic bronchitis. It is administered by mouth or by inhalation and may cause nausea and vomiting, insomnia, headache, and nervousness.

epi- *prefix denoting* above or upon.

epiblepharon *n.* an abnormal fold of skin, present from birth, stretching across the eye just above the lashes of the upper eyelid or in front of them in the lower lid. It may cause the lower lashes to turn upwards or inwards against the eye. It usually disappears within the first year of life.

epicanthus (epicanthic fold) *n.* a vertical fold of skin from the upper eyelid that covers the inner corner of the eye. It is normal in Mongolian races and occurs abnormally in certain congenital conditions, e.g. *Down's syndrome. —**epicanthal, epicanthic** *adj.*

epicardia *n.* the part of the *oesophagus, about 2 cm long, that extends from the level of the diaphragm to the stomach.

epicardium *n.* the outermost layer of the heart wall, enveloping the myocardium. It is a serous membrane that forms the inner layer of the serous *pericardium. —**epicardial** *adj.*

epicondyle *n.* the protuberance above a *condyle at the end of an articulating bone.

epicranium *n.* the structures that cover the cranium, i.e. all layers of the scalp.

epicranius *n.* the muscle of the scalp. The *frontal* portion, at the forehead, is responsible for raising the eyebrows and wrinkling the forehead; the *occipital* portion, at the base of the skull, draws the scalp backwards.

epicritic *adj.* describing or relating to sensory nerve fibres responsible for the fine degrees of sensation, as of temperature and touch. *Compare* protopathic.

epidemic *n.* a sudden outbreak of infectious disease that spreads rapidly through the population, affecting a large proportion of people. The commonest epidemics today are of influenza. *Compare* endemic, pandemic. —**epidemic** *adj.*

epidemiology *n.* the study of epidemic disease, with a view to finding means of control and future prevention. This not only applies to the study of such classical epidemics as plague, smallpox, and cholera but also includes all forms of disease that relate to the environment and ways of life. It thus includes the study of the links between smoking and cancer, and diet and coronary disease, as well as *communicable diseases.

epidermis *n.* the outer layer of the *skin, which is divided into four layers (see illustration). The innermost *Malpighian* or *germinative layer* (*stratum germinativum*) consists of continuously dividing cells. The other three layers are continually renewed as cells from the germinative layer are gradually pushed outwards and become progressively impregnated with keratin (*see* keratinization). The outermost layer (*stratum corneum*) consists of dead cells whose cytoplasm has been entirely replaced by keratin. It is thickest on the soles of the feet and palms of the hands. —**epidermal** *adj.*

epidermoid *adj.* having the appearance of epidermis (the outer layer of the skin): used to describe certain tumours of tissues other than the skin.

epidermolysis *n.* loosening of the outer layer of the skin (epidermis), with the development of large blisters, occurring either spontaneously or after injury.

Epidermophyton *n.* a genus of fungi that grow on the skin and produce the skin infections *athlete's foot and *dhobie itch.

epidiascope *n.* an apparatus for projecting a greatly magnified image of an object, such as a specimen on a microscope slide, on to a screen.

epididymis *n.* (*pl.* **epididymides**) a highly convoluted tube, about seven metres long, that connects the *testis to the vas deferens. The spermatozoa are moved passively along the tube over a period of several days, during which time they mature and become capable of fertilization. They are concentrated and stored in the lower part of the epididymis until ejaculation. —**epididymal** *adj.*

epididymitis *n.* inflammation of the epididymis. The usual cause is infection spreading down the vas deferens from the bladder or urethra, resulting in pain, swelling, and redness of the affected half of the scrotum. The inflammation may spread to the testicle (*epididymo-orchitis*). Treatment is by administration of antibiotics and analgesics.

epidural (extradural) *adj.* on or over the dura mater (the outermost of the three membranes covering the brain and spinal cord). The *epidural space* is the space between the dura mater of the spinal cord and the vertebral canal. *See also* spinal anaesthesia.

epigastrium *n.* the upper central region of the *abdomen. —**epigastric** *adj.*

epigastrocele *n.* a *hernia through the upper central abdominal wall.

epiglottis *n.* a thin leaf-shaped flap of cartilage, covered with mucous membrane, situated immediately behind the root of the tongue. It covers the entrance to the *larynx during swallowing.

epiglottitis *n.* inflammation of the mucous membrane of the epiglottis.

A section of epidermis

207

Swelling and inflammation of the tissues at the laryngeal entrance obstructs the air flow to the lungs, causing a dangerous form of *croup.

epilation *n.* the removal of a hair by its roots. This can be done mechanically (by pulling the hairs individually or using wax to strip an area of hair) or by electrolysis, which removes the hair permanently.

epilepsy *n.* any one of a group of disorders of brain function characterized by recurrent attacks that have a sudden onset. *Idiopathic epilepsy* is not associated with structural damage to the brain. It includes *grand mal and *petit mal, which can be controlled by the use of different *anticonvulsant drugs.
Focal (or *symptomatic*) *epilepsy* is a symptom of structural disease of the brain, and the nature of the fit depends upon the location of the disease in the brain. In *Jacksonian epilepsy* the epileptic discharge spreads over the cerebral cortex, with the resulting manifestations spreading throughout the body. In a Jacksonian motor fit the convulsive movements might spread from the thumb to the hand, arm, and face (this spread of symptoms is called the *march*). *Temporal lobe* (or *psychomotor*) *epilepsy* is caused by disease in the cortex of the temporal lobe or the adjacent parietal lobe of the brain. Its symptoms include *hallucinations of smell, taste, sight, and hearing, paroxysmal disorders of memory, and *automatism. Throughout an attack the patient is in a state of clouded awareness and afterwards he may have no recollection of the event (*see also* déja vu, jamais vu). —**epileptic** *adj., n.*

epileptogenic *adj.* having the capacity to provoke epileptic fits.

epiloia *n. see* tuberous sclerosis.

epimenorrhagia *n. see* menorrhagia.

epimenorrhoea *n.* menstruation at shorter intervals than is normal.

epimysium *n.* the fibrous elastic tissue that surrounds a *muscle.

epinephrine *n. see* adrenaline.

epineural *adj.* derived from or situated on the neural arch of a vertebra.

epineurium *n.* the outer sheath of connective tissue that encloses the bundles (fascicles) of fibres that make up a *nerve.

epiphenomenon *n.* an unusual symptom or event that may occur simultaneously with a disease but is not necessarily directly related to it. *Compare* complication.

epiphora *n.* watering of the eye, in which tears flow onto the cheek. It is due to some abnormality of the tear drainage system (*see* lacrimal apparatus).

epiphysis *n.* **1.** the end of a long bone, which is initially separated by cartilage from the shaft (diaphysis) of the bone and develops separately. It eventually fuses with the diaphysis to form a complete bone. **2.** *see* pineal body.

epiphysitis *n.* inflammation of the end (epiphysis) of a long bone. It may result in retardation of growth and deformity of the affected bone.

epiplo- *prefix denoting* the omentum. Example: *epiplocele* (hernia containing omentum).

epiploon *n. see* omentum.

episio- *prefix denoting* the vulva. Example: *episioplasty* (plastic surgery of).

episiorrhaphy *n.* stitching together the margins of a tear in the tissues around the vaginal opening.

episiotomy *n.* an incision into the tissues surrounding the opening of the vagina (perineum) during a difficult birth, at the stage when the infant's head has partly emerged through the opening of the birth passage. The aim is to enlarge the opening in a controlled manner so as to make delivery easier and to avoid extensive tearing of adjacent tissues.

epispadias *n.* a congenital abnormality in which the opening of the *urethra is on the dorsal (upper) surface of the penis. Surgical correction is carried out in infancy.

epispastic *n. see* vesicant.

epistasis *n.* a type of gene action in which one gene suppresses the action of another (nonallelic) gene. The term is sometimes used for any interaction between nonallelic genes. —**epistatic** *adj.*

epistaxis *n. see* nosebleed.

epithalamus *n.* part of the forebrain, consisting of a narrow band of nerve tissue in the roof of the third ventricle (including the region where the choroid plexus is attached) and the *pineal body. *See also* brain.

epithalaxia *n.* loss of layers of epithelial cells from the skin or the lining of the intestine.

epithelioma *n.* a tumour of *epithelium, the covering of internal and external surfaces of the body: a former term for *carcinoma, but now also used to describe benign tumours.

epithelium *n.* the tissue that covers the external surface of the body and lines hollow structures (except blood and lymphatic vessels). It is derived from embryonic ectoderm and endoderm. Epithelial cells may be flat and scalelike (*squamous*), *cuboidal*, or *columnar*. The latter may bear cilia or brush borders or secrete mucus or other substances (*see* goblet cell). The cells rest on a common *basement membrane*, which separates epithelium from underlying *connective tissue. Epithelium may be either

simple, consisting of a single layer of cells; *stratified*, consisting of several layers; or *pseudostratified*, in which the cells appear to be arranged in layers but in fact share a common basement membrane (see illustration). *See also*

Stratified squamous epithelium, surface view above and sectional view below

basement membrane
Simple cuboidal epithelium

goblet cell

Ciliated columnar epithelium

basement membrane
Pseudostratified ciliated epithelium

Types of epithelium

endothelium, mesothelium. —**epithelial** *adj.*

epitrichium (periderm) *n.* the most superficial layer of the skin, one cell in thickness, that is only present early in embryonic development. It protects the underlying *epidermis until it is fully formed.

epituberculosis *n.* enlargement of a lymph node in the thorax due to tuberculosis infection, causing the gland to press upon and occlude a bronchiole, which may result in the collapse of a lung segment (*see* atelectasis).

eponychium *n. see* nail.

eponym *n.* a disease, structure, or species named after a particular person, usually the person who first discovered or described it. Eponyms are widespread in medicine, but they are being replaced as more descriptive terms become necessary. Thus the eponyms islets of Langerhans, aqueduct of Sylvius, and Hashimoto's disease are more likely to be designated in text books as pancreatic islands, cerebral aqueduct, and autoimmune thyroiditis, respectively. —**eponymous** *adj.*

epoophoron *n. see* paroophoron.

Epstein-Barr virus the virus thought to be the causative agent of *glandular fever.

epulis *n.* a swelling on the gum. Most such swellings are due to fibrous hyperplasia.

equi- *prefix denoting* equality.

equinia *n. see* glanders.

Erb's palsy a partial paralysis of the arm caused by injury to a baby's *brachial plexus during birth. This may happen if – during a difficult delivery – excess traction applied to the head damages the fifth cervical root of the spinal cord. The muscles of the shoulder and the flexors of the elbow are paralysed and the arm hangs at the side internally rotated at the shoulder.

ERCP (endoscopic retrograde cholangiopancreatography) a technique in which a catheter is passed through a *duodenoscope into the *ampulla of Vater of the common bile duct and injected with a radio-opaque medium to outline the pancreatic duct and bile ducts radiologically. It is now widely used in the diagnosis of obstructive jaundice and pancreatic disease. *See also* papillotomy.

erectile *adj.* capable of causing erection or becoming erect. The penis is composed largely of erectile tissue.

erection *n.* the sexually active state of the penis, which becomes enlarged and rigid (due to the erectile tissue being swollen with blood) and capable of penetrating the vagina. The term is also applied to the clitoris in a state of sexual arousal.

erepsin *n.* a mixture of protein-digesting enzymes (*see* peptidase) secreted by the intestinal glands. It is part of the *succus entericus.

erethism *n.* **1.** a state of abnormal mental excitement or irritation. **2.** rapid response to a stimulus.

erg *n.* a unit of work or energy equal to the work done when the point of application of a force of 1 dyne is displaced through a distance of 1 centimetre in the direction of the force. 1 erg = 10^{7} joule.

erg- (ergo-) *prefix denoting* work or activity.

ergocalciferol *n. see* vitamin D.

ergograph *n.* an apparatus for recording the work performed by the muscles of the body when undergoing activity. Ergographs are useful for assessment of the capabilities of athletes undergoing training.

ergometrine *n.* a drug that stimulates contractions of the womb. It is administered by injection to assist labour and to control bleeding following delivery.

ergonomics *n.* the study of man in relation to his work and working surroundings. This broad science involves the application of psychological as well as physiological principles to the design of buildings, machinery, vehicles, packaging, implements, and anything else with which man comes into contact.

ergosterol *n.* a plant sterol that, when irradiated with ultraviolet light, is converted to ergocalciferol (vitamin D_2). *See* vitamin D.

ergot *n.* a fungus (*Claviceps purpurea*) that grows on rye. It produces several important alkaloids, chemically related to LSD, including *ergotamine and *ergometrine, which are used in medicine in the treatment of migraine and in childbirth. Eating bread made with rye infected with the fungus has led to sporadic outbreaks of *ergotism over the centuries.

ergotamine *n.* a drug that causes constriction of blood vessels and is used to relieve migraine. It is administered by mouth, injection, inhalation, or in suppositories. Common side-effects are nausea and vomiting, and ergotism may develop as a result of high doses. Trade names: **Femergin**, **Lingraine**.

ergotism *n.* poisoning caused by eating rye infected with the fungus *ergot. The chief symptom is gangrene of the fingers and toes, with diarrhoea and vomiting, nausea, and headache. In the Middle Ages the disease was known as *St. Anthony's fire*, because of the inflamed appearance of the tissues afflicted with gangrene and the belief that a pilgrimage to St. Anthony's tomb would result in cure.

erogenous *adj.* describing certain parts of the body, the physical stimulation of which leads to sexual arousal.

erosion *n.* **1.** an eating away of surface tissue by physical or chemical processes, including those associated with inflammation. A *cervical erosion* is an abnormal area of epithelium that may develop at the neck of the womb due to tissue damage caused at childbirth or by attempts at abortion. **2.** (in dentistry) loss of surface tooth substance, usually caused by repeated application of acid, as may occur with excessive intake of citrus fruits.

erot- (eroto-) *prefix denoting* sexual desire or love. Example: *erotophobia* (morbid dread of).

erotomania *n.* a delusion that the individual is loved by some person, often a person of importance. Sometimes, but not always, this progresses to schizophrenia.

eructation *n.* belching: the sudden raising of gas from the stomach.

eruption *n.* **1.** any lesion that appears at the surface of the skin and is characterized by its prominence and redness. A *bullous eruption* is an eruption of blisters. **2.** (in dentistry) the emergence of a growing tooth from the gum into the mouth.

erysipelas *n.* an infection of the skin and underlying tissues with the bacterium *Streptococcus pyogenes*. The affected areas, usually the face and scalp, become inflamed and swollen, with the development of raised patches that may be several inches across. The patient is ill, with a high temperature. Attacks may recur in certain individuals, possibly because of a defect in their lymphatic systems. Treatment is with antibiotics.

erysipeloid (erythema serpens) *n.* an infection of the skin and underlying tissues with *Erysipelothrix rhusiopathiae*, developing usually in people handling fish, poultry, or meat. Infection enters through scratches or cuts on the hands, and is normally confined to

Erysipelothrix

a finger or hand, which becomes reddened; sometimes systemic illness develops. Treatment is with antibiotics.

Erysipelothrix *n.* a genus of Gram-positive non-motile rod-shaped bacteria with a tendency to form filaments. They are parasites of mammals, birds, and fish. *E. rhusiopathiae* is a widely distributed species causing the disease *erysipelas in swine, which is transmissible to man.

erythema *n.* abnormal flushing of the skin caused by dilation of the blood capillaries. Erythema may be produced by various conditions – it is often a sign of inflammation and infection. For example, *erythema nodosum* is a disease of sudden onset, characterized by fever, joint pains, and an eruption of painful swellings on the legs. In *erythema multiforme*, a disease caused by toxins in the blood, the eruption consists of circular or irregular red patches, commonly occurring on the backs of the arms and hands and sometimes accompanied by systemic disease.

erythr- (erythro-) *prefix denoting* **1.** redness. Example: *erythuria* (excretion of red urine). **2.** erythrocytes.

erythraemia *n. see* polycythaemia vera.

erythrasma *n.* a chronic skin infection due to the bacterium *Corynebacterium minutissimum*, occurring in such areas as the armpits, groin, and toes, where skin surfaces are in contact.

erythritol *n.* a drug that has a mild prolonged action in reducing blood pressure by dilating blood vessels (*see* vasodilator) and is used to treat hypertension and angina. It is administered by mouth and high doses may cause flushing, headache, fainting, and increased heart rate.

erythroblast *n.* any of a series of nucleated cells (*see* normoblast, proerythroblast) that pass through a succession of stages of maturation to form red blood cells (*erythrocytes). Erythroblasts are normally present in the blood-forming tissue of the bone marrow, but they may appear in the circulation in a variety of diseases, (*see* erythroblastosis). *See also* erythropoiesis.

erythroblastosis *n.* the presence in the blood of the nucleated precursors of the red blood cells (*erythroblasts). This may occur when there is an increase in the rate of red cell production, as in haemorrhagic or haemolytic *anaemia, or in infiltrations of the bone marrow by tumours, etc.

erythroblastosis foetalis a severe but rare haemolytic *anaemia affecting newborn infants due to destruction of the infant's red blood cells by factors present in the mother's serum. It is usually caused by incompatibility of the rhesus blood groups between mother and infant (*see* rhesus factor).

erythrocyanosis *n.* mottled purplish discoloration on the legs and thighs, usually of adolescent girls or fat boys before puberty. The disorder sometimes occurs in older women. The condition is worse in cold weather and there is no satisfactory treatment.

erythrocyte (red blood cell) *n.* a *blood cell containing the pigment *haemoglobin, the principal function of which is the transport of oxygen. A mature erythrocyte has no nucleus and its shape is that of a biconcave disc, approximately 7 μm in diameter. There are normally about 5×10^{12} erythrocytes per litre of blood. *See also* erythropoiesis.

erythrocyte sedimentation rate *see* ESR.

erythrocytic *adj.* describing those stages in the life cycle of the malarial parasite (*see* Plasmodium) that develop inside the red blood cells (*see* trophozoite). *Compare* exoerythrocytic.

erythroderma (exfoliative dermatitis) *n.* abnormal reddening, flaking, and thickening of the skin, typically affecting a wide area of the body. Commoner after the age of 50, erythroderma affects men three times as often as women and it frequently develops from a preceding skin disease, such as psoriasis.

erythroedema *n. see* pink disease.

erythrogenesis *n. see* erythropoiesis.

erythromelalgia *n.* painful paroxysmal dilation of the blood vessels of the skin, usually affecting the feet and extremities.

erythromycin *n.* an *antibiotic used to treat infections caused by a wide range of bacteria and other microorganisms. It is administered by mouth or injection. Side-effects are rare and mild, though nausea, vomiting, and diarrhoea occur occasionally. Trade names: **Erycen, Erythromia, Erythropea, Ilotycin**.

erythron *n.* that part of the blood-forming system of the body that is directed towards the production of red blood cells. The erythron is not a single organ but is dispersed throughout the blood-forming tissue of the *bone marrow. See also* erythropoiesis.

erythropenia *n.* a reduction in the number of red blood cells (*erythrocytes) in the blood. This usually, but not invariably, occurs in *anaemia.

erythropoiesis (erythrogenesis) *n.* the process of red blood cell (*erythrocyte) production, which normally occurs in the blood-forming tissue of the *bone marrow. The ultimate precursor of the red cell is the *haemopoietic stem cell, but the earliest precursor that can be identified microscopically is the *proerythroblast. This divides and passes through a series of stages of maturation termed respectively early, intermediate, and late *normoblasts,

the latter finally losing its nucleus to become a mature red cell. *See also* haemopoiesis.

erythropoietin *n.* a hormone secreted by certain cells in the kidney in response to a reduction in the amount of oxygen reaching the tissues. Erythropoietin increases the rate of red cell production (*erythropoiesis) and is the mechanism by which the rate of erythropoiesis is controlled.

erythropsia *n.* red vision: a rare symptom sometimes experienced after removal of a cataract and also in snow blindness.

eschar *n.* a scab or slough, as produced by the action of heat or a corrosive substance on living tissue.

escharotic *n.* a *caustic agent that produces a dry scab, or slough, when applied to the skin.

Escherichia *n.* a genus of Gram-negative, generally motile, rodlike bacteria that have the ability to ferment carbohydrates, usually with production of gas, and are found in the intestines of man and many animals. *E. coli* – a lactose-fermenting species – is usually not harmful but under certain conditions can cause infection of the urinogenital tract and diarrhoea in children. It is also widely used in laboratory experiments for bacteriological and genetic studies.

eserine *n. see* physostigmine.

esophoria *n.* a tendency to squint in which the eye, when covered, tends to turn inwards towards the nose. *See also* heterophoria.

esotropia *n.* convergent *strabismus: a type of squint.

espundia (mucocutaneous leishmaniasis) *n.* a disease of the skin and mucous membranes caused by the parasitic protozoan *Leishmania braziliensis* (*see* leishmaniasis). Occurring in

South and Central America, espundia takes the form of ulcerating lesions on the arms and legs; the infection may also spread to the mucous membranes of the nose and mouth, causing serious destruction of the tissues.

ESR (erythrocyte sedimentation rate) the rate at which red blood cells (erythrocytes) settle out of suspension in blood plasma, measured under standardized conditions. The ESR increases if the level of certain proteins in the plasma rises, as in rheumatic diseases, chronic infections, and malignant disease, and thus provides a simple but valuable screening test for the latter condition.

essence *n.* a solution consisting of an essential oil dissolved in alcohol.

essential *adj.* describing a disorder that is not apparently attributable to an outside cause; for example, essential *hypertension.

essential amino acid an *amino acid that is essential for normal growth and development but cannot be synthesized by the body. Essential amino acids are normally obtained from protein-rich foods in the diet, such as liver, eggs, and dairy products. There are eight essential amino acids: tryptophan, lysine, phenylalanine, threonine, valine, methionine, leucine, and isoleucine.

essential fatty acid one of a group of unsaturated fatty acids that are essential for growth but cannot be synthesized by the body. The essential fatty acids are *linoleic, linolenic,* and *arachidonic acids*; of these, only linoleic acid need be included in the diet as the other two can be synthesized from it in the body. Large amounts of linoleic acid occur in maize (corn) oil and soya bean oil; smaller amounts in pork fat.

essential oil a volatile oil derived from an aromatic plant. Essential oils are used in various pharmaceutical preparations.

esterase *n.* an enzyme that catalyses the hydrolysis of esters into their constituent acids and alcohols. For example, fatty-acid esters are broken down to form fatty acids plus alcohol.

ethacrynic acid a *diuretic used to treat fluid retention (oedema), such as that associated with heart failure and kidney and liver disorders. It is administered by mouth or injection. Common side-effects are loss of appetite, difficulty in swallowing, nausea, vomiting, and diarrhoea. Trade name: **Edecrin**.

ethambutol *n.* a drug used in the treatment of tuberculosis, in conjunction with other drugs. It is administered by mouth and occasionally causes visual disturbances, which cease when the drug is withdrawn. Allergic rashes and digestive upsets may also occur. Trade name: **Myambutol**.

ethamivan *n.* an *analeptic drug that stimulates breathing and is used to treat reduced or abnormal breathing, particularly in newborn babies and in cases of drug overdosage. It is administered by mouth or injection; high doses may cause restlessness, sneezing, and gasping. Trade name: **Clairvan**.

ethanol (ethyl alcohol) *n. see* alcohol.

ethchlorvynol *n.* a drug used to treat insomnia (*see* hypnotic). It is administered by mouth; side-effects include temporary giddiness, muscle incoordination, nausea, and vomiting. Trade name: **Serenesil**.

ethebenecid *n.* a *uricosuric drug used to treat gout and other conditions involving high blood levels of uric acid. It is administered by mouth and may cause skin rashes, digestive discomfort, and sedation.

ether *n.* a volatile liquid formerly used as an anaesthetic administered by inhalation, though now largely replaced by safer and more efficient drugs. It also has laxative action when administered by mouth. Ether irritates the respiratory tract and affects the circulation.

ethical committee (in Britain) a group of consultants and other experts set up (especially in a hospital) to monitor investigations, concerned with teaching or research, that involve the use of human subjects. It is responsible for ensuring that patients are adequately informed of the procedures involved in a research project (including the use of dummy or placebo treatments as controls), that the tests and/or therapies are safe, and that no-one is pressurized into participating.

ethinamate *n.* a mild *sedative used to treat insomnia. It is administered by mouth and may cause digestive discomfort.

ethinyloestradiol *n.* a synthetic female sex hormone (*see* oestrogen) administered by mouth to treat symptoms of the menopause and menstrual disorders, to suppress lactation in mothers not breast-feeding, and to treat cancer of the prostate gland. It is also used, in combination with a progestogen, in *oral contraceptives. Trade name: **Lynoral**.

ethionamide *n.* a drug used to treat tuberculosis, usually in conjunction with other drugs. It is administered by mouth or in suppositories. Loss of appetite, nausea, and vomiting are common side-effects. Trade name: **Trescatyl**.

ethisterone *n.* a synthetic female sex hormone (*see* progestogen) used, often in combination with an *oestrogen, to treat menstrual disorders, particularly amenorrhoea. It was formerly used in hormone pregnancy tests. It is administered by mouth.

ethmoid bone a bone in the floor of the cranium that contributes to the nasal cavity and orbits. The part of the ethmoid forming the roof of the nasal

cavity – the *cribriform plate* – is pierced with many small holes through which the olfactory nerves pass. *See also* nasal concha, skull.

ethnology *n.* the study of the different races of mankind and their variations: a branch of anthropology that deals mainly with cultural and social differences between groups and the problems, medical and otherwise, that arise from their particular ways of life. —**ethnic** *adj.*

ethoglucid *n.* a drug that prevents the growth of tumours and is used to treat various cancers. It is administered by injection; side-effects commonly include nausea and vomiting. Trade name: **Epodyl**.

ethopropazine *n.* a drug that has effects similar to those of *atropine and is used to treat parkinsonism. It is administered by mouth and may cause lethargy and drowsiness in the early stages of treatment. Trade name: **Lysivane**.

ethosuximide *n.* an *anticonvulsant drug used to treat petit mal epileptic fits. It is administered by mouth; side-effects such as drowsiness, depression, and digestive disturbances may occur but are usually temporary. Trade names: **Emeside, Zarontin**.

ethotoin *n.* an *anticonvulsant drug used, usually in conjunction with other anticonvulsants, to treat grand mal epileptic fits. It is administered by mouth; side-effects can include digestive and visual disturbances and drowsiness. Trade name: **Peganone**.

ethyl biscoumacetate an *anticoagulant drug used to prevent blood clotting. It is administered by mouth and may cause nausea and vomiting, hair loss, and skin rash. Trade name: **Tromexan**.

ethylene *n.* an inflammable gas sometimes used as an anaesthetic administered by inhalation. There are usually no toxic effects, but nausea and vomiting commonly occur after its use.

ethyloestrenol *n.* a steroid drug with *anabolic properties, used to treat conditions involving wasting of protein and bone, such as osteoporosis. It is administered by mouth and sometimes causes nausea, water retention, and menstrual disturbances at high doses. Trade name: **Orabolin**.

ethynodiol *n.* a synthetic female sex hormone (*see* progestogen) that is used to treat menstrual disorders and in *oral contraceptives. It is administered by mouth, usually in combination with an *oestrogen. Side-effects can include nausea, vomiting, headache, breast swelling, weight gain, fluid retention, and breakthrough bleeding.

etiology *n. see* aetiology.

etoposide (VP16-213) *n.* a *cytotoxic drug derived from an extract of the mandrake plant. It is administered intravenously or by mouth, primarily in the treatment of bronchial carcinoma and lymphomas. Side-effects include alopecia, nausea, and marrow suppression. Trade name: **Vepesid**.

eu- *prefix denoting* **1.** good, well, or easy. **2.** normal.

eubacteria *pl. n.* a very large group of bacteria with rigid cell walls and – typically – flagella for movement. The group comprises the so-called 'true' bacteria, excluding those, such as spirochaetes and mycoplasmas, with flexible cell walls.

eucalyptol *n.* a volatile oil that has a mild irritant effect on the mucous membranes of the mouth and digestive system. It is taken as pastilles or inhaled as vapour to relieve catarrh. Large doses may cause nausea, vomiting, and diarrhoea.

euchromatin *n.* chromosome material (*see* chromatin) that stains most deeply during mitosis and represents the major genes. *Compare* heterochromatin.

eugenics *n.* the science that is concerned with the improvement of the human race by means of the principles of genetics. It is mainly concerned with the detection and, where possible, the elimination of genetic disease in man.

eupepsia *n.* the state of normal or good digestion: freedom from digestive symptoms.

euphoria *n.* a state of optimism, cheerfulness, and well-being. A morbid degree of euphoria is characteristic of *mania and *hypomania. *See also* ecstasy, elation.

euplastic *adj.* describing a tissue that heals quickly after injury.

euploidy *n.* the condition of cells, tissues, or organisms in which there is one complete set of chromosomes or a whole multiple of this set in each cell. *Compare* aneuploidy. —**euploid** *adj., n.*

Eustachian tube the tube that connects the middle *ear to the pharynx. It allows the pressure on the inner side of the eardrum to remain equal to the external pressure.

euthanasia *n.* the act of taking life to relieve suffering. In *voluntary euthanasia* the sufferer asks for measures to be taken to end his life. This may be accomplished by active steps, usually the administration of a drug, or by *passive euthanasia* – the deliberate withholding of treatment. In *compulsory euthanasia* society or a person acting on authority gives instructions to terminate the life of a person, such as an infant, who cannot express his wishes. In no country is either voluntary or compulsory euthanasia legal, although many societies exist to promote the cause of voluntary euthanasia.

euthyroid *adj.* having a normally functioning thyroid gland. *Compare* hyperthyroidism, hypothyroidism. —**euthyroidism** n.

eutocia n. natural uncomplicated labour and childbirth.

evacuator n. a device for sucking fluid out of a cavity. In its simplest form it consists of a hollow rubber bulb that is attached, via a valve system, to a tube inserted into the cavity. Another valve leads to a discharge tube. Evacuators may be used to empty the bladder of unwanted material during such operations as the removal of a calculus.

evagination n. the protrusion of a part or organ from a sheathlike covering or by eversion of its inner surface.

eventration n. **1.** protrusion of the intestines through the abdominal wall. **2.** (of the diaphragm) abnormal elevation of part of the diaphragm due to a congenital weakness (but without true herniation), as observed by X-ray.

event sampling (in psychology) a way of recording behaviour in which the presence of a particular kind of behaviour is noted whenever it occurs. It is used for precise descriptions of behaviour and for following the course of *behaviour modification. *See also* time sampling.

eversion n. a turning outward; in *eversion of the cervix* the edges of the neck of the womb turn outward after having been torn during childbirth.

evisceration n. (in ophthalmology) an operation in which the contents of the eyeball are removed, the empty outer envelope (sclera) being left behind. *Compare* enucleation.

evulsion n. *see* avulsion.

Ewing's sarcoma a highly malignant tumour of bone occurring in children and young adults. Distinguished from *osteosarcoma by J. Ewing in 1921, it commonly arises in the limbs but may affect any bone. It is sensitive to radi-

otherapy, and systemic therapy with *cytotoxic drugs has improved its prognosis.

ex- (exo-) *prefix denoting* outside or outer.

exaltation n. *see* elation.

exanthem n. **1.** a skin rash accompanying any eruptive disease or fever. **2.** any disease characterized by a skin rash. —**exanthematous** adj.

excavator n. **1.** a spoon-shaped surgical instrument that is used to scrape out diseased tissue, usually for laboratory examination. **2.** a type of hand instrument with spoon ends used for removing decayed dentine from teeth. It may also be used as a *curette.

exchange transfusion a technique for treating *haemolytic disease in newborn infants. Using a 20-ml syringe with a three-way tap, Rh positive blood is withdrawn from the baby (via the umbilical vein), ejected, and replaced by 20 ml Rh negative donor blood, without detaching the syringe. By many repetitions of this exchange, red blood cells liable to be destroyed and bilirubin released from those already destroyed are removed, while keeping the baby's blood volume and number of red cells constant.

excipient n. a substance that is combined with a drug in order to render it suitable for administration; for example in the form of pills. Excipients should have no pharmacological action themselves.

excise vb. to cut out tissue, an organ, or a tumour from the body. —**excision** n.

excitation n. (in neurophysiology) the triggering of a conducted impulse in the membrane of a muscle cell or nerve fibre. During excitation a polarized membrane becomes momentarily depolarized and an *action potential is set up.

excoriation *n.* the destruction and removal of the surface of the skin or the covering of an organ by scraping, the application of a chemical, or other means.

excrescence *n.* an abnormal outgrowth on the surface of the body, such as a wart.

excreta *n.* any waste material discharged from the body, especially faeces.

excretion *n.* the removal of the waste products of metabolism from the body, mainly through the action of the *kidneys. Excretion also includes the loss of water, salts, and some urea through the sweat glands and carbon dioxide and water vapour from the lungs, and the term is also used to include the egestion of faeces.

exenteration *n.* (in ophthalmology) an operation in which all the contents of the eye socket (orbit) are removed, leaving only the bony walls intact. The bone is covered by a skin graft. This operation is sometimes necessary when there is a malignant tumour in the orbit.

exflagellation *n.* the formation and release of mature flagellated male sex cells (*see* microgamete) by the *microgametocytes of the malarial parasite (*see* Plasmodium). The process, which is completed in 10–15 minutes, occurs after the microgametocytes have been transferred from man to the stomach of a mosquito.

exfoliation *n.* **1.** flaking off of the upper layers of the skin. **2.** separation of a surface epithelium from the underlying tissue. **3.** the natural shedding of deciduous teeth. —**exfoliative** *adj.*

exhalation (expiration) *n.* the act of breathing air from the lungs out through the mouth and nose. *See* breathing.

exhibitionism *n.* exposure of the genitals to another person, as a sexually deviant act. The word is often broadened to mean public flaunting of any quality of the individual.

exo- *prefix. see* ex-.

exocoelom *n. see* extraembryonic coelom.

exocrine gland a gland that discharges its secretion by means of a duct, which opens onto an epithelial surface. An exocrine gland may be *simple*, with a single unbranched duct, or *compound*, with branched ducts and multiple secretory sacs. The illustration shows some different types of these glands. Examples of exocrine glands are the sebaceous and sweat glands. *See also* secretion.

simple tubular   simple alveolar

compound tubular   compound alveolar   compound tubulo-alveolar

Types of exocrine gland

exoenzyme *n.* an *enzyme that acts outside the cell that produced it. Examples of exoenzymes are the digestive enzymes.

exoerythrocytic *adj.* describing those stages in the life cycle of the malarial parasite (*see* Plasmodium) that develop in the cells of the liver. Each parasite (*sporozoite) divides repeatedly to produce a schizont containing many merozoites.

exogenous *adj.* originating outside the body or part of the body: applied particularly to substances in the body that are derived from the diet rather than built up by the body's own processes of metabolism. *Compare* endogenous.

exomphalos *n.* an umbilical *hernia.

exopeptidase *n.* an enzyme (e.g. *trypsin) that takes part in the digestion of proteins by splitting off the terminal amino acids of a polypeptide chain. *Compare* endopeptidase. *See also* peptidase.

exophoria *n.* a tendency to squint in which the eye, when covered, tends to turn outwards. *See also* heterophoria.

exophthalmic goitre (Graves's disease) *see* thyrotoxicosis.

exophthalmometer (proptometer) *n.* an instrument for measuring the degree of protrusion of the eyeball. The distance measured is that from the rim of bone at the outer edge of the eye, forwards to the surface of the front of the cornea.

exophthalmos *n.* protrusion of the eyeballs in their sockets. This can result from injury or disease of the eyeball or socket but is most commonly associated with overactivity of the thyroid gland (*see* thyrotoxicosis).

exosmosis *n.* outward osmotic flow. *See also* osmosis.

exostosis *n.* a benign cartilaginous outgrowth from a bone. *See* osteoma.

exothermic *adj.* describing a chemical reaction in which energy is released in the form of heat. *Compare* endothermic.

exotic *adj.* describing a disease occurring in a region of the world far from where it might be expected. Thus malaria and leishmaniasis are regarded as exotic when they are diagnosed in patients in Britain.

exotoxin *n.* a highly potent poison, often harmful to only a limited range of tissues, that is produced by a bacterial cell and secreted into its surrounding medium. It is generally unstable, being rendered inactive by heat, light, and chemicals. Exotoxins are produced by such bacteria as those causing *botulism, *diphtheria, and *tetanus. *Compare* endotoxin.

exotropia *n.* divergent *strabismus: a type of squint.

expectorant *n.* a drug that enhances the secretion of sputum by the air passages so that it is easier to cough up. Expectorants are used in cough mixtures; they act by increasing the bronchial secretion or make it less viscous (*see* mucolytic). Drugs such as *ipecacuanha are *stimulant expectorants* in small quantities: they irritate the lining of the stomach, which provides a stimulus for the reflex production of sputum by the glands in the bronchial mucous membrane. At higher doses they produce vomiting.

expectoration *n.* the act of spitting out material brought into the mouth by coughing.

expiration *n.* **1.** the act of breathing out air from the lungs: exhalation. **2.** dying.

explant **1.** *n.* live tissue transferred from the body (or any organism) to a suitable artificial medium for culture. The tissue grows in the artificial medium and can be studied for diagnostic or experimental purposes. Tumour growths are sometimes examined in this way. **2.** *vb.* to transfer live tissue for culture outside the body. —**explantation** *n.*

exploration *n.* (in surgery) an investigative operation to determine the cause of symptoms. —**exploratory** *adj.*

exposure *n.* (in behaviour therapy) a method of treating fears and phobias that involves confronting the individual with the situation he has been avoiding, so allowing the fears to wane by *extinction. It can be achieved gradually by *desensitization or suddenly by *flooding.

exsanguinate *vb.* to deprive the body of blood; for example, as a result of an accident causing severe bleeding or – very rarely – through uncontrollable bleeding during a surgical operation. —**exsanguination** *n.*

exsiccation *n.* drying up, as may occur in tissues deprived of an adequate supply of water during dehydration or starvation.

exsufflation *n.* the forcible removal of secretions from the air passages by some form of suction apparatus.

extension *n.* **1.** the act of extending or stretching, especially the muscular movement by which a limb is straightened. **2.** the application of *traction to a fractured or dislocated limb in order to restore it to its normal position.

extensor *n.* any muscle that causes the straightening of a limb or other part.

exteriorization *n.* a surgical procedure in which an organ is brought from its normal site to the surface of the body. This may be done as a temporary or permanent measure; for example, the intestine may be brought to the surface of the abdomen (*see* colostomy). The process is also sometimes used in physiological experiments on animals.

exteroceptor *n.* a sensory nerve, ending in the skin or a mucous membrane, that is responsive to stimuli from outside the body. *See also* chemoreceptor, receptor.

extinction *n.* (in psychology) the weakening of a conditioned reflex that takes place if it is not maintained by *reinforcement. This is used as a method of treatment when undesirable behaviour (e.g. destructiveness) is reduced simply by withdrawing whatever rewards it (e.g. the fuss made by other people).

extirpation *n.* the complete surgical removal of tissue, an organ, or a growth.

extra- *prefix denoting* outside or beyond.

extracellular *adj.* situated or occurring outside cells; for example, *extracellular fluid* is the fluid surrounding cells.

extract *n.* a preparation containing the pharmacologically active principles of a drug, made by evaporating a solution of the drug in water, alcohol, or ether.

extraction *n.* **1.** the surgical removal of a part of the body. Extraction of teeth is usually achieved by applying extraction *forceps to the crown or root of the tooth to dislocate it from its socket. When this is not possible, for example because the tooth or root is deeply buried within the bone, extraction is performed surgically by removing bone and dividing the tooth. **2.** the act of pulling out a baby from the body of its mother during childbirth.

extractor *n.* an instrument used to pull out a natural part of the body, to remove a foreign object, or to assist delivery of a baby (*see* vacuum extractor).

extradural *adj. see* epidural.

extraembryonic coelom (exocoelom) the cavity, lined with mesoderm, that surrounds the embryo from the earliest stages of development. It communicates temporarily with the coelomic cavity within the embryo (peritoneal cavity). Late in pregnancy it becomes almost entirely obliterated by the growth of the *amnion, which fuses with the *chorion.

extraembryonic membranes the membranous structures that surround the embryo and contribute to the placenta and umbilical cord. They include the *amnion, *chorion, *allantois, and *yolk sac. In man the allantois is always very small and by the end of pregnancy the amnion and chorion have fused into a single membrane and the yolk sac has disappeared.

extrapleural adj. relating to the tissues of the chest wall outside the parietal *pleura.

extrapyramidal system the system of nerve tracts and pathways connecting the cerebral cortex, basal ganglia, thalamus, cerebellum, reticular formation, and spinal neurones in complex circuits not included in the *pyramidal system. The extrapyramidal system is mainly concerned with the regulation of stereotyped reflex muscular movements.

extrasensory perception (ESP) a supposed way of perceiving that involves none of the known senses. *Clairvoyance* is the extrasensory perception of current events; *precognition* is extrasensory perception of future events; *telepathy* is extrasensory perception of the thoughts of others.

extrasystole n. see ectopic beat.

extrauterine adj. outside the womb.

extravasation n. the leakage and spread of blood or fluid from vessels into the surrounding tissues, which follows injury, burns, inflammation, and allergy.

extraversion n. see extroversion.

extrinsic muscle a muscle, such as any of those controlling movements of the eyeball, that has its origin some distance from the part it acts on. *See also* eye.

extroversion n. **1.** (or **extraversion**) an enduring personality trait characterized by interest in the outside world rather than the self. People high in extroversion (*extroverts*), as measured by questionnaires and tests, are gregarious and outgoing, prefer to change activities frequently, and are not susceptible to permanent *conditioning. Extroversion was first described by Carl Jung as a tendency to action rather than thought, to scientific rather than philosophical interests, and to emotional rather than intellectual reactions. *Compare* introversion. **2.** a turning inside out of a hollow organ, such as the womb (which sometimes occurs after childbirth).

extrovert n. see extroversion.

extrusion n. (in dentistry) the movement of a tooth beyond its normal alignment.

exudation n. the slow escape of liquid (called the *exudate*) containing proteins and white cells through the walls of intact blood vessels, usually as a result of inflammation. Exudation is a normal part of the body's defence mechanisms.

eye n. the organ of sight: a three-layered roughly spherical structure specialized for receiving and responding to light (see illustration).
Light enters the eye through the cornea, which refracts it through the aqueous humour onto the lens. By adjustment of the shape of the lens (*see* accommodation) light is focused through the vitreous humour onto the retina. In the retina light-sensitive cells (*see* cone, rod) send nerve impulses to the brain via the optic nerve. The arrangement of the two eyes at the front of the head provides *binocular vision. Each eye is contained in an *orbit, and movement

eyeball

The eye (sagittal section)

of the eye within the orbit is controlled by extrinsic eye muscles (see illustration).

eyeball *n.* the body of the *eye, which is roughly spherical, is bounded by the *sclera, and lies in the *orbit. It is closely associated with accessory structures – the eyelids, conjunctiva, and lacrimal (tear-producing) apparatus – and its movements are controlled by three pairs of extrinsic eye muscles (see illustration).

Extrinsic muscles of the eye

eyebrow *n.* the small fringe of hair on the bony ridge just above the eye. It helps to prevent moisture from running into the eye. Anatomical name: **supercilium**.

eyeground *n.* the inside of the eye as seen through an ophthalmoscope; the ocular fundus.

eyelash *n.* one of the long stiff hairs that form a row projecting outwards from the front edge of the upper and lower eyelids. The eyelashes help keep dust away from the eye. Anatomical name: **cilium**.

eyelid *n.* the protective covering of the eye. Each eye has two eyelids consisting of skin, muscle, and connective tissue. Each eyelid is lined with membrane (*conjunctiva) and fringed with eyelashes. Stimulation of the pain receptors in the cornea causes the eyelids to close in a reflex action. Anatomical names: **blepharon, palpebra**.

eyepiece *n.* the part of an optical instrument, such as a microscope, that is nearest to the eye of the examiner. *Compare* objective.

eyestrain *n.* a sense of fatigue brought on by use of the eyes for prolonged close work or in persons who have an uncorrected error of *refraction or an imbalance of the muscles that move the eyes. Symptoms are usually aching or burning of the eyes, accompanied by headache and even general fatigue if the eyes are not rested. Medical name: **asthenopia**.

F

Fabry's disease *see* angiokeratoma.

face-bow *n.* (in dentistry) an instrument for transferring the jaw relationship of a patient to an *articulator to allow reproduction of the lateral and protrusive movements of the lower jaw.

facet *n.* a small flat surface on a bone or tooth, especially a surface of articulation.

facial nerve the seventh *cranial nerve (VII): a mixed sensory and motor nerve that supplies the muscles of facial expression, the taste buds of the front part of the tongue, the sublingual salivary glands, and the lacrimal glands. A small branch to the middle ear regulates the tension on the ear ossicles.

-facient *suffix denoting* causing or making. Example: *abortifacient* (causing abortion).

facies *n.* facial expression, often a guide to a patient's state of health as well as his emotions. The typical facies seen in adenoids is the vacant look, with the mouth drooping open. A *Hippocratic facies* is the sallow face, sagging and with listless staring eyes, that some read as the expression of approaching death.

facilitation *n.* (in neurology) the phenomenon that occurs when a neurone receives, through a number of different synapses, impulses that are not powerful enough individually to start an *action potential but whose combined activity brings about some *depolarization of the membrane. In this facilitated

state a small additional depolarization will suffice to trigger off an impulse in the cell.

factitious *adj.* produced artificially, either deliberately or by accident, and therefore not to be taken into account when the results of an experiment are considered or a diagnosis is being made.

Factory Inspectorate the largest and oldest of the statutory bodies responsible for monitoring the health and safety of factory workers. It is administered by the Department of Employment through the Health and Safety Commission under the terms of the Health and Safety at Work Act. Requirements include a routine examination of young persons and those exposed to toxic hazards (e.g. lead) and the adequate guarding of machinery. Ensuring that the atmosphere inside the factory is free from poisonous fumes and chemicals may cause conflict with local authorities, whose *Environmental Health Officers have responsibility to prevent atmospheric pollution.

facultative *adj.* describing an organism that is not restricted to one way of life. A *facultative parasite* can live either as a parasite or, in different conditions, as a nonparasite able to survive without a host. *Compare* obligate.

FAD (flavin adenine dinucleotide) a *coenzyme, derived from riboflavin, that takes part in many important oxidation-reduction reactions. It consists of two phosphate groups, adenine, and ribose.

fading *n.* (in behaviour modification) *see* prompting.

faecalith *n.* a small hard mass of faeces, found particularly in the vermiform appendix: a cause of inflammation.

faeces *n.* the waste material that is eliminated through the anus. It is formed in the *colon and consists of a solid or semisolid mass of undigested food remains (chiefly cellulose) mixed with *bile pigments (which are responsible for the colour), bacteria, various secretions (e.g. mucus), and some water. **—faecal** *adj.*

Fahrenheit temperature temperature expressed on a scale in which the melting point of ice is assigned a temperature of 32° and the boiling point of water a temperature of 212°. For most medical purposes the Celsius (centigrade) scale has replaced the Fahrenheit scale. The formula for converting from Fahrenheit (F) to Celsius (C) is: $C = \frac{5}{9}(F - 32)$. *See also* Celsius temperature.

fainting *n. see* syncope.

falciform ligament a fold of peritoneum separating the right and left lobes of the liver and attaching it to the diaphragm and the anterior abdominal wall as far as the umbilicus.

Fallopian tube (oviduct; uterine tube) either of a pair of tubes that conduct ova (egg cells) from the ovary to the womb (*see* reproductive system). The ovarian end opens into the abdominal cavity via a funnel-shaped structure with finger-like projections (*fimbriae*) surrounding the opening. Movements of the fimbriae at ovulation assist in directing the ovum to the Fallopian tube. The ovum is fertilized near the ovarian end of the tube.

Fallot's tetralogy *see* tetralogy of Fallot.

falx (falx cerebri) *n.* a sickle-shaped fold of the *dura mater that dips inwards from the skull in the midline, between the cerebral hemispheres.

familial *adj.* describing a condition or character that is found in some families but not in others. It is often inherited.

family planning 1. the use of *contraception to limit or space out the num-bers of children born to a couple. **2.** provision of contraceptive methods within a community or nation.

Family Practitioner Committee (FPC) (in Britain) an authority responsible for running general medical services (general practitioners, dentists, pharmacists, and opticians) for the population served by one or more District Health Authorities. Members of the FPC are appointed by the District Health Authority, local authority, local *medical committee, local dental committee, local pharmaceutical committee and local optical committee. The general practitioners have independent contracts (as distinct from salaries) with the FPC, which must approve all names included on the *medical list* (a special list of general practitioners working in the National Health Service). Such inclusion is subject to overall monitoring of the *Medical Practices Committee*, which advises the Department of Health and Social Security; similar arrangements exist for the other three services (*see* general dental services). Refusal to include a suitable registered practitioner is usually the result of there being a surplus for the population being served. However the FPC must also approve the premises and the hours of service. The committee meets regularly (e.g. every two months) and has separate subcommittees for each of the four services as well as those concerned with vacancies, hours of availability, and allocation of patients who are refused acceptance by all general practitioners in the vicinity.

Fanconi syndrome a disorder of the proximal kidney tubules, which may be inherited or acquired and is most common in children. It is characterized by the urinary excretion of large amounts of amino acids, glucose, and phosphates (though blood levels of these substances are normal). Symptoms may include osteomalacia, rickets, muscle weakness, and *cystinosis. Treatment is directed to the cause.

fantasy (phantasy) *n.* a complex sequence of imagination in which several imaginary elements are woven together into a story. An excessive preoccupation with one's own imaginings may be symptomatic of a difficulty in coping with reality. In psychoanalytic psychology, *unconscious fantasies* are supposed to control behaviour, so that psychological symptoms can be symbols of or defences against such fantasies (*see* symbolism).

farad *n.* the *SI unit of capacitance, equal to the capacitance of a capacitor between the plates of which a potential difference of 1 volt appears when it is charged with 1 coulomb of electricity. Symbol: F.

faradism *n.* the use of induced rapidly alternating electric currents to stimulate nerve and muscle activity. *See also* electrotherapy.

farcy *n. see* glanders.

farmer's lung an occupational lung disease caused by allergy to fungal spores that grow in inadequately dried stored hay. It is an allergic *alveolitis, such as also results from sensitivity to many other allergens. An acute reversible form can develop a few hours after exposure; a chronic form, with the gradual development of irreversible breathlessness, occurs with or without preceding acute attacks. Avoidance of the allergen is the main principle of treatment.

fascia *n.* (*pl.* **fasciae**) connective tissue forming membranous layers of variable thickness in all regions of the body. Fascia surrounds the softer or more delicate organs and is divided into *superficial fascia* (found immediately beneath the skin) and *deep fascia* (which forms sheaths for muscles).

fasciculation *n.* brief spontaneous contraction of a few muscle fibres, which is seen as a flicker of movement under the skin. It is most often associated with disease of the motor neurones in the spinal cord or of the nerve fibres.

fasciculus (fascicle) *n.* a bundle, e.g. of nerve or muscle fibres.

fasciitis *n.* inflammation of *fascia. It may result from bacterial infection or from a rheumatic disease, such as *Reiter's syndrome or ankylosing spondylitis.

Fasciola *n.* a genus of *flukes. *F. hepatica*, the liver fluke, normally lives as a parasite of sheep and other herbivorous animals but sometimes infects man (*see* fascioliasis).

fascioliasis *n.* an infestation of the bile ducts and liver with the liver fluke, *Fasciola hepatica*. Man acquires the infection through eating wild watercress on which the larval stages of the parasite are present. Symptoms include fever, dyspepsia, vomiting, loss of appetite, abdominal pain, and coughing; the liver may also be extensively damaged (causing *liver rot*). *Emetine and *chloroquine have been used in the treatment of fascioliasis.

fasciolopsiasis *n.* a disease, common in the Far East, caused by the fluke *Fasciolopsis buski* in the small intestine. At the site of attachment of the adult flukes in the intestine there may be inflammation with some ulceration and bleeding. Symptoms include diarrhoea, and in heavy infections the patient may experience loss of appetite, vomiting, and (later) swelling of the face, abdomen, and legs. Death may follow in cases of severe ill health and malnutrition. The flukes can be removed with an anthelmintic.

Fasciolopsis *n.* a genus of large parasitic flukes widely distributed throughout eastern Asia and especially common in China. The adults of *F. buski*, the giant intestinal fluke, live in the human small intestine. Man becomes infected with the fluke on eating uncooked water chestnuts contaminated with fluke larvae and the resulting symptoms can be serious (*see* fasciolopsiasis).

fastigium *n.* the highest point of a fever.

fat *n.* a substance that contains one or more fatty acids (in the form of *triglycerides) and is the principal form in which energy is stored by the body (in *adipose tissue). It also serves as an insulating material beneath the skin (in the subcutaneous tissue) and around certain organs (including the kidneys). Much of the carbohydrate of the diet is converted to fat before it is used for providing energy. However, a certain amount of fat is necessary in the diet to provide an adequate supply of *essential fatty acids and for the efficient absorption of fat-soluble vitamins from the intestine. Excessive deposition of fat in the body leads to *obesity. *See also* brown fat, lipid.

fatigue *n.* **1.** mental or physical tiredness, following prolonged or intense activity. Muscle fatigue may be due to the waste products of metabolism accumulating in the muscles faster than they can be removed by the venous blood. Incorrect or inadequate food intake or disease may predispose a person to fatigue. **2.** the inability of an organism, an organ, or a tissue to give a normal response to a stimulus until a certain recovery period has elapsed.

fatty acid an organic acid with a long straight hydrocarbon chain and an even number of carbon atoms. Fatty acids are the fundamental constituents of many important lipids, including *triglycerides. Some fatty acids can be synthesized by the body; others, the *essential fatty acids, must be obtained from the diet. Examples of fatty acids are *palmitic acid*, *oleic acid*, and *stearic acid*. *See also* fat.

fatty degeneration deterioration in the health of a tissue due to the deposition of abnormally large amounts of fat in its cells. The accumulation of fat in the liver and heart may seriously impair their functioning. The deposition of fat may be linked with incorrect diet, excessive alcohol consumption, or a shortage of oxygen in the tissues caused by poor circulation or a deficiency of haemoglobin.

fauces *n.* the opening leading from the mouth into the pharynx. It is surrounded by the *glossopalatine arch* (which forms the anterior pillars of the fauces) and the *pharyngopalatine arch* (the posterior pillars).

favism *n.* an inherited allergy to a chemical substance found in broad beans; it occurs in parts of the Mediterranean and Iran. Destruction of red blood cells may lead to severe anaemia, requiring blood transfusion.

favus *n.* a type of *ringworm of the scalp, caused by the fungus *Trichophyton schoenleini*. Favus, which is rare in Europe, is typified by yellow crusts made up of the threads of fungus and skin debris, which form honeycomb-like masses.

fear *n.* an emotional state evoked by threat of danger and usually characterized by unpleasant subjective experiences and physiological and behavioural changes. Fear is often distinguished from *anxiety in having a specific object. Physiological changes can include increases in heart rate, blood pressure, sweating, etc. Behavioural changes can include an avoidance of fear-producing objects or situations and may be extremely disabling; for example, fear of open spaces. These specific disabling fears are known as *phobias. Treatment of short-term fears, such as the fear of hearing the results of an examination, can be relieved by tranquillizers, such as diazepam.

febricula *n.* a fever of low intensity or short duration.

febrifuge *n.* a treatment or drug that reduces or prevents fever. *See* antipyretic.

febrile *adj.* relating to or affected with fever.

feeblemindedness *n.* a mild degree of mental *subnormality, corresponding roughly to an *intelligence quotient of 50–70. It is usually caused by an interaction of genetic and environmental factors, the nature of the psychological environment being of much importance.

feedback *n.* the coupling of the output of a process to the input. Feedback mechanisms are important in regulating many physiological processes; for example, hormone output and enzyme-mediated reactions. In *negative feedback*, a rise in the output of a substance (e.g. a hormone) will inhibit a further increase in its production, either directly or indirectly. In *positive feedback*, a rise in the output of a substance is associated with an increase in the output of another substance, either directly or indirectly.

Fehling's solution a solution used for detecting the presence of sugar in urine. There are two components: Fehling's I (a copper sulphate solution) and Fehling's II (a solution of potassium sodium tartrate and sodium hydroxide), which are kept separate until required for use. Boiling Fehling's solution (equal amounts of Fehling's I and II) is added to an equal volume of boiling urine; a yellowish or brownish coloration indicates the presence of sugar.

Feingold diet a diet that purports to treat many illnesses by the elimination of artificial food colourings, preserva-

tives, and salicylates from the diet. It is particularly recommended for the treatment of *hyperkinetic syndrome, but is of unproved value.

felon *n. see* whitlow.

feminization *n.* the development of female secondary sexual characteristics (enlargement of the breasts, loss of facial hair, and fat beneath the skin) in the male, either as a result of an endocrine disorder or of hormone therapy.

femoral *adj.* of or relating to the thigh or to the femur.

femoral artery an artery arising from the external iliac artery at the inguinal ligament. It is situated superficially, running down the front medial aspect of the thigh. Two-thirds of the way down it passes into the back of the thigh, continuing downward behind the knee as the *popliteal artery*.

femoral nerve the nerve that supplies the quadriceps muscle at the front of the thigh and receives sensation from the front and inner sides of the thigh. It arises from the second, third, and fourth lumbar nerves.

femoral triangle (Scarpa's triangle) a triangular depression on the inner side of the thigh bounded by the sartorius and adductor longus muscles and the inguinal ligament. The pulse can be felt here as the femoral artery lies over the depression.

femur (thigh bone) *n.* a long bone between the hip and the knee (see illustration). The head of the femur articulates with the acetabulum of the *hip bone. The *greater* and *lesser trochanters* are protuberances on which the gluteus and psoas major muscles, respectively, are inserted. The *lateral* and *medial condyles* articulate with the *tibia and the concave grooved *patellar surface* accommodates the kneecap (patella).

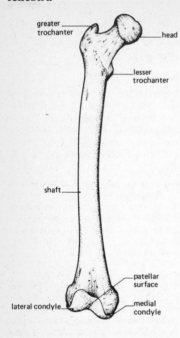

greater trochanter

head

lesser trochanter

shaft

patellar surface

lateral condyle

medial condyle

The femur (front view)

fenestra n. (in anatomy) an opening resembling a window. The *fenestra ovalis* (*fenestra vestibuli*) – the oval window – is the opening between the middle *ear and the vestibule of the inner ear. It is closed by a membrane to which the stapes is attached. The *fenestra rotunda* (*fenestra cochleae*) – the round window – is the opening between the scala tympani of the cochlea and the middle ear. Sound vibrations leave the cochlea through the fenestra rotunda which, like the fenestra ovalis, is closed by a membrane.

fenestration n. a surgical operation in which a new opening is formed in the bony *labyrinth of the inner ear as part of the treatment of deafness due to *otosclerosis.

fenfluramine n. a drug, similar to *amphetamine, that reduces the appe-

tite and is used in the treatment of obesity. It is administered by mouth; common side-effects are drowsiness and diarrhoea. Trade name: **Ponderax**.

fenoprofen n. an *analgesic drug that also reduces inflammation and is used to treat arthritic conditions. It is administered by mouth and may cause digestive upsets, drowsiness, dizziness, sweating, and headache. Trade name: **Fenopron**.

fermentation n. the biochemical process by which organic substances, particularly carbohydrates, are decomposed by the action of enzymes to provide chemical energy. An example is *alcoholic fermentation*, in which enzymes in yeast decompose sugar to form ethyl alcohol and carbon dioxide.

ferri- (ferro-) *prefix denoting* iron.

ferritin n. an iron-protein complex that is one of the forms in which iron is stored in the tissues.

ferrous sulphate an *iron salt administered by mouth to treat or prevent iron-deficiency anaemia. There are few serious side-effects; stomach upsets and diarrhoea may be prevented by taking the drug with meals. Similar preparations used to treat anaemia include ferrous fumarate and ferrous succinate.

fertility rate the number of live births occurring in a year per 1000 women of child-bearing age (usually 15 to 44 years of age). A less reliable measure of fertility can be obtained from the *live birth rate* (the number of live births per 1000 of the population) or the *natural increase* (the excess of live births over deaths). More rarely quoted are the *gross reproduction rate* (the rate at which the child-bearing female population is reproducing itself) and the *net reproduction rate*, which takes into account female mortality before the age of reproduction. Other measures of fertility include the *legitimate birth rate* (the number of live births per 1000 women married once and aged 16 to 44) and the *illegitimate birth rate* (the number of illegitimate births per 1000 unmarried women and widows aged 15 to 44).

fertilization *n.* the fusion of a spermatozoon and an ovum. Rapid changes in the membrane of the ovum prevent other spermatozoa from penetrating. Penetration stimulates the completion of meiosis and the formation of the second polar body. Once the male and female pronuclei have fused the zygote starts to divide by cleavage.

festination *n.* the short tottering steps that characterize the gait of a patient with *parkinsonism.

fetishism *n.* sexual attraction to an inappropriate object (known as a *fetish*). This may be a part of the body (e.g. the foot or the hair), clothing (e.g. underwear or shoes), or other objects (e.g. leather handbags or rubber sheets). In all these cases the fetish has replaced the normal object of sexual love, in some cases to the point at which sexual relationships with another person are impossible or are possible only if the fetish is either present or fantasized. Treatment can involve *psychotherapy or behaviour therapy using *aversion therapy and masturbatory conditioning of desirable sexual behaviour. *See also* perversion.

feto- *prefix denoting* a fetus.

fetor (foetor) *n.* an unpleasant smell. *Fetor oris* is bad breath (*halitosis).

fetoscopy *n.* a technique in which a hollow needle is inserted through the abdomen of a pregnant woman and fetal blood is withdrawn from a blood vessel on the placenta, close to the umbilical cord. Fetoscopy, usually performed in the 18th–20th week of gestation, enables the blood of a fetus to be examined for the presence of abnormal cells and hence the *prenatal diagnosis of blood disorders (such as *thalassaemia, haemophilia, and *sickle-cell disease) and Duchenne *muscular dystrophy.

fetus (foetus) *n.* a mammalian *embryo during the later stages of development within the womb. In man it refers to the products of conception from the beginning of the third month of pregnancy until birth. —**fetal** *adj.*

Feulgen reaction a method of demonstrating the presence of DNA in cell nuclei. The tissue section under investigation, after hydrolysis with dilute hydrochloric acid, is treated with *Schiff's reagent. A purple coloration develops in the presence of DNA.

fever (pyrexia) *n.* a rise in body temperature above the normal, i.e. above an oral temperature of 98.6°F (37°C) or a rectal temperature of 99°F (37.2°C). Fever is generally accompanied by shivering, headache, nausea, constipation, or diarrhoea. A rise in temperature above 105°F (40.5°C) may cause delirium and, in young children, *convulsions too. Fevers are usually caused by bacterial or viral infections and can accompany any infectious illness, from the common cold to *malaria. An *intermittent fever* is a periodic rise and fall in body temperature, often returning to normal during the day and reaching its peak at night, as in malaria. A *remittent fever* is one in which body temperature fluctuates but does not return to normal. *See also* relapsing fever.

fibr- (fibro-) *prefix denoting* fibres or fibrous tissue.

fibre *n.* **1.** (in anatomy) a threadlike structure, such as a muscle cell, a nerve fibre, or a collagen fibre. **2.** (in dietetics) *see* dietary fibre. —**fibrous** *adj.*

fibre optics the use of fibres for the transmission of light images. Synthetic fibres with special optical properties can be used in instruments to relay pictures of the inside of the body for direct observation or photography. *See* fibrescope.

fibrescope *n.* an *endoscope that uses *fibre optics for the transmission of images from the interior of the body. Fibrescopes have a great advantage over the older endoscopes as they are flexible and can be introduced into relatively inaccessible cavities of the body.

fibril *n.* a very small fibre or a constituent thread of a fibre (for example, a *myofibril of a muscle fibre). —**fibrillar, fibrillary** *adj.*

fibrillation *n.* a rapid and chaotic beating of the many individual muscle fibres of the heart, which is consequently unable to maintain effective synchronous contraction. The affected part of the heart then ceases to pump blood.
Fibrillation may affect the atria or ventricles independently. *Atrial fibrillation*, a common type of *arrhythmia, results in rapid and irregular heart and pulse rates. The main causes are atherosclerosis, chronic rheumatic heart disease, and hypertensive heart disease. It may also complicate various other conditions, including chest infections and thyroid overactivity. The heart rate is controlled by the administration of *digoxin; in some cases the heart rhythm can be restored to normal by *cardioversion.
When *ventricular fibrillation* occurs the heart stops beating (*see* cardiac arrest). It is most commonly the result of *myocardial infarction.

fibrin *n.* the final product of the process of *blood coagulation, produced by the action of the enzyme thrombin on a soluble precursor fibrinogen. The product thus formed (*fibrin monomer*) links up (polymerizes) with similar molecules to give a fibrous meshwork that forms the basis of a blood clot, which seals off the damaged blood vessel.

fibrinogen *n.* a substance (*coagulation factor), present in blood plasma, that is acted upon by the enzyme thrombin to produce the insoluble protein fibrin in the final stage of *blood coagulation. The normal level of fibrinogen in plasma is 2–4 g/l.

fibrinogenopenia *n.* *see* hypofibrinogenaemia.

fibrinoid *adj.* resembling the protein fibrin. Fibrinoid material is found in the placenta in increasing amounts as pregnancy advances.

fibrinokinase *n.* one of a group of substances (activators) that convert the inactive substance plasminogen to the active enzyme *plasmin, which digests blood clots (*see* fibrinolysis). Fibrinokinase is insoluble in water and can be extracted from animal tissue.

fibrinolysin *n.* *see* plasmin.

fibrinolysis *n.* the process by which blood clots are removed from the circulation, involving digestion of the insoluble protein *fibrin by the enzyme *plasmin. The latter exists in the plasma as an inactive precursor (plasminogen), which is activated in parallel with the *blood coagulation process. Normally a balance is maintained between the processes of coagulation and fibrinolysis in the body; an abnormal increase in fibrinolysis leads to excessive bleeding.

fibroadenoma *n.* *see* adenoma.

fibroblast *n.* a widely distributed cell in *connective tissue that is responsible for the production of both the ground substance and of the precursors of collagen, elastic fibres, and reticular fibres.

fibrocartilage *n.* a tough kind of *cartilage in which there are dense bundles of fibres in the matrix. It is found in the intervertebral discs and pubic symphysis.

fibrocyst *n.* a benign tumour of fibrous connective tissue containing cystic spaces. —**fibrocystic** *adj.*

fibrocystic disease of the pancreas *see* cystic fibrosis.

fibrocyte *n.* an inactive cell present in fully differentiated *connective tissue. It is derived from a *fibroblast.

fibrodysplasia *n.* abnormal development affecting connective tissue.

fibroelastosis *n.* overgrowth or disturbed growth of the yellow (elastic) fibres in *connective tissue, especially *endocardial fibroelastosis*, overgrowth and thickening of the wall of the heart's left ventricle.

fibroepithelial polyp a fibrous overgrowth covered by epithelium, often occurring in the mouth in response to chronic irritation. It is sometimes called an *epulis*.

fibroid 1. *n.* (**fibromyoma, uterine fibroma**) a benign tumour of fibrous and muscular tissue, one or more of which may develop in the muscular wall of the womb. Fibroids often cause pain and excessive menstrual bleeding and they may become extremely large. They do not threaten life, but render pregnancy unlikely. It is usually women over 30 years of age who are affected. Fibroids can be removed surgically; in some cases removal of the womb (hysterectomy) may be necessary. If, as frequently happens, discomfort and other symptoms are absent, surgery is not required. **2.** *adj.* resembling or containing fibres.

fibroma *n.* (*pl.* **fibromas** or **fibromata**) a nonmalignant tumour of connective tissue.

fibromyoma *n.* a tumour of muscular and fibrous material, usually occurring in the womb (*see* fibroid).

fibroplasia *n.* the production of fibrous tissue, occurring normally during the healing of wounds. *Retrolental fibroplasia* is the abnormal proliferation of fibrous tissue immediately behind the lens of the eye, leading to blindness. It was formerly seen in newborn premature infants due to overadministration of oxygen.

fibrosarcoma *n.* a malignant tumour of connective tissue, derived from *fibroblasts. Fibrosarcomas may arise in soft tissue or bone; they can affect any organ but are most common in the limbs, particularly the leg. They occur in people of all ages and may be congenital. The cells of these tumours show varying degrees of differentiation; the less well differentiated tumours containing elements of histiocytes have been recently reclassified as *malignant fibrous histiocytomas*. Tumours arising in soft tissue have a considerably better prognosis than those arising in bone.

fibrosis *n.* thickening and scarring of connective tissue, most often a consequence of inflammation or injury. *Pulmonary interstitial fibrosis* is thickening and stiffening of the lining of the air sacs (alveoli) of the lungs, causing progressive breathlessness. *See also* cystic fibrosis.

fibrositis *n.* inflammation of fibrous connective tissue, especially an acute inflammation of back muscles and their sheaths, causing pain and stiffness. *See also* muscular rheumatism.

fibrous dysplasia a developmental abnormality in which changes occur in bony tissue, resulting in aching and a tendency to pathological fracture. In *monostotic fibrous dysplasia* one bone is affected; *polyostotic fibrous dysplasia* involves many bones.

fibula *n.* the long thin outer bone of the lower leg. The head of the fibula articulates with the *tibia just below the knee; the lower end projects laterally as the *lateral malleolus*, which articulates with one side of the *talus.

field of vision

field of vision *see* visual field.

figlu test a test for folic acid or vitamin B_{12} deficiency. A dose of the amino acid histidine, which requires the presence of folic acid or vitamin B_{12} for its complete breakdown, is given by mouth. In the absence of these vitamins, *form*imino*glu*tamic acid (figlu) – an intermediate product in histidine metabolism – accumulates and can be detected in the urine.

filament *n.* a very fine threadlike structure, such as a chain of bacterial cells. —**filamentous** *adj.*

filaria *n.* (*pl.* **filariae**) any of the long threadlike nematode worms that, as adults, are parasites of the connective and lymphatic tissues of man capable of causing disease. They include the genera *Brugia, *Loa, *Onchocerca, and *Wuchereria. Filariae differ from the intestinal nematodes (*see* hookworm) in that they undergo part of their development in the body of a bloodsucking insect, e.g. a mosquito, on which they subsequently depend for their transmission to another human host. *See also* microfilaria. —**filarial** *adj.*

filariasis *n.* a disease, common in the tropics and subtropics, caused by the presence in the lymph vessels of the parasitic nematode worms *Wuchereria bancrofti* and *Brugia malayi* (*see* filaria). The worms, transmitted to man by various mosquitoes (including *Aëdes, Culex, Anopheles,* and *Mansonia*), bring about inflammation and eventual blocking of lymph vessels, which causes the surrounding tissues to swell (*see* elephantiasis). The rupture of urinary lymphatics may lead to the presence of *chyle in the urine. Filariasis is treated with the drug *diethylcarbamazine.

filiform *adj.* shaped like a thread; for example, the threadlike *filiform papillae* of the *tongue.

filling *n.* (in dentistry) the operation of inserting a specially prepared substance into a cavity drilled in a carious tooth. The filling may be *temporary* or *permanent*, and various materials may be used (*see* amalgam, cement, composite resin, gold).

filum *n.* a threadlike structure. The *filum terminale* is the slender tapering terminal section of the spinal cord.

fimbria *n.* (*pl.* **fimbriae**) a fringe or fringelike process, such as any of the finger-like projections that surround the opening of the ovarian end of the *Fallopian tube.

fingerprint *n.* the distinctive pattern of minute ridges in the outer horny layer of the skin. Every individual has his or her own unique pattern, though there are six basic fingerprint formations: *double loop, tented loop, radial loop, arch, whorl,* and *ulnar loop* (see illustration). Fingerprint patterns can show the presence of inherited disorders. *See also* dermatoglyphics.

firedamp *n.* (in mining) an explosive mixture of gases, usually containing a high proportion of methane, occasionally encountered in pockets underground. It is distinguished from *blackdamp (chokedamp), which does not ignite.

first aid procedures used in an emergency to help a wounded or ill patient before the arrival of a doctor or admission to hospital.

first intention *see* intention.

fission *n.* a method of asexual reproduction in which the body of a protozoan or bacterium splits into two equal parts (*binary fission*), as in the *amoebae, or more than two equal parts (*multiple fission*), for example sporozoite formation in the malarial parasite (*see* Plasmodium). The resulting products of fission eventually grow into complete organisms.

Ridges on the hand, with details of the most common fingerprints

double loop tented loop radial loop

arch whorl ulnar loop

ionomer cements have been used as fissure sealants.

fistula *n.* an abnormal communication between two hollow organs or between a hollow organ and the exterior. Many fistulas are due to infection or injury. For example, an *anal fistula* may develop after an abscess in the rectum has burst, creating an opening between the anal canal and the surface of the skin. Some fistulas result from malignant growths or ulceration: a carcinoma of the colon may invade and ulcerate the adjacent wall of the stomach, causing a *gastrocolic fistula*. Other fistulas develop as complications of surgery: after gall-bladder surgery, for example, bile may continually escape to the surface through the wound producing a *biliary fistula*. Fistulas may also be a form of congenital abnormality; examples include a *tracheo-oesophageal fistula* (between the windpipe and gullet) and a *rectovaginal fistula* (between the rectum and vagina).

fit *n.* a sudden attack. The term is usually reserved for the attacks of *epilepsy but it is also used more generally, e.g. a fit of coughing.

fixation *n.* **1.** (in psychoanalysis) a failure of psychological development, in which traumatic events prevent a child from progressing to the next developmental stage. This is said to be a cause of mental illness and of personality disorder. *See also* psychosexual development. **2.** a procedure for the hardening and preservation of tissues or microorganisms to be examined under a microscope. Fixation kills the tissues and ensures that their original shape and structure are retained as closely as possible. It also prepares them for sectioning and staining. The specimens can be immersed in a chemical *fixative or subjected to *freeze-drying.

fixative (fixing agent) *n.* a chemical agent, e.g. alcohol or osmium tetroxide,

fissure *n.* **1.** (in anatomy) a groove or cleft; e.g. the *fissure of Sylvius* is the groove that separates the temporal lobe of the brain from the frontal and parietal lobes. **2.** (in pathology) a cleft-like defect in the skin or mucous membrane caused by some disease process; e.g. an *anal fissure* is a break in the skin lining the anal canal. **3.** (in dentistry) a naturally occurring groove in the enamel on the surface of a tooth, especially a molar.

fissure sealant (in dentistry) a material that is bonded to the enamel surface of teeth to seal the fissures, in order to prevent dental caries. Composite resins, unfilled resins, and glass used for the preservation and hardening of tissues for microscopical study. *See* fixation (def. 2).

flaccid *adj.* **1.** flabby and lacking in firmness. **2.** characterized by a decrease in muscle tone (e.g. flaccid *paralysis). —**flaccidity** *n.*

flagellate *n.* a type of *protozoan with one or more fine whiplike threads (*see* flagellum) projecting from its body surface, by means of which it is able to swim. Some flagellates are parasites of man and are therefore of medical importance. *See* Trypanosoma, Leishmania, Giardia, Trichomonas.

flagellation *n.* the act of whipping oneself or others as a means of obtaining sexual pleasure (*see* masochism, sadism). A person displaying this sexual deviation is called a *flagellant* or *flagellomane*.

flagellum *n.* (*pl.* **flagella**) a fine long whiplike thread attached to certain types of cell (e.g. spermatozoa and some unicellular organisms). Flagella are responsible for the movement of the organisms to which they are attached.

flap *n.* **1.** (in surgery) a strip of tissue dissected away from the underlying structures but left attached at one end so that it retains its blood and nerve supply. The flap is then used to repair a defect in another part of the body. The free end of the flap is sewn into the area to be repaired and after about three weeks, when the flap has 'healed into' its new site, the other end is detached and the remainder of the flap is sewn in. Flaps are commonly used by plastic surgeons in treating patients who have suffered severe skin and tissue loss after burns or injuries not amenable to repair by split skin grafting (*see* skin graft). Skin flaps are also used to cover the end of a bone in an amputated limb. **2.** (in dentistry) a piece of mucous membrane and periosteum attached by a broad base. It is lifted back to expose the underlying bone and enable a procedure such as surgical *extraction to be performed. It is subsequently replaced.

flare *n.* **1.** reddening of the skin that spreads outwards from a focus of infection or irritation in the skin. **2.** the red outside part of an urticarial wheal – the skin's response in an allergic or hypersensitivity reaction (*see* urticaria).

flat-foot *n.* absence of the arching of the foot, so that the sole lies flat upon the ground. It may be present in infancy or be acquired in adult life, usually either from prolonged standing or from excessive weight. Flat feet need treatment (exercises) only if they cause pain. Medical name: **pes planus**.

flatulence *n.* **1.** the expulsion of gas or air from the stomach through the mouth; belching. **2.** a sensation of abdominal distension. —**flatulent** *adj.*

flatus *n.* intestinal gas, composed partly of swallowed air and partly of gas produced by bacterial fermentation of intestinal contents. It consists of hydrogen, carbon dioxide, and methane in varying proportions.

flatworm (platyhelminth) *n.* any of the flat-bodied worms, including the *flukes and *tapeworms. Both these groups contain many parasites of medical importance.

flav- (flavo-) *prefix denoting* yellow.

flavin adenine dinucleotide *see* FAD.

flavin mononucleotide *see* FMN.

flavoprotein *n.* a compound consisting of a protein bound to either *FAD or *FMN (called *flavins*). Flavoproteins are constituents of several enzyme systems involved in intermediary metabolism.

flea *n.* a small wingless bloodsucking insect with a laterally compressed body and long legs adapted for jumping. Adult fleas are temporary parasites on birds and mammals and those species that attack man (*Pulex*, *Xenopsylla*, and *Nosopsyllus*) may be important in the transmission of various diseases. Their bites are not only a nuisance but may become a focus of infection. *DDT and pyrethrum powders are used to destroy fleas in the home.

flexibilitas cerea a disorder of posture in which a patient's limbs offer a continuous mild resistance to being moved passively by the examiner and remain for long periods in the position into which the examiner has moved them. It is a feature of *catatonia. *See also* catalepsy.

flexion *n.* the bending of a joint so that the bones forming it are brought to-wards each other. *Plantar flexion* is the bending of the toes (or fingers) down-wards, towards the sole (or palm). *See also* dorsiflexion.

flexor *n.* any muscle that causes bend-ing of a limb or other part.

flexure *n.* a bend in an organ or part, such as the *hepatic* and *splenic flexures* of the *colon.

floccillation *n. see* carphology.

flocculation *n.* a reaction in which normally invisible material leaves solu-tion to form a coarse suspension or precipitate as a result of a change in physical or chemical conditions. Floc-culation tests using serum and special reagents are useful in diagnosing liver abnormalities. *See also* agglutination.

flocculus *n.* a small ovoid lobe of the *cerebellum, overhung by the posterior lobe and connected centrally with the nodulus in the midline.

flooding *n.* **1.** excessive bleeding from the womb, as in *menorrhagia or mis-carriage. **2.** (also called **implosion**) a method of treating *phobias in which the patient is exposed intensively and at length to the feared object, either in reality or fantasy. Although it is dis-tressing and needs good motivation if

treatment is to be completed, it is an effective and rapid therapy.

floppy baby syndrome *see* amyotonia congenita.

flowmeter *n.* an instrument for mea-suring the flow of a liquid or gas. Anaesthetic equipment is fitted with flowmeters so that the administration of anaesthetic gases in different propor-tions can be controlled.

floxuridine *n.* a drug, similar in its action and side-effects to *fluorouracil, used to treat cancers of the digestive system. It is administered by injection.

fluctuation *n.* the characteristic feeling of a wave motion produced in a fluid-filled part of the body by an examiner's fingers. If fluctuation is present when a swelling is examined, this is an indica-tion that there is fluid within and that the swelling is not due to a solid growth.

fludrocortisone *n.* a synthetic *corti-costeroid used to treat disorders of the adrenal glands. It is administered by mouth and side-effects include muscle weakness, bone disorders, digestive and skin disorders, and fluid retention. Trade name: **Florinef**.

flufenamic acid an *analgesic drug used to relieve moderate pain, such as headache, rheumatic conditions, and toothache. It is administered by mouth and may cause indigestion, nausea, and diarrhoea. Trade name: **Arlef**.

fluke *n.* any of the parasitic flatworms belonging to the group Trematoda. Adult flukes, which have suckers for attachment to their host, are parasites of man, occurring in the liver (*liver flukes; see* Fasciola), lungs (*see* Para-gonimus), gut (*see* Heterophyes), and blood vessels (*blood flukes; see* Schisto-soma) and often cause serious disease. Eggs, passed out with the stools, hatch into larvae called *miracidia, which penetrate an intermediate snail host. Miracidia give rise asexually to *redia larvae and finally *cercariae in the snail's tissues. The released cercariae may enter a second intermediate host (such as a fish or crustacean); form a cyst (*metacercaria) on vegetation; or directly penetrate the human skin.

fluorescein sodium a water-soluble dye that glows with a brilliant green colour when light is shone on it. A dilute solution is used to detect defects in the surface of the cornea, since it stains areas where the *epithelium is not intact. In retinal *angiography it is injected into a vein and its circulation through the blood vessels of the retina is viewed and photographed by a special camera.

fluorescence *n.* the emission of light by a material as it absorbs radiation from outside. The radiation absorbed may be visible or invisible (e.g. ultraviolet rays or X-rays). *See* fluoroscope. —**fluorescent** *adj.*

fluoridation *n.* the addition of *fluoride to drinking water in order to reduce *dental caries. Drinking water with a fluoride ion content of one part per million is effective in reducing caries throughout life when given during the years of tooth development. *See also* fluorosis.

fluoride *n.* a compound of fluorine. The incorporation of fluoride ions in the enamel of teeth makes them more resistant to *dental caries. The ions enter enamel during its formation, by surface absorption. The addition of fluoride to public water supplies is called *fluoridation. Fluoride may also be applied topically in toothpaste or by a dentist. If the water supply contains too little fluoride, fluoride salts may be given to children in the form of drops or tablets.

fluoroscope *n.* an instrument on which X-ray images may be viewed directly, without taking and developing X-ray photographs. It consists basically of a

fluorescent screen, which is coated with chemicals that exhibit the property of *fluorescence when exposed to X-rays. Fluoroscopes are used for mass chest X-ray examinations.

fluorosis *n.* the effects of high *fluoride intake. Dental fluorosis is characterized by mottled enamel, which is opaque and may be stained. Its incidence increases when the level of fluoride in the water supply is above 2 parts per million. The mottled enamel is resistant to dental caries. When the level is over 8 parts per million systemic fluorosis may occur, with calcification of ligaments.

fluorouracil *n.* a drug that prevents cell growth (*see* antimetabolite) and is used in the treatment of cancers of the digestive system and breast. It is administered by mouth or injection. Side-effects, which may be severe, include digestive and skin disorders, mouth ulcers, hair loss, nail changes, and blood disorders. Fluorouracil is also applied as a cream to treat certain skin conditions, including skin cancer.

fluphenazine *n.* a *tranquillizer used to relieve anxiety and tension and to treat nausea and vomiting following anaesthesia. It is administered by mouth or injection. High doses may cause drowsiness, restlessness, and abnormal muscular movements. Trade names: **Modecate**, **Moditen**.

flurazepam *n.* a sedative drug used to treat insomnia and sleep disturbances (*see* hypnotic). It is administered by mouth and sometimes causes morning drowsiness, dizziness, and muscle incoordination. Trade name: **Dalmane**.

flush *n.* reddening of the face and/or neck. *Hectic flush* occurs in such wasting diseases as pulmonary tuberculosis. A *hot flush*, accompanied by a feeling of heat, occurs in some emotional disorders and during the menopause.

fluspirilene *n.* a major *tranquillizer used to treat schizophrenia. It is administered by injection; side-effects can include fatigue, digestive upsets, and drowsiness. Trade name: **Redeptin**.

flutter *n.* a disturbance of normal heart rhythm that – like *fibrillation – may affect the atria or ventricles. However, the arrhythmia is less rapid and less chaotic. The causes and treatment are similar to those of fibrillation. *See also* cardiac arrest, defibrillation.

flux *n.* an abnormally copious flow from an organ or cavity. *Alvine flux* is *diarrhoea.

fly *n.* a two-winged insect belonging to a large group called the Diptera. The mouthparts of flies are adapted for sucking and sometimes also for piercing and biting. Fly larvae (maggots) may infest human tissues and cause disease (*see* myiasis).

FMN (flavin monucleotide) a derivative of riboflavin (vitamin B_2) that is the immediate precursor of *FAD and functions as a *coenzyme in various oxidation-reduction reactions.

focal distance (of the eye) the distance between the lens and the point behind the lens at which light from a distant object is focused. In a normal-sighted person this point of focus is on the retina, but distortion of the shape of the eyeball may result in *myopia (short-sightedness) or *hypermetropia (long-sightedness).

focus 1. *n.* the point at which rays of light converge after passing through a lens. **2.** *n.* the principal site of an infection or other disease. **3.** *vb.* (in ophthalmology) to accommodate (*see* accommodation).

foetus *n. see* fetus.

fold *n.* (in anatomy and embryology) the infolding of two surfaces of membranes.

folic acid (pteroylglutamic acid) a B vitamin that is important in the synthesis of nucleic acids. The metabolic role of folic acid is interdependent with that of *vitamin B_{12} (both are required by rapidly dividing cells) and a deficiency of one may lead to deficiency of the other. A deficiency of folic acid results in the condition of megaloblastic anaemia. Good sources of folic acid are liver and vegetables. The actual daily requirement of folate is not known but the suggested daily intake is $200 \mu g$/day for an adult, which should be doubled during pregnancy.

folie à deux (communicated insanity) a condition in which two people who are closely involved with each other share a system of *delusions. Sometimes one member of the pair has developed a *psychosis and has imposed it on the other by a process of suggestion; sometimes both members are schizophrenic and elaborate their delusions or hallucinations together. More than two people may be involved (*folie à trois, folie à quatre*, etc.). Treatment usually involves separation of the affected people and management according to their individual requirements.

folinic acid a derivative of folic acid involved in purine synthesis. Administered by mouth or by injection, it is used to reverse the biological effects of *methotrexate and so to prevent excessive toxicity. This action is termed *folinic acid rescue*. Trade name: **Leucovorin**.

folium *n.* (*pl.* **folia**) a thin leaflike structure, such as any of the folds on the surface of the cerebellum.

follicle *n.* a small secretory cavity, sac, or gland, such as any of the cavities in the *ovary in which the ova are formed. *See also* Graafian follicle, hair follicle. —**follicular** *adj.*

follicle-stimulating hormone

follicle-stimulating hormone (FSH)
a hormone (*see* gonadotrophin) synthesized and released by the anterior pituitary gland. FSH stimulates ripening of the follicles in the ovary and formation of sperm in the testes. It is administered by injection to treat sterility due to lack of ovulation, amenorrhoea, and decreased sperm production. Stimulation of ovulation by FSH may, in some cases, lead to multiple pregnancy.

folliculitis *n.* inflammation of hair follicles in the skin, commonly caused by infection. *See also* sycosis.

fomentation *n. see* poultice.

fomes *n.* (*pl.* **fomites**) any object that is used or handled by a person with a *communicable disease and may therefore become contaminated with the infective organisms and transmit the disease to a subsequent user. Common fomites are towels, bed-clothes, cups, and money.

fontanelle *n.* an opening in the skull of a fetus or young infant due to incomplete *ossification of the cranial bones and the resulting incomplete closure of the *sutures. The *anterior fontanelle* occurs where the coronal, frontal, and sagittal sutures meet; the *posterior fontanelle* occurs where the sagittal and lambdoidal sutures meet (see illustration).

food handler a person engaged in the preparation, storage, cooking, and serving of food. Such people should be free from infectious conditions, either in the form of disease or as carriers. They may be subject to inspection to prove freedom from infection, particularly those who handle food that is either to be eaten raw or has previously been subjected to cooking (e.g. meat pies, paté).

food poisoning an illness affecting the digestive system that results from eating food contaminated either by bacteria or bacterial toxins or, less commonly, by

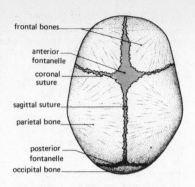

Fontanelles in the skull of a newborn infant (from above)

residues of insecticides (on fruit and vegetables) or poisonous chemicals such as lead or mercury. It can also be caused by eating poisonous fungi, berries, etc. Symptoms commence 1–24 hours after ingestion and include vomiting, diarrhoea, abdominal pain, and nausea. Food-borne infections are caused by bacteria of the genus *Salmonella* in foods of animal origin. The disease is transmitted by human carriers who handle the food, by shellfish growing in sewage-polluted waters, or by vegetables fertilized by manure. Toxin-producing bacteria causing food poisoning include those of the genus *Staphylococcus*, which rapidly multiply in warm foods, and the species *Clostridium welchii*, which multiplies in reheated cooked meals. A rare form of food poisoning – *botulism – is caused by toxins produced by the bacterium *Clostridium botulinum*, which may contaminate badly preserved canned foods. *See also* gastroenteritis.

foramen *n.* (*pl.* **foramina**) an opening or hole, particularly in a bone. The *apical foramen* is the small opening at the apex of a tooth. The *foramen magnum* is a large hole in the occipital bone through which the spinal cord passes. The *foramen ovale* is the opening between the two atria of the fetal heart, which allows blood to flow from the right to the left side of the heart by displacing a membranous valve.

forceps *n.* a pincer-like instrument designed to grasp an object so that it can be held firm or pulled. Specially designed forceps – of which there are many varieties – are used by surgeons and dentists in operations (see illustration). The forceps used in childbirth are so designed as to fit firmly round the baby's head without damaging it. Dental *extraction forceps* are specially designed to fit the various shapes of teeth. By having long handles and short beaks they provide considerable leverage.

forebrain *n.* the furthest forward division of the *brain, consisting of the *diencephalon and the two cerebral hemispheres.

foregut *n.* the front part of the embryonic gut, which gives rise to the oesophagus (gullet), stomach, and part of the small intestine (from which the liver and pancreas develop).

forensic medicine the branch of medicine concerned with the scientific investigation of the causes of injury and death in unexplained circumstances, particularly when criminal activity is suspected. Such investigations are carried out chiefly by pathologists at the request of a *coroner, in conjunction with other experts and police investigators.

forequarter amputation an operation involving removal of an entire arm, including the scapula and clavicle. It is usually performed for soft tissue or bone sarcomas arising from the upper arm or shoulder. *Compare* hindquarter amputation.

foreskin *n. see* prepuce.

forewaters *n.* fluid that comes out of the vaginal opening when the bag

bone-holding forceps

volsella

sinus forceps

dissecting forceps

dressing forceps

obstetrical forceps

dental extraction forceps

Types of forceps

(amnion) around the fetus bursts during labour.

formaldehyde *n.* the aldehyde derivative of formic acid, used as a vapour to sterilize and disinfect rooms and such items as mattresses and blankets. The toxic vapour is produced by boiling *formalin in an open container or using it in a sealed autoclave.

formalin

formalin *n.* a solution containing 40% formaldehyde in water, used as a sterilizing agent. It is lethal to bacteria, viruses, fungi, and spores. It is used to treat wools and hides to kill anthrax spores. Heating the solution produces the irritating vapour of *formaldehyde, which is also used for disinfection.

forme fruste an atypical form of a disease in which the usual symptoms fail to appear and its progress is stopped at an earlier stage than would ordinarily be expected.

formication *n.* a prickling sensation said to resemble the feeling of ants crawling over the skin. It is a form of *paraesthesiae and it is sometimes a symptom of drug intoxication.

formulary *n.* a compendium of formulae used in the preparation of medicinal drugs.

fornix *n.* (*pl.* **fornices**) an arched or vaultlike structure, especially the *fornix cerebri*, a triangular structure of white matter in the brain, situated between the hippocampus and hypothalamus. The *fornix of the vagina* is any of three vaulted spaces at the top of the vagina, around the cervix of the womb.

fossa *n.* (*pl.* **fossae**) a depression or hollow. The *cubital fossa* is the triangular hollow at the front of the elbow joint; the *iliac fossa* is the depression in the inner surface of the ilium; the *pituitary fossa* is the hollow in the sphenoid bone in which the pituitary gland is situated; a *tooth fossa* is a pit in the enamel on the surface of a tooth.

fovea *n.* (in anatomy) a small depression, especially the shallow pit in the retina at the back of the eye. It contains a large number of *cones and is therefore the area of greatest acuity of vision: when the eye is directed at an object, the part of the image that is focused on the fovea is the part that is most accurately registered by the brain. *See also* macula (lutea).

foveola *n.* (in anatomy) a small depression.

fracture *n.* breakage of a bone, either complete or incomplete. A *simple fracture* involves a clean break with little damage to surrounding tissues and no break in the overlying skin. If a bone end pierces the overlying skin the fracture is *compound*, and there is a risk of infection (*see* osteomyelitis). Fracture of an already diseased bone is termed a *pathological fracture* and may occur after minor injuries. Treatment of a simple fracture includes realignment of the bone ends where there is displacement, immobilization by external splints or internal fixation, followed by *rehabilitation. *See also* comminuted fracture, greenstick fracture.

fraenectomy *n.* an operation to remove the fraenum, including the underlying fibrous tissue.

fraenum (frenum, frenulum) *n.* **1.** any of the folds of mucous membrane under the tongue or between the gums and the upper or lower lips. **2.** any of several other structures of similar appearance.

fragile-X syndrome an inherited cause of mental subnormality, and possibly of autism, associated with easily damaged *X chromosomes.

fragilitas *n.* abnormal brittleness or fragility, for example of the hair (*fragilitas crinium*) or the bones (*fragilitas ossium*; *see* osteogenesis imperfecta).

framboesia *n. see* yaws.

framycetin *n.* an *antibiotic used in the form of an ointment, cream, or solution to treat skin, eye, and ear infections. It is also administered by mouth to treat gastroenteritis and food poisoning. Skin sensitivity sometimes occurs and when taken by mouth the drug may cause diarrhoea and diseases due to growth of resistant organisms. Trade names: **Framygen, Soframycin**.

fraternal twins *see* twins.

freckle *n.* a brown spot on the skin commonly found on the arms and face of young people with a fair complexion. Freckles, which are harmless, appear where there is excessive production of the pigment melanin in discrete areas of the skin after exposure to sunlight.

free association (in *psychoanalysis) a technique in which the patient is encouraged to pursue a particular train of ideas as they enter consciousness. *See also* association of ideas.

freeze drying a method for the *fixation of histological specimens, involving a minimum of chemical and physical change. Specimens are immersed in isopentane cooled to −190°C in liquid air. This fixes the tissue instantly, without the formation of large ice crystals (which would cause structural changes). The tissue is then dehydrated in a vacuum for about 72 hours at −32.5°C.

freeze etching a technique for preparing specimens for electron microscopy. The unfixed tissue is frozen and then split with a knife and a layer of ice is sublimed from the exposed surface. The resultant image is thus not distorted by chemical fixatives.

Frei test a diagnostic test for the venereal disease *lymphogranuloma venereum. A small quantity of the virus, inactivated by heat, is injected into the patient's skin. If the disease is present a small red swelling appears at the site of injection within 48 hours.

fremitus *n.* vibrations or tremors in a part of the body, detected by feeling with the fingers or hand (*palpation) or by listening (*auscultation). The term is most commonly applied to vibrations perceived through the chest when a patient breathes, speaks (*vocal fremitus*), or coughs. The nature of the fremitus gives an indication as to whether the chest is affected by disease.

For example, loss of vocal fremitus suggests the presence of fluid in the pleural cavity; its increase suggests consolidation of the underlying lung.

frenulum *n. see* fraenum.

frenum *n. see* fraenum.

frequency distribution (in statistics) presentation of the characteristics (*variables) of a series of individuals (e.g. their heights, weights, or blood pressures) in tabular form or as a histogram so as to indicate the proportion of the series that have different measurements. In a *normal* or *Gaussian distribution* the number of readings and their range on either side of the *mean value is symmetrical; in a *skewed distribution* (e.g. *Poisson*) the measurements are bunched on one side of the mean and spread out over a wider range on the other.

Freudian *adj.* relating to or describing the work and ideas of Sigmund Freud (1856–1939): applied particularly to the school of psychiatry based on his teachings (*see* psychoanalysis).

friction murmur (friction rub) a scratching sound, heard over the heart with the aid of the stethoscope, in patients who have *pericarditis. It results from the two inflamed layers of the pericardium rubbing together during activity of the heart.

Friedman's test a pregnancy test in which a sample of the woman's urine is injected into an unmated female rabbit. After two days the rabbit is killed and its ovaries examined. If the woman is pregnant her urine will contain enough ovary-stimulating hormone (*chorionic gonadotrophin) to induce the development of corpora lutea in the ovaries of the rabbit.

Friedreich's ataxia *see* ataxia.

frigidity *n.* lack of sexual desire or inability to reach the climax of sexual excitement. Frigidity may affect either sex, but the term is almost always applied to women only. In some cases the woman feels revulsion towards sexual activity.

fringe medicine the various systems of healing that are not regarded as part of orthodox treatment by the medical profession. Some of these are based on theories that coincide to some extent with more orthodox medical ideas; others are based on ideas that bear no relation to standard medicine. Among the more reputable systems of fringe medicine are *osteopathy, *acupuncture, *homeopathy, *naturopathy, and *chiropractic.

Fröhlich's syndrome a disorder of the *hypothalamus (part of the brain) affecting males: the boy is overweight with sexual development absent and disturbances of sleep and appetite. Medical name: **dystrophia adiposogenitalis**.

frontal *adj.* **1.** of or relating to the forehead (*see* frontal bone). **2.** denoting the *anterior part of a body or organ.

frontal bone the bone forming the forehead and the upper parts of the orbits; it contains several air spaces (*frontal sinuses: see* paranasal sinuses). At birth it consists of right and left halves, joined by a suture that usually closes during infancy. *See* skull.

frontal lobe the anterior part of each cerebral hemisphere (*see* cerebrum), extending as far back as the deep central sulcus (cleft) of its upper and outer surface. Immediately anterior to the central sulcus lies the motor cortex, responsible for the control of voluntary movement; the area further forward – the *prefrontal lobe – is concerned with behaviour, learning, judgment, and personality.

frontal sinus *see* paranasal sinuses.

frostbite *n.* damage to the tissues caused by freezing. The affected parts,

usually the nose, fingers, or toes, become pale and numb. Ice forms in the tissues, which may thus be destroyed, and amputation may become necessary. Frostbitten parts should not be rubbed, since there is no blood circulation in the tissues, but they may be gently warmed in tepid water. Precautions must be taken against bacterial infection, to which frostbitten skin is highly susceptible.

frottage *n.* rubbing up against somebody (usually in a crowd) as a means of obtaining sexual pleasure. A person displaying this sexual deviation is called a *frotteur*.

frozen shoulder chronic painful stiffness of the shoulder joint. This may follow injury, a stroke, or *myocardial infarction or may gradually develop for no apparent reason. Treatment is by gentle stretching and exercises, sometimes combined with *corticosteroid injection into the joint. *See also* capsulitis.

fructose *n.* a simple sugar found in honey and in such fruit as figs. Fructose is one of the two sugars in *sucrose. Fructose from the diet can be used to produce energy by the process known as *glycolysis, which takes place in the liver. Fructose is important in the diet of diabetics since, unlike glucose, fructose metabolism is not dependent on insulin.

fructosuria (levulosuria) *n.* the presence of fructose (levulose) in the urine.

frusemide *n.* a *diuretic used to treat fluid retention (oedema) associated with heart, liver, or kidney disease and also high blood pressure. It is administered by mouth or injection; common side-effects are nausea and vomiting. Trade name: **Lasix**.

FSH *see* follicle-stimulating hormone.

fuchsin (magenta) *n.* any one of a group of reddish to purplish dyes used in staining bacteria for microscopic observation and capable of killing various disease-causing microorganisms. *Acid fuchsin* (*acid magenta*) is a mixture of sulphonated fuchsins; *basic fuchsin* (*basic magenta*) and *new* (*trimethyl*) *fuchsin* are basic histological dyes (basic fuchsin is also an antifungal agent).

-fuge *suffix denoting* an agent that drives away, repels, or eliminates. Example: *febrifuge* (a drug that reduces fever).

fugue *n.* a period of memory loss during which the patient leaves his usual surroundings and wanders aimlessly or starts a new life elsewhere. It is often preceded by psychological conflict and depression, and may be associated with hysteria or organic mental disease. *See also* dissociation.

fulguration (electrodesiccation) *n.* the destruction with a *diathermy instrument of warts, growths, or unwanted areas of tissue, particularly inside the bladder. This latter operation is performed via the urethra and viewed through a cystoscope.

fulminating (fulminant, fulgurant) *adj.* describing a condition or symptom that is of very sudden onset, severe, and of short duration.

fumigation *n.* the use of gases or vapours to bring about *disinfestation of clothing, buildings, etc. Sulphur dioxide, formaldehyde, and chlorine are common fumigating agents.

functional disorder a condition in which a patient complains of symptoms for which no physical cause can be found. Such a condition is frequently an indication of a psychiatric disorder. *Compare* organic disorder.

fundus *n.* 1. the base of a hollow organ: the part farthest from the opening; e.g. the fundus of the stomach, bladder, or uterus. 2. part of the interior of the eye that is situated opposite the pupil.

fungicide *n.* an agent that kills fungi. *See also* antimycotic.

fungoid 1. *adj.* resembling a fungus. 2. *n.* a fungus-like growth.

fungus *n.* (*pl.* **fungi**) a simple plant that lacks the green pigment chlorophyll. Fungi include the *yeasts, rusts, moulds, and mushrooms. They live either as *saprophytes or as *parasites of plants and animals; some species infect and cause disease in man (*see* blastomycosis). The single-celled microscopic yeasts are a good source of vitamin B and many antibiotics are obtained from the moulds (*see* penicillin). —**fungal** *adj.*

funiculitis *n.* inflammation of the spermatic cord. This usually arises in association with *epididymitis and causes pain and swelling of the involved cord. Treatment is by administration of antibiotics and analgesics.

funiculus *n.* 1. any of the three main columns of white matter found in each lateral half of the spinal cord. 2. a bundle of nerve fibres enclosed in a sheath; a fasciculus. 3. (formerly) the spermatic cord or umbilical cord.

funis *n.* (in anatomy) any cordlike structure, especially the umbilical cord.

furcation *n.* the place where the roots fork on a multirooted tooth.

furfuraceous *adj.* describing scaling of skin in which the scales resemble bran or dandruff.

furor *n.* indiscriminate violence and destructiveness, occurring especially during a period of mental confusion due to *epilepsy.

furuncle *n. see* boil.

furunculosis *n.* 1. the occurrence of several *boils (furuncles) at the same time. 2. the recurrence of boils in the skin over a period of weeks or months. This occurs because of persistence of the infecting bacteria (usually *Staphylo-*

fusiform

coccus aureus) in the skin. Treatment includes thorough daily disinfection of the skin as well as antibiotic therapy.

fusiform *adj.* spindle-shaped; tapering at both ends.

fusion *n.* (in surgery) the joining together of two structures. For example, fusion of two or more vertebra is performed to produce a stable spine.

Fusobacterium *n.* a genus of Gramnegative rodlike bacteria with tapering ends. Most species are normal inhabitants of the mouth of animals and man and produce no harmful effects, but *F. fusiformis* (*Bacteroides fusiformis*), an anaerobic species, is associated with *Borrelia vincentii* in *ulcerative gingivitis.

G

GABA *see* gamma-aminobutyric acid.

Gaffkya *n.* a genus of bacteria now classified as *Micrococcus.*

gag *n.* (in medicine) an instrument that is placed between a patient's teeth to keep his mouth open.

galact- (galacto-) *prefix denoting* 1. milk. Example: *galactosis* (formation of). 2. galactose.

galactagogue *n.* an agent that stimulates the secretion of milk or increases milk flow.

galactocele *n.* 1. a breast tumour containing milk, caused by closure of a milk duct. 2. an accumulation of milky liquid in the sac surrounding the testis (*see* hydrocele).

galactorrhoea *n.* 1. abnormally copious milk secretion. 2. secretion of milk after breast feeding has been stopped.

galactosaemia *n.* an inborn inability to utilize the sugar galactose, which in

consequence accumulates in the blood. Untreated, affected infants fail to thrive and become mentally retarded, but if galactose is eliminated from the diet growth and development may be normal.

galactose *n.* a simple sugar and a constituent of the milk sugar *lactose. Galactose is converted to glucose in the liver. The enzyme necessary for this conversion is missing in infants with a rare inherited metabolic disease called *galactosaemia.

galea *n.* 1. a helmet-shaped part, especially the *galea aponeurotica*, a flat sheet of fibrous tissue (*see* aponeurosis) that caps the skull and links the two parts of the *epicranius muscle. 2. a type of head bandage.

galenical *n.* a pharmaceutical preparation of a drug of animal or plant origin.

gallamine *n.* a drug administered by injection to produce muscle relaxation during anaesthesia (*see* muscle relaxant). It is also used in a diagnostic test for *myasthenia gravis. Trade name: **Flaxedil**.

gall bladder a pear-shaped sac (7–10 cm long), lying underneath the right lobe of the liver, in which *bile is stored (see illustration). Bile passes (via the hepatic duct) to the gall bladder from the liver, where it is formed, and is released into the duodenum (through the common bile duct) under the influence of the hormone *cholecystokininpancreozymin, which is secreted when food is present in the duodenum.

gallstone *n.* a hard mass composed of bile pigments, cholesterol, and calcium salts, in varying proportions, that can form in the gall bladder. The formation of gallstones (*cholelithiasis*) occurs when the physical characteristics of bile alter so that cholesterol is less soluble, though chronic inflammation of the gall bladder (*see* cholecystitis) may also be a contributory factor. Gallstones

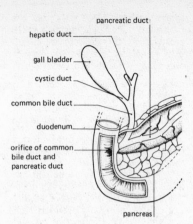

pancreatic duct

hepatic duct

gall bladder

cystic duct

common bile duct

duodenum

orifice of common
bile duct and
pancreatic duct

pancreas

The gall bladder and pancreas and their
associated ducts

may exist for many years without causing symptoms. However, they may cause severe pain (*see* biliary colic) or they may pass into the common bile duct and cause obstructive *jaundice or *cholangitis. Gallstones containing calcium may be seen as a plain X-ray (opaque stones), but if their calcium content is low they can be seen only by *cholecystography. Cholelithiasis is treated by surgical removal of the gall bladder or the stones themselves.

galvanism *n.* (formerly) any form of medical treatment using electricity. *Interrupted galvanism* is a form of *electrotherapy in which direct current, in impulses lasting for 30 to 100 milliseconds, is used to stimulate the activity of nerves or the muscles they supply. *See also* faradism.

galvanocautery *n. see* electrocautery.

Gamblers Anonymous an organization, founded in the US in 1957 and established in the UK in 1964, that seeks to assist compulsive gamblers. The despair, humiliation, and loneliness of compulsive gamblers is neither widely known nor understood. Invari-

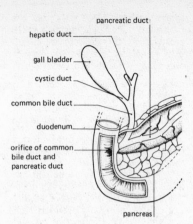

ably their addiction leads to bankruptcy, loss of jobs, rejection by family and friends, and ultimately to criminal means of obtaining money with which to gamble. G.A. offers a form of group therapy similar to that provided by *Alcoholics Anonymous. Senior members help the new members to face their creditors and to work out repayment budgets that will eventually free them from their obligations. The sister organization, Gam-Anon, provides advice and encouragement for the families of compulsive gamblers.

gamete *n.* a mature sex cell: the *ovum of the female or the *spermatozoon of the male. Gametes are haploid, containing half the normal number of chromosomes.

gametocide *n.* a drug that kills *gametocytes. Drugs such as *primaquine destroy gametocytes of the malaria parasite (*see* Plasmodium), so interrupting the life cycle and preventing infection of the mosquito.

gametocyte *n.* any of the cells that are in the process of developing into gametes by undergoing *gametogenesis. *See also* oocyte, spermatocyte.

gametogenesis *n.* the process by which spermatozoa and ova are formed. In both sexes the precursor cells undergo *meiosis, which halves the number of chromosomes. However, the timing of events and the size and number of gametes produced are very different in the male and female. *See* oogenesis, spermatogenesis.

gamma aminobutyric acid (GABA) an amino acid found in the central nervous system, predominantly in the brain, where it acts as an inhibitory *neurotransmitter.

gamma benzene hexachloride a drug used in creams, lotions, solutions, or shampoos to treat infestations caused by scabies, mites, and lice (including head lice). Mild skin reactions occasionally occur. Trade names: **Lorexane, Quellada.**

gamma camera a piece of apparatus for taking photographs of parts of the body into which radioactive isotopes that give off *gamma rays have been introduced as *tracers.

gamma globulin any of a class of proteins, present in the blood *plasma, identified by their characteristic rate of movement in an electric field (*see* electrophoresis). Almost all gamma globulins are *immunoglobulins. *See also* globulin.

gamma rays electromagnetic radiation of wavelengths shorter than X-rays, given off by certain radioactive substances. Gamma rays have greater penetration than X-rays; they are harmful to living tissues and can be used to sterilize certain materials. Carefully controlled doses are used in *radiotherapy.

gamo- *prefix denoting* marriage.

gangli- (ganglio-) *prefix denoting* a ganglion.

ganglion *n.* (*pl.* **ganglia**) **1.** (in neurology) any structure containing a collection of nerve cell bodies and often also numbers of synapses. In the *sympathetic nervous system chains of ganglia are found on each side of the spinal cord, while in the *parasympathetic system ganglia are situated in or nearer to the organs innervated. Swellings in the posterior sensory *roots of the spinal nerves are termed ganglia; these contain cell bodies but no synapses. Within the central nervous system certain well-defined masses of nerve cells are called ganglia (or *nuclei*); for example, the *basal ganglia. **2.** an abnormal but harmless swelling (cyst) that sometimes forms in tendon sheaths, especially at the wrist.

ganglioside *n.* one of a group of *glycolipids found in the brain, liver,

spleen, and red blood cells (they are particularly abundant in nerve cell membranes). Gangliosides are chemically similar to *cerebrosides but contain additional carbohydrate groups.

gangosa *n.* a lesion that occasionally appears in the final stage of *yaws, involving considerable destruction of the tissues of both the hard palate and the nose.

gangrene *n.* death and decay of part of the body due to deficiency or cessation of blood supply. The causes include disease, injury, or *atheroma in major blood vessels, frostbite or severe burns, and diseases such as *diabetes mellitus and *Raynaud's disease. *Dry gangrene* is death and withering of tissues caused simply by a cessation of local blood circulation. *Moist gangrene* is death and putrefactive decay of tissue caused by bacterial infection. *See also* gas gangrene.

Ganser state (pseudodementia) a syndrome characterized by *approximate answers*, i.e. the patient gives grossly and absurdly false replies to questions, but the reply shows that the question has been understood. For example, the question "What colour is snow?" may elicit the reply "Green". This can be accompanied by odd behaviour or episodes of *stupor. The condition is due to *hysteria or to conscious malingering.

gargoylism *n. see* Hurler's syndrome.

gas gangrene death and decay of wound tissue infected by the soil bacterium *Clostridium welchii.* Toxins produced by the bacterium cause putrefactive decay of connective tissue with the generation of gas. Treatment is usually by surgery.

Gasterophilus *n.* a genus of widely distributed non-bloodsucking beelike flies. The parasitic maggots normally live in the alimentary canal of horses but, rarely, can also infect man and cause an inflamed itching eruption of the skin (*see* creeping eruption).

gastr- (gastro-) *prefix denoting* the stomach. Examples: *gastralgia* (pain in); *gastrocolic* (relating to the stomach and colon).

gastrectasia *n.* dilatation of the stomach. This may be caused by *pyloric stenosis or it may occur as a complication of abdominal operations or trauma.

gastrectomy *n.* a surgical operation in which the whole or a part of the stomach is removed. *Total gastrectomy*, in which the oesophagus is joined to the duodenum, is usually performed for stomach cancer but occasionally for the *Zollinger-Ellison syndrome. In *partial* (or *subtotal*) *gastrectomy* the upper third or half of the stomach is joined to the duodenum or small intestine (*gastroenterostomy*): an operation usually carried out in severe cases of *peptic ulcers. After gastrectomy capacity for food is reduced, sometimes leading to weight loss. Other complications of gastrectomy include *dumping syndrome, anaemia, and *malabsorption.

gastric *adj.* relating to or affecting the stomach.

gastric glands tubular glands that lie in the mucous membrane of the stomach wall. There are three varieties: the *cardiac*, *fundic* (*oxyntic*), and *pyloric glands*, and they secrete *gastric juice.

gastric juice the liquid secreted by the *gastric glands of the stomach. Its main digestive constituents are hydrochloric acid, mucin, *rennin, and pepsinogen. The acid acts on pepsinogen to produce *pepsin, which functions best in an acid medium. The acidity of the stomach contents also kills unwanted bacteria and other organisms that have been ingested with the food. Gastric juice also contains *intrinsic factor, which is necessary for the absorption of vitamin B_{12}.

gastric ulcer an ulcer in the stomach, caused by the action of acid, pepsin, and bile on the stomach lining (mucosa). The output of stomach acid is not usually increased. Symptoms include vomiting and pain in the upper abdomen soon after eating, and such complications as bleeding, *perforation, and obstruction due to scarring may occur. Symptoms are relieved by antacid medicines, but surgery may be required if the ulcer persists. Since stomach cancer may mimic a gastric ulcer, all gastric ulcers should be examined by a *gastroscope to aid in their differentiation.

gastrin *n.* a hormone produced in the mucous membrane of the pyloric region of the *stomach. Its secretion is stimulated by the presence of food. It is circulated in the blood to the rest of the stomach, where it stimulates the production of *gastric juice.

gastritis *n.* inflammation of the lining (mucosa) of the stomach. *Acute gastritis* is caused by ingesting excess alcohol or other irritating or corrosive substances and causes vomiting. *Chronic gastritis* is associated with smoking and chronic alcoholism and may be caused by bile entering the stomach from the duodenum. It has no definite symptoms, but the patient is liable to develop gastric ulcers. *Atrophic gastritis*, in which the stomach lining is atrophied, may succeed chronic gastritis but may occur spontaneously as an *autoimmune disease. Dyspeptic symptoms such as nausea, vomiting, loss of appetite, and abdominal discomfort, popularly ascribed to gastritis, are not due to inflammation of the stomach.

gastrocele *n.* a *hernia of the stomach.

gastrocnemius *n.* a muscle that forms the greater part of the calf of the leg (see illustration). It flexes the knee and foot (so that the toes point downwards).

femur

fibula

tibia

gastrocnemius

soleus

Achilles tendon

Gastrocnemius and soleus muscles

gastrocolic reflex a wave of peristalsis produced in the colon by introducing food into a fasting stomach.

gastroduodenostomy *n.* a surgical operation in which the *duodenum (usually the third or fourth part) is joined to an opening made in the stomach in order to bypass an obstruction (such as *pyloric stenosis) or to facilitate the exit of food from the stomach after vagotomy. *See also* duodenostomy.

gastroenteritis *n.* inflammation of the stomach and intestine. It is usually due to acute infection by viruses or bacteria or to food-poisoning toxins and causes vomiting and diarrhoea. The illness usually lasts 3–5 days. Fluid loss is sometimes severe, especially in infants, and intravenous fluid replacement may be necessary.

gastroenterology *n.* the study of gastrointestinal disease, which includes disease of any part of the digestive tract and also of the liver, biliary tract, and pancreas.

gastroenterostomy *n.* a surgical operation in which the small intestine is joined to an opening made in the stomach. The usual technique is *gastroduodenostomy.

gastroileac reflex the relaxation of the *ileocaecal valve caused by the presence of food in the stomach.

gastrojejunostomy *n.* a surgical operation in which the *jejunum is joined to an opening made in the stomach. This is done in preference to *gastroduodenostomy if the latter operation is technically difficult or in special operations to avoid a backflow of bile into the stomach.

gastrolith *n.* a stone in the stomach, which usually builds up around a *bezoar.

gastro-oesophagostomy *n.* a surgical operation in which the *oesophagus (gullet) is joined to the stomach, bypassing the natural junction when this is obstructed by *achalasia, *stricture (narrowing) of the oesophagus, or cancer. This operation is rarely performed, because gastric juices entering the oesophagus through the artificial junction cause inflammation and stricture.

gastropexy *n.* surgical attachment of the stomach to the abdominal wall.

gastroplasty *n.* surgical treatment of a deformity of the stomach, e.g. a deformity due to peptic ulcers.

gastroptosis *n.* a condition in which the stomach hangs low in the abdomen. Although the diagnosis was once used to explain various abdominal complaints, it is now known that the stomach may assume various anatomical positions without causing any symptoms.

gastrorrhoea *n.* excessive secretion of gastric juice. *See* hyperchlorhydria.

gastroscope *n.* an illuminated optical instrument used to inspect the interior of the stomach. For many years these were rigid or semi-rigid instruments affording only limited views, but modern fully flexible *fibreoptic instruments allow all areas of the stomach to be seen and photographed and specimens taken for microscopic examination. As the same instruments can usually be introduced into the duodenum they are also known as *gastroduodenoscopes* or *oesophagogastroduodenoscopes*. —**gastroscopy** *n.*

gastrostaxis *n.* an old term for *haematemesis (bleeding from the stomach).

gastrostomy *n.* a surgical operation in which the stomach is brought through the abdominal wall and an opening made into it. It is usually performed to allow food and fluid to be poured directly into the stomach when swallowing is impossible because of disease or obstruction of the oesophagus. Sometimes it is used temporarily after operations on the oesophagus, until healing has occurred.

gastrotomy *n.* a procedure during abdominal surgery in which the stomach is opened, usually to allow inspection of the interior (e.g. to find a point of bleeding), to remove a foreign body, or to allow the oesophagus to be approached from below (e.g. to pull down a tube through a constricting growth).

gastrula *n.* an early stage in the development of many animal embryos. It consists of a double-layered ball of cells formed by invagination and movement of cells in the preceding single-layered stage (blastula) in the process of *gastrulation*. It contains a central cavity, the *archenteron, which opens through the *blastopore* to the outside. True gastrulation only occurs in the embryos of amphibians and certain fish, but a similar process occurs in the embryonic disc in other vertebrates, including man.

Gaucher's disease an inborn chemical defect causing accumulation of fatty compounds (*cerebrosides) in the liver, spleen, lymph nodes, and nervous system. The disease is fatal in infancy; a less severe form may become apparent only in adult life.

gauss *n.* a unit of magnetic flux density equal to 1 maxwell per square centimetre. 1 gauss = 10^{-4} tesla.

Gaussian distribution *see* frequency distribution, significance.

gauze *n.* thin open-woven material used in several layers for the preparation of dressings and swabs.

gavage *n.* forced feeding: any means used to get an unwilling or incapacitated patient to take in food by mouth, especially via a stomach tube.

gel *n.* a colloidal suspension that has set to form a jelly. Some insoluble drugs are administered in the form of gels.

gelatin *n.* a jelly-like substance formed when tendons, ligaments, etc. containing *collagen (a protein) are boiled in water. Gelatin has been used in medicine as a source of protein in the treatment of malnutrition, in pharmacy for the manufacture of capsules and suppositories, and in bacteriology for preparing culture media.

gemmule *n.* one of the minute spines or surface extensions of a *dendrite, through which contact is made with another neurone at a *synapse.

gene *n.* the basic unit of genetic material, which is carried at a particular place on a *chromosome. Originally it was regarded as the unit of inheritance and mutation but is now usually defined as a piece of *DNA or *RNA that acts as the unit controlling the formation of a single polypeptide chain (*see* cistron). In diploid organisms, including man, genes occur as pairs of *alleles. Various kinds of gene have been discovered: *structural genes* determine the biochemical makeup of the proteins; *regulator genes* control the rate of protein production (*see* operon). *Architectural genes* are responsible for the integration of the protein into the structure of the cell, and *temporal genes* control the time and place of action of the other genes and largely control the *differentiation of the cells and tissues of the body.

general dental services a part of the NHS dental service. Dentists are included on the dental list of the appropriate *Family Practitioner Committee and are independent contractors. They are paid by item of service and the contract with a patient is for a course of treatment only. They are entirely responsible for the financial management of their own practices.

general paralysis of the insane (GPI) a late consequence of syphilitic infection. The symptoms are those of a *dementia and spastic weakness of the limbs. Deafness, epilepsy, and *dysarthria (defective pronunciation) may occur. The infecting organism can be detected in the brain cells and the *Wasserman reaction is usually positive in blood and cerebrospinal fluid. When the symptoms are combined with those of *tabes dorsalis, the condition is called *tabo-paresis*. Vigorous treatment with procaine penicillin is required.

general practitioner (GP) a doctor who is the main agent of *primary medical care*, through whom patients make first contact with health services for a new episode of illness or fresh developments of chronic diseases. Advice and treatment are provided for those who do not require the expertise of a consultant or other specialist services of hospitals (*secondary medical care*). In the British *National Health Service patients on the practice list of a GP receive care without payment on an open-access basis. A practitioner may have private patients in addition to

NHS patients; a few have exclusively private practices. No NHS patient may be charged for a NHS prescription or for a medical certificate; conversely no private patient may receive a NHS prescription. Two or more practitioners may form a partnership sharing fees and work loads, including cross-cover for each other's NHS patients. When they share premises, secretarial help, and other resources this constitutes a *group practice* and the premises from which they operate may be privately owned or may be a publicly owned *health centre. Remuneration of GPs is based on a quarterly capitation fee for each registered patient (higher for those over 65 years of age) regardless of the number of consultations; however, additional claims can be made for a few services (e.g. antenatal care and household calls during sleeping hours).

generic *adj.* of or relating to a *genus.

-genesis *suffix denoting* origin or development. Example: *spermatogenesis* (development of spermatozoa).

genetic code the information carried by *DNA and *messenger RNA that determines the sequence of amino acids in every protein and thereby controls the nature of all proteins made by the cell. The genetic code is expressed by the sequence of *nucleotide bases in the nucleic acid molecule, a unit of three consecutive bases (a *codon*) coding for each amino acid. The code is translated into protein at the ribosomes (*see* transcription, translation). Changes in the genetic code result in the insertion of incorrect amino acids in a protein chain, giving a *mutation.

genetic drift the tendency for variations to occur in the genetic composition of small isolated inbreeding populations by chance. Such populations become genetically rather different from the original population from which they were derived.

genetics *n.* the science of inheritance. It attempts to explain the differences and similarities between related organisms and the ways in which characters are passed from parents to their offspring. *Human* and *medical genetics* are concerned with the study of inherited diseases. *See also* cytogenetics, Mendel's laws.

geni- (genio-) *prefix denoting* the chin.

-genic *suffix denoting* **1.** producing. **2.** produced by.

genicular *adj.* relating to the knee joint: applied to arteries that supply the knee.

geniculum *n.* a sharp bend in an anatomical structure, such as the bend in the facial nerve in the medial wall of the middle ear.

genion *n.* (in *craniometry) the tip of the protuberance of the chin.

genioplasty *n.* an operation performed in plastic surgery to build up the cheek bone with grafted bone, cartilage, or artificial material.

genital *adj.* relating to the reproductive organs or to reproduction.

genital herpes *see* herpes.

genitalia *pl. n.* the reproductive organs of either the male or the female. However, the term is usually used in reference to the external parts of the reproductive system. *See also* vulva.

genito- *prefix denoting* the reproductive organs. Examples: *genitoplasty* (plastic surgery of); *genitourinary* (relating to the reproductive and excretory systems).

genogram *n.* a technique of family *psychotherapy, in which a family tree and family history are constructed in view of the whole family to help them understand each other better.

genome *n.* the basic *haploid set of chromosomes of an organism. Man has a genome of 23 chromosomes.

genotype *n.* **1.** the genetic constitution of an individual or group, as determined by the particular set of genes it possesses. **2.** the genetic information carried by a pair of alleles, which determines a particular characteristic. *Compare* phenotype.

gentamicin *n.* an *antibiotic used to treat infections caused by a wide range of bacteria. It can be administered by injection or applied in a cream to the skin or in drops to the ears and eyes. Kidney and ear damage may occur at high doses. Trade names: **Cidomycin, Genticin**.

gentian violet 1. *see* crystal violet. **2.** *see* methyl violet.

genu *n.* **1.** the knee. **2.** any bent anatomical structure resembling the knee. —**genual** *adj.*

genus *n.* (*pl.* **genera**) a category used in the classification of animals and plants. A genus consists of several closely related and similar species; for example the genus *Canis* includes the dog, wolf, and jackal.

genu valgum abnormal in-curving of the legs, resulting in excessive separation of the feet when the knees are in contact. *See* knock-knee.

genu varum abnormal outward curving of the legs, resulting in separation of the knees. *See* bow-legs.

geo- *prefix denoting* the earth or soil.

geophagia *n.* the eating of dirt. *See* pica.

ger- (gero-, geront(o)-) *prefix denoting* old age.

geriatrics *n.* the branch of medicine concerned with the diagnosis and treatment of disorders that occur in old age

germ

and with the care of the aged. *See also* gerontology.

germ *n.* any microorganism, especially one that causes disease. *See also* infection.

German measles a mild highly contagious virus infection, mainly of childhood, causing enlargement of lymph nodes in the neck and a widespread pink rash. The disease is spread by close contact with a patient. After an incubation period of 2–3 weeks a headache, sore throat, and slight fever develop, followed by swelling and soreness of the neck and the eruption of a rash of minute pink spots, spreading from the face and neck to the rest of the body. The spots disappear within seven days but the patient remains infectious for a further 3–4 days. An infection usually confers immunity. As German measles can cause fetal malformations during early pregnancy, girls should be immunized against the disease before puberty. Medical name: **rubella**. *Compare* scarlet fever.

germ cell (gonocyte) any of the embryonic cells that have the potential to develop into spermatozoa or ova. The term is also applied to any of the cells undergoing gametogenesis and to the gametes themselves.

germicide *n.* an agent that destroys microorganisms, particularly those causing disease. *See* antibiotic, antimycotic, antiseptic, disinfectant.

germinal *adj.* **1.** relating to the early developmental stages of an embryo or tissue. **2.** relating to a germ.

germinal epithelium the epithelial covering of the ovary, which was formerly thought to be the site of formation of *oogonia. It is now thought that oogonia persist in a dormant state from the prenatal period until required in reproductive life.

germinal vesicle the nucleus of a mature *oocyte, prior to fertilization. It is considerably larger than the nucleus of other cells.

germ layer any of the three distinct types of tissue found in the very early stages of embryonic development (*see* ectoderm, endoderm, mesoderm). The germ layers can be traced throughout embryonic development as they differentiate to form the entire range of body tissues.

germ plasm the substance postulated by 19th century biologists (notably Weismann) to be transmitted via the gametes from one generation to the next and to give rise to the body cells.

gerontology *n.* the study of the changes in the mind and body that accompany ageing and the problems associated with them.

Gerstmann's syndrome a group of symptoms that represent a partial disintegration of the patient's recognition of his *body image. It consists of an inability to name the individual fingers, misidentification of the right and left sides of the body, and inability to write or make mathematical calculations (*see* acalculia, agraphia). It is caused by disease in the association area of the left parietal lobe of the brain.

gestaltism *n.* a school of psychology that regards mental processes as wholes (*gestalts*) that cannot be broken down into constituent parts. From this was developed *gestalt therapy*, which aims at achieving a suitable gestalt within the patient that includes all facets of functioning.

gestation *n.* the period during which a fertilized egg cell develops into a baby that is ready to be delivered. Gestation averages 266 days in humans (or 280 days from the first day of the last menstrual period). *See also* pregnancy.

Ghon's focus the lesion produced in the lung of a previously uninfected person by tubercle bacilli. It is a small focus of granulomatous inflammation, which may become visible on a chest X-ray if it grows large enough or if it calcifies. A Ghon focus usually heals without further trouble, but in some patients tuberculosis spreads from it via the lymphatics, the air spaces, or the bloodstream.

giant cell any large cell, such as a *megakaryocyte. Giant cells may have one or many nuclei.

giant-cell arteritis *see* arteritis.

Giardia *n.* a genus of parasitic pear-shaped protozoa inhabiting the small intestine of man. They have four pairs of *flagella, two nuclei, and two sucking discs used for attachment to the intestinal wall. *Giardia* is usually harmless but may occasionally cause diarrhoea (*see* giardiasis).

giardiasis (lambliasis) *n.* a disease caused by the parasitic protozoan *Giardia lamblia* in the small intestine. Man becomes infected by eating food contaminated with cysts containing the parasite. Symptoms include diarrhoea, nausea, bellyache, flatulence, and the passage of pale fatty stools (steatorrhoea). Large numbers of the parasite may interfere with the absorption of food through the gut wall. The disease occurs throughout the world and is particularly common in children; it responds well to oral doses of quinacrine and *metronidazole.

gibbus (gibbosity) *n.* a sharply angled curvature of the backbone, resulting from collapse of a vertebra. Infection with tuberculosis was a common cause.

Giemsa's stain a mixture of *methylene blue and *eosin, used for distinguishing different types of white blood cell and for detecting parasitic microorganisms in blood smears. It is one of the *Romanowsky stains.

gigantism *n.* abnormal growth causing excessive height, most commonly due to oversecretion during childhood of *growth hormone (somatotrophin) by the pituitary gland. In *eunuchoid gigantism* the tall stature is due to delayed puberty, which results in continued growth of the long bones before their growing ends (epiphyses) fuse. *See also* acromegaly.

Gilbert's syndrome familial unconjugated hyperbilirubinaemia: a condition due to an inherited congenital deficiency of the enzyme UDP glucuronyl transferase in the liver cells. Patients become mildly jaundiced, especially if they fast or have some minor infection. Occasionally they have mild abdominal discomfort. The jaundice can be diminished by small doses of phenobarbitone, which stimulates enzyme activity. The condition is harmless.

Gilles de la Tourette syndrome a condition of severe and multiple *tics, including vocal tics and involuntary obscene speech (*coprolalia). The patient may also involuntarily repeat the words or imitate the actions of others (*see* palilalia). The condition usually starts in childhood and becomes chronic; the causes are unknown. Drug treatment (for example, with *haloperidol) is sometimes successful.

gingiv- (gingivo-) *prefix denoting* the gums. Example: *gingivoplasty* (plastic surgery of).

gingiva *n.* (*pl.* **gingivae**) the gum: the layer of dense connective tissue and overlying mucous membrane that covers the alveolar bone and necks of the teeth. —**gingival** *adj.*

gingivectomy *n.* the surgical removal of excess gum tissue.

gingivitis *n.* inflammation of the gums (*see* gingiva) caused by *plaque on the surfaces of the teeth at their necks. The gums are swollen and bleed easily. *Chronic gingivitis* is an early stage of *periodontal disease but is reversible with good oral hygiene. *Ulcerative gingivitis is painful and destructive.

ginglymus (hinge joint) *n.* a form of *diarthrosis (freely movable joint) that allows angular movement in one plane only, increasing or decreasing the angle between the bones. Examples are the knee joint and the elbow joint.

girdle *n.* (in anatomy) an encircling or arching arrangement of bones. *See also* pelvic girdle, shoulder girdle.

glabella *n.* the smooth rounded surface of the *frontal bone in the middle of the forehead, between the two eyebrows.

gladiolus *n.* the middle and largest segment of the *sternum.

gland *n.* an organ or group of cells that is specialized for synthesizing and secreting certain fluids, either for use in the body or for excretion. There are two main groups of glands: the *exocrine glands, which discharge their secretions by means of ducts, and the *endocrine glands, which secrete their products – hormones – directly into the bloodstream. *See also* secretion.

glanders (equinia) *n.* an infectious disease of horses, donkeys, and mules that is caused by the bacterium *Actinobacillus mallei* and can be transmitted to man. Symptoms include fever and inflammation (with possible ulceration) of the lymph nodes (a form of the disease known as *farcy*), skin, and nasal mucous membranes. In the untreated acute form death may follow in 2–20 days. In the more common chronic form, many patients survive without treatment. Administration of sulphonamides or streptomycin is usually effective.

glandular fever an infectious disease, thought to be caused by the Epstein-Barr virus, that affects the lymph nodes in the neck, armpits, and groin; it mainly affects adolescents and young adults. After an incubation period of up to seven weeks, symptoms commence with swelling and tenderness of the lymph nodes, fever, headache, a sore throat, and loss of appetite. In some cases the liver is affected, causing *hepatitis, or the spleen is enlarged. Glandular fever is diagnosed by the presence of large numbers of *monocytes in the blood. Complications are rare but symptoms may persist for weeks before recovery. Medical name: **infectious mononucleosis**.

glans (glans penis) *n.* the acorn-shaped end part of the *penis, formed by the expanded end of the corpus spongiosum (erectile tissue). It is normally covered by the prepuce (foreskin), unless this has been removed by circumcision. The term glans is also applied to the end of the *clitoris.

glaucoma *n.* a condition in which loss of vision occurs because of an abnormally high pressure in the eye. In most cases there is no other ocular disease. This is known as *primary glaucoma* and there are two pathologically distinct types: *acute congestive glaucoma*, in which a sudden rise in pressure is accompanied by pain and marked blurring of vision; and *chronic simple glaucoma*, in which the pressure increases gradually, usually without producing pain, and the visual loss is insidious. The same type of visual loss may occur in eyes with a normal pressure: this is called *low-tension glaucoma*. Primary glaucoma occurs increasingly with age and is an important cause of blindness. *Secondary glaucoma* may occur when other ocular disease impairs the normal circulation of the aqueous humour and causes the intraocular pressure to rise.

In all types of glaucoma the eventual problem is to reduce the intraocular pressure. Drops are put into the eye at regular intervals to improve the outflow of aqueous humour from the eye, and drops and tablets (e.g. diuretics) are used to reduce the production of aqueous humour. If this treatment is inadequate surgery may be performed to make an accessory channel through which the aqueous humour may drain from the eye in sufficient quantities to allow the pressure to return to normal. Such operations are known as *drainage* or *fistularizing operations.*

gleet *n.* a discharge of purulent mucus from the penis or vagina resulting from chronic *gonorrhoea.

glenohumeral *adj.* relating to the glenoid cavity and the humerus: the region of the shoulder joint.

glenoid cavity (glenoid fossa) the socket of the shoulder joint: the pear-shaped cavity at the top of the *scapula into which the head of the humerus fits.

gli- (glio-) *prefix denoting* 1. glia. 2. a glutinous substance.

glia (neuroglia) *n.* the special connective tissue of the central nervous system, composed of different cells, including the *oligodendrocytes, *astrocytes, ependymal cells (*see* ependyma), and *microglia, with various supportive and nutritive functions (see illustration). Glial cells outnumber the neurones by between five and ten to one, and make up some 40% of the total volume of the brain and spinal cord. —**glial** *adj.*

gliadin *n.* a protein, soluble in alcohol, that is obtained from wheat. It is one of the constituents of *gluten.

glibenclamide *n.* a drug that reduces the level of sugar in the blood and is used to treat diabetes. It is administered by mouth. Side-effects include mild digestive upsets and skin reactions. Trade name: **Daonil, Euglucon.**

gliding joint *see* arthrodic joint.

glioblastoma (spongioblastoma) *n.* the most malignant type of brain tumour derived from non-nervous (glial)

Ependymal cells

Protoplasmic astrocyte

Fibrous astrocyte

Microglia

Oligodendroglia

Types of glia

tissue (*see* astrocytoma). Its rapid enlargement destroys normal brain cells, with a progressive loss of function, and raises the intracranial pressure, causing headache, vomiting, and drowsiness.

glioma *n.* any tumour of non-nervous cells (*glia) in the nervous system. The term is sometimes used for all tumours that arise in the central nervous system, including *astrocytomas, *oligodendrogliomas, medulloblastomas, and ependymomas. Tumours of low-grade malignancy produce symptoms by pressure on surrounding structures; those of high-grade malignancy may be invasive.

gliosome *n.* a *lysosome in an *astrocyte.

globin *n.* a protein, found in the body, that can combine with iron-containing groups to form *haemoglobin (found in red blood cells) and *myoglobin (found in muscle).

globulin *n.* one of a group of simple proteins that are soluble in dilute salt solutions and can be coagulated by heat. A range of different globulins is present in the blood (the *serum globulins*, including alpha (α), beta (β), and *gamma (γ) globulins). Some globulins have important functions as antibodies (*see* immunoglobulin); others are responsible for the transport of lipids, iron, or copper in the blood.

globulinuria *n.* the presence in the urine of globulins.

globus *n.* a spherical or globe-shaped structure; for example the *globus pallidus*, part of the lenticular nucleus in the brain (*see* basal ganglia).

glomangioma *n.* a harmless but often painful tumour usually occurring in the skin at the ends of the fingers and toes. It arises from nerve tissue in the blood vessels.

glomerulitis *n.* any one of a variety of lesions of the glomeruli (*see* glomerulus) associated with acute or chronic kidney disease. Such lesions are recognized by electron microscopic examination, using immunofluorescent staining techniques, of kidney biopsy specimens taken during the course of the disease.

glomerulonephritis *n.* a disease of the kidneys resulting in the syndrome of *acute nephritis*: the passage of blood in the urine and occasionally fluid retention and swelling (*see* oedema). The exact cause of acute glomerulonephritis is obscure, but in most cases it is thought to represent an abnormal allergic response following a streptococcal sore throat. The acute form of the disease usually settles completely, with rapid return to normal kidney function. Occasionally, it progresses to chronic glomerulonephritis and kidney failure, sometimes via the *nephrotic syndrome.

glomerulus *n.* (*pl.* **glomeruli**) **1.** the network of blood capillaries contained within the cuplike end (*Bowman's capsule*) of a *nephron. It is the site of primary filtration of waste products from the blood into the kidney tubule. **2.** any other small rounded mass.

glomus *n.* (*pl.* **glomera**) a small communication between a tiny artery and vein in the skin of the limbs. It is concerned with the regulation of temperature. Occasionally its malformation and overgrowth produces a small painful tender red swelling (*glomus tumour*). This may be cauterized or removed surgically.

gloss- (glosso-) *prefix denoting* the tongue. Examples: *glossopharyngeal* (relating to the tongue and pharynx); *glossoplasty* (plastic surgery of).

glossa *n. see* tongue.

glossectomy *n.* surgical removal of the tongue, an operation usually carried out for cancer in this structure.

Glossina *n. see* tsetse.

glossitis *n.* inflammation of the tongue. This can be caused by anaemia, candidiasis, vitamin deficiency, or lichen planus.

glossolalia *n.* nonsense speech that mimics normal speech in that it is appropriately formed into an imitation of syllables, words, and sentences. It can be uttered in *trance states and during sleep.

glossopharyngeal nerve the ninth *cranial nerve (IX), which supplies motor fibres to part of the pharynx and to the parotid salivary glands and sensory fibres to the posterior third of the tongue and the soft palate.

glossoplegia *n.* paralysis of the tongue.

glottis *n.* the space between the two *vocal cords. The term is often applied to the vocal cords themselves or to that part of the larynx associated with the production of sound.

gluc- (gluco-) *prefix denoting* glucose. Example: *glucosuria* (urinary excretion of).

glucagon *n.* a hormone, produced by the pancreas, that causes an increase in the blood sugar level and thus has an effect opposite to that of *insulin. Glucagon is administered by injection to counteract diabetic *hypoglycaemia.

glucocorticoid *n. see* corticosteroid.

glucokinase *n.* an enzyme, found in the liver, that catalyses the conversion of glucose to glucose-6-phosphate. This is the first stage of *glycolysis.

gluconeogenesis *n.* the biochemical process in which glucose, an important source of energy, is synthesized from non-carbohydrate sources, such as amino acids. Gluconeogenesis occurs mainly in the liver and kidney and meets the needs of the body for glucose when carbohydrate is not available in sufficient amounts in the diet.

glucosamine *n.* the amino sugar of glucose, i.e. glucose in which the hydroxyl group is replaced by an amino group. Glucosamine is a component of *mucopolysaccharides and *glycoproteins: for example, hyaluronic acid, a mucopolysaccharide found in synovial fluid, and *heparin.

glucose (dextrose) *n.* a simple sugar containing six carbon atoms (a hexose). Glucose is an important source of energy in the body and the sole source of energy for the brain. Free glucose is not found in many foods (grapes are an exception); however, glucose is one of the constituents of both sucrose and starch, both of which yield glucose after digestion. Glucose is stored in the body in the form of *glycogen. The concen-

tration of glucose in the blood is maintained at around 5 mmol/l by a variety of hormones, principally *insulin and *glucagon. If the blood-glucose concentration falls below this level neurological and other symptoms may result (*see* hypoglycaemia). Conversely, if the blood-glucose level is raised above its normal level, to 10 mmol/l, the condition of *hyperglycaemia develops. This is a symptom of *diabetes mellitus.

glucose tolerance test a test used in the diagnosis of *diabetes mellitus. A quantity of glucose is given to the patient by mouth, after a period of fasting, and the concentration of sugar in the blood and urine is estimated at regular intervals during the next few hours. These readings indicate the ability of the patient's body to utilize glucose.

glucoside *n. see* glycoside.

glucuronic acid a sugar acid derived from glucose. Glucuronic acid is an important constituent of *chondroitin sulphate (found in cartilage) and *hyaluronic acid (found in synovial fluid).

glutamate dehydrogenase (glutamic acid dehydrogenase) an important enzyme involved in the *deamination of amino acids.

glutamic acid (glutamate) *see* amino acid.

glutamic oxaloacetic transaminase (GOT) an enzyme involved in the *transamination of amino acids. This enzyme is present in blood serum (*serum GOT, SGOT*); measurement of SGOT may be used in the diagnosis of acute *myocardial infarction and acute liver disease.

glutamic pyruvic transaminase (GPT) an enzyme involved in the *transamination of amino acids. High levels of this enzyme are found in the liver, and measurement of GPT in the serum (*serum GPT, SGPT*) is of use in the diagnosis and study of acute liver disease.

glutaminase n. an enzyme, found in the kidney, that catalyses the breakdown of the amino acid glutamine to ammonia and glutamic acid: a stage in the production of urea.

glutamine n. *see* amino acid.

glutathione n. a peptide containing the amino acids glutamic acid, cysteine, and glycine. It functions as a *coenzyme in several oxidation-reduction reactions.

glutelin n. one of a group of simple proteins found in plants and soluble only in dilute acids and bases. An example is *glutenin*, found in wheat (*see* gluten).

gluten n. a mixture of the two proteins *gliadin* and *glutenin*. Gluten is present in wheat and rye and is important for its baking properties: when mixed with water it becomes sticky and enables air to be trapped and dough to be formed. Sensitivity to gluten leads to *coeliac disease in children.

glutethimide n. a drug used to treat insomnia and other sleep disturbances (*see* hypnotic). It is administered by mouth. Side-effects can include nausea, mental excitement, and skin rashes, and prolonged use may lead to dependence of the *barbiturate type. Trade name: **Doriden**.

gluteus n. one of three paired muscles of the buttocks (*gluteus maximus, gluteus medius* and *gluteus minimus*). They are responsible for movements of the thigh. —**gluteal** *adj.*

glyc- (glyco-) *prefix denoting* sugar.

glyceride n. a *lipid consisting of glycerol (an alcohol) combined with one or more fatty acids. *See also* triglyceride.

glycerin (glycerol) n. a clear viscous liquid obtained by hydrolysis of fats and mixed oils and produced as a by-product in the manufacture of soap. It is used as an *emollient in many skin preparations, as a laxative (particularly in the form of *suppositories), and as a sweetening agent in the pharmaceutical industry.

glyceryl trinitrate (nitroglycerin) a drug that dilates blood vessels and is used to prevent and treat angina (*see* vasodilator). It is administered by mouth and large doses may cause flushing, headache, and fainting. Trade names: **Nitrocontin, Sustac**.

glycine n. *see* amino acid.

glycocholic acid *see* bile acids.

glycogen n. a carbohydrate consisting of branched chains of glucose units. Glycogen is the principal form in which carbohydrate is stored in the body: it is the counterpart of starch in plants. Glycogen is stored in the liver and muscles and may be readily broken down to glucose.

glycogenesis n. the biochemical process, occurring chiefly in the liver and in muscle, by which glucose is converted into glycogen.

glycogenolysis n. a biochemical process, occurring chiefly in the liver and in muscle, by which glycogen is broken down into glucose-1-phosphate. Glycogenolysis forms the first stage of *glycolysis.

glycolipid n. a *lipid containing a sugar molecule (usually galactose or glucose). The *cerebrosides are examples of glycolipids.

glycolysis n. the conversion of glucose, by a series of ten enzyme-catalysed reactions, to lactic acid. Glycolysis takes place in the cytoplasm of cells and the first nine reactions (converting glucose to pyruvate) form the first stage of cellular *respiration. The process involves the production of a small amount of energy (in the form of ATP), gold

which is used for biochemical work. The final reaction of glycolysis (converting pyruvate to lactic acid) provides energy for short periods of time when oxygen consumption exceeds demand; for example, during bursts of intense muscular activity. *See also* lactic acid.

glycoprotein *n.* one of a group of compounds consisting of a protein combined with a carbohydrate (such as galactose or mannose). Examples of glycoproteins are certain enzymes, hormones, and antigens.

glycoside *n.* a compound formed by replacing the hydroxyl (–OH) group of a sugar by another group. (If the sugar is glucose the compound is known as a *glucoside*.) Glycosides found in plants include some pharmacologically important products (such as *digitalis). Other plant glycosides are natural food toxins, present in cassava, almonds, and other plant products, and may yield hydrogen cyanide if the plant is not prepared properly before eating.

glycosuria *n.* the presence of glucose in the urine in abnormally large amounts. Only very minute quantities of this sugar may be found normally in the urine. Higher levels may be associated with diabetes mellitus, kidney disease, and some other conditions.

glymidine *n.* a drug that reduces the level of sugar in the blood and is used to treat diabetes. It is administered by mouth; the commonest side-effects are digestive upsets and skin reactions. Trade name: **Gondafon.**

gnath- (gnatho-) *prefix denoting* the jaw. Example: *gnathoplasty* (plastic surgery of).

gnathion *n.* the lowest point of the midline of the lower jaw (mandible).

Gnathostoma *n.* a genus of parasitic nematodes. Adult worms are commonly found in the intestines of tigers, leopards, and dogs. The presence of the larval stage of *G. spinigerum* in man, who is not the normal host, causes a skin condition called *creeping eruption.

gnotobiotic *adj.* describing germ-free conditions or a germ-free animal that has been inoculated with known microorganisms.

goblet cell a column-shaped secretory cell found in the *epithelium of the respiratory and intestinal tracts. Goblet cells secrete the principal constituents of mucus.

goitre *n.* a swelling of the neck due to enlargement of the thyroid gland. This may be due to lack of dietary iodine, which is necessary for the production of thyroid hormone: the gland enlarges in an attempt to increase the output of hormone. This was the cause of *endemic goitre*, formerly common in regions where the diet lacked iodine. *Sporadic goitre* may be due to simple overgrowth (hyperplasia) of the gland or to a tumour. In *exophthalmic goitre (Graves's disease)* the swelling is associated with overactivity of the gland and is accompanied by other symptoms (*see* thyrotoxicosis).

gold *n.* **1.** a bright yellow metal that is very malleable. In dentistry pure gold is occasionally used as a filling. Alloys are used extensively for *crowns, *inlays, and *bridges, either alone or veneered with a tooth-coloured material. Gold alloys are now only rarely used as the metal framework for partial dentures, *cobalt-chromium alloys being used instead. **2.** (in pharmacology) any of several compounds of the metal gold, used in the treatment of rheumatoid arthritis. It is administered by injection. Common side-effects include mouth ulcers, itching, blood disorders, skin reactions, and inflammation of the colon and kidneys. Trade name: **Myocrisin.**

Golgi apparatus

Golgi apparatus a collection of vesicles and folded membranes in a cell, usually connected to the *endoplasmic reticulum. It stores and later transports the proteins manufactured in the endoplasmic reticulum. The Golgi apparatus is well developed in cells that produce secretions, e.g. pancreatic cells producing digestive enzymes.

Golgi cells types of *neurones (nerve cells) within the central nervous system. *Golgi type I neurones* have very long axons that connect different parts of the system; *Golgi type II neurones*, also known as *microneurones*, have only short axons or sometimes none.

Golgi tendon organ *see* tendon organ.

Gomori's method a method of staining for the demonstration of enzymes, especially phosphatases and lipases, in histological specimens.

gomphosis *n.* a form of *synarthrosis (immovable joint) in which a conical process fits into a socket. An example is the joint between the root of a tooth and the socket in the jawbone.

gonad *n.* a male or female reproductive organ, which produces the gametes. *See* ovary, testis.

gonadotrophin (gonadotrophic hormone) *n.* any of several hormones synthesized and released by the pituitary gland that act on the testes or ovaries (gonads) to promote production of sex hormones and either sperm or ova. The main gonadotrophins are *follicle-stimulating hormone and *luteinizing hormone. They may be given by injection to treat infertility. *See also* chorionic gonadotrophin.

gonagra *n.* gout in the knee.

goni- (gonio-) *prefix denoting* an anatomical angle or corner.

goniometer *n.* an instrument for measuring angles, such as those made in joint movements.

gonion *n.* the point of the angle of the lower jawbone (mandible).

goniopuncture *n.* an operation for congenital glaucoma (*see* buphthalmos) to enable fluid to be drawn from the eye. Using a fine knife, an incision is made from within the eye into Schlemm's canal, at the junction of the cornea and sclera, and continued outwards until the knife appears beneath the conjunctiva. This creates a pathway for fluid to drain from the anterior chamber of the eye to the subconjunctival tissue. The tip of the knife within the eye is observed through a special contact lens.

gonioscope *n.* a special lens used for viewing the structures around the edge of the anterior chamber of the eye (in front of the lens). These structures are hidden behind the sclera just beyond the edge of the cornea and are not accessible to direct viewing.

goniotomy (trabeculotomy) *n.* an operation for congenital glaucoma (*see* buphthalmos) in which a fine knife is used to make an incision into Schlemm's canal from within the eye. It is the first stage of *goniopuncture.

gonococcus *n.* (*pl.* **gonococci**) the causative agent of gonorrhoea: the bacterium *Neisseria gonorrhoeae*. —**gonococcal** *adj.*

gonocyte *n. see* germ cell.

gonorrhoea *n.* a venereal disease, caused by the bacterium *Neisseria gonorrhoeae*, that affects the genital mucous membranes of either sex. Symptoms develop about a week after infection and include pain on passing water and discharge of pus (known as *gleet*) from the penis (in men) or vagina (in women); some infected women, however, experience no symptoms. If a pregnant woman has gonorrhoea, her baby's eyes may become infected during passage through the birth canal (*see* ophthalmia neonatorum). In untreated cases, the infection may spread throughout the reproductive system, causing sterility; severe inflammation of the urethra in men can prevent passage of water (a condition known as *stricture*). Later complications include arthritis, inflammation of the heart valves (*endocarditis), and infection of the eyes, causing conjunctivitis. Treatment with sulphonamides, penicillin, or tetracycline in the early stages of the disease is usually effective. *Compare* syphilis.

good neighbour scheme (in Britain) a voluntary experimental scheme organized by Social Service Departments of local authorities to bridge the gap in the care of the elderly between total independence and the provision of a home help. *See also* social services.

goose flesh the reaction of the skin to cold or fear. The blood vessels contract and the small muscle attached to the base of each hair follicle also contracts, causing the hairs to stand up: this gives the skin an appearance of plucked goose skin. Medical name: **cutis anserina**.

gorget *n.* an instrument used in the operation for removal of stones from the bladder. It is a *director or guide with a wide groove.

gouge *n.* a curved chisel used in orthopaedic operations to cut and remove bone (see illustration).

A gouge

goundou (**anákhré**) *n.* a condition following an infection with *yaws in which the nasal processes of the upper jaw bone thicken (*see* hyperostosis) to form two large bony swellings, about 7 cm in diameter, on either side of the nose. The swellings not only obstruct the nostrils but also interfere with the

field of vision. Initial symptoms include persistent headache and a bloody purulent discharge from the nose. Early cases can be treated with injections of neosalvarsan; otherwise surgical removal of the growths is necessary. Goundou occurs in central Africa and South America.

gout *n.* a disease in which a defect in uric acid metabolism causes an excess of the acid and its salts (urates) to accumulate in the bloodstream and the joints. It results in attacks of acute gouty arthritis and chronic destruction of the joints and deposits of urates (*tophi*) in the skin and cartilage, especially of the ears. The excess of urates also damages the kidneys, in which stones may form. Treatment with drugs that increase the excretion of urates (*uricosuric drugs) or with *allopurinol, which slows their formation, has largely controlled the disease. *See also* podagra.

Graafian follicle a mature follicle in the ovary prior to ovulation, containing a large fluid-filled cavity that distends the surface of the ovary. The *oocyte develops inside the follicle, attached to one side.

graft 1. *n.* any organ, tissue, or object used for *transplantation to replace a faulty part of the body. A *skin graft is a piece of skin cut from a healthy part of the body and used to heal a damaged area of skin. A healthy kidney removed from one person and transplanted to another individual is described as a *kidney* (or *renal*) *graft*. Corneal grafts are taken from a recently dead individual to repair corneal opacity (*see* keratoplasty). Artificial valve grafts are used to replace faulty heart valves. **2.** *vb.* to transplant an organ or tissue.

graft-versus-host disease a condition that occurs following bone marrow transplantation, in which lymphocytes from the grafted marrow reject the host tissues. The skin, gut, and liver are the most severely affected. Drugs that suppress the immune reaction, such as steroids and *cyclosporin A, reduce the severity of the rejection.

grain *n.* a unit of mass equal to 1/7000 of a pound (avoirdupois). 1 grain = 0.0648 gram.

gram *n.* a unit of mass equal to one thousandth of a kilogram. Symbol: g.

-gram *suffix denoting* a record; tracing. Example: *electrocardiogram* (record of an electrocardiograph).

gramicidin *n.* an *antibiotic that acts against a wide range of bacteria. It is used alone or in combination with other antibiotics or antiseptics in ointments, solutions, or sprays for the treatment of infected ulcers, wounds, and burns.

Gram's stain a method of staining bacterial cells, used as a primary means of identification. A film of bacteria spread onto a glass slide is dried and heat-fixed, stained with a violet dye, treated with decolourizer (e.g. alcohol), and then counterstained with red dye. *Gram-negative* bacteria lose the initial stain but take up the counterstain, so that they appear red microscopically. *Gram-positive* bacteria retain the initial stain, appearing violet microscopically. These staining differences are based on variations in the structure of the cell wall in the two groups.

grand mal (major epilepsy) an epileptic fit, sometimes called the *tonic-clonic fit*. At the onset the patient falls to the ground unconscious with his muscles in a state of spasm. The lack of any respiratory movement results in a bluish discoloration of the skin and lips (cyanosis). This – the tonic phase – is replaced by convulsive movements, when the tongue may be bitten and urinary incontinence may occur (the clonic phase). Movements die away and the patient may rouse in a state of confusion, complaining of headache, or he may fall asleep. *See also* epilepsy.

granular cast a cellular *cast derived from a kidney tubule. In certain kidney diseases, notably acute *glomerulonephritis, abnormal collections of renal tubular cells are shed from the kidney, often as a cast of the tubule. The casts can be observed on microscopic examination of the centrifuged deposit of a specimen of urine. Their presence in the urine indicates continued activity of the disease.

granulation *n.* the growth of small rounded outgrowths, made up of small blood vessels and connective tissue, on the healing surface of a wound (when the edges do not fit closely together) or an ulcer. Granulation is a normal stage in the healing process.

granulocyte *n.* any of a group of white blood cells that, when stained with *Romanowsky stains, are seen to contain granules in their cytoplasm. They can be subclassified on the basis of the colour of the stained granules into *neutrophils, *eosinophils, and *basophils.

granulocytopenia *n.* a reduction in the number of *granulocytes (a type of white cell) in the blood. *See* neutropenia.

granuloma *n.* (*pl.* **granulomata** or **granulomas**) a mass of *granulation tissue produced in response to chronic infection, inflammation, a foreign body, or to unknown causes. Infections giving rise to granulomata include tuberculosis, syphilis, *granuloma inguinale, *Wegener's granuloma, leprosy, and some fungal diseases, such as coccidiodomycosis. Granulomata may occur as reactions to such foreign bodies as starch and talc following surgical procedures or to some metals, such as beryllium and zirconium. Sarcoidosis and Crohn's disease are granulomatous diseases of which the causes are not known. A granuloma may occur around the apex of a tooth root as a result of inflammation or infection of its pulp. —**granulomatous** *adj.*

granuloma inguinale an infectious disease caused by the bacterium *Donovania granulomatis*, usually transmitted during sexual intercourse. It is marked by a pimply rash on and around the genital organs, which develops into a granulomatous ulcer. The disease responds to treatment with tetracyclines and streptomycin.

granulomatosis *n.* any condition marked by multiple widespread *granulomas.

granulopoiesis *n.* the process of production of *granulocytes, which normally occurs in the blood-forming tissue of the *bone marrow. Granulocytes are ultimately derived from a *haemopoietic stem cell, but the earliest precursor that can be identified microscopically is the *myeloblast. This divides and passes through a series of stages of maturation termed respectively *promyelocyte, *myelocyte, and *metamyelocyte, before becoming a mature granulocyte. *See also* haemopoiesis.

graph- (grapho-) *prefix denoting* handwriting.

-graph *suffix denoting* an instrument that records. Example: *electrocardiograph* (instrument recording heart activity).

graphology *n.* the study of the characteristics of handwriting to obtain indications about a person's psychological make-up or state of health. It is possible to detect certain signs of physical disease, such as fine nervous tremors or irregularity of the pulse.

grattage *n.* the process of brushing or scraping the surface of a slowly healing ulcer or wound to stimulate healing. Grattage removes *granulation tissue, which – though a stage in the healing

process – sometimes overgrows or becomes infected and therefore delays healing.

gravel *n.* small stones formed in the urinary tract. The stones usually consist of calcareous debris or aggregations of other crystalline material. The passage of gravel from the kidneys is usually associated with severe pain (*ureteric colic*) and may cause blood in the urine. *See also* calculus.

Graves's disease (exophthalmic goitre) *see* thyrotoxicosis.

gravid *adj.* pregnant.

Grawitz tumour *see* hypernephroma.

gray *n.* the *SI unit of absorbed dose of ionizing radiation, being the absorbed dose when the energy per unit mass imparted to matter by ionizing radiation is 1 joule per kilogram. It has replaced the rad. Symbol: Gy.

green monkey disease *see* Marburg disease.

greenstick fracture an incomplete break in a long bone occurring in children, whose bones have greater flexibility. *See also* fracture.

grey matter the darker coloured tissues of the central nervous system, composed mainly of the cell bodies of neurones, branching dendrites, and glial cells (*compare* white matter). In the brain grey matter forms the *cerebral cortex and the outer layer of the cerebellum; in the spinal cord the grey matter lies centrally and is surrounded by white matter.

gripe *n.* severe abdominal pain (*see* colic).

griseofulvin *n.* an *antibiotic administered by mouth to treat fungal infections of the hair, skin, and nails, such as ringworm. Mild and temporary side-effects such as headache, skin rashes, and digestive upsets may occur. Trade names: **Fulcin, Grisovin**.

groin *n.* the external depression on the front of the body that marks the junction of the abdomen with either of the thighs. *See also* inguinal.

grommet *n.* a double-cuffed tube that is inserted in the eardrum to allow drainage of fluid from the middle ear in secretory *otitis media (glue ear).

ground substance the matrix of *connective tissue, in which various cells and fibres are embedded.

group practice *see* general practitioner.

group therapy 1. (**group psychotherapy**) *psychotherapy involving at least two patients and a therapist. The patients are encouraged to understand and analyse their own and one another's problems. *See also* encounter group, psychodrama. 2. therapy in which people with the same problem, such as *alcoholism, meet and discuss together their difficulties and possible ways of overcoming them.

growth hormone (GH, somatotrophin) a hormone, synthesized and stored in the anterior pituitary gland, that promotes growth of the long bones in the limbs and increases protein synthesis. Excessive production of growth hormone results in *gigantism before puberty and *acromegaly in adults. Lack of growth hormone in children causes *dwarfism.

grumous *adj.* coarse; lumpy; clotted; often used to describe the appearance of the centre of wounds or diseased cells or the surface of a bacterial culture.

guaiphenesin *n.* an *expectorant used in cough mixtures and tablets.

guanethidine *n.* a drug that is used to reduce high blood pressure (*see* sympatholytic). It is administered by mouth; common side-effects are diarrhoea, faintness, and dizziness. Trade name: **Ismelin**.

guanine *n.* one of the nitrogen-containing bases (*see* purine) that occurs in the nucleic acids DNA and RNA.

guanosine *n.* a compound containing guanine and the sugar ribose. *See also* nucleotide.

gubernaculum *n.* (*pl.* **gubernacula**) either of a pair of fibrous strands of tissue that connect the gonads to the inguinal region in the fetus. In the male they guide and possibly move the testes into the scrotum before birth. In the female the ovaries descend only slightly within the abdominal cavity and the gubernacula persist as the round ligaments connecting the ovaries and uterus (womb) to the abdominal wall.

Guillain-Barré syndrome a disease of the peripheral nerves in which there is numbness and weakness in the limbs. It usually develops 10–20 days after a respiratory infection that provokes an allergic response in the peripheral nerves. A rapidly progressive form of the disease is called *Landry's paralysis*. *See* polyradiculitis.

guillotine *n.* a surgical instrument used for removing the tonsils. It is loop-shaped and contains a sliding knife blade (see illustration).

A tonsil guillotine

guinea worm a nematode worm, *Dracunculus medinensis*, that is a parasite of man. The white threadlike adult female, 60–120 cm long, lives in the connective tissues beneath the skin. It releases its larvae into a large blister on the legs or arms; when the limbs are immersed in water the larvae escape and are subsequently eaten by tiny water fleas (*Cyclops*), in which their development continues. The disease *dracontiasis results from drinking water contaminated with *Cyclops*.

gullet *n. see* oesophagus.

gum *n.* (in anatomy) *see* gingiva.

gumboil *n.* the opening on the surface of the gum of a chronic abscess associated with the roots of a tooth. It may be accompanied by varying degrees of swelling, pain, and discharge and is more often related to deciduous than to permanent teeth.

gumma *n.* a small soft tumour, characteristic of the tertiary stage of *syphilis, that occurs in connective tissue, the liver, brain, testes, heart, or bone.

gumshield *n.* a soft flexible cover that fits over the teeth for protection in contact sports. The best type is specially made to fit the individual.

gustation *n.* the sense of taste or the act of tasting.

gustatory *adj.* relating to the sense of taste or to the organs of taste.

gut *n.* **1.** *see* intestine. **2.** *see* catgut.

Guthrie test examination of blood obtained from a heel stab to exclude the presence of *phenylketonuria. This rare metabolic disorder (estimated incidence 1/20,000) has severe consequences in terms of mental handicap unless the child receives a special diet from an early age.

gutta *n.* (*pl.* **guttae**) (in pharmacy) a drop. Drops are the form in which medicines are applied to the eyes and ears.

gutta percha the juice of an evergreen Malaysian tree, which is hard at room temperature but becomes soft and elastic when heated in boiling water. On cooling gutta percha will retain any deformity imparted to it when hot; thus it was used in dentistry as an impression material and as a temporary filling material. It has been superseded by better materials but is still used as the core of *root fillings.

guttate *adj.* describing lesions in the skin that are shaped like drops.

gyn- (gyno-, gynaec(o)-) *prefix denoting* women or the female reproductive organs.

gynaecology *n.* the study of diseases of women and girls, particularly those affecting the female reproductive system. *Compare* obstetrics. —**gynaecological** *adj.* —**gynaecologist** *n.*

gynaecomastia *n.* enlargement of the breasts in the male, due either to hormone imbalance or to hormone therapy.

gypsum *n. see* plaster of Paris.

gyr- (gyro-) *prefix denoting* **1.** a gyrus. **2.** a ring or circle.

gyrus *n.* (*pl.* **gyri**) a raised convolution of the *cerebral cortex, between two sulci (clefts).

H

habituation *n.* (in pharmacology) the condition of being psychologically dependent on a drug, following repeated consumption, marked by a craving for the drug if it is withdrawn. *See also* dependence.

habitus *n.* an individual's general physical appearance, especially when this is associated with a constitutional tendency to a particular disease.

haem *n.* an iron-containing compound (a *porphyrin) that combines with the protein globin to form *haemoglobin, found in the red blood cells.

haem- (haema-, haemo-, haemat(o)-) *prefix denoting* blood. Examples: *haematogenesis* (formation of); *haemophobia* (fear of).

haemangioblastoma (Lindau's tumour) *n.* a tumour of the brain or spinal cord arising in the blood vessels of the meninges or brain. It is often associated with *phaeochromocytoma and *syringomyelia. *See also* von Hippel-Lindau disease.

haemangioma *n.* a benign tumour of blood vessels. It often appears on the skin as a type of birthmark (*see* naevus). For example, a *strawberry haemangioma* is seen in newborn babies and infants, usually on the face; it is red and may attain a very large size, but usually disappears spontaneously within the first year of life. *Senile haemangiomas* occur in the elderly. *See also* angioma.

Haemaphysalis *n.* a genus of hard *ticks. Certain species transmit tick *typhus in the Old World; *H. spinigera* transmits the virus causing *Kyasanur Forest disease in India.

haemarthrosis *n.* joint pain and swelling caused by bleeding into a joint. This may follow injury or may occur spontaneously in a disease of the blood, such as *haemophilia. Treatment is by immobilization, cold compresses, and correction of the blood disorder (if present). Removal of blood from the joint may relieve the pain.

haematemesis *n.* the act of vomiting blood. The blood may have been swallowed (e.g. following nosebleed or tonsillectomy) but more often arises from bleeding in the oesophagus, stomach, or duodenum. Common causes are gastric and duodenal ulcers, gastritis brought on by irritating food or drink, and varicose veins in the oesophagus. If much blood is lost, it is usually replaced by blood transfusion.

haemathidrosis (haematidrosis) *n.* *see* haematohidrosis.

haematin *n.* a chemical derivative of *haemoglobin formed by removal of the protein part of the molecule and oxidation of the iron atom from the ferrous to the ferric form.

haematinic *n.* a drug that increases the amount of *haemoglobin in the blood, e.g. ferrous sulphate and other iron-containing compounds. Haematinics are used, often in combination with vitamins and *folic acid, to prevent and treat anaemia due to iron deficiency. They are used particularly to prevent anaemia during pregnancy. Digestive disturbances sometimes occur with haematinics.

haematocoele *n.* a swelling caused by leakage of blood into a cavity, especially that of the membrane overlying the front and sides of the testis. A *parametric* (*pelvic*) *haematocoele* is a swelling near the womb formed by the escape of blood, usually from a Fallopian tube in ectopic pregnancy.

haematocolpos *n.* the accumulation of menstrual blood in the vagina because the hymen at the entrance to the vagina lacks an opening. *See* cryptomenorrhoea.

haematocrit *n.* *see* packed cell volume.

haematocyst *n.* a cyst containing blood.

haematogenous (haematogenic) *adj.* **1.** relating to the production of blood or its constituents; haematopoietic. **2.** produced by, originating in, or carried by the blood.

haematohidrosis (haemathidrosis, haematidrosis) *n.* the secretion of sweat containing blood.

haematology n. the study of blood and blood-forming tissues and the disorders associated with them. —**haematological** adj. —**haematologist** n.

haematoma n. an accumulation of blood within the tissues that clots to form a solid swelling. Injury, disease of the blood vessels, or a clotting disorder of the blood are the usual causative factors. An *intracranial haematoma* causes symptoms by compressing the brain and by raising the pressure within the skull. Injury to the head may tear the middle meningeal artery, giving rise to a rapidly accumulating *extradural haematoma* requiring urgent surgical treatment. In elderly people a relatively slight head injury may tear the veins where they cross the space beneath the dura, giving rise to a *subdural haematoma*. Excellent results are obtained by surgical treatment. An *intracerebral haematoma* may be a consequence of severe head injury but is more often due to *atherosclerosis of the cerebral arteries and high blood pressure. *See also* perianal haematoma.

haematometra n. **1.** accumulation of menstrual blood in the womb. **2.** abnormally copious bleeding in the womb.

haematomyelia n. bleeding into the tissue of the spinal cord. This has been thought to be the cause of acutely developing symptoms that mimic *syringomyelia.

haematopoiesis n. *see* haemopoiesis.

haematoporphyrin n. a type of *porphyrin produced during the metabolism of haemoglobin.

haematosalpinx (haemosalpinx) n. the accumulation of menstrual blood in the *Fallopian tubes.

haematoxylin n. a colourless crystalline compound extracted from logwood (*Haematoxylon campechianum*) and used in various histological stains. When oxidized haematoxylin is converted to *haematein*, which imparts a blue colour to certain parts of cells, especially cell nuclei. *Heidenhain's iron haematoxylin* is used to stain sections that are to be photographed, since it gives great clarity at high magnification.

haematuria n. the presence of blood in the urine. The blood may come from the kidneys, one or both ureters, the bladder, or the urethra, as a result of injury or disease.

haemin n. a chemical derivative of haemoglobin formed by removal of the protein part of the molecule, oxidation of the iron atom, and combination with an acid to form a salt (*compare* haematin). *Chlorohaemin* forms characteristic crystals, the identification of which provides the basis of a chemical test for blood stains.

haemo- *prefix. see* haem-.

haemochromatosis (bronze diabetes, iron-storage disease) n. a hereditary disorder in which there is excessive absorption and storage of iron. This leads to damage and functional impairment of many organs, including the liver, pancreas, and endocrine glands. The main features are a bronze colour of the skin, diabetes, and liver failure. Iron may be removed from the body by blood letting or an iron *chelating agent may be administered. *Compare* haemosiderosis.

haemoconcentration n. an increase in the proportion of red blood cells relative to the plasma, brought about by a decrease in the volume of plasma. Haemoconcentration may occur in any condition in which there is a severe loss of water from the body. *Compare* haemodilution.

haemocytoblast n. *Obsolete.* a type of cell, found in the bone marrow, that was thought by early microscopists to be the ultimate precursor from which all blood cells were derived. *See also* haemopoietic stem cell.

haemocytometer *n.* a special glass chamber of known volume into which diluted blood is introduced. The numbers of the various blood cells present are then counted visually, through a microscope. Haemocytometers have been largely replaced by electronic cell counters.

haemodialysis *n.* a technique of removing waste materials or poisons from the blood using the principle of *dialysis. Haemodialysis is performed on patients whose kidneys have ceased to function; the process takes place in an *artificial kidney*, or *dialyser*. A stream of blood taken from an artery is circulated through the dialyser on one side of a semipermeable membrane, while a solution of similar electrolytic composition to the patient's blood circulates on the other side. Water and waste products from the patient's blood filter through the membrane, whose pores are too small to allow passage of blood cells and proteins. The purified blood is then returned to the patient's body through a vein.

haemodilution *n.* a decrease in the proportion of red blood cells relative to the plasma, brought about by an increase in the total volume of plasma. This may occur in a variety of conditions, including pregnancy and enlargement of the spleen. *Compare* haemoconcentration.

haemoglobin *n.* a substance contained within the red blood cells (*erythrocytes) and responsible for their colour, composed of the pigment *haem* (an iron-containing *porphyrin) linked to the protein *globin*. Haemoglobin has the unique property of combining reversibly with oxygen and is the medium by which oxygen is transported within the body. It takes up oxygen as blood passes through the lungs and releases it as blood passes through the tissues.

Blood normally contains 12–18 g/dl of haemoglobin. *See also* oxyhaemoglobin.

haemoglobinometer *n.* an instrument for determining the concentration of *haemoglobin in a sample of blood, which is a measure of its oxygen-carrying power.

haemoglobinopathy *n.* any of a group of inherited diseases, including *thalassaemia and *sickle-cell disease, in which there is an abnormality in the production of haemoglobin.

haemoglobinuria *n.* the presence in the urine of free haemoglobin. Haemoglobinuria occurs if haemoglobin, released from disintegrating red blood cells, cannot be taken up rapidly enough by blood proteins. The condition sometimes follows strenuous exercise. It is also associated with certain infectious diseases (such as blackwater fever), ingestion of certain chemicals (such as arsenic), and injury.

haemogram *n.* the results of a routine blood test, including an estimate of the blood haemoglobin level, the *packed cell volume, and the numbers of red and white blood cells (*see* blood count). Any abnormalities seen in microscopic examination of the blood are also noted.

haemolysin *n.* a substance capable of bringing about destruction of red blood cells (*haemolysis). It may be an antibody or a bacterial toxin.

haemolysis *n.* the destruction of red blood cells (*erythrocytes). Within the body, haemolysis may result from defects within the red cells or from poisoning, infection, or the action of antibodies in mismatched blood transfusions and it leads to anaemia. Haemolysis of blood specimens may result from unsatisfactory collection or storage or be brought about intentionally as part of an analytical procedure (*see* laking).

haemolytic *adj.* causing, associated with, or resulting from destruction of red blood cells (*erythrocytes). For example, a *haemolytic antibody* is one that causes destruction of red cells; a *haemolytic anaemia* is due to red-cell destruction (*see* anaemia).

haemolytic disease of the newborn the condition resulting from destruction (haemolysis) of the red blood cells of the fetus by antibodies in the mother's blood passing through the placenta. This most commonly happens when the red blood cells of the fetus are Rh positive (i.e. they have the *rhesus factor) but the mother's red cells are Rh negative. The fetal cells are therefore incompatible in her circulation and evoke the production of antibodies. This may result in very severe anaemia of the fetus, leading to heart failure with oedema (*hydrops foetalis) or stillbirth. When the anaemia is less severe the fetus may reach term in good condition, but the accumulation of the bile pigment bilirubin from the destroyed cells causes severe jaundice after birth, which may require *exchange transfusion. If untreated it may cause serious brain damage (*see* kernicterus).

A blood test early in pregnancy enables the detection of antibodies in the mother's blood and the adoption of various precautions for the infant's safety. Some cases of predictably very severe haemolytic disease have been successfully treated by intrauterine transfusion. The incidence of the disease has been greatly reduced by preventing the formation of antibodies in a Rh negative mother. If fetal cells are detected in a woman's blood soon after delivery or after an abortion (using the *Kleihauer technique*), she is given an injection of Rh antibody (anti-D immunoglobulin). This rapidly destroys any Rh positive fetal cells so that they do not remain long enough to stimulate antibody production in her blood (which could affect her next pregnancy).

haemolytic uraemic syndrome a condition in which sudden rapid destruction of red blood cells (*see* haemolysis) causes acute renal failure due partly to obstruction of small arteries in the kidneys. The haemolysis also causes a reduction in the number of platelets, which can lead to severe haemorrhage. The syndrome may occur as a result of septicaemia, eclamptic fits in pregnancy (*see* eclampsia), or as a reaction to certain drugs. There may also be small sporadic outbreaks of the condition without any obvious cause.

haemopericardium *n.* the presence of blood within the membranous sac (pericardium) surrounding the heart, which may result from injury, tumours, rupture of the heart (e.g. following myocardial infarction), or a leaking aneurysm. The heart is compressed (*cardiac tamponade*) and the circulation impaired; a large fall in blood pressure and cardiac arrest may result. Surgical drainage of the blood may be life saving.

haemoperitoneum *n.* the presence of blood in the peritoneal cavity, between the lining of the abdomen or pelvis and the membrane covering the organs within.

haemophilia *n.* a hereditary disorder in which the blood clots very slowly, due to a deficiency of one of the *coagulation factors (*antihaemophilic factor* or *Factor VIII*). The patient may experience prolonged bleeding following any injury or wound, and in severe cases there is spontaneous bleeding into muscles and joints. Bleeding in haemophilia may be treated by transfusions of plasma (which contains Factor VIII). Alternatively concentrated preparations of Factor VIII, obtained by freezing fresh plasma, may be administered (*see* cryoprecipitate). Haemophilia is controlled by a *sex-linked gene, which means that it is almost exclusively restricted to males: women can carry the disease – and pass it on to their sons – without being affected themselves.

Haemophilus *n.* a genus of Gram-negative aerobic nonmotile parasitic rodlike bacteria frequently found in the respiratory tract. They can grow only in the presence of certain factors in the blood and/or certain coenzymes: they are cultured on fresh blood *agar. Most species are pathogenic: *H. aegyptius* causes conjunctivitis, and *H. ducreyi* soft sore (chancroid). *H. influenzae* is associated with acute and chronic respiratory infections and is a common secondary cause of influenza infections.

haemophthalmia *n.* bleeding into the *vitreous humour of the eye.

haemopneumothorax (pneumohaemothorax) *n.* the presence of blood and air in the pleural cavity, usually as a result of injury. Both must be drained out to allow the lung to expand normally. *See also* haemothorax.

haemopoiesis *n.* the process of production of blood cells and platelets which continues throughout life, replacing aged cells (which are removed from the circulation). In healthy adults, haemopoiesis is confined to the *bone marrow, but in embryonic life and in early infancy, as well as in certain diseases,. it may occur in other sites (*extramedullary haemopoiesis*). *See also* erythropoiesis, leucopoiesis, thrombopoiesis. —**haemopoietic** *adj.*

haemopoietic stem cell the cell from which all classes of blood cells are derived. It cannot be identified microscopically, although some workers believe that it is identical in appearance with a *lymphocyte. It can be demonstrated by *tissue culture of the blood-forming tissue of the bone marrow, as well as in certain other sites. *See also* haemopoiesis.

haemoptysis *n.* the coughing up of blood. This symptom should always be taken seriously, however small the amount. In some patients the cause is not serious; in others it is never found. But it should always be reported to a doctor.

haemorrhage (bleeding) *n.* the escape of blood from a ruptured blood vessel, externally or internally. Arterial blood is bright red and emerges in spurts, venous blood is dark red and flows steadily, while damage to minor vessels may produce only an oozing. Rupture of a major blood vessel such as the femoral artery can lead to the loss of several litres of blood in a few minutes, resulting in *shock, collapse, and death, if untreated. *See also* haematemesis, haematuria, haemoptysis.

haemorrhagic *adj.* associated with or resulting from blood loss. (*See* haemorrhage.) For example, *haemorrhagic anaemia* is due to blood loss (*see* anaemia).

haemorrhoidectomy *n.* the surgical operation for removing *haemorrhoids, which are tied and then excised. Possible complications are bleeding or, later, anal stricture (narrowing). The operation is usually performed only for second- or third-degree haemorrhoids.

haemorrhoids (piles) *pl. n.* enlarged (varicose) veins in the wall of the anus (*internal haemorrhoids*), usually a consequence of prolonged constipation or, occasionally, diarrhoea. They most commonly occur at three main points equidistant around the circumference of the anus. Uncomplicated haemorrhoids are seldom painful; pain is usually caused by a *fissure. The main symptom is bleeding, and in *first-degree haemorrhoids*, which never appear at the anus, bleeding at the end of defaecation is the only symptom. *Second-degree haemorrhoids* protrude beyond the anus as an uncomfortable swelling but return spontaneously; *third-degree haemorrhoids* remain outside the anus and need to be returned by pressure.

First- and second-degree haemorrhoids may respond to bowel regulation using a high-fibre diet with faecal softening agents. If bleeding persists, an irritant fluid (a sclerosing agent) may be injected around the swollen veins to make them shrivel up. Forceful dilation of the anus under general anaesthesia is also effective. Third-degree haemorrhoids often require surgery (see haemorrhoidectomy), especially if they become *strangulated (producing severe pain and further enlargement).

External haemorrhoids are either prolapsed internal haemorrhoids or – more often – *perianal haematomas or the residual skin tags remaining after a perianal haematoma has healed.

haemosalpinx *n. see* haematosalpinx.

haemosiderin *n.* a substance composed of a protein shell containing iron salts which may be present inside certain cells, being one of the forms in which iron is stored within the body. It is insoluble and may be demonstrated microscopically in suitably stained tissue preparations.

haemosiderosis *n.* a disorder caused by excessive deposition of iron, which in turn results from excessive intake or administration of iron, usually in the form of blood transfusions. It results in damage to various organs, including the heart and liver. *Compare* haemochromatosis.

haemostasis *n.* the arrest of bleeding, involving the physiological processes of *blood coagulation and the contraction of damaged blood vessels. The term is also applied to various surgical procedures (for example the application of *ligatures or *diathermy to cut vessels) used to stop bleeding.

haemostatic (styptic) *n.* an agent that stops or prevents haemorrhage; for example, *phytomenadione and *thromboplastin. Haemostatics are used to control bleeding due to various causes and may be used in treating bleeding disorders, such as haemophilia.

haemothorax *n.* blood in the pleural cavity, usually due to injury. If the blood is not drained dense fibrous *adhesions occur between the pleural surfaces, which can impair the normal movement of the lung. The blood may also become infected (see empyema).

haemozoin *n.* an iron-containing pigment present in the organisms that cause malaria (*Plasmodium species).

hair *n.* a threadlike keratinized outgrowth of the epidermis of the *skin. It develops inside a tubular *hair follicle*. The part above the skin consists of three layers: an outer *cuticle*; a *cortex*, forming the bulk of the hair and containing the pigment that gives the hair its colour; and a central core (*medulla*), which may be hollow. The *root* of the hair, beneath the surface of the skin, is expanded at its base to form the *bulb*, which contains a matrix of dividing cells. As new cells are formed the older ones are pushed upwards and become keratinized to form the root and shaft. A hair may be raised by a small erector muscle in the dermis, attached to the hair follicle.

hair follicle a sheath of epidermal cells and connective tissue that surrounds the root of a *hair.

hair papilla a projection of the dermis that is surrounded by the base of the hair bulb. It contains the capillaries that supply blood to the growing *hair.

hairy cell an abnormal white blood cell that has the appearance of an immature lymphocyte with fine hairlike cytoplasmic projections around the perimeter of the cell. It is found in a rare form of leukaemia most commonly occurring in young men.

halfway house a residential home for a group of people where some professional supervision is available. It is used as a stage in the rehabilitation of the mentally ill, usually when they have just been discharged from hospital and are able to work but are not yet ready for independent life.

halitosis *n.* bad breath. Causes of temporary halitosis include recently eaten strongly flavoured food, such as garlic or onions, and drugs such as paraldehyde. Other causes include mouth breathing, *periodontal disease, and infective conditions of the nose, throat, and lungs (especially *bronchiectasis). Constipation, indigestion, and some liver diseases may also cause the condition.

hallucination *n.* a false perception of something that is not really there. Hallucinations may be visual, auditory, tactile, gustatory (of taste), or olfactory (of smell). They may be provoked by psychological illness (such as *schizophrenia) or physical disorders in the brain (such as temporal lobe *epilepsy) or they may be caused by drugs or sensory deprivation. Hallucinations should be distinguished from dreams and from *illusions (since they occur at the same time as real perceptions).

hallucinogen *n.* a drug that produces hallucinations, e.g. *cannabis and *lysergic acid diethylamide. Hallucinogens were formerly used to treat certain types of mental illness. —**hallucinogenic** *adj.*

hallux *n.* (*pl.* **halluces**) the big toe.

haloperidol *n.* a *tranquillizer used to relieve anxiety and tension in the treatment of schizophrenia and other psychiatric disorders. It is administered by mouth or injection; muscular incoordination and restlessness are common side-effects. Trade names: **Haldol, Serenace**.

halophilic *adj.* requiring solutions of high salt concentration for healthy growth. Certain bacteria are halophilic. —**halophile** *n.*

halos *pl. n.* coloured rings seen around lights by people with acute congestive glaucoma and sometimes by people with cataract.

halothane *n.* a potent general *anaesthetic administered by inhalation, used for inducing and maintaining anaesthesia in all types of surgical operations. Reduced blood pressure and irregular heartbeat may occur during halothane anaesthesia. Trade name: **Fluothane**.

hamartoma *n.* an overgrowth of mature tissue in which the elements show disordered arrangement and proportion in comparison to normal. The overgrowth is benign but malignancy may occur in any of the constituent tissue elements.

hamate bone (**unciform bone**) a hook-shaped bone of the wrist (*see* carpus). It articulates with the pisiform and triquetral bones behind and with the fourth and fifth metacarpal bones in front.

hammer *n.* (in anatomy) *see* malleus.

hammer toe a deformity of a toe, most often the second, caused by fixed flexion of the first joint. A corn often forms over the deformity, which may be painful. If severe pain does not respond to strapping or corrective footwear, it may be necessary to perform *arthrodesis at the affected joint.

hamstring *n.* any of the tendons at the back of the knee. They attach the *hamstring muscles* (the biceps femoris, semitendinosus, and semimembranosus) to their insertions in the tibia and fibula.

hamulus *n.* (*pl.* **hamuli**) any hooklike process, such as occurs on the hamate, lacrimal, and sphenoid bones and on the cochlea.

handicap *n.* partial or total inability to perform a social, occupational, or other activity. It reflects the extent to which an individual is disadvantaged by some partial or total *disability* when compared with those in a peer group who have no such disability. A handicap is usually related to an identifiable structural *impairment*, often based on a range of two standard deviations from the *mean observation obtained from studying a large number of apparently healthy subjects. It may also reflect functional impairment, which may be unsuspected by the individual and discovered by clinical observation or testing. The alternative terms *abnormality*, *defect*, or *malformation* (for impairment) and *malfunction* (for disability) are used by many authorities but this may sometimes cause confusion.

Hand-Schüller-Christian disease *see* reticuloendotheliosis.

Hansen's bacillus *see* Mycobacterium.

haploid (monoploid) *adj.* describing cells, nuclei, or organisms with a single set of unpaired chromosomes. In man the gametes are haploid following *meiosis. *Compare* diploid, triploid. —**haploid** *n.*

hapt- (hapto-) *prefix denoting* touch.

hapten *n. see* antigen.

haptoglobin *n.* a protein present in blood plasma that binds with free haemoglobin to form a complex that is rapidly removed from the circulation. Depletion of plasma haptoglobin is a feature of anaemias in which red blood cells are destroyed inside the circulation with the release of haemoglobin into the plasma.

harara *n.* a severe and itchy inflammation of the skin occurring in people continuously subjected to the bites of the *sandfly *Phlebotomus papatasii*. The incidence of this allergic skin reaction,

prevalent in the Middle East, may be checked by controlling the numbers of sandflies.

harelip *n.* the congenital deformity of a cleft in the upper lip, on one or both sides of the midline. It occurs when the three blocks of embryonic tissue that go to form the upper lip fail to fuse and it is often associated with a *cleft palate. Medical name: **cheiloschisis**.

Harrison's sulcus a depression on both sides of the chest wall of a child between the pectoral muscles and the lower margin of the ribcage. It is caused by exaggerated suction of the diaphragm when breathing in and develops in conditions in which the airways are partially obstructed or when the lungs are abnormally congested due to some congenital abnormality of the heart.

Hartnup disease a hereditary defect in the metabolism of the amino acid tryptophan, leading to mental retardation, thickening and roughening of the skin, and lack of muscular coordination.

harvest mite *see* Trombicula.

Hashimoto's disease chronic inflammation of the thyroid gland (*thyroiditis*) due to the formation of antibodies against normal thyroid tissue (autoantibodies). Its features include a firm swelling of the thyroid and partial or total failure of secretion of thyroid hormones; often there are autoantibodies to other organs, such as the stomach.

hashish *n. see* cannabis.

haustrum *n.* one of the pouches on the external surface of the *colon.

Haversian canal one of the small canals (diameter about 50 μm) that ramify throughout compact *bone. *See also* Haversian system.

Haversian system one of the cylindrical units of which compact *bone is made. A *Haversian canal* forms a central tube, around which are alternate layers of bone matrix (*lamellae*) and *lacunae* containing bone cells. The lacunae are linked by minute channels (*canaliculi*).

hay fever a form of *allergy due to the pollen of grasses, trees, and other plants, characterized by inflammation of the membrane lining the nose and sometimes of the conjunctiva. The symptoms of sneezing, running or blocked nose, and watering eyes are due to histamine release and often respond to treatment with *antihistamines. If the allergen is identified, it may be possible to undertake *desensitization. Medical name: **allergic rhinitis**.

HCG *see* chorionic gonadotrophin.

head *n*. 1. the part of the body that contains the brain and the organs of sight, hearing, smell, and taste. 2. the rounded portion of a bone, which fits into a groove of another to form a joint; for example, the head of humerus or femur.

headache *n*. pain felt deep within the skull. Most headaches are caused by emotional stress or fatigue but some are symptoms of serious intracranial disease. *See also* migraine.

health centre (in Britain) a building, owned or leased by a District Health Authority, that houses personnel and/or services from one or several sections of the National Health Service (e.g. general practitioners, *community nurses, dentists, *child health clinics, and facilities for X-rays, laboratory tests, and electrocardiography). Services provided by local authorities, such as social services, chiropody, and child psychology, may also operate from such a centre.

health education persuasive methods used to encourage people (either individually or collectively) to adopt life styles that the educators believe will improve health and to reject habits regarded as harmful to health or likely to shorten life expectancy. The term is also used in a broader sense to include instruction about bodily function, etc., so that the public is better informed about health issues.

health service commissioner (ombudsman) an official responsible to Parliament and appointed to protect the interests of patients in relation to administration of the *National Health Service. He can investigate complaints and allegations of maladministration but not of professional negligence.

health visitor a trained nurse with experience in midwifery and special training in preventive medicine (including health education). The training usually takes place at a technical college over three academic terms, the course being approved by the *United Kingdom Central Council for Nursing, Midwifery, and Health Visiting*. All births are notified to the appropriate health visitor, most of whose work is concerned with routine visiting of selected preschool children (though the elderly and chronic sick also receive routine visits). Health visitors do not carry out practical nursing care but seek to educate parents or relatives how best to care for their charges, in particular by drawing attention to unmet needs in terms of health care and those of the social services likely to improve health. A few health visitors have specialist roles (e.g. handicapped children, the elderly, or the tuberculous). Many belong to a professional body known as the *Health Visitors Association* but membership is not obligatory.

hearing aid an electronic device to enable a deaf person to hear, consisting of a miniature sound receiver, an amplifier, and either an earpiece or a vibrator to transfer the amplified sound to the ear. The earpiece fits into the ear; the vibrator (used in cases of conductive *deafness) fits behind the ear and transmits through the bone directly to the inner ear. The aid is powered by a battery, and the whole unit is usually small enough to fit behind the ear inconspicuously.

heart *n.* a hollow muscular cone-shaped organ, lying between the lungs, with the pointed end (*apex*) directed downwards, forwards, and to the left. The heart is about the size of a closed fist. Its wall consists largely of *cardiac muscle (myocardium), lined and surrounded by membranes (*see* endocardium, pericardium). It is divided by a *septum* into separate right and left halves, each of which is divided into an upper *atrium and a lower *ventricle (see illustration). Deoxygenated blood from the *venae cavae passes through the right atrium to the right ventricle. This contracts and pumps blood to the lungs via the *pulmonary artery. The newly oxygenated blood returns to the left atrium via the pulmonary veins and passes through to the left ventricle. This forcefully contracts, pumping blood out

to the body via the *aorta. The direction of blood flow within the heart is controlled by *valves.

heart attack *see* myocardial infarction.

heart block a condition in which conduction of the electrical impulses generated by the natural pacemaker of the heart (the *sinoatrial node) is impaired, so that the pumping action of the heart is slowed down. In *partial* or *incomplete heart block* conduction between atria and ventricles is delayed (*first degree heart block*) or not all the impulses are conducted from the atria to the ventricles (*second degree heart block*). In *third degree* or *complete heart block* no impulses are conducted and the ventricles beat at their own slow intrinsic rate (20–40 per minute).
Heart block may be congenital or it may be due to heart disease, including myocardial infarction, myocarditis, cardiomyopathy, and disease of the valves. It is most frequently seen in the elderly as the result of chronic degenerative scarring around the conducting tissue. There may be no symptoms, but when very slow heart and pulse rates occur the patient may develop heart failure or *Stokes-Adams syndrome. Symptoms

semilunar valve
superior vena cava
inferior vena cava
right atrium
tricuspid valve
right ventricle
septum

pulmonary artery
aorta
pulmonary vein
left atrium
bicuspid valve
chorda tendina (tendon)
left ventricle

→ direction of blood flow through the heart

Vertical section through the heart

may be abolished by the use of an artificial *pacemaker.

heartburn (pyrosis) *n.* discomfort or pain, usually burning in character, that is felt behind the breastbone and often appears to rise from the abdomen towards or into the throat. It may be accompanied by the appearance of acid or bitter fluid in the mouth and is usually caused by regurgitation of the stomach contents into the gullet or by *oesophagitis.

heart failure a condition in which the pumping action of the ventricle of the heart is inadequate. This results in back pressure of blood, with congestion of the lungs and liver. The veins in the neck becomed engorged and fluid accumulates in the tissues (*see* oedema). There is a reduced flow of arterial blood from the heart, which in extreme cases results in peripheral circulatory failure (cardiogenic shock). Heart failure may result from any condition that overloads, damages, or reduces the efficiency of the heart muscle. Common causes are coronary thrombosis, hypertension, chronic disease of the valves, and arrhythmias. The patient experiences breathlessness, even when lying flat, and oedema of the legs.
Treatment consists of rest, a low salt diet, diuretic drugs (e.g. frusemide), and digitalis derivatives (e.g. digoxin). Structural abnormalities, such as defective valves, may be corrected surgically.

heart-lung machine an apparatus for taking over temporarily the functions of both the heart and the lungs during heart surgery. It incorporates a pump, to maintain the circulation, and equipment to oxygenate the blood. Blood is taken from the body by tubes inserted into the superior and inferior venae cavae, and the oxygenated blood is returned under pressure into a large artery, such as the femoral artery. The surgeon is therefore able to undertake the repair or replacement of heart valves or perform other surgical operations involving the heart and great blood vessels.

heat exhaustion fatigue and collapse due to the low blood pressure and blood volume that result from loss of body fluids and salts after prolonged or unaccustomed exposure to heat. It is most common in new arrivals in a hot climate and is treated by giving drinks or intravenous injections of salted water.

heat rash *see* prickly heat.

heatstroke (sunstroke) *n.* raised body temperature (pyrexia), absence of sweating, and eventual loss of consciousness due to failure or exhaustion of the temperature-regulating mechanism of the body. It is potentially fatal unless treated immediately: the body should be cooled by applying damp cloths and body fluids restored by giving drinks or intravenous injections of salted water.

hebephrenia *n.* a form of *schizophrenia. It is typically a chronic condition, and the most prominent features are disordered thinking; inappropriate emotions with thoughtless cheerfulness, apathy, or querulousness; and silly behaviour. It typically starts in adolescence or young adulthood. Social and occupational rehabilitation are the most important therapies for most patients; drugs such as the *phenothiazines or butyrophenones can also help. —**hebephrenic** *adj.*

Heberden's node a lump of cartilage-covered bone arising at the terminal joint of a finger in *osteoarthritis. It is often inherited.

hebetude *n.* apathy and emotional dullness. This is not a symptom specific to any one condition; extreme degrees are found in *schizophrenia and *dementia.

hectic *adj.* occurring regularly. A *hectic fever* typically develops in the afternoons, in cases of pulmonary tuberculosis.

hecto- *prefix denoting* a hundred.

heel *n.* the part of the foot that extends behind the ankle joint, formed by the *heel bone* (*see* calcaneus).

Hegar's sign an indication of pregnancy that may be detectable during the second and third months. If fingers of one hand are inserted into the vagina and those of the other are placed over the pelvic cavity, the lower part of the womb, including the neck, can easily be compressed between the two hands. *See also* Jacquemier's sign.

helc- (helco-) *prefix denoting* an ulcer.

helcoplasty *n.* the surgical repair of ulcers by skin grafting. *See* skin graft.

helicotrema *n.* the narrow opening between the scala vestibuli and the scala tympani at the tip of the *cochlea in the ear.

helio- *prefix denoting* the sun.

heliotherapy *n.* the use of sunlight to promote healing; sunbathing.

helix *n.* the outer curved fleshy ridge of the *pinna of the outer ear.

Heller's syndrome (disintegrative psychosis) a rare mental illness of childhood. Abnormalities of behaviour may be the only sign at first but the condition progresses to psychotic manifestations, such as *stereotypies and hallucinations, and ultimately to dementia. Nearly always a physical cause can be found. The illness progresses to severe incapacity or death.

Heller's test a test for the presence of protein (albumin) in the urine. A quantity of urine is carefully poured onto the same quantity of pure nitric acid in a test tube. A white ring forms at the junction of the liquids if albumin is present. However, a similar result may be obtained if the urine contains certain drugs or is very concentrated. A dark brown ring indicates the presence of an abnormally high level of potassium indoxyl sulphate in the urine (*see* indicanuria).

Helly's fluid a mixture of potassium bichromate, sodium sulphate, mercuric chloride, formaldehyde, and distilled water, used in the preservation of bone marrow.

helminth *n.* any of the various parasitic worms, including the *flukes, *tapeworms, and *nematodes.

helminthiasis *n.* the diseased condition resulting from an infestation with parasitic worms (helminths).

helminthology *n.* the study of parasitic worms.

heloma *n.* a *callosity or *corn on the foot or hand.

hemeralopia *n. see* day blindness.

hemi- *prefix denoting* (in medicine) the right or left half of the body. Example: *hemianaesthesia* (anaesthesia of one side of the body).

hemiachromatopsia *n.* loss of colour appreciation in one half of the visual field.

hemianopia *n.* absence of half of the normal field of vision. The commonest type is *homonymous hemianopia*, in which the same half (right or left) in lost in both eyes. Sometimes the inner halves of the visual field are lost in both eyes, producing a *binasal hemianopia*, while in others the outer halves are lost, producing a *bitemporal hemianopia*. Very rarely both upper halves or both lower halves are lost, producing an *altitudinal hemianopia*.

hemiballismus *n.* a violent involuntary movement usually restricted to one arm and primarily involving the proximal muscles. It is a symptom of disease of the *basal ganglia.

hemicolectomy *n*. surgical removal of about half the *colon (large intestine), usually the right section (*right hemicolectomy*) with subsequent joining of the *ileum to the transverse colon. This is performed for disease of the terminal part of the ileum (such as *Crohn's disease) or of the caecum or ascending colon (such as cancer or Crohn's disease).

hemicrania *n*. **1.** a headache affecting only one side of the head, usually *migraine. **2.** absence of half of the skull in a developing fetus.

hemimelia *n*. congenital absence or gross shortening (aplasia) of the distal portion of the arms or legs. Sometimes only one of the two bones of the distal arm (radius and ulna) or leg (tibia and fibula) may be affected. *See also* ectromelia.

hemiparesis *n*. *see* hemiplegia.

hemiplegia (hemiparesis) *n*. paralysis of one side of the body. Movements of the face and arm are often more severely affected than those of the leg. It is caused by disease of the opposite (contralateral) hemisphere of the brain.

hemisacralization *n*. fusion of the fifth lumbar vertebra to one side only of the sacrum. *See* sacralization.

hemisphere *n*. one of the two halves of the *cerebrum, not in fact hemispherical but more nearly quarter-spherical.

hemizygous *adj*. describing genes that are carried on an unpaired chromosome, for example the genes on the X chromosome in man. —**hemizygote** *n*.

hemlock *n*. the plant *Conium maculatum*, found in Britain and central Europe. It is a source of the poisonous alkaloid *coniine.

hemp *n*. *see* cannabis.

Henle's loop the part of a kidney tubule that forms a loop extending towards the centre of the kidney. It is surrounded by blood capillaries, which reabsorb water and selected soluble substances back into the bloodstream.

henry *n*. the *SI unit of inductance, equal to the inductance of a closed circuit with a magnetic flux of 1 weber per ampere of current. Symbol: H.

Hensen's node (primitive knot) the rounded front end of the embryonic *primitive streak.

heparin *n*. an *anticoagulant produced in liver cells, some white blood cells, and certain other sites, which acts by inhibiting the action of the enzyme *thrombin in the final stage of *blood coagulation. An extracted purified form of heparin is widely used for the prevention of blood coagulation both in patients with thrombosis and similar conditions and in blood collected for examination. The drug is usually administered by injection and the most important side-effect is bleeding.

hepat- (hepato-) *prefix denoting* the liver. Examples: *hepatopexy* (surgical fixation of); *hepatorenal* (relating to the liver and kidney).

hepatalgia *n*. pain in or over the liver. It is caused by liver inflammation (especially an abscess) or swelling (as in cardiac failure).

hepatectomy *n*. the operation of removing the liver. *Partial hepatectomy* is the removal of one or more lobes of the liver; it may be carried out after severe injury or to remove a tumour localized in one part of the liver.

hepatic *adj*. relating to the liver.

hepatic duct *see* bile duct.

hepatic encephalopathy (portosystemic encephalopathy) a condition in which brain function is impaired by the presence of toxic substances, absorbed from the colon, which are normally removed or detoxified by the liver. It occurs when the liver is severely damaged (as in cirrhosis) or bypassed. Symptoms include drowsiness, confusion, difficulty in performing tasks (e.g. writing), and coma. Treatment consists of stopping protein intake and giving antibiotics (to prevent bacterial production of toxins) and enemas and cathartics (to remove colonic toxins).

hepatic flexure the bend in the *colon, just underneath the liver, where the ascending colon joins the transverse colon.

hepaticostomy *n.* a surgical operation in which a temporary or permanent opening is made into the main duct carrying bile from the liver.

hepatic vein one of several short veins originating within the lobes of the liver as small branches, which unite to form the hepatic veins. These lead directly to the inferior vena cava, draining blood from the liver.

hepatitis *n.* inflammation of the liver due to a virus infection or such diseases as amoebic dysentery and lupus. *Infectious hepatitis* (*epidemic hepatitis, epidemic jaundice*) is transmitted by food or drink contaminated by a carrier or patient and commonly occurs where sanitation is poor. After an incubation period of 15–40 days, the patient develops fever and sickness. Yellow discoloration of the skin (*see* jaundice) appears about a week later and persists for up to three weeks. The patient may be infectious throughout this period. Serious complications are unusual and an attack often confers immunity. Injection of *gamma globulin provides temporary protection.
Serum hepatitis is transmitted by infected blood or blood products contaminating hypodermic needles, blood transfusions, or tattooing needles: it often occurs in drug addicts. Symptoms, which develop suddenly after an incubation period of 1–6 months, include headache, fever, chills, general weakness, and jaundice. Most patients make a gradual recovery but the mortality rate is 5–20%. Patients may be detected by identification of the *Australia antigen in their blood.

hepatization *n.* the conversion of lung tissue, which normally holds air, into a solid liver-like mass during the course of acute lobar pneumonia.

hepato- *prefix. see* hepat-.

hepatoblastoma *n.* a malignant tumour of the liver occurring in children, made up of embryonic liver cells. It is often confined to one lobe of the liver; such cases may be treated by partial *hepatectomy.

hepatocellular *adj.* relating to or affecting the cells of the liver.

hepatocyte *n.* the principal cell type in the *liver: a large cell with many metabolic functions, including synthesis, storage, detoxification, and bile production.

hepatoma *n.* a malignant tumour of the liver, originating in mature liver cells. In Western countries it is rare in normal livers, but often develops in patients with cirrhosis. In Africa and other tropical countries it is frequent, possible causes including fungi (*see* aflatoxin) and other ingested toxins. Hepatomas often synthesize *alpha-fetoprotein, which circulates in the blood and is a useful indicator of these tumours.
The term hepatoma is often, though incorrectly, used to include malignant tumours arising in the bile duct (*cholangiocarcinomas*).

hepatomegaly *n.* enlargement of the liver to such an extent that it can be felt below the rib margin. This may be due to congestion (as in heart failure), inflammation, infiltration (e.g. by fat), or tumour.

hepatotoxic *adj.* damaging or destroying liver cells. Drugs such as *paracetamol and *phenacemide can cause liver damage at high doses or with prolonged use.

hept- (hepta-) *prefix denoting* seven.

heptabarbitone *n.* a *barbiturate administered by mouth to treat insomnia. A common side-effect is drowsiness, and prolonged use can lead to dependence. Trade name: **Medomin**.

hereditary *adj.* transmitted from parents to their offspring; inherited.

heredity *n.* the process that causes the biological similarity between parents and their offspring. *Genetics is the study of heredity.

heredo- *prefix denoting* heredity.

hermaphrodite *n.* an individual in which both male and female sex organs are present or in which the sex organs contain both ovarian and testicular cells. Human hermaphrodites are very rare. —**hermaphroditism** *n.*

hernia *n.* the protrusion of an organ or tissue out of the body cavity in which it normally lies. An *inguinal hernia* (or *rupture*) occurs in the lower abdomen; a sac of peritoneum, containing fat or part of the bowel, bulges through a weak part (*inguinal canal*) of the abdominal wall. It may result from physical straining or coughing. A *scrotal hernia* is an inguinal hernia so large that it passes into the scrotum; a *femoral hernia* is similar to an inguinal hernia but protrudes at the top of the thigh, through the point at which the femoral artery passes from the abdomen to the thigh. A *diaphragmatic hernia* is the protrusion of an abdominal organ through the diaphragm into the chest cavity; the most common type is the *hiatus hernia,* in which the stomach passes partly or completely into the chest cavity through the hole (*hiatus*) for the oesophagus (gullet). An *umbilical hernia*, most common in young children, appears as a bulge at the navel.

Hernias may be complicated by becoming impossible to return to their normal site (*irreducible*); swollen and fixed within their sac (*incarcerated*); or cut off from their blood supply, becoming painful and eventually gangrenous (*strangulated*). The best treatment for hernias, especially if they are painful, is surgical repair (*see* hernioplasty).

hernio- *prefix denoting* a hernia.

hernioplasty *n.* the surgical operation to repair a hernia, in which the abnormal opening is sewn up and/or the weakness strengthened with suture material.

herniorrhaphy *n.* surgical repair of a hernia.

heroin (diamorphine) *n.* a white crystalline powder derived from *morphine but with a shorter duration of action. Like morphine it is a powerful narcotic analgesic whose continued use leads to *dependence.

herpangina *n.* a viral infectious disease of sudden onset that causes fever, blisters, and ulceration of the soft palate and tonsillar area.

herpes *n.* inflammation of the skin caused by viruses and characterized by collections of small blisters. *Herpes simplex* (*cold sore*) can cause an acute *conjunctivitis or inflammation of the mouth or vagina, but many people contract the virus without showing any symptoms. The disease may recur. *Genital herpes*, caused by herpes simplex II virus, is a sexually transmitted disease characterized by painful blisters in the genital region. It is recurrent and extremely contagious as the blisters burst to release viruses that infect the sexual partner. *Herpes zoster* (*shingles*) usually starts with pain along the distribution of a nerve (often in the face, chest, or abdomen), followed by the development of vesicles. The disease subsides in about three weeks, though sometimes severe pain may persist for many months in the area of the affected nerve. The virus that causes herpes zoster can also cause chickenpox in children. *See also* Ramsay Hunt syndrome.

herpesvirus *n.* one of a group of DNA-containing viruses causing latent infections in man and animals. The herpesviruses are the causative agents of *herpes and chickenpox. The group also includes the *cytomegalovirus and *Epstein-Barr virus. *Herpesvirus simiae (virus B)* causes an infection in monkeys similar to herpes simplex, but when transmitted to man it can produce fatal encephalitis.

hertz *n.* the *SI unit of frequency, equal to one cycle per second. Symbol: Hz.

heter- (hetero-) *prefix denoting* difference; dissimilarity.

heterochromatin *n.* chromosome material (*see* chromatin) that stains most deeply when the cell is not dividing. It is thought not to represent major genes but may be involved in controlling these genes, and also in controlling mitosis and development. *Compare* euchromatin.

heterochromia *n.* colour difference in the iris of the eye, which is usually congenital but is occasionally secondary to inflammation of the iris. In *heterochromia iridis* one iris differs in colour from the other; in *heterochromia iridum* one part of the iris differs in colour from the rest.

heterogametic *adj.* describing the sex that produces two different kinds of gamete, which carry different *sex chromosomes, and that therefore determines the sex of the offspring. In humans men are the heterogametic sex: the sperm cells carry either an X or a Y chromosome. *Compare* homogametic.

heterograft (xenograft) *n.* a living tissue graft that is made from one animal species to another. For example, attempts have been made to graft animal organs into humans.

heterophoria *n.* a tendency to squint. Under normal circumstances both the eyes work together and look at the same point simultaneously, but if one eye is covered it will move out of alignment with the object the other eye is still viewing. When the cover is removed the eye immediately returns to its normal position. Most people have a small degree of the type of heterophoria known as *exophoria,* in which the covered eye turns outwards, away from the nose (*compare* esophoria). Heterophoria often produces eyestrain because of the unconscious effort required to keep the two eyes coordinated. *See also* strabismus.

Heterophyes *n.* a genus of small parasitic *flukes occurring in Egypt and the Far East. Adult flukes of the species *H. heterophyes* live in the small intestine of man and other fish-eating animals; in man the flukes can produce serious symptoms (*see* heterophyiasis). The fluke has two intermediate hosts, a snail and a mullet fish.

heterophyiasis *n.* an infestation of the small intestine with the parasitic fluke *Heterophyes heterophyes.* Man becomes infected on eating raw or salted fish that contains the larval stage of the fluke. The presence of adult flukes may provoke symptoms of abdominal pain and diarrhoea; if the eggs reach the brain, spinal cord, and heart (via the bloodstream) they produce serious lesions. *Tetrachloroethylene is used in treatment of the infection.

heteroplasty *n.* the grafting of tissue from an animal of one species to another.

heteropsia *n.* different vision in each eye.

heterosexuality *n.* the pattern of sexuality in which sexual behaviour and thinking are directed towards people of the opposite sex. It includes both normal and deviant forms of sexual activity. —**heterosexual** *adj., n.*

heterosis *n.* hybrid vigour: the increased sturdiness, resistance to disease, etc., of individuals whose parents are of different races or species compared both with their parents and with the offspring of genetically similar parents.

heterotopia (heterotopy) *n.* the displacement of an organ or part of the body from its normal position.

heterotrophic (organotrophic) *adj.* describing organisms (known as heterotrophs) that use complex organic compounds to synthesize their own organic materials. Most are *chemoheterotrophic*, i.e. they use the organic compounds as an energy source. This group includes the majority of bacteria and all animals and fungi. *Compare* autotrophic.

heterotropia *n. see* strabismus.

heterozygous *adj.* describing an individual in whom the members of a pair of genes determining a particular characteristic are dissimilar. *See* allele. *Compare* homozygous. —**heterozygote** *n.*

hex- (hexa-) *prefix denoting* six.

hexacanth *n. see* oncosphere.

hexachlorophane *n.* a disinfectant similar to *phenol, formerly used in soaps and creams to treat skin disorders. Its use in medicinal products was limited by law in 1973 because of the toxic effects it might produce when absorbed into the body.

hexachromia *n.* the ability to distinguish only six of the seven colours of the spectrum, the exception being indigo. Most people cannot distinguish indigo from blue or violet.

hexamine (methenamine) *n.* an *antiseptic with a wide range of antibacterial activity, used to treat infections and inflammation of the urinary tract, such as cystitis. High doses may cause irritation of the stomach or bladder. Trade names: **Hiprex, Mandelamine**.

hexobarbitone *n.* an intermediate-acting *barbiturate administered by mouth to treat insomnia. Prolonged use can lead to dependence.

hexokinase *n.* an enzyme that catalyses the conversion of glucose to glucose-6-phosphate. This is the first stage of *glycolysis.

hexosamine *n.* the amino derivative of a *hexose sugar. The two most important hexosamines are *glucosamine and galactosamine.

hexose *n.* a simple sugar with six carbon atoms. Hexose sugars are the sugars most frequently found in food. The most important hexose is *glucose.

hiatus *n.* an opening or aperture. For example, the diaphragm contains hiatuses for the oesophagus and aorta.

hiatus hernia *see* hernia.

hiccup *n.* abrupt involuntary lowering of the diaphragm and closure of the sound-producing folds at the upper end of the trachea, producing a characteristic sound as the breath is drawn in. Hiccups, which usually occur repeatedly, may be caused by indigestion or more serious disorders, such as alcoholism. Medical name: **singultus**.

hidr- (hidro-) *prefix denoting* sweat. Example: *hidropoiesis* (formation of).

hidradenitis (hidrosadenitis) *n.* inflammation of the sweat glands, usually occurring when the glands become blocked. This may occur in the armpit, around the nipple or umbilicus, or in the groin; if infection develops the condition is called *hidradenitis suppurativa*.

hidroa *n. see* hydroa.

hidrosis *n.* **1.** the excretion of sweat. **2.** excessive sweating.

hidrotic *n.* an agent that causes sweating. *Parasympathomimetic drugs are hidrotics.

hilus *n.* (*pl.* **hila**) a hollow situated on the surface of an organ, such as the kidney or spleen, at which structures such as blood vessels, nerve fibres, and ducts enter or leave it.

hindbrain *n.* the part of the *brain comprising the cerebellum, pons, and medulla oblongata. The pons and medulla contain the nuclei of many of the cranial nerves, which issue from their surfaces, and the reticular formation. The fluid-filled cavity in the midline is the fourth *ventricle.

hindgut *n.* the back part of the embryonic gut, which gives rise to part of the large intestine, the rectum, bladder, and urinary ducts. *See also* cloaca.

hindquarter amputation an operation involving removal of an entire leg and part or all of the pelvis associated with it. It is usually performed for soft tissue or bone sarcomas arising from the upper thigh, hip, or buttock. *Compare* forequarter amputation.

hinge joint *see* ginglymus.

hip *n.* the region of the body where the thigh bone (femur) articulates with the *pelvis: the region on each side of the pelvis.

hip bone (innominate bone) a bone formed by the fusion of the ilium, ischium, and pubis. It articulates with the femur by the *acetabulum*, a deep socket into which the head of the femur fits. Between the pubis and ischium, below and slightly in front of the acetabulum, is a large opening – the *obturator foramen*. The right and left hip bones form part of the *pelvis.

hip girdle *see* pelvic girdle.

Hippelates *n.* a genus of small flies. The adults of *H. pallipes* are suspected of transmitting *yaws in the West Indies. Other species of *Hippelates* may be involved in the transmission of conjunctivitis.

hippocampal formation a curved band of cortex lying within each cerebral hemisphere: in evolutionary terms one of the brain's most primitive parts. It forms a portion of the *limbic system and is involved in the complex physical aspects of behaviour governed by emotion and instinct.

hippocampus *n.* a swelling in the floor of the lateral *ventricle of the brain. It contains complex foldings of cortical tissue and is involved, with other connections of the *hippocampal formation, in the workings of the *limbic system. —**hippocampal** *adj.*

Hippocratic oath the oath taken by a doctor that binds him to observe the code of behaviour and practice followed by the Greek physician Hippocrates (460–370 BC), called the 'Father of Medicine', and the students of the medical school in Cos where he taught.

hippus *n.* abnormal rhythmical variations in the size of the pupils, independent of the intensity of the light falling on the eyes. It is occasionally seen in various diseases of the nervous system.

Hirschsprung's disease a congenital condition in which the rectum and sometimes part of the lower colon have failed to develop a normal nerve network. The affected portion does not expand or conduct the contents of the bowel, which accumulate in and distend the upper colon. Symptoms, which are usually apparent in the first weeks of life, are abdominal pain and swelling and severe or complete constipation. Diagnosis is by X-ray and by microscopic examination of samples of the bowel wall, which shows the absence of nerve cells. Treatment is by surgery to remove the affected segment and join the remaining (normal) colon to the anus. *See also* megacolon.

hirsutism *n.* excessive hairiness, particularly in women. Rarely, the cause may be a disturbance of the hormone systems but usually the cause is not known.

hirudin *n.* an *anticoagulant present in the salivary glands of leeches and in certain snake venoms, that prevents *blood coagulation by inhibiting the action of the enzyme *thrombin.

hist- (histio-, histo-) *prefix denoting* tissue.

histaminase *n.* an enzyme, widely distributed in the body, that is responsible for the inactivation of histamine.

histamine *n.* a compound derived from the amino acid histidine. It is found in nearly all tissues of the body, associated mainly with the *mast cells. Histamine has pronounced pharmacological activity, causing dilation of blood vessels and contraction of smooth muscle (for example, in the lungs). It is an important mediator of inflammation and is released in large amounts after skin damage (such as that due to animal venoms and toxins), producing a characteristic skin reaction (consisting of flushing, a flare, and a wheal). Histamine is also released in anaphylactic reactions and allergic conditions, including asthma, and gives rise to some of the symptoms of these conditions. *See also* anaphylaxis.

histamine acid phosphate a derivative of *histamine used to test for acid secretion in the stomach in conditions involving abnormal gastric secretion, such as *Zollinger-Ellison syndrome. It is administered by injection and can cause headache, wheezing, rapid heart beat, disturbed vision, and digestive upsets.

histidine *n.* an *amino acid from which *histamine is derived.

histiocyte *n.* a fixed *macrophage, i.e. one that is stationary within connective tissue.

histiocytoma *n.* a tumour that contains *macrophages or *histiocytes, large cells with the ability to engulf foreign matter and bacteria. *See also* fibrosarcoma (malignant fibrous histiocytoma).

histiocytosis *n.* any of a group of diseases in which there are abnormalities in certain large phagocytic cells (*histiocytes), leading to biochemical defects, such as abnormal storage of fats (as in *Gaucher's disease), and other poorly understood conditions, such as Letterer-Siwe disease and Hand-Schüller-Christian disease (*see* reticuloendotheliosis).

histochemistry *n.* the study of the identification and distribution of chemical compounds within and between cells, by means of stains, indicators, and light and electron microscopy. —**histochemical** *adj.*

histocompatibility *n.* the form of *compatibility that depends upon tissue components, mainly specific glycoprotein antigens in cell membranes. A high degree of histocompatibility is necessary for a tissue graft or organ transplant to be successful. —**histocompatible** *adj.*

histogenesis *n.* the formation of tissues.

histogram *n.* a form of statistical graph in which values are plotted in the form of rectangles on a chart; a bar-chart.

histoid *adj.* 1. resembling normal tissue. 2. composed of one type of tissue.

histology *n.* the study of the structure of tissues by means of special staining techniques combined with light and electron microscopy. —**histological** *adj.*

histone *n.* a simple protein that combines with a nucleic acid to form a *nucleoprotein.

Histoplasma *n.* a genus of parasitic yeastlike fungi. The species *H. capsulatum* causes the respiratory infection *histoplasmosis.

histoplasmin *n.* a preparation of antigenic material from a culture of the fungus *Histoplasma capsulatum*, used to test for the presence of the disease *histoplasmosis by subcutaneous injection.

histoplasmosis *n.* an infection caused by inhaling spores of the fungus *Histoplasma capsulatum*. The primary pulmonary form usually produces no symptoms or harmful effects and is recognized retrospectively by X-rays and positive *histoplasmin skin testing. Occasionally, progressive histoplasmosis, which resembles tuberculosis, develops. Symptomatic disease is treated with intravenous amphotericin-B. The spores are found in soil contaminated by faeces, especially from chickens and bats. The disease is endemic in the northern and central US, Argentina, Brazil, Venezuela, and parts of Africa.

histotoxic *adj.* poisonous to tissues: applied to certain substances and conditions.

hives *n. see* urticaria.

HL-A system histocompatibility lymphocyte-A system: a group of eight antigens that are the most important of the 20 or more antigens responsible for *histocompatibility. Successful tissue transplantation requires a minimum number of HL-A differences between donor's and recipient's tissues.

hobnail liver the liver of a patient with cirrhosis, which has a knobbly appearance caused by regenerating nodules separated by bands of fibrous tissue.

Hodgkin's disease a malignant disease of lymphatic tissues, usually characterized by painless enlargement of one or more groups of lymph nodes in the neck, armpits, groin, chest, or abdomen; the spleen, liver, bone marrow, and bones may also be involved. Apart from the enlarging glands, there may also be weight loss, fever, profuse sweating at night, and itching (known as *B symptoms*). Treatment depends on the extent of disease and may include surgery, radiotherapy, drug therapy, or a combination of these. Drugs used in the treatment of the disease include nitrogen mustard, vincristine, procarbazine, prednisone, chlorambucil, and vinblastine. Many patients can be cured; in the early stages of the disease this may be in the order of 85% or more.

holistic *adj.* describing an approach to patient care in which the physical, mental, and social factors in the patient's condition are taken into account, rather than just the diagnosed disease.

Holmes-Adie syndrome *see* Adie's syndrome.

holo- *prefix denoting* complete or entire.

holocrine *adj.* describing a gland or type of secretion in which the entire cell disintegrates when the product is released.

home help *see* social services.

home nurse (district nurse) (in Britain) a trained nurse with special training in *domiciliary services. Formerly all home nurses were State Registered, but in recent years increasing numbers of State Enrolled Nurses are working in this field. Prior to 1974 they were employed either by voluntary agencies on repayment from local health authorities or by these authorities directly. The home nursing service is now the responsibility of District Health Authorities; normally day care only is provided but under special circumstances out of hours nursing can be arranged. Formerly each nurse was allocated to a geographic district and doctors requiring the services for their patients had to contact the local headquarters. However, it is now common for nurses to be allocated to a designated general practice, an arrangement sometimes known as *attachment*.

homeo- (homoeo-) *prefix denoting* similar; like.

homeopathic (homoeopathic) *adj.* 1. of or relating to *homeopathy. 2. infinitesimally small, as applied to the dose of a drug.

homeopathy (homoeopathy) *n.* a system of medicine based on the theory that 'like cures like'. The patient is treated with extremely small quantities of drugs that are themselves capable of producing symptoms of his particular disease. The system was founded by Samuel Hahnemann (1755–1843) at the end of the 18th century and is followed by a minority of doctors in the UK. There is a Royal London Homeopathic Hospital. *See also* fringe medicine. —**homeopathist** *n.*

homeostasis *n.* the physiological process by which the internal systems of the body (e.g. blood pressure, body temperature, *acid-base balance) are maintained at equilibrium, despite variations in the external conditions. —**homeostatic** *adj.*

homo- *prefix denoting* the same or common.

homoeopathy *n. see* homeopathy.

homogametic *adj.* describing the sex that produces only one kind of gamete, which carries the same *sex chromosome, and that therefore does not determine the sex of the offspring. In humans women are the homogametic sex: each egg cell carries an X chromosome. *Compare* heterogametic.

homogenize *vb.* to reduce material to a uniform consistency, e.g. by crushing and mixing. Organs and tissues are homogenized to determine their overall content of a particular enzyme or other substance. —**homogenization** *n.*

homogentisic acid a product formed during the metabolism of the amino acids phenylalanine and tyrosine. In normal individuals homogentisic acid is oxidized by the enzyme *homogentisic acid oxidase*. In rare cases this enzyme is lacking and a condition known as *alcaptonuria, in which large amounts of homogentisic acid are excreted in the urine, results.

homograft (allograft) *n.* a living tissue or organ graft between two members of the same species; for example, a heart transplant from one person to another. Such grafts will not survive unless the recipient is treated to suppress his body's automatic rejection of the foreign tissue.

homoiothermic *adj.* warm-blooded: able to maintain a constant body temperature independently of, and despite variations in, the temperature of the surroundings. Mammals (including man) and birds are homoiothermic. *Compare* poikilothermic. —**homoiothermy** *n.*

homolateral *adj. see* ipsilateral.

homologous *adj.* 1. (in anatomy) describing organs or parts that have the same basic structure and evolutionary origin, but not necessarily the same function or superficial structure. *Compare* analogous. 2. (in genetics) describing a pair of chromosomes of similar shape and size and having identical gene loci. One member of the pair is derived from the mother; the other from the father.

homoplasty *n.* surgical repair of defective or damaged tissues or organs with a *homograft.

homosexuality *n.* the condition of being sexually attracted, covertly or overtly, by members of one's own sex: it can affect either sex (*see also* lesbianism). The cause of homosexuality remains unclear, although explanations in terms of either a deviant family structure or an environment with limited opportunities for heterosexual contacts are increasingly accepted. Homosexuality is no longer generally regarded as a psychological disorder but therapy may be offered to individuals wishing to change their sexual orientation. There are no drugs available for changing sexual orientation, although it is possible to depress the sexual drive. Treatment consists of psychotherapy or specific *behaviour therapy designed to eliminate homosexual behaviour and fantasy and to increase heterosexual behaviour. Persons seeking help for their homosexuality may benefit from *counselling to reduce their anxiety and guilt, rather than trying to change their sexual behaviour. —**homosexual** *adj.*, *n.*

homozygous *adj.* describing an individual in whom the members of a pair of genes determining a particular characteristic are identical. *See* allele. *Compare* heterozygous. —**homozygote** *n.*

homunculus *n.* **1. (manikin)** a dwarf with no deformity or abnormality other than small size. **2. (manikin)** a small jointed anatomical model of a man. **3.** (in early biological theory) a miniature human being thought to be contained within each of the reproductive cells.

hook *n.* a surgical instrument with a bent or curved tip, used to hold, lift, or retract tissue at operation.

hookworm *n.* either of two nematode worms, *Necator americanus* or *Ancylostoma duodenale*, which live as parasites in the intestine of man. Both species, also known as the New and Old World hookworms respectively, are of great medical importance (*see* hookworm disease).

hookworm disease a condition resulting from an infestation of the small intestine by hookworms. Hookworm larvae live in the soil and infect man by penetrating the skin. The worms travel to the lungs in the bloodstream and from there pass via the windpipe and gullet to the small intestine. Heavy hookworm infections may cause considerable damage to the wall of the intestine, leading to a serious loss of blood; this, in conjunction with malnutrition, can provoke severe anaemia. Symptoms include abdominal pain, diarrhoea, debility, and mental inertia. The disease occurs throughout the tropics and subtropics and is prevalent in areas of poor personal hygiene and sanitation. Bephenium hydroxynaphthoate, reliable and easy to administer, is used in treatment.

hordeolum *n. see* stye.

hormone *n.* a substance that is produced in one part of the body (by an *endocrine gland, such as the thyroid, adrenal, or pituitary), passes into the bloodstream and is carried to other (distant) organs or tissues, where it acts to modify their structure or function. Examples of hormones are corticosteroids (from the adrenal cortex), growth hormone (from the pituitary gland), and androgens (from the testes).

horn *n.* (in anatomy) a process, outgrowth, or extension of an organ or other structure. It is often paired. In the spinal cord crescent-shaped areas of grey matter (seen in cross section) are known as the dorsal and ventral horns.

Horner's syndrome a group of symptoms that are due to a disorder of the sympathetic nerves in the cervical (neck) region. The syndrome consists of a constricted pupil, drooping of the upper eyelid (*ptosis), and an absence of sweating over the affected side of the face.

horseshoe kidney an anatomical variation in kidney development whereby the lower poles of both kidneys are joined together. This usually causes no trouble but it may be associated with impaired drainage of urine from the kidney by the ureters, which cross in front of the united lower segment.

hospice *n.* an institution that specializes in the care of terminally ill patients, using narcotic drugs in carefully controlled doses for the relief of pain.

hospital *n.* an institution offering residential, investigatory, and/or therapeutic care regarded as too complex or specialized for provision as a *domiciliary service. Such care may be residential (in-patient), including the care of patients for a whole day and their return home at night (*day hospital*). Out-patient services include consultation with designated specialists by prior appointment, X-rays, laboratory tests, physiotherapy, and accident and emergency services for those requiring urgent care. Most Health Districts have a *general hospital* (*DGH*), which provides sufficient basic services for the population of the District. Some larger hospitals have resources that are more highly specialized, to meet the needs of a wider population, providing so-called *regional* or *supra-regional* (*national*) services. Such hospitals often provide training for medical students (*teaching* or *university hospitals*) and for postgraduate education. Some smaller hospitals – known as *community hospitals* – are staffed mainly or exclusively by general practitioners and are intended for patients for whom home care is impracticable on social grounds.

Hospital Activity Analysis *see* Hospital In-patient Enquiry.

hospital fatality ratio *see* case fatality ratio.

Hospital In-patient Enquiry (in Britain) a statistical review, organized jointly by the *Department of Health and Social Security and the *Office of Population Censuses and Surveys, providing information about in-patients treated in National Health Service hospitals. The data, based on a sample of episodes of illness (as distinct from individual patients), include diagnosis on discharge or death, duration on the waiting list, and length of stay. More detailed information, including aspects of therapy while in the hospital, are included in *Hospital Activity Analysis*. *Compare* record linkage.

host *n.* an animal or plant in or upon which a *parasite lives. An *intermediate host* is one in which the parasite passes its larval or asexual stages; a *definitive* host is one in which the parasite develops to its sexual stage.

hourglass contraction constriction of an organ at its centre as a result of abnormal muscular contraction. Hourglass contraction may be a complication of labour, tending to trap the placenta in the upper part of the constricted womb and possibly leading to excessive blood loss after delivery.

housemaid's knee a fluid-filled swelling of the bursa in front of the kneecap, often resulting from frequent kneeling. Treatment – and prevention – is by avoidance of kneeling. *See also* bursitis.

house physician/surgeon *see* doctor.

humectant 1. *n.* a substance that is used for moistening. **2.** *adj.* causing moistening.

humerus *n.* the bone of the upper arm. The *head* of the humerus articulates with the *scapula at the shoulder joint. At the lower end of the shaft the *trochlea* articulates with the *ulna and part of the radius. The radius also articulates with a rounded protuberance (*capitulum*) close to the trochlea. Depressions (*fossae*) at the front and back of the humerus accommodate the ulna and radius, respectively, when the arm is flexed or straightened.

humour *n.* a body fluid. *See* aqueous humour, vitreous humour.

Hurler's syndrome an inborn defect of metabolism causing the accumulation of mucopolysaccharides and lipids in the cells of the body. This leads to mental retardation, enlargement of the liver and spleen, deformities of the bones, and coarsening and thickening of the features (*gargoylism*).

Hutchinson's teeth narrowed and notched permanent incisor teeth: a sign of congenital *syphilis.

hyal- (hyalo-) *prefix denoting* **1.** glassy; transparent. **2.** hyalin. **3.** the vitreous humour of the eye.

hyalin *n.* a clear glassy material produced as the result of degeneration in certain tissues, particularly connective tissue and epithelial cells.

hyaline cartilage the most common type of *cartilage: a bluish-white elastic material with a matrix of chondroitin sulphate in which fine collagen fibrils are embedded.

hyaline membrane disease *see* respiratory distress syndrome.

hyalitis *n.* inflammation of the *vitreous body of the eye. *Asteroid hyalitis* is a degenerative condition (rather than an inflammation), in which the vitreous contains many small white opacities.

hyaloid artery a fetal artery lying in the *hyaloid canal of the eye and supplying the lens.

hyaloid canal a channel within the vitreous humour of the *eye. It extends from the centre of the optic disc, where it communicates with the lymph spaces of the optic nerve, to the posterior wall of the lens.

hyaloid membrane the transparent membrane that surrounds the *vitreous humour of the eye, separating it from the retina.

hyaluronic acid an acid *mucopolysaccharide that acts as the binding and protective agent of the ground substance of connective tissue. It is also present in the synovial fluid around joints and in the vitreous and aqueous humours of the eye.

hyaluronidase *n.* an enzyme that depolymerizes *hyaluronic acid and therefore increases the permeability of connective tissue. Hyaluronidase is found in the testes, in semen, and in other tissues.

hybrid *n.* the offspring of a cross between two genetically unlike individuals. A hybrid, whose parents are usually of different species or varieties, is often sterile.

hydatid *n.* a bladder-like cyst formed in various human tissues following the growth of the larval stage of an *Echinococcus* tapeworm. *E. granulosus* produces a single large fluid-filled cyst, called *unilocular hydatid*, which gives rise internally to smaller daughter cysts. The entire hydatid is bound by a fibrous capsule. *E. multilocularis* forms aggregates of many smaller cysts with a jelly-like matrix, called an *alveolar hydatid*, and enlarges by budding off external daughter cysts. Alveolar hydatids are not delimited by fibrous capsules and produce malignant tumours, which invade and destroy human tissues. *See also* hydatid disease.

hydatid disease (hydatidosis, echinococciasis, echinococcosis) a condition resulting from the presence in the liver, lungs, or brain of the *hydatid cysts. The cysts of *Echinococcus multilocularis* form malignant tumours; those of *E. granulosus* exert pressure as they grow and thereby damage surrounding tissues. The presence of hydatids in the brain may result in blindness and epilepsy, and the rupture of any cyst can cause severe allergic reactions including fever and *urticaria. Treatment may necessitate surgical removal of the cysts. Spread of hydatid disease, particularly common in sheep-raising countries, can be prevented by the deworming of dogs.

hydatidiform mole (hydatid mole, vesicular mole) a collection of fluid-filled sacs that develop when the membrane (chorion) surrounding the embryo degenerates in early pregnancy. These sacs give the placenta the appearance of a bunch of grapes. The embryo dies, the womb enlarges, and there is a discharge of pinkish liquid and cysts from the vagina. A malignant condition may subsequently develop (*see* chorionepithelioma).

hydatidosis *n. see* hydatid disease.

hydr- (hydro-) *prefix denoting* water or a watery fluid.

hydraemia *n.* the presence in the blood of more than the normal proportion of water.

hydragogue *n.* an agent that produces a watery discharge, particularly a laxative that produces watery stools.

hydrallazine *n.* a drug that lowers blood pressure and is used, usually in conjunction with *diuretics, to treat hypertension. It is given by mouth or injection; side-effects, including rapid heart rate, headache, faintness, and digestive upsets, can occur, especially at high doses. Trade name: **Apresoline**.

hydramnios (hydramnion) *n.* the presence of an abnormally large amount of *amniotic fluid surrounding the fetus from about the fifth month of pregnancy. The womb becomes swollen, which causes breathlessness, excess fluid in the body tissues, and other symptoms in the woman, and there may be a difficult birth. Most cases of hydramnios are associated with twin pregnancies.

hydrargaphen *n.* a mercury-containing drug with antibacterial and antifungal activity, used to treat skin and ear infections. It is applied in a cream, solution, dusting powder, or pessary and has the toxic effects of *mercury.

hydrargyria *n. see* mercurialism.

hydrarthrosis *n.* swelling at a joint caused by excessive synovial fluid. The condition usually involves the knees and may be recurrent. Often no cause is apparent; in some cases rheumatoid arthritis develops later.

hydroa (hidroa) *n.* an eruption of small blisters accompanied by intense itching, occurring (usually in preadolescent boys) on skin surfaces exposed to sunlight. Hydroa is a severe form of light-sensitive dermatitis, described as *polymorphic light eruptions*.

hydrocele *n.* the accumulation of watery liquid in a sac, usually the sac surrounding the testes. This condition is characterized by painless enlargement of the scrotum; it is treated surgically, by drainage of the fluid or removal of the sac.

hydrocephalus *n.* an abnormal increase in the amount of cerebrospinal fluid within the ventricles of the brain. In childhood, before the sutures of the skull have fused, hydrocephalus makes the head enlarge. In adults, because of the unyielding nature of the skull, hydrocephalus raises the intracranial pressure with consequent drowsiness and vomiting. Hydrocephalus may be caused by obstruction to the outflow of cerebrospinal fluid from the ventricles or a failure of its reabsorption into the cerebral sinuses. *Spina bifida is commonly associated with hydrocephalus.

hydrochloric acid a strong acid present, in a very dilute form, in gastric juice. The secretion of excess hydrochloric acid by the stomach results in the condition *hyperchlorhydria.

hydrochlorothiazide *n.* a *diuretic used to treat fluid retention (oedema) and high blood pressure. It is administered by mouth, and side-effects can include digestive upsets, skin reactions, and dizziness. Trade names: **Direma, Esidrex, Hydrosaluric**.

hydrocolpos *n.* a cyst containing watery liquid or mucus formed in the vagina.

hydrocortisone (cortisol) *n.* a steroid hormone: the major glucocorticoid synthesized and released by the human adrenal cortex (*see* corticosteroid). It is important for normal carbohydrate metabolism and for the normal response to any stress. Hydrocortisone is used to treat adrenal failure (*Addison's disease) and inflammatory, allergic, and rheumatic conditions (including rheumatoid arthritis, colitis, and eczema). It may be given by mouth, by injection, or in the form of a cream or ointment. Possible side-effects of hydrocortisone therapy include peptic ulcers, bone and muscle damage, suppression of growth in children, and the signs of *Cushing's syndrome.

hydrocyanic acid (prussic acid) an intensely poisonous volatile acid that can cause death within a minute if inhaled. It smells of bitter almonds. *See* cyanide.

hydroflumethiazide *n.* a *diuretic used to treat fluid retention (oedema) and high blood pressure. It is administered by mouth and may cause skin reactions, digestive upsets, dizziness, and weakness. Trade name: **Hydrenox**.

hydrogenase *n.* an enzyme that catalyses the addition of hydrogen to a compound in reduction reactions.

hydrogen bond a weak electrostatic bond formed by linking a hydrogen atom between two electronegative atoms (e.g. nitrogen or oxygen). The large number of hydrogen bonds in proteins and nucleic acids are respon-

sible for maintaining the stable molecular structure of these compounds.

hydrogen peroxide a colourless liquid used as a disinfectant for cleansing wounds and, diluted, as a deodorant mouthwash or as ear drops for removing wax. Strong solutions irritate the skin.

hydrolase *n.* an enzyme that catalyses the hydrolysis of compounds. Examples are the *peptidases.

hydroma *n. see* hygroma.

hydromyelia *n.* a dilatation of the central canal of the spinal cord (which is a continuation of the ventricular system of the brain). It has been suggested that the canal is distended by a rise in the pressure of the ventricular cerebrospinal fluid caused by a blockage to its normal outflow to the surface of the brain. The patient's symptoms are those of *syringomyelia.

hydronephrosis *n.* distension and dilatation of the pelvis of the kidney. This is due to an obstruction to the free flow of urine from the kidney. An obstruction at or below the neck of the bladder will cause hydronephrosis of both kidneys. The term *primary pelvic hydronephrosis* is used when the obstruction, usually functional, is at the junction of the renal pelvis and ureter. Surgical relief by *pyeloplasty is advisable to avoid the back pressure atrophy of the kidney and the complications of infection and stone formation. —**hydronephrotic** *adj.*

hydropericarditis *n. see* hydropericardium.

hydropericardium *n.* accumulation of a clear serous fluid within the membranous sac surrounding the heart. It occurs in many cases of *pericarditis (*hydropericarditis*). If the heart is compressed the fluid is withdrawn (aspirated) via a needle inserted into the pericardial sac through the chest wall (*pericardiocentesis*). *See also* hydropneumopericardium.

hydroperitoneum *n. see* ascites.

hydrophobia *n. see* rabies.

hydrophthalmos *n. see* buphthalmos.

hydropneumopericardium *n.* the presence of air and clear fluid within the pericardial sac around the heart, which is most commonly due to entry of air during pericardiocentesis (*see* hydropericardium). The presence of air does not affect the management of the patient.

hydropneumoperitoneum *n.* the presence of fluid and gas in the peritoneal cavity. This may be due either to the introduction of air through an instrument being used to remove the fluid; because a perforation in the digestive tract has allowed the escape of fluid and gas; or because gas-forming bacteria are growing in the peritoneal fluid.

hydropneumothorax (pneumohydrothorax) *n.* air and fluid in the pleural cavity. If the patient is shaken the fluid makes a splashing sound (called a *succussion splash*). An *effusion of serous fluid commonly complicates a *pneumothorax, and must be drained.

hydrops foetalis the state of certain infants severely affected by *haemolytic disease. Fluid accumulates in the body cavities, especially in the peritoneal and pleural cavities (*see* oedema, ascites) and the liver becomes enlarged: these are features of chronic heart failure due to profound anaemia. Repeated intrauterine transfusions into the fetal peritoneum during pregnancy have saved some infants in whom hydrops foetalis was predicted.

hydrorrhoea *n.* a watery discharge. *Hydrorrhoea gravidarum* occurs during pregnancy: excessive secretion by the glands of the womb leads to a discharge from the vagina.

hydrosalpinx (hydrops tubae) *n.* the accumulation of watery fluid in one of the *Fallopian tubes, which becomes swollen. In *intermittent hydrosalpinx* so much fluid accumulates that some of it is forced into the womb.

hydrotherapy *n.* the use of water in the treatment of disorders: today restricted in orthodox medicine to exercises in remedial swimming pools for the *rehabilitation of arthritic or partially paralysed patients.

hydrothorax *n.* fluid in the pleural cavity. *See also* hydropneumothorax.

hydroureter *n.* an accumulation of urine in one of the tubes (ureters) leading from the kidneys to the bladder. The ureter becomes swollen and the condition usually results from obstruction of the ureter by a stone or a misplaced artery.

hydrovarium *n.* the accumulation of watery fluid in an ovary.

hydroxocobalamine *n.* a cobalt-containing drug administered by injection to treat conditions involving vitamin B_{12} deficiency, such as pernicious anaemia. Trade names: **Cobalin-H, Neo-Cytamen**.

hydroxyamphetamine *n.* a *sympathomimetic drug used in solution or sprays for the relief of nasal symptoms such as congestion, inflammation, and sinusitis. It is also used to dilate the pupil of the eye for eye examinations. Side-effects can include headache, nausea, vomiting, and palpitations.

hydroxychloroquine *n.* a drug similar to *chloroquine, used mainly to treat lupus erythematosus and rheumatoid arthritis. Side-effects such as skin reactions, hair loss, and digestive upsets may occur and prolonged use can lead to eye damage. Trade name: **Plaquenil**.

hydroxyprogesterone *n.* a synthetic female sex hormone (*see* progestogen) administered by injection to prevent miscarriage and to treat menstrual disorders. There may be pain at the injection site, and progestogens taken by mouth are often preferred. Trade name: **Primolut**.

hydroxyproline *n.* a compound, similar in structure to the *amino acids, found only in *collagen.

hydroxystilbamidine *n.* a drug used to treat infections caused by fungi and protozoa, such as blastomycosis. It is administered by injection and may cause dizziness, headache, nausea, and fainting if injected too quickly.

hydroxytryptamine *n. see* serotonin.

hydroxyurea *n.* a drug that prevents cell growth and is used to treat some types of leukaemia. It is administered by mouth. Hydroxyurea may lower the white cell content of the blood due to its effects on the bone marrow. Trade name: **Hydrea**.

hydroxyzine *n.* an *antihistamine drug with sedative properties, used to relieve anxiety, tension, and agitation and to treat nausea and vomiting. It is administered by mouth and may cause drowsiness, headache, dry mouth, and itching. Trade name: **Atarax**.

hygiene *n.* the science of health and the study of ways of preserving it, particularly by promoting cleanliness.

hygr- (hygro-) *prefix denoting* moisture.

hygroma (hydroma) *n.* a type of cyst. It may develop from a *lymphangioma (*cystic hygroma*) or from the liquified remains of a subdural *haematoma (*subdural hygroma*).

hymen *n.* the membrane that covers the opening of the vagina at birth but usually perforates spontaneously before puberty. If the initial opening is small it may tear, with slight loss of blood, at the first occasion of sexual intercourse.

Hymenolepis *n.* a genus of small widely distributed parasitic tapeworms. The dwarf tapeworm, *H. nana*, only 40 mm in length, lives in the human intestine. Fleas can be important vectors of this species, and children in close contact with flea-infested dogs are particularly prone to infection. *H. diminuta* is a common parasite of rodents; man occasionally becomes infected on swallowing stored cereals contaminated with insect pests – the intermediate hosts for this parasite. Symptoms of abdominal pain, diarrhoea, loss of appetite, and headache are obvious only in heavy infections of either species. Treatment involves a course of *anthelmintics.

hymenorrhaphy *n.* a tissue-grafting operation on the hymen at the entrance to the vagina in order to partially or completely close the vagina.

hymenotomy *n.* incision of the hymen at the entrance to the vagina. This operation may be performed on a young girl if the membrane completely closes the vagina and thus impedes the flow of menstrual blood.

hyo- *prefix denoting* the hyoid bone. Example: *hyoglossal* (relating to the hyoid bone and tongue).

hyoglossus *n.* a muscle that serves to depress the tongue. It has its origin in the hyoid bone.

hyoid bone a small isolated U-shaped bone in the neck, below and supporting the tongue. It is held in position by muscles and ligaments between it and the styloid process of the temporal bone.

hyoscine (scopolamine) *n.* a drug that prevents muscle spasm (*see* parasympatholytic). It is used in the treatment of gastric or duodenal ulcers, spasm in the digestive system, and difficult or painful menstruation and also to relax the womb in labour. It can also be used to calm excitement in some psychiatric conditions, for preoperative medication, for travel sickness, and to dilate the pupil and paralyse the muscles of the eye for examination. It is administered by mouth or injection. Side-effects are rare but can include dry mouth, blurred vision, difficulty in urination, and increased heart rate. Trade names: **Buscospan, Pamine.**

hyoscyamine *n.* a drug with similar activity to *hyoscine, used, often in mixtures, to treat muscle spasm. It is administered by mouth. Trade name: **Peptard**.

hyp- (hypo-) *prefix denoting* **1.** deficiency, lack, or small size. Example: *hypognathous* (having a small lower jaw). **2.** (in anatomy) below; beneath. Example: *hypoglossal* (under the tongue).

hypalgesia *n.* an abnormally low sensitivity to pain.

hyper- *prefix denoting* **1.** excessive; abnormally increased. **2.** (in anatomy) above.

hyperacusis *n.* abnormally acute hearing or painful sensitivity to sounds.

hyperadrenalism *n.* overactivity of the adrenal glands. *See* Cushing's syndrome.

hyperaemia *n.* the presence of excess blood in the vessels supplying a part of the body. In *active hyperaemia* (*arterial hyperaemia*) the arterioles are relaxed and there is an increased blood flow. In *passive hyperaemia* the blood flow from the affected part is obstructed.

hyperaesthesia *n.* excessive sensibility, especially of the skin.

hyperalgesia *n.* an abnormal state of increased sensitivity to painful stimuli.

hyperbaric *adj.* at a pressure greater than atmospheric pressure.

hyperbaric oxygenation a technique for exposing a patient to oxygen at high pressure. It is used to treat carbon monoxide poisoning, gas gangrene, and acute breathing difficulties. It is also used in some cases during heart surgery.

hypercalcaemia *n.* the presence in the blood of an abnormally high concentration of calcium. *Idiopathic hypercalcaemia*, which affects infants who have received too much vitamin D, leads to mental disorder. *Compare* hypocalcaemia.

hypercalcinuria (hypercalcuria) *n.* the presence in the urine of an abnormally high concentration of calcium.

hypercapnia (hypercarbia) the presence in the blood of an abnormally high concentration of carbon dioxide.

hyperchloraemia *n.* the presence in the blood of an abnormally high concentration of chloride.

hyperchlorhydria *n.* a greater than normal secretion of hydrochloric acid by the stomach, usually associated with a *duodenal ulcer. Extremely high levels of acid secretion are found in the *Zollinger-Ellison syndrome.

hyperchromatism *n.* the property of the nuclei of certain cells (for example, those of tumours) to stain more deeply than normal. —**hyperchromatic** *adj.*

hyperdactylism (polydactylism) *n.* the condition of having more than the normal number of fingers or toes. The extra digits are commonly undersized (rudimentary) and are usually removed surgically shortly after birth.

hyperdynamia *n.* excessive activity of muscles.

hyperemesis *n.* severe vomiting. *Hyperemesis gravidarum* affects pregnant women: the stomach contents and bile are vomited, and the acidity of the arterial blood increases. If the vomiting is allowed to continue for a long time, liver disease may develop. If rest, restriction of liquid intake, controlled diet, and drugs aimed at stopping the vomiting fail to cure the condition, it may be necessary to terminate the pregnancy. *Hyperemesis lactentium* is vomiting by babies at the breast-feeding stage.

hyperextension *n.* excessive and forceful extension of a limb beyond the normal limits, usually as part of an orthopaedic procedure to correct deformity.

hyperglycaemia *n.* an excess of glucose in the bloodstream. It may occur in a variety of diseases, most notably in *diabetes mellitus, due to insufficient insulin in the blood and excessive intake of carbohydrates. Untreated it may progress to diabetic coma.

hyperidrosis (hyperhidrosis) *n.* excessive sweating, which may occur in certain diseases, such as fevers or thyrotoxicosis, or following the use of certain drugs.

hyperinsulinism *n.* **1.** excessive secretion of the hormone insulin by the islet cells of the pancreas. **2.** metabolic disturbance due to administration of too much insulin.

hyperinvolution (superinvolution) *n.* **1.** excessive shrinkage of the womb and associated structures after childbirth. The condition may become extreme if breast-feeding continues for a very long time or if the reproductive tract becomes seriously infected shortly after delivery. **2.** excessive reduction in the size of any organ after it has attained an extremely large size.

hyperkalaemia *n.* the presence in the blood of an abnormally high concentration of potassium. *See* electrolyte.

hyperkeratosis *n.* thickening of the outer horny layer of the skin. It may occur as an inherited disorder, affecting the palms and soles. Another inherited

disorder in which hyperkeratosis occurs is *ichthyosis.

hyperkinesia *n.* a state of overactive restlessness in children. *See* hyperkinetic syndrome. —**hyperkinetic** *adj.*

hyperkinetic syndrome a mental disorder, usually of children, characterized by a grossly excessive level of activity and a marked impairment of the ability to attend. Learning is impaired as a result, and behaviour is disruptive and may be defiant or aggressive. The syndrome is most common in the intellectually subnormal, the epileptic, and the brain-damaged. Treatment usually involves drugs (such as amphetamines or haloperidol) and behaviour therapy; the family usually needs advice.

hyperlipaemia *n.* the presence in the blood of an abnormally high concentration of fats.

hyperlipoproteinaemia *n.* the presence in the blood of abnormally high concentrations of *lipoproteins.

hypermetropia   **(long-sightedness)**

focusing point is beyond the retina

Uncorrected

Corrected

convex lens converges light rays falling on the eye

Hypermetropia (long-sightedness)

hypermotility

n. the condition in which parallel light rays are brought to a focus behind the retina when the *accommodation is relaxed (see illustration). Objects closer than six metres from the eye appear blurred, and objects further than six metres from the eye are not seen clearly but in many cases can be made sharp by an effort of accommodation. Normal vision can be restored by wearing spectacles with convex lenses. *Compare* emmetropia, myopia.

hypermotility *n.* excessive movement or activity, especially of the stomach or intestine.

hypernatraemia *n.* the presence in the blood of an abnormally high concentration of *sodium. *See also* electrolyte.

hypernephroma (Grawitz tumour, renal cell carcinoma) *n.* a malignant tumour of kidney cells, so called because it is said to resemble part of the adrenal gland and at one time was thought to originate from this site. It may be present for some years before giving rise to symptoms, which include fever, loin pain, and blood in the urine. Treatment is by surgery but tumours are apt to recur locally. The tumour spreads via the bloodstream and can often be seen growing along the renal vein. Secondary growths from a renal cell carcinoma in the lung have a characteristic 'cannon-ball' appearance. These tumours are relatively insensitive to radiotherapy and cytotoxic drugs but some respond to such hormones as progestogens and testosterone.

hyperopia *n.* the usual US term for *hypermetropia.

hyperosmia *n.* an abnormally acute sense of smell.

hyperostosis *n.* excessive enlargement of the outer layer of a bone. The condition is harmless and is usually recognized as an incidental finding on X-ray. It commonly affects the frontal bone of the skull (*hyperostosis frontalis*).

hyperparathyroidism *n.* overactivity of the parathyroid glands. *See* von Recklinghausen's disease.

hyperpiesia *n. see* hypertension.

hyperplasia *n.* the increased production and growth of normal cells in a tissue or organ. The affected part becomes larger but retains its normal form. During pregnancy the breasts grow in this manner. *Compare* hypertrophy, neoplasm.

hyperpnoea *n.* an increase in the rate of breathing that is proportional to an increase in metabolism; for example, on exercise. *Compare* hyperventilation.

hyperpraxia *n.* excessive motor activity, such as is seen in *mania and the *hyperkinetic syndrome.

hyperpyrexia *n.* a rise in body temperature above $106°F$ ($41.1°C$). *See* fever.

hypersensitive *adj.* prone to respond abnormally to the presence of a particular antigen, which may cause a variety of tissue reactions ranging from *serum sickness to an allergy (such as hay fever) or, at the severest, to anaphylactic shock (*see* anaphylaxis). It is thought that when the normal antigen-antibody defence reaction is followed by tissue damage this may be due to an abnormality in the working of the *complement system. *See also* allergy, immunity. —**hypersensitivity** *n.*

hypersomnia *n.* sleep lasting for exceptionally long periods, as occurs in some cases of brain inflammation.

hypersplenism *n.* a decrease in the numbers of red cells, white cells, and platelets in the blood resulting from destruction or pooling of these cells by an enlarged spleen. Hypersplenism may occur in any condition in which there is enlargement of the spleen (*see* splenomegaly).

hypersthenia *n.* an abnormally high degree of strength or physical tension in all or part of the body.

hypertension *n.* high *blood pressure, i.e. elevation of the arterial blood pressure above the normal range expected in a particular age group. Hypertension may be of unknown cause (*essential hypertension* or *hyperpiesia*). It may also result from kidney disease, including narrowing (stenosis) of the renal artery (*renal hypertension*), endocrine diseases (such as Cushing's disease or phaeochromocytoma) or disease of the arteries (such as coarctation of the aorta), when it is known as *secondary* or *symptomatic hypertension*.

Complications that may arise from hypertension include atherosclerosis, heart failure, cerebral haemorrhage, and kidney failure, but treatment may prevent their development. Hypertension is symptomless until the symptoms of its complications develop. Some cases of hypertension may be cured by eradicating the cause. Most cases, however, depend upon long-term drug therapy to lower the blood pressure and maintain it within the normal range. The drugs used include thiazide *diuretics, *beta blockers, *methyldopa, *guanethidine, and many others. Combinations of drugs may be needed to obtain optimum control. *See also* portal hypertension, pulmonary hypertension.

hyperthermia (hyperthermy) *n.* **1.** exceptionally high body temperature (about 41°C or above). *See* fever. **2.** treatment of disease by inducing fever. *Compare* hypothermia.

hyperthyroidism *n.* overactivity of the thyroid gland, either due to a tumour, overgrowth of the gland, or Graves's disease. *See* thyrotoxicosis.

hypertonia (hypertonicity) *n.* exceptionally high tension in muscles.

hypertonic *adj.* **1.** describing a solution that has a greater osmotic pressure than another solution. *See* osmosis. **2.** describing muscles that demonstrate an abnormal increase in *tonicity.

hypertrichosis *n.* excessive growth of hair (*see* hirsutism).

hypertrophy (hypertrophia) *n.* increase in the size of a tissue or organ brought about by the enlargement of its cells rather than by cell multiplication (as during normal growth and tumour formation). Muscles undergo this change in response to increased work. *Compare* hyperplasia.

hypertropia *n. see* strabismus.

hyperuricaemia (lithaemia) *n.* the presence in the blood of an abnormally high concentration of uric acid. *See* gout.

hyperuricuria (lithuria) *n.* the presence in the urine of an abnormally high concentration of uric acid.

hyperventilation *n.* breathing at an abnormally rapid rate at rest. This can be done deliberately and causes unconsciousness by lowering the carbon dioxide concentration in the blood. It occurs clinically if the carbon dioxide level is abnormally high as a result of impaired gas exchange in the lungs, which occurs, for example, in pneumonia.

hypervitaminosis *n.* the condition resulting from excessive consumption of vitamins. This is not serious in the case of water-soluble vitamins, when any intake in excess of requirements is easily excreted in the urine. However, fat-soluble vitamins A and D are toxic if taken in excessive amounts.

hypervolaemia *n.* an increase in the volume of circulating blood.

hyphaema *n.* bleeding into the chamber of the eye that lies in front of the lens.

hyphedonia *n.* a lower than normal capacity for achieving enjoyment.

hypn- (hypno-) *prefix denoting* 1. sleep. 2. hypnosis.

hypnagogic *adj. see* imagery.

hypnopompic *adj. see* imagery.

hypnosis *n.* a sleeplike state, artificially induced in a person by a *hypnotist*, in which the mind is more than usually receptive to suggestion and memories of past events – apparently forgotten – may be elicited by questioning. Hypnotic suggestion has been used for a variety of purposes in medicine, for example as a cure for addiction and in other forms of *psychotherapy.

hypnotic (soporific) *n.* a drug that produces sleep by depressing brain function. Hypnotics include *barbiturates, *chloral hydrate, *methaqualone, and *nitrazepam. Hypnotics are used for insomnia and sleep disturbances, especially in mental illnesses and in the elderly. They often cause hangover effects in the morning and the barbiturate hypnotics can lead to *dependence.

hypnotism *n.* the induction of *hypnosis.

hypo- *prefix. see* hyp-.

hypoaesthesia *n.* a condition in which the sense of touch is diminished; uncommonly this may be extended to include other forms of sensation.

hypobaric *adj.* at a pressure lower than that of the atmosphere.

hypobulia *n.* mild deficiency of will power. *See* abulia.

hypocalcaemia *n.* the presence in the blood of an abnormally low concentration of calcium. *See* tetany. *Compare* hypercalcaemia.

hypocapnia *n.* the presence in the blood of an abnormally low concentration of carbon dioxide.

hypochloraemia *n.* the presence in the blood of an abnormally low concentration of chloride.

hypochlorhydria *n.* reduced secretion of hydrochloric acid by the stomach. *See* achlorhydria.

hypochondria *n.* preoccupation with the physical functioning of the body and with fancied ill health. It may amount to a handicapping neurosis and dominate a person's life. In the most severe form there are delusions of ill health, usually due to underlying *depression. Treatment with reassurance, *antidepressant drugs, and/or psychotherapy is usual, but the condition is often chronic. —**hypochondriac** *adj., n.*

hypochondrium *n.* the upper lateral portion of the *abdomen, situated beneath the lower ribs. —**hypochondriac** *adj.*

Hypoderma *n.* a genus of non-bloodsucking beelike insects – the warble flies – widely distributed in Europe, North America, and Asia. Cattle are the usual hosts for the parasitic maggots, but rare and accidental infections of man have occurred (*see* myiasis), especially in farm workers. The maggots migrate beneath the skin surface, producing an inflamed linear lesion similar to that of *creeping eruption.

hypodermic *adj.* beneath the skin: usually applied to subcutaneous *injections. The term is also applied to the syringe used for such injections, and sometimes – loosely – to any injection.

hypodermoclysis *n.* the continuous infusion under the skin of saline or other medicated solution to clean away blood, pus, and foreign matter from a wound.

hypodontia *n.* a reduction in the normal number of teeth through congenital absence.

hypofibrinogenaemia (fibrinogenopenia) *n.* a deficiency of the clotting factor *fibrinogen in the blood, which results in an increased tendency to bleed. It may occur as an inherited disorder in which either production of fibrinogen is impaired or the fibrinogen produced does not function in the normal way (*dysfibrinogenaemia*). Alternatively, it may be acquired.

hypogammaglobulinaemia *n.* a deficiency of the protein *gamma globulin in the blood. It may occur in a variety of inherited disorders or as an acquired defect, as in certain *lymphomas. Since gamma globulin consists mainly of defensive antibodies (*immunoglobulins), hypogammaglobulinaemia results in an increased susceptibility to infections.

hypogastrium *n.* that part of the central *abdomen situated below the region of the stomach. —**hypogastric** *adj.*

hypogeusia *n.* a condition in which the sense of taste is abnormally weak. *See also* hypoaesthesia.

hypoglossal nerve the twelfth *cranial nerve (XII), which supplies the muscles of the tongue and is therefore responsible for the movements of talking and swallowing.

hypoglycaemia *n.* a deficiency of glucose in the bloodstream, causing muscular weakness and incoordination, mental confusion, and sweating. If severe it may lead to *hypoglycaemic coma*. Hypoglycaemia most commonly occurs in *diabetes mellitus, as a result of insulin overdosage and insufficient intake of carbohydrates. It is treated by administration of glucose, by injection if the patient is in a coma; by mouth otherwise. —**hypoglycaemic** *adj.*

hypogonadism *n.* impaired function of the testes or ovaries, causing absence or impairment of the *secondary sexual characteristics.

hypoidrosis (hypohidrosis) *n.* the production of an abnormally small amount of sweat relative to the environ-mental temperature, bodily activity, or other relevant circumstances.

hypoinsulinism *n.* a deficiency of insulin due either to inadequate secretion of the hormone by the pancreas or to inadequate treatment of diabetes mellitus.

hypokalaemia *n.* the presence of abnormally low levels of potassium in the blood: occurs in dehydration. *See* electrolyte.

hypomania *n.* a mild degree of *mania. Elated mood leads to faulty judgment; behaviour lacks the usual social restraints and the sexual drive is increased; speech is rapid and animated; the individual is energetic but not persistent and tends to be irritable. The abnormality is not so great as in mania and the patient may appear normal and 'a bit of a character' to those who do not know him (*see* elation, euphoria). Treatment follows the same principles as for mania, and it may be difficult to prevent an individual from damaging his own interests with extravagant behaviour. —**hypomanic** *adj.*, *n.*

hypomenorrhoea *n.* the release of an abnormally small quantity of blood at menstruation. The duration of bleeding may be normal or less than normal.

hyponatraemia *n.* the presence in the blood of an abnormally low concentration of *sodium: occurs in dehydration. *See* electrolyte.

hypoparathyroidism *n.* subnormal activity of the parathyroid glands, causing a fall in the blood concentration of calcium and muscular spasms (*see* tetany).

hypophysectomy *n.* the surgical removal or destruction of the pituitary gland (hypophysis) in the brain. The operation may be conducted by opening the skull or by inserting special needles that produce a very low temperature (*see* cryosurgery).

hypophysis *n. see* pituitary gland.

hypopiesis *n.* abnormally reduced blood pressure in the absence of organic disease (*see* hypotension).

hypopituitarism *n.* subnormal activity of the pituitary gland, causing *dwarfism in childhood and a syndrome of impaired sexual function, pallor, and premature ageing in adult life (*see* Simmond's disease).

hypoplasia *n.* underdevelopment of an organ or tissue. *Dental hypoplasia* is the defective formation of parts of a tooth due to illnesses such as measles or starvation while the tooth is being formed. It is marked by transverse lines of brown defective enamel, which define the date of the illness.

hypopnoea *n.* a decrease in breathing rate which indicates that the body is attempting to compensate for metabolic disturbances due to disease in nonrespiratory organs by retaining acid in the form of carbon dioxide.

hypopraxia *n.* **1.** a condition of diminished and enfeebled activity. **2.** a lack of interest in, or a disinclination for, activity; listlessness.

hypoproteinaemia *n.* a decrease in the quantity of protein in the blood. It may result from malnutrition, impaired protein production (as in liver disease), or increased loss of protein from the body (as in the *nephrotic syndrome). It results in swelling (*oedema), because of the accumulation of fluid in the tissues, and increased susceptibility to infections. *See also* hypogammaglobulinaemia.

hypoprothrombinaemia *n.* a deficiency of the clotting factor *prothrombin in the blood, which results in an increased tendency to bleed. It may occur as an inherited defect, as the result of liver disease, vitamin K deficiency, or anticoagulant treatment.

hypopyon *n.* pus in the chamber of the eye that lies in front of the lens.

hyposensitive *adj.* less than normally responsive to the presence of antigenic material. *Compare* hypersensitive. —**hyposensitivity** *n.*

hyposensitization *n. see* desensitization.

hyposmia *n.* a condition in which the sense of smell is exceptionally weak. *See also* hypoaesthesia.

hypospadias *n.* a congenital abnormality in which the opening of the *urethra is on the underside of the penis: either on the glans penis (*glandular hypospadias*), at the junction of the glans with the shaft (*coronal hypospadias*), or on the shaft itself (*penile hypospadias*). All varieties can be treated surgically, and neither micturition nor sexual function need be impaired.

hypostasis *n.* accumulation of fluid or blood in a dependent part of the body, under the influence of gravity, in cases of poor circulation. Hypostatic congestion of the lung bases may be seen in debilitated patients who are confined to bed. It predisposes to pneumonia (hypostatic pneumonia) but may be prevented by careful nursing and physiotherapy. A similar condition affects the dependent parts of the body after death. —**hypostatic** *adj.*

hyposthenia *n.* a state of physical weakness or abnormally low muscular tension.

hyposthenuria *n.* the secretion of urine of low specific gravity. The inability to concentrate the urine occurs in patients at the final stage of chronic renal failure.

hypotension *n.* a condition in which the arterial *blood pressure is abnormally low. It occurs after excessive fluid loss (e.g. through diarrhoea, burns, or vomiting) or following severe blood loss (haemorrhage) from any cause. Other causes include myocardial infarction, pulmonary embolism, severe infections, allergic reactions, arrhythmias, acute abdominal conditions (e.g. pancreatitis), Addison's disease, and drugs (e.g. an overdose of the drugs used to treat hypertension).

Some people experience a temporary fall in blood pressure when rising from a horizontal position (*orthostatic hypotension*). Temporary hypotension may result in a simple faint (syncope). The patient becomes light-headed, sweats, and may develop impaired consciousness. In severe cases peripheral circulatory failure (cardiogenic shock) develops, with unrecordable blood pressure, weak pulses, and suppression of urine production. The patient is placed flat, with legs elevated, and given oxygen. Fluid and blood are replaced by an intravenous infusion as required. Specific treatment of the cause is provided (e.g. corticosteroids in Addison's disease).

hypothalamus *n.* the region of the forebrain in the floor of the third ventricle, linked with the thalamus above and the *pituitary gland below (*see* brain). It contains several important centres controlling body temperature, thirst, hunger, and eating, water balance, and sexual function. It is also closely connected with emotional activity and sleep and functions as a centre for the integration of hormonal and autonomic nervous activity through its control of pituitary secretions (*see* neuroendocrine system, pituitary gland). —**hypothalamic** *adj.*

hypothenar *adj.* describing or relating to the fleshy prominent part of the palm of the hand below the little finger. *Compare* thenar.

hypothermia *n.* **1.** accidental reduction of body temperature below the normal range in the absence of protective reflex actions, such as shivering. Often insidious in onset, it is particularly liable to occur in babies and the elderly if they are living in poorly heated homes and have inadequate clothing. **2.** deliberate lowering of body temperature for therapeutic purposes. This may be done during surgery, in order to reduce the patient's requirement for oxygen.

hypothymia *n.* a diminished intensity of emotional response. It is a feature of *asthenic personalities, of some chronic schizophrenics, and of some depressives.

hypothyroidism *n.* subnormal activity of the thyroid gland. If present at birth and untreated it leads to *cretinism. In adult life it causes mental and physical slowing, undue sensitivity to cold, slowing of the pulse, weight gain, and coarsening of the skin (*myxoedema*). The condition can be treated by administration of thyroxine.

hypotonia *n.* a state of reduced tension in muscle.

hypotonic *adj.* **1.** describing a solution that has a lower osmotic pressure than another solution. *See* osmosis. **2.** describing muscles that demonstrate diminished *tonicity.

hypotrichosis *n.* a condition in which less hair develops than normal.

hypotropia *n. see* strabismus.

hypoventilation *n.* breathing at an abnormally slow rate, which results in an increased amount of carbon dioxide in the blood.

hypovitaminosis *n.* a deficiency of a vitamin caused either through lack of the vitamin in the diet or from an inability to absorb or utilize it.

hypovolaemia (oligaemia) *n.* a decrease in the volume of circulating blood. *See* shock.

hypoxaemia *n.* the presence in the blood of an abnormally low concentration of oxygen, usually as a result of inadequate uptake of oxygen in the lungs because of lung disease. *See also* anoxia.

hypoxia *n.* a deficiency of oxygen in the tissues. *See also* anoxia, hypoxaemia.

hypsarrhythmia *n.* an abnormal and chaotic pattern of brain activity, demonstrated by *encephalography, that is usually associated with *infantile spasms.

hyster- (hystero-) *prefix denoting* **1.** the womb. **2.** hysteria.

hysteralgia (hysterodynia, uteralgia) *n.* pain in the womb.

hysterectomy *n.* the surgical removal of the womb, either through an incision in the abdominal wall or through the vagina. *Subtotal hysterectomy* involves removing the body of the womb but leaving the neck (cervix); in *total hysterectomy* (*panhysterectomy*) the entire womb is removed. The operation is most commonly performed if the womb contains large *fibroids; other cases requiring hysterectomy include cervical cancer, malignant tumours or precancerous cells in the womb, or severe damage to the womb following a *Caesarean section. Although pregnancy is no longer possible, hysterectomy does not affect sexual desire or activity.

hysteria *n.* **1.** a neurosis whose principal features consist of emotional instability, repression, *dissociation, physical symptoms, and vulnerability to suggestion. Freud postulated that hysteria arose as the result of frustrated libidinous impulses. Two types are usually described: *conversion hysteria*, characterized mainly by physical symptoms, such as paralysis; and *dissociative hysteria*, in which patients show changes in thinking, such as multiple personality states or amnesia. There is doubt as to whether hysteria constitutes a clinical entity. Patients with such symptoms are usually treated with psychotherapy. *See also* hysterical. **2.** a state of great emotional excitement.

hysterical *adj.* **1.** describing a symptom that is not due to organic disease, is produced unconsciously, and from which the individual derives some gain. For example paralysis can be a hysterical symptom. **2.** describing a kind of *personality disorder characterized by instability and shallowness of feelings and by superficiality and a tendency to manipulate in personal relationships.

hysterocele (uterocele) *n.* hernia (rupture) of the womb, usually during pregnancy.

hysterocleisis *n.* surgical closure of the passage from the womb to the vagina at the mouth of the womb.

hysteropexy *n.* stitching the womb to the abdominal wall to prevent its downward displacement. *See* prolapse.

hysterorrhaphy *n.* stitching the womb. *See also* hysteropexy.

hysterorrhexis (metrorrhexis) *n.* rupture of the womb.

hysterosalpingography *n. see* uterosalpingography.

hysteroscope (uteroscope) *n.* a tubular instrument with a light source for observing the interior of the womb. *See also* endoscope.

hysterotomy *n.* incision of the womb, either through the abdominal wall or the vagina. *See* Caesarean section.

I

-iasis *suffix denoting* a diseased condition. Example: *leishmaniasis* (disease caused by *Leishmania* species).

iatro- *prefix denoting* 1. medicine. 2. doctors.

iatrogenic *adj.* describing a condition that has resulted from treatment, as either an unforeseen or inevitable side-effect.

ibuprofen *n.* an *analgesic that relieves inflammation, used in the treatment of arthritic conditions. It is administered by mouth and sometimes causes skin rashes and digestive upsets. Trade name: **Brufen**.

ichor *n.* a watery material oozing from wounds or ulcers.

ichthyosis *n.* a congenital condition, usually present at birth, in which the skin is dry, rough, and scaly because of a defect in *keratinization. Ichthyosis varies in severity from slight skin dryness to a severe condition in which an infant is born, usually dead, with skin like armour plate.

ICSH (interstitial-cell-stimulating hormone) *see* luteinizing hormone.

icterus *n. see* jaundice.

ictus *n.* a stroke or any sudden attack. The term is often used for an epileptic fit, stressing the suddenness of its onset.

id *n.* (in psychoanalysis) a part of the unconscious mind governed by the instinctive forces of *libido and the death wish. These violent forces seek immediate release in action or in symbolic form. The id is therefore said to be governed by the pleasure principle and not by the demands of reality or of logic. In the course of individual devel-

opment some of the functions of the id are taken over by the *ego.

-id *suffix denoting* relationship or resemblance to. Example: *spermatid* (a stage of sperm formation).

ideation *n.* the process of thinking or of having *imagery or ideas.

identical twins *see* twins.

identification *n.* (in psychological development) the process of adopting other people's characteristics more or less permanently. Identification with a parent is important in personality formation, and has been especially implicated in the development of a moral sense and of an appropriate sex role.

ideo- *prefix denoting* 1. the mind or mental activity. 2. ideas.

ideomotor *adj.* describing or relating to a motor action that is evoked by an idea. *Ideomotor apraxia* is the inability to translate the idea of a complex behaviour into action.

idio- *prefix denoting* peculiarity to the individual.

idiocy *n.* a profound degree of intellectual *subnormality in which the affected individual can do nothing for himself and cannot speak. The term is now obsolete, but roughly corresponds to an *intelligence quotient of less than 20. There are usually associated physical handicaps and there is always physical damage of the brain.

idiopathic *adj.* denoting a disease or condition the cause of which is not known or that arises spontaneously. —**idiopathy** *n.*

idiosyncrasy *n.* an unusual and unexpected sensitivity exhibited by an individual to a particular drug or food. —**idiosyncratic** *adj.*

idiot savant an individual whose overall functioning is at the level of mental *subnormality but who has one or more special intellectual abilities that are advanced to a high level. Musical ability, calculating ability, and rote memory are examples of abilities that may be highly developed. Many such individuals suffer from *autism.

idioventricular *adj.* affecting or peculiar to the ventricles of the heart. The term is most often used to describe the very slow beat of the ventricles under the influence of their own natural subsidiary pacemaker (*idioventricular rhythm*).

idoxuridine *n.* an iodine-containing drug that inhibits the growth of viruses and is used to treat viral infections of the eye (such as keratitis). It is administered in eye drops or ointment and may cause irritation and stinging on application. Trade names: **Dendrid, Kerecid**.

ifosfamide *n.* a *cytotoxic drug used in the treatment of malignant disease, particularly sarcomas, testicular tumours, and lymphomas. It is administered intravenously by injection or infusion. Side-effects include nausea, vomiting, alopecia, and haemorrhagic cystitis; concomitant administration of *mesna is recommended to prevent cystitis. Trade name: **Mitoxana.**

ile- (ileo-) *prefix denoting* the ileum. Examples: *ileocaecal* (relating to the ileum and caecum); *ileocolic* (relating to the ileum and colon).

ileal conduit a segment of small intestine (ileum) used to convey urine from the ureters to the exterior into an appliance. The ureters are implanted into an isolated segment of bowel, usually ileum but sometimes sigmoid colon, one end of which is brought through the abdominal wall to the skin surface. This end forms a spout, or *stoma*, which projects into a suitable urinary appliance. The ureters themselves cannot be used for this purpose as they tend to narrow and retract if brought through the skin. The oper-

ation is performed if the bladder has to be removed or bypassed; for example, because of cancer.

ileectomy *n.* surgical removal of the ileum (small intestine) or part of the ileum.

ileitis *n.* inflammation of the ileum (small intestine). It may be caused by *Crohn's disease, tuberculosis, or typhoid or it may occur in association with ulcerative *colitis (when it is known as *backwash ileitis*).

ileocaecal valve a valve at the junction of the small and large intestines consisting of two membranous folds that close to prevent the backflow of food from the colon and caecum to the ileum.

ileocolitis *n.* inflammation of the ileum and the colon (small and large intestines). The commonest causes are *Crohn's disease and tuberculosis.

ileocolostomy *n.* a surgical operation in which the ileum is joined to some part of the colon. It is usually performed when the right side of the colon has been removed or if it is desired to bypass either the terminal part of the ileum or right side of the colon.

ileoproctostomy (ileorectal anastomosis) *n.* a surgical operation in which the ileum is joined to the rectum, usually after surgical removal of the colon (*see* colectomy).

ileostomy *n.* a surgical operation in which the ileum is brought through the abdominal wall to create an artificial opening (*stoma*) through which the intestinal contents can discharge, thus bypassing the colon. Various types of bag may be worn to collect the effluent. The operation is usually performed in association with *colectomy; or to allow the colon to rest and heal in cases of colitis; or following injury or surgery to the colon.

ileum *n.* the lowest of the three portions of the small *intestine. It runs from the jejunum to the *ileocaecal valve. —**ileal**, **ileac** *adj.*

ileus *n.* intestinal obstruction, usually obstruction of the small intestine (ileum). *Paralytic* or *adynamic ileus* is functional obstruction of the ileum due to loss of intestinal movement (peristalsis), which may be caused by abdominal surgery (*see* laparotomy), spinal injuries, deficiency of potassium in the blood (hypokalaemia), or peritonitis. Treatment consists of intravenous administration of fluid and nutrients and removal of excess stomach secretions by tube until peristalsis returns. If possible, the underlying condition is treated. Mechanical obstruction of the ileum may be caused by a gallstone entering the bowel through a fistula or widened bile duct (*gallstone ileus*); thickened *meconium in newborn babies with *cystic fibrosis (*meconium ileus*); or intestinal worms, usually the threadworm *Enterobius vermicularis* (*verminous ileus*).

ili- (ilio-) *prefix denoting* the ilium.

iliac arteries the arteries that supply most of the blood to the lower limbs and pelvic region. The right and left *common iliac arteries* form the terminal branches of the abdominal aorta. Each branches into the *external iliac artery* and the smaller *internal iliac artery*.

iliacus *n.* a flat triangular muscle situated in the area of the groin. This muscle acts in conjunction with the *psoas muscle to flex the thigh.

iliac veins the veins draining most of the blood from the lower limbs and pelvic region. The right and left *common iliac veins* unite to form the inferior vena cava. They are each formed by the union of the *internal* and *external iliac veins*.

iliopsoas *n.* a composite muscle made up of the *iliacus and *psoas muscles, which have a common tendon.

ilium *n.* the haunch bone: a wide bone forming the upper part of each side of the *hip bone (*see also* pelvis). There is a concave depression (*iliac fossa*) on the inside of the pelvis; the right iliac fossa provides space for the vermiform appendix. —**iliac** *adj.*

illusion *n.* a false perception due to misinterpretation of the stimuli arising from an object. For example, a patient may misinterpret the conversation of others as the voices of enemies conspiring to destroy him. Illusions can occur in quite normal people, when they are usually spontaneously corrected. They may also occur in almost any psychiatric syndrome, especially *depression. *Compare* hallucination.
Optical illusions are perceptions that do not agree with the actual object in the external world. They are produced by deceptive qualities of the stimulus and are in no way pathological.

imagery *n.* the production of vivid mental representations by the normal processes of thought. *Hypnagogic imagery* occurs just before falling asleep, and the images are often very distinct. *Hypnopompic imagery* occurs in the state between sleep and full wakefulness. Like hypnagogic imagery, the experiences may be very vivid. *Eidetic imagery*, commoner in children than adults, is the production of images of exceptional clarity, which may be recalled long after being first experienced.

imago *n.* (in psychoanalysis) the internal unconscious representation of an important person in the individual's life, particularly a parent.

imbecility *n.* a moderate to severe degree of intellectual *subnormality that falls short of *idiocy. The term is now obsolete, but roughly corresponds to an *intelligence quotient of between

20 and 50. It is almost always caused by physical damage to the brain, and affected individuals usually require help and supervision throughout their lives.

imipramine *n.* a drug administered by mouth or injection to treat depression (*see* antidepressant). Its effects may be slow to develop; common side-effects include dry mouth, blurred vision, constipation, sweating, and rapid heart beat. Trade names: **Berkomine**, **Dimipressin**, **Tofranil**.

imitation *n.* acting in the same way as another person, either temporarily or permanently. This is one of the mechanisms of *identification. It can be used in therapy (*see* modelling).

immersion foot *see* trench foot.

immobilization *n.* the procedure of making a normally movable part of the body, such as a joint, immovable. This helps an infected, diseased, or injured tissue (bone, joint, or muscle) to heal. Immobilization may be temporary (for example, by means of a plaster of Paris cast on a limb) or it may be permanent. Permanent immobilization of a joint is achieved by the operation of *arthrodesis.

immune *adj.* protected against a particular infection by the presence of specific antibodies against the organisms concerned. *See* immunity.

immunity *n.* the body's ability to resist infection, afforded by the presence of circulating *antibodies and white blood cells. Antibodies are manufactured specifically to deal with the antigens associated with different diseases as they are encountered. *Active immunity* arises when the body's own cells produce, and remain able to produce, appropriate antibodies following an attack of a disease or deliberate stimulation (*see* immunization). *Passive immunity*, which is only short-lived, is provided by injecting ready-made antibodies in *an-

tiserum taken from another person or animal already immune. Babies have passive immunity, conferred by antibodies from the maternal blood and *colostrum, to common diseases for several weeks after birth.

immunization *n.* the production of *immunity by artificial means. Passive immunity, which is temporary, may be conferred by the injection of an *antiserum, but the production of active immunity calls for the use of treated antigens, to stimulate the body to produce its own antibodies: this is the procedure of *vaccination (also called *inoculation*). The material used for immunization (the *vaccine) may consist of live bacteria or viruses so treated that they are harmless while remaining antigenic or completely dead organisms or their products (e.g. toxins) chemically or physically altered to produce the same effect.

immuno- *prefix denoting* immunity or immunological response.

immunoelectrophoresis *n.* a technique for identifying antigenic fractions in a serum. The components of the serum are separated by *electrophoresis and allowed to diffuse through agar gel towards a particular antiserum. Where the antibody meets its antigen, a band of precipitation occurs. *See also* precipitin.

immunofluorescence *n.* a technique for observing the amount and/or distribution of antibody or antigen in a tissue section. The antibodies are labelled (directly or indirectly) with a fluorescent dye (e.g. fluorescein) and applied to the tissue, which is observed through an ultraviolet microscope. In *direct immunofluorescence* the antibody is labelled before being applied to the tissue. In *indirect immunofluorescence* the antibody is labelled after it has bound to the antigen, by means of fluorescein-labelled anti-immunoglobulin serum. —**immunofluorescent** *adj.*

immunoglobulin (Ig) *n.* one of a group of structurally related proteins (gamma *globulins) that act as antibodies. Several classes of Ig with different functions are distinguished – IgA, IgD, IgE, IgG, and IgM. They can be separated by *immunoelectrophoresis. *See* antibody.

immunological tolerance a failure of the body to distinguish between materials that are 'self', and therefore to be tolerated, and those that are 'not self', against which antibodies are produced. For example, the body fails to produce antibodies against foreign materials if an antigen has previously been introduced into the body before the antibody-producing system is mature; apparently the presence of antigen within the growing cells inhibits antibody formation.

immunology *n.* the study of *immunity and all of the phenomena connected with the defence mechanisms of the body. —**immunological** *adj.*

immunophoresis *n.* a technique, relying upon the *precipitin reaction, for identifying an unknown antigen or testing for an antibody in a serum. Antibody and antigen are allowed to diffuse towards each other in agar gel.

immunosuppressive *n.* a drug, such as *azathioprine or *cyclophosphamide, that reduces the body's resistance to infection and other foreign bodies by suppressing the immune system. Immunosuppressives are used to maintain the survival of organ and tissue transplants and to treat various *autoimmune diseases, including rheumatoid arthritis. Because immunity is lowered during treatment with immunosuppressives, there is an increased risk of infection.

immunotherapy *n.* the prevention or treatment of disease using agents that may modify the immune response. It is a largely experimental approach, stud-

ied most widely in the treatment of cancer.

immunotransfusion *n.* the transfusion of an *antiserum to treat or give temporary protection against a disease.

impacted *adj.* firmly wedged. An *impacted tooth* (usually a wisdom tooth) is one that cannot erupt into a normal position because it is obstructed by other tissues. *Impacted faeces* are so hard and dry that they cannot pass through the anus without special measures being taken (*see* constipation). An *impacted fracture* is one in which the bone ends are driven into each other. —**impaction** *n.*

impairment *n. see* handicap.

impalpable *adj.* describing a structure within the body that cannot be detected (or that can be detected only with difficulty) by feeling with the hand.

imperforate *adj.* lacking an opening. Occasionally girls at puberty are found to have an *imperforate hymen* (a fold of membrane close to the vaginal orifice), which impedes the flow of menstrual blood.

imperforate anus (proctatresia) partial or complete obstruction of the anus: a condition, discovered at birth, due to failure of the anus to develop normally in the embryo. There are several different types of imperforate anus, including *developmental anal stenosis*, *persistent anal membrane*, and *covered anus* (due to fused genital folds). If the anal canal fails to develop, the rectum ends blindly above the muscles of the perineum. Most mild cases of imperforate anus can be treated by a simple operation. If the defect is extensive a temporary opening is made in the colon (*see* colostomy), with later surgical reconstruction of the rectum and anus.

impetigo *n.* a bacterial skin infection usually caused by staphylococci,

implant

though occasionally by streptococci. Impetigo is particularly common in babies and children, occurring mainly on the face and limbs. The infection, which spreads quickly over the body, starts as a red patch and develops into small pustules that join together, forming crusty yellow sores. Impetigo is very contagious, especially in communities of children, being readily spread by contact and via towels and face cloths. The condition usually responds to treatment with antibiotics, applied locally, within 7 to 10 days. Impetigo of the newborn is rare today but an outbreak may spread rapidly in a maternity unit.

implant *n.* **1.** a substance (such as a drug) or a tissue graft inserted into the skin. **2.** (in dentistry) a rigid structure that is embedded in bone or under its periosteum to provide support for replacement teeth on a *denture or a *bridge. Another type protrudes through the end of a shortened tooth root to stabilize it.

implantation *n.* **1.** (*or* **nidation**) the attachment of the early embryo to the lining of the womb, which occurs at the *blastocyst stage of development, six to eight days after ovulation. The site of implantation determines the position of the placenta. **2.** the placing of a substance (e.g. a drug) or an object (e.g. an artificial pacemaker) within a tissue. **3.** the surgical replacement of damaged tissue with healthy tissue (*see* transplantation).

implosion *n. see* flooding.

impotence *n.* inability in a man to have sexual intercourse. Impotence may be *erectile*, in which the penis does not become firm enough to enter the vagina, or *ejaculatory*, in which penetration occurs but there is no ejaculation of semen (orgasm). Either kind of impotence may be due to a physical disease, such as diabetes (*organic*) or to

a psychological or emotional problem (*psychogenic*).

impression *n.* (in dentistry) an elastic mould made of the teeth and surrounding soft tissues or of a toothless jaw. A soft impression material is placed over the teeth or jaw and sets within several minutes. After removal from the mouth a plaster model is made; on this are constructed *restorations of teeth, *dentures, or *orthodontic appliances.

imprinting *n.* (in animal behaviour) a rapid and irreversible form of learning that takes place in some animals during the first hours of life. Animals attach themselves in this way to members of their own species, but if they are exposed to creatures of a different species during this short period, they become attached to this species instead.

impulse *n.* (in neurology) *see* nerve impulse.

in- (im-) *prefix denoting* **1.** not. **2.** in; within; into.

inanition *n.* a condition of exhaustion caused by lack of nutrients in the blood. This may arise through starvation, malnutrition, or intestinal disease.

inappetence *n.* lack of desire, usually for food.

in articulo mortis Latin: at the moment of death.

inbreeding *n.* the production of offspring by parents who are closely related; for example, who are first cousins or siblings. The amount of inbreeding in a population is largely controlled by culture and tradition. *Compare* outbreeding.

incarcerated *adj.* confined or constricted so as to be immovable: applied particularly to a type of *hernia.

incidence rate (inception rate) a measure of morbidity based on the number of new episodes of illness arising in a population over an estimated period. It can be expressed in terms of sick persons or episodes per 1000 individuals at risk. *Compare* prevalence rate.

incision *n.* **1.** the surgical cutting of soft tissues, such as skin or muscle, with a knife or scalpel. **2.** the cut so made.

incisor *n.* any of the four front teeth in each jaw, two on each side of the midline. *See also* dentition.

incisure *n.* (in anatomy) a notch, small hollow, or depression.

inclusion bodies particles occurring in the nucleus and cytoplasm of cells usually as a result of virus infection. Their presence can sometimes be used to diagnose such an infection.

incompatibility *n. see* compatibility.

incompetence *n.* impaired function of the valves of the heart or veins, which allows backward leakage of blood. *See* aortic regurgitation, mitral incompetence, varicose veins.

incontinence *n.* **1.** the inappropriate involuntary passage of urine, resulting in wetting. *Stress incontinence* is the leak of urine on coughing and straining. It is common in women in whom the muscles of the pelvic floor are weakened after childbirth. *Overflow incontinence* is leakage from a full bladder, which occurs most commonly in old men with bladder outflow obstruction or in patients with neurological conditions affecting bladder control. *Urge incontinence* is leakage of urine that accompanies an intense desire to pass water with failure of restraint. *See also* enuresis. **2.** inability to control bowel movements (*faecal incontinence*).

incoordination *n.* (in neurology) an impairment in the performance of precise rapid movements. These are dependent upon the normal function of the whole nervous system, and incoordination may result from a disorder in

any part of it. *See* apraxia, ataxia, dyssynergia.

incubation *n.* **1.** the process of development of an egg or a culture of bacteria. **2.** the care of a premature baby in an *incubator.

incubation period (latent period) 1. the interval between exposure to an infection and the appearance of the first symptoms. **2.** (in bacteriology) the period of development of a bacterial culture.

incubator *n.* a transparent container for keeping premature babies in controlled conditions and protecting them from infection. Other forms of incubator are used for cultivating bacteria in Petri dishes and for hatching eggs.

incudectomy *n.* surgical removal of the second ear ossicle, the incus, as in the treatment of chronic middle ear infection (*otitis media).

incus *n.* a small anvil-shaped bone in the middle *ear that articulates with the malleus and the stapes. *See* ossicle.

Inderal *n. see* propranolol.

indican *n.* a compound excreted in the urine as a detoxification product of *indoxyl. Indican is formed by the conjugation of indoxyl with sulphuric acid.

indicanuria *n.* the presence in the urine of an abnormally high concentration of *indican. This may be a sign that the intestine is obstructed.

indication *n.* (in medicine) a strong reason for believing that a particular course of action is desirable. In a wounded patient, the loss of blood, which would lead to circulatory collapse, is an indication for blood transfusion. *Compare* contraindication.

indigestion *n. see* dyspepsia.

indole *n.* a derivative of the amino acid tryptophan, excreted in the urine and faeces. Abnormal patterns of urinary indole excretion are found in some mentally retarded patients.

indolent *adj.* describing a disease process that is failing to heal or has persisted. The term is applied particularly to ulcers of skin or mucous membrane.

indomethacin *n.* an *analgesic that relieves inflammation, used in the treatment of arthritic conditions. It is administered by mouth or in suppositories; common side-effects are headache, dizziness, and digestive upsets. Trade names: **Imbrilon**, **Indocid**.

indoxyl *n.* an alcohol derived from *indole by bacterial action. It is excreted in the urine as *indican.

induction *n.* **1.** (in obstetrics) the artificial starting of childbirth. Labour can often be reduced by giving the pregnant woman a warm bath followed by an enema. If necessary the muscles of the womb may be stimulated to contract by injections of *oxytocin or by puncturing the sac surrounding the baby to release some of the amniotic fluid in which it is bathed. Induction of labour is attempted if pregnancy has continued considerably beyond the expected date of birth or if there is a risk to the health of mother or infant. If induction is not successful it may be necessary to perform a *Caesarean section. **2.** (in anaesthetics) initiation of *anaesthesia. General anaesthesia is usually induced by injecting certain drugs, usually barbiturates, into the bloodstream. In acupuncture, anaesthesia is induced by the manipulation of needles in a specified area of skin. **3.** (in embryology) the process by which a chemical released from one part of an embryo causes another part to develop in a particular way. Also called: **evocation**.

induration *n.* abnormal hardening of a tissue or organ. *See also* sclerosis.

indusium *n.* a thin layer of grey matter covering the upper surface of the *corpus callosum between the two cerebral hemispheres.

industrial disease *see* occupational disease.

inertia *n.* (in physiology) sluggishness or absence of activity in certain smooth muscles. In *uterine inertia* the muscular wall of the womb fails to contract adequately during labour, making the process excessively long. This inertia may be present from the start of labour or it may develop because of exhaustion following strong contractions.

in extremis Latin: at the point of death.

infant *n.* a child incapable of any form of independence from its mother: a child under one year of age, especially a premature or newborn child. In legal use the term denotes a child up to the age of seven years.

infanticide *n.* (in Britain) under the terms of the Infanticide Act (1938), the felony of child destruction by the natural mother within 12 months of birth when the balance of her mind is disturbed because she has not fully recovered from childbirth and/or lactation. Under such circumstances a charge that would have been one of murder is reduced to manslaughter.

infantile *adj.* **1.** denoting conditions occurring in adults that are recognizable in childhood, e.g. poliomyelitis (*infantile paralysis*) and *infantile scurvy*. **2.** of, relating to, or affecting infants.

infantile spasms a serious brain disorder of infants, usually beginning under the age of six months. The spasms are involuntary flexing movements of the arms, legs, neck, and trunk; each spasm lasts 1–3 seconds and is associated with flushing of the face, and runs of spasms occur over a period of several minutes. The baby fails to respond to human contact and development is profoundly slowed. An EEG pattern of *hypsarrhythmia is sometimes seen. Interpretation of the spasms as wind has often delayed diagnosis, but immediate recognition and treatment with corticosteroids and ACTH offers a chance of arresting the disease.

infantilism *n.* persistence of childlike physical or psychological characteristics into adult life.

infant mortality rate (IMR) the number of deaths of infants under one year of age per 1000 live births in a given year. Included in the IMR are the *neonatal death rate* (calculated from deaths occurring in the first four weeks of life) and *postneonatal death rate* (from deaths in the remainder of the first year). Neonatal deaths are further subdivided into *early* (first week) and *late* (second, third, and fourth weeks). In prosperous countries neonatal deaths account for about two-thirds of infant mortalities, the majority being in the first week. The IMR is usually regarded more as a measure of social affluence than a measure of the quality of antenatal and/or obstetric care; the latter is more truly reflected in the *perinatal mortality rate* (the sum of stillbirths and first-week or neonatal deaths per 1000 total births).

infarct *n. see* infarction.

infarction *n.* the death of part or the whole of an organ that occurs when the artery carrying its blood supply is obstructed by a blood clot (thrombus) or an *embolus. For example, *myocardial infarction, affecting the muscle of the heart, follows coronary thrombosis. A small localized area of dead tissue produced as a result of an inadequate blood supply is known as an *infarct*.

infection *n.* invasion of the body by harmful organisms (pathogens), such as bacteria, fungi, protozoa, rickettsiae, or viruses. The infective agent may be transmitted by a patient or *carrier in airborne droplets expelled during coughing and sneezing or by direct contact, such as kissing or sexual intercourse (*see* venereal disease); by animal or insect *vectors; by ingestion of contaminated food or drink; or from an infected mother to the fetus during pregnancy or birth. Pathogenic organisms present in soil, organisms from animal intermediate hosts, or those living as *commensals on the body can also cause infections. Organisms may invade via a wound or bite or through mucous membranes. After an *incubation period symptoms appear, usually consisting of either localized inflammation and pain or more remote effects. Treatment with drugs is usually effective against all but the viral infections (there is no specific treatment for most of the common viral infections, including the common cold and influenza).

infectious disease *see* communicable disease.

infectious mononucleosis *see* glandular fever.

inferior *adj.* (in anatomy) lower in the body in relation to another structure or surface.

inferior dental block a type of injection to anaesthetize the inferior *dental nerve. Inferior dental block is routinely performed to allow dental procedures to be carried out on the lower teeth on one side of the mouth.

inferior dental canal a bony canal in the *mandible on each side. It carries the inferior *dental nerve and vessels and for part of its length its outline is visible on a radiograph.

inferiority complex 1. an unconscious and extreme exaggeration of feelings of insignificance or inferiority, which is shown by behaviour that is defensive or compensatory (such as aggression). **2.** (in psychoanalysis) a *complex resulting from the conflict between Oedipal wishes (*see* Oedipus complex) and the reality of the child's lack of power. This gives rise to repressed feelings of personal inferiority.

infertility *n.* inability in a woman to conceive or in a man to induce conception. Female infertility may be due to failure to ovulate, to obstruction of the *Fallopian tubes, or to disease of the lining of the uterus (endometrium). Male infertility may be due to spermatozoa in the ejaculate being defective either in motility (necrospermia) or in numbers (*see* oligospermia) or to a total absence of sperm (*see* azoospermia).

infestation *n.* the presence of animal parasites either on the skin (for example ticks) or inside the body (for example tapeworms).

infiltration *n.* **1.** the abnormal entry of a substance (*infiltrate*) into a cell, tissue, or organ. Examples of infiltrates are blood cells, cancer cells, fat, starch, or calcium and magnesium salts. **2.** the injection of a local anaesthetic solution into the tissues to cause local *anaesthesia. Infiltration anaesthesia is routinely used to anaesthetize upper teeth to allow dental procedures to be carried out.

inflammation *n.* the body's response to injury, which may be acute or chronic. *Acute inflammation* is the immediate defensive reaction of tissue to any injury, which may be caused by infection, chemicals, or physical agents. It involves pain, heat, redness, swelling, and loss of function of the affected part. Blood vessels near the site of injury are dilated, so that blood flow is locally increased. White blood cells enter the tissue and begin to engulf bacteria and other foreign particles. Similar cells from the tissues remove and consume the dead cells, sometimes with the production of pus, and the process of healing commences. In certain circumstances healing does not occur and *chronic inflammation* ensues.

influenza *n.* a highly contagious virus infection that affects the respiratory system. The viruses are transmitted by coughing and sneezing. Symptoms commence after an incubation period of 1–4 days and include headache, fever, loss of appetite, weakness, and general aches and pains. They may continue for about a week. After bed rest and aspirin most patients recover, but a secondary infection of the lungs is a common serious complication. An infection – and immunization too – provides protection only against the specific strain of virus concerned.

infra- *prefix denoting* below.

infrared radiation the band of electromagnetic radiation that is longer in wavelength than the red of the visible spectrum. Infrared radiation is responsible for the transmission of radiant heat. It may be used in physiotherapy to warm tissues, reduce pain, and improve circulation, but is not as effective as *diathermy for deep structures. Special photographic film sensitive to infrared radiation is used in *thermography.

infundibulum *n.* any funnel-shaped channel or passage, particularly the hollow conical stalk that extends downwards from the hypothalamus and is continuous with the posterior lobe of the pituitary gland.

infusion *n.* **1.** a slow injection of a substance (e.g. saline or dextrose) into a vein or subcutaneous tissue. **2.** the process whereby the active principles are extracted from plant material by steeping it in water that has been heated to boiling point (as in the making of tea). **3.** the solution produced by this process.

ingesta *pl. n.* food and drink that is taken into the alimentary canal through the mouth.

ingestion *n.* **1.** the process by which food is taken into the alimentary canal.

It involves chewing and swallowing. **2.** the process by which a phagocytic cell takes in solid material, such as bacteria.

ingravescent *adj.* gradually increasing in severity.

inguinal *adj.* relating to or affecting the region of the groin (inguen).

inguinal canal either of a pair of openings that connect the abdominal cavity with the scrotum in the male fetus. The inguinal canals provide a route for the descent of the testes into the scrotum, after which they normally become obliterated.

inguinal hernia *see* hernia.

inguinal ligament (Poupart's ligament) a ligament in the groin that extends from the anterior superior iliac spine to the pubic tubercle. It is part of the *aponeurosis of the external oblique muscle of the abdomen.

INH *see* isoniazid.

inhalation *n.* **1.** (*or* **inspiration**) the act of breathing air into the lungs through the mouth and nose. *See* breathing. **2.** a gas, vapour, or aerosol breathed in for the treatment of conditions of the respiratory tract.

inhibition *n.* **1.** (in physiology) the prevention or reduction of the functioning of an organ, muscle, etc., by the action of certain nerve impulses. **2.** (in psychoanalysis) an inner command that prevents one from doing something forbidden. Some inhibitions are essential for social adjustment, but excessive inhibitions can severely restrict one's life. **3.** (in psychology) a tendency not to carry out a specific action, produced each time the action is carried out.

inhibitor *n.* a substance that prevents the occurrence of a given process or reaction. *See also* MAO inhibitor.

inion *n.* the projection of the occipital bone that can be felt at the base of the skull.

injection *n.* introduction into the body of drugs or other fluids by means of a syringe, usually drugs that would be destroyed by the digestive processes if taken by mouth. Common routes for injection are into the skin (*intracutaneous* or *intradermal*); below the skin (*subcutaneous*), e.g. for insulin; into a muscle (*intramuscular*), for drugs that are slowly absorbed; and into a vein (*intravenous*), for drugs to be rapidly absorbed. *Enemas are also regarded as injections.

inlay *n.* **1.** a substance or piece of tissue inserted to replace a defect in a tissue. For example, a bone graft may be inlaid into an area of missing or damaged bone. **2.** (in dentistry) a rigid restoration inserted into a tapered cavity in a tooth. It is held in place with a cement *lute. The material most widely used is cast gold.

inlet *n.* an aperture providing the entrance to a cavity, such as that of the pelvis.

innate *adj.* describing a condition or characteristic that is present in an individual at birth and is inherited from his parents. *See also* congenital.

inner ear *see* labyrinth.

innervation *n.* the nerve supply to an area or organ of the body, which can carry either motor impulses to the structure or sensory impulses away from it towards the brain.

innocent *adj.* (of a tumour) benign; not malignant.

innominate artery (brachiocephalic artery) a short artery originating as the first large branch of the *aortic arch, passing upwards to the right, and ending at the lower neck near the right sternoclavicular joint. Here it divides into the right common carotid and the right subclavian arteries.

innominate bone *see* hip bone.

innominate vein (brachiocephalic vein) either of two veins, one on each side of the neck, formed by the junction of the external jugular and subclavian veins. The two veins join to form the superior vena cava.

ino- *prefix denoting* **1.** fibrous tissue. **2.** muscle.

inoculation *n.* the introduction of a small quantity of vaccine in the process of *immunization: a more general name for *vaccination.

inoculum *n.* any material that is used for inoculation.

inositol *n.* a compound similar to a hexose sugar. Inositol is present in many foods, in particular in the bran of cereal grain. It is sometimes classified as a vitamin but it can be synthesized by most animals and there is no evidence that it is essential to man.

inotropic *adj.* affecting the contraction of heart muscle. Drugs such as *digitalis have positive inotropic action, stimulating heart muscle contractions and causing the heart rate to increase. *Beta-blocker drugs, such as *propranolol, have negative inotropic action, reducing heart muscle contractions and causing the heart rate to decrease.

in-patient *n.* a patient who is admitted to a bed in a hospital ward and remains there for a period of time for treatment, examination, or observation. *Compare* out-patient.

inquest *n.* an official judicial enquiry into the cause of a person's death: carried out when the death is sudden or takes place under suspicious circumstances. The results of medical and legal investigations that have been carried out are considered by a *coroner, sitting with or without a jury, and made publicly known. *See also* autopsy.

insanity *n.* a degree of mental illness such that the affected individual is not responsible for his actions or is not capable of entering into a legal contract. The term is used in legal rather than medical contexts.

insect *n.* a member of a large group of mainly land-dwelling *arthropods. The body of the adult is divided into a head, thorax, and abdomen. The head bears a single pair of sensory antennae; the thorax bears three pairs of legs and, in most insects, wings (these are absent in some parasitic groups, such as lice and fleas). Some insects are of medical importance. Various bloodsucking insects transmit tropical diseases, for example the female *Anopheles* mosquito transmits malaria and the tsetse fly transmits sleeping sickness. The bites of lice can cause intense irritation and, secondarily, bacterial infection. The organisms causing diarrhoea and dysentery can be conveyed to food on the bodies of flies. *See also* myiasis.

insecticide *n.* a preparation used to kill destructive or disease-carrying insects. Ideally, an insecticide should have no toxic effects when ingested by human beings or animals, but modern powerful compounds have inherent dangers and have caused fatalities. Some insect powders contain organic phosphorus compounds and fluorides; when ingested accidentally they may cause damage to the nervous system. The use of such compounds is generally under strict control. *See also* DDT, dieldrin.

insemination *n.* introduction of semen into the vagina. *See also* artificial insemination.

insertion *n.* (in anatomy) the point of attachment of a muscle (e.g. to a bone) that is relatively movable when the muscle contracts. *Compare* origin.

insight *n.* (in psychology) knowledge of oneself. The term is applied particularly to a patient's recognition that he has psychological problems; in this sense absence of insight is a feature of psychosis. The term is also applied to the patient's accuracy of understanding the development of his personality and his problems; in this sense insight is enhanced by psychotherapy.

insolation *n.* exposure to the sun's rays. *See also* heatstroke.

insomnia *n.* inability to fall asleep or to remain asleep for an adequate length of time, so that tiredness is virtually permanent. Insomnia may be associated with disease, particularly if there are painful symptoms, but is more often caused by worry.

inspiration *n. see* inhalation.

instillation *n.* **1.** the application of liquid medication drop by drop, as into the eye. **2.** the medication, such as eye drops, applied in this way.

instinct *n.* **1.** a complex pattern of behaviour innately determined, which is characteristic of all individuals of the same species. The behaviour is released and modified by environmental stimuli, but its pattern is relatively uniform and predetermined. **2.** an innate drive that urges the individual towards a particular goal (for example, *libido in psychoanalytic psychology).

institutionalization *n.* a condition produced by residence in an unstimulating impersonal institution (such as some mental hospitals and orphanages). The individual adapts to the behaviour characteristic of the institution to such an extent that he is handicapped in other environments. The features often include apathy, dependence, and a lack of personal responsibility. Some symptoms, such as *stereotypy, are commoner in the institutionalized.

insufficiency *n.* inability of an organ or part, such as the heart or kidney, to carry out its normal function.

insufflation *n.* the act of blowing gas or a powder, such as a medication, into a body cavity.

insula *n.* an area of the *cerebral cortex that is overlapped by the sides of the deep lateral sulcus (cleft) in each hemisphere.

insulin *n.* a protein hormone, produced in the pancreas by the beta cells of the *islets of Langerhans, that is important for regulating the amount of sugar (glucose) in the blood. Insulin secretion is stimulated by a high concentration of blood sugar. Lack of this hormone gives rise to *diabetes mellitus, in which large amounts of sugar are present in the blood and urine. This condition may be treated successfully by insulin injections.

insulinase *n.* an enzyme, found in such tissues as the liver and kidney, that is responsible for the normal breakdown of insulin in the body.

insulinoma *n.* an insulin-producing tumour of the beta cells in the *islets of Langerhans of the pancreas. Symptoms include sweating, faintness, episodic loss of consciousness, and other features of *hypoglycaemia. Single tumours can be removed surgically. Multiple very small tumours scattered throughout the pancreas cannot be treated by surgery but do respond to drugs that poison the beta cells, including *diazoxide.

Intal *n. see* cromolyn sodium.

integration *n.* the blending together of the *nerve impulses that arrive through the thousands of synapses at a nerve cell body. Impulses from some synapses cause *excitation, and from others *inhibition; the overall pattern decides whether an individual nerve cell is activated to transmit a message or not.

integument *n.* **1.** the skin. **2.** a membrane or layer of tissue covering any organ of the body.

315

intelligence quotient (IQ) an index of intellectual development. In childhood and adult life it represents intellectual ability relative to the rest of the population; in children it can also represent rate of development (*mental age as a percentage of chronological age). Most *intelligence tests are constructed so that the resulting intelligence quotients in the general population have a *mean of about 100 and a *standard deviation of about 15.

intelligence test a standardized assessment procedure for the determination of intellectual ability. The score produced is usually expressed as an *intelligence quotient. Most tests present a series of different kinds of problems to be solved. The best known are the Wechsler Adult Intelligence Scale (WAIS), the Wechsler Intelligence Scale for Children (WISC), and the Stanford Binet Intelligence Scale. Scores on intelligence tests are used for such purposes as the diagnosis of *subnormality and the assessment of intellectual deterioration.

intention n. a process of healing. Healing by *first intention* is the natural healing of a wound or surgical incision when the edges are brought together under aseptic conditions and *granulation tissue forms.

intention tremor *see* tremor.

inter- *prefix denoting* between. Examples: *intercostal* (between the ribs); *intertrochanteric* (between the trochanters).

intercalated *adj.* describing structures, tissues, etc., that are inserted or situated between other structures.

intercellular *adj.* situated or occurring between cells.

intercostal muscles muscles that occupy the spaces between the ribs and are responsible for controlling some of the movements of the ribs. The superfi-

cial *external intercostals* lift the ribs during inspiration; the deep *internal intercostals* draw the ribs together during expiration.

intercurrent *adj.* going on at the same time: applied to an infection contracted by a patient who is already suffering from an infection or other disease.

interferon n. a substance that is produced by cells infected with a virus and has the ability to inhibit viral growth. Interferon is active against many different viruses, but particular interferons are effective only in the species that produces them. Attempts are being made to produce human interferon in large quantities in bacterial host cells.

interkinesis n. **1.** the resting stage between the two divisions of *meiosis. **2.** *see* interphase.

intermittent claudication *see* claudication.

intermittent fever a fever that rises, subsides, then returns again. *See* malaria.

intern n. *see* Doctor.

International Classification of Diseases a list of all known diseases and syndromes published by the World Health Organization every ten years (approximately). Diseases are grouped either according to system (e.g. cardiovascular, respiratory) or type (e.g. malignant growths, accidents); each is allocated a three-digit number for computerization and hence comparison of mortality and morbidity rates, both regionally and nationally. Agreed simplified groupings exist, and some rubrics are subdivided by the use of a fourth digit.

interneurone n. a neurone in the central nervous system that acts as a link between the different neurones in a *reflex arc. It usually possesses numerous branching processes (dendrites) that make possible extensive and complex circuits and pathways within the brain and spinal cord.

internode *n.* the length of *axon covered with a myelin sheath. Internodes are separated by nodes of Ranvier, where the sheath is absent.

interoceptor *n.* any *receptor organ composed of sensory nerve cells that respond to and monitor changes within the body, such as the stretching of muscles or the acidity of the blood.

interparietal bone (inca bone, incarial bone) the bone lying between the *parietal bones, at the back of the skull.

interpeduncular *adj.* situated between the peduncles of the cerebrum or cerebellum.

interphase (interkinesis) *n.* the period when a cell is not undergoing division (mitosis), during which activities such as DNA synthesis occur.

intersex *n.* an individual who shows anatomical characteristics of both sexes. *See* hermaphrodite, pseudohermaphroditism. —**intersexuality** *n.*

interstice *n.* a small space in a tissue or between parts of the body. —**interstitial** *adj.*

interstitial cells (Leydig cells) the cells interspersed between the seminiferous tubules of the *testis. They secrete *androgens in response to stimulation by *luteinizing hormone from the anterior pituitary gland.

interstitial-cell-stimulating hormone *see* luteinizing hormone.

intertrigo *n.* superficial inflammation (dermatitis) of two skin surfaces that are in contact, such as between the thighs or under the breasts, particularly in obese people. The dermatitis is caused by friction, warmth, moisture, and sweat and is often aggravated by infection.

intervention study a comparison of the outcome between two or more groups of patients that are deliberately subjected to different regimes (usually of treatment but sometimes of a preventive measure, such as vaccination). Wherever possible those entering the trial should be allocated to their respective groups by means of random numbers, and one such group (*controls*) should have no active treatment (*randomized controlled trial*). Ideally neither the patient nor the person assessing the outcome should be aware of which therapy is allocated to which patient (*blind trial*), nor should the doctor responsible for treatment (*double-blind trial*), and groups should exchange treatment after a prearranged period (*cross-over trial*).

intervertebral disc the flexible plate of fibrocartilage that connects any two adjacent vertebrae in the backbone. At birth the central part of the disc – the *nucleus pulposus* – consists of a gelatinous substance, which becomes replaced by cartilage with age. The intervertebral discs account for one quarter of the total length of the backbone; they act as shock absorbers, protecting the brain and spinal cord from the impact produced by running and other movements. *See also* prolapsed intervertebral disc.

intestinal flora bacteria normally present in the intestinal tract. Some are responsible for the synthesis of *vitamin K. By producing a highly acidic environment in the intestine they may also prevent infection by pathogenic bacteria that cannot tolerate such conditions.

intestinal juice *see* succus entericus.

intestine (bowel, gut) *n.* the part of the *alimentary canal that extends from the stomach to the anus. It is divided into two main parts – the small intestine and the large intestine. The *small intestine* is divided into the *duodenum, *jejunum, and *ileum. It is here that most of the processes of digestion and absorption of food take place. The surface area of the inside of the small intestine is increased by the presence of finger-like projections called *villi* (see illustration). Glands in the mucous layer of the intestine secrete digestive enzymes and mucus. The *large intestine* consists of the *caecum, vermiform *appendix, *colon, and *rectum. It is largely concerned with the absorption of water from the material passed from the small intestine. The contents of the intestines are propelled forwards by means of rhythmic muscular contractions (*see* peristalsis). —**intestinal** *adj.*

villi
lacteal
smooth muscle fibres
goblet cells
mucous membrane
crypts of Lieberkühn (intestinal glands)
Paneth cells
muscularis mucosa
blood vessel
circular muscle layer
connective tissue
longitudinal muscle layer
serosa

mucosa
submucosa
myenteron

Longitudinal section through the ileum

intima (tunica intima) *n.* **1.** the inner layer of the wall of an *artery or *vein. It is composed of a lining of endothelial cells and an elastic membrane. **2.** the inner layer of various other organs or parts.

intolerance *n.* the inability of a patient to tolerate a particular drug, manifested by various adverse reactions.

intoxication *n.* the symptoms of poisoning due to ingestion of any toxic material, including alcohol and heavy metals.

intra- *prefix denoting* inside; within. Examples: *intralobular* (within a lobule); *intrauterine* (within the womb).

intracellular *adj.* situated or occurring inside a cell or cells.

intracranial *adj.* within the skull.

intradermal *adj.* within the skin. An *intradermal injection* is made into the skin.

intramuscular *adj.* within a muscle. An *intramuscular injection* is made into a muscle.

intraocular *adj.* of or relating to the area within the eyeball.

intrathecal *adj.* within the *meninges of the spinal cord. An *intrathecal injection* is made into the meninges.

intrauterine device *see* IUD.

intravenous *adj.* into or within a vein. An *intravenous injection* is made into a vein.

intravenous pyelogram (IVP) a succession of X-ray films of the urinary tract following the injection into a vein of an iodine-containing substance (which is opaque to X-rays). This material is concentrated and excreted by the kidneys, and the IVP reveals details of the kidneys, the ureters, and subsequently the bladder. An IVP tests kidney function and reveals the presence of stones in the kidneys or ureters and other abnormalities of the urinary tract. *See also* pyelography.

intraversion *n. see* introversion.

intra vitam Latin: during life.

intrinsic factor a glycoprotein secreted in the stomach. The secretion of intrinsic factor is necessary for the absorption of *vitamin B$_{12}$; a failure of secretion of intrinsic factor leads to a deficiency of the vitamin and the condition of *pernicious anaemia.

intrinsic muscle a muscle that is contained entirely within the organ or part it acts on. For example, there are intrinsic muscles of the tongue, whose contractions change the shape of the tongue.

intro- *prefix denoting* in; into.

introitus *n.* (in anatomy) an entrance into a hollow organ or cavity.

introjection *n.* (in psychoanalysis) the process of adopting, or of believing that one possesses, the qualities of another person. This can be a form of *defence mechanism. *See also* identification.

intromission *n.* the introduction of one organ or part into another, e.g. the penis into the vagina.

introversion *n.* **1.** (*or* **intraversion**) an enduring personality trait characterized by interest in the self rather than the outside world. People high in introversion (*introverts*), as measured by questionnaires and psychological tests, tend to have a small circle of friends, like to persist in activities once they have started, and are highly susceptible to permanent *conditioning. Introversion was first described by Carl Jung as a tendency to distancing oneself from others, to philosophical interests, and to reserved defensive reactions. *Compare* extroversion. **2.** a turning inwards of a hollow organ (such as the womb) on itself.

introvert *n. see* introversion.

intubation *n.* the introduction of a tube into part of the body for the purpose of diagnosis or treatment. Thus *gastric intubation* may be performed to remove a sample of the stomach contents for analysis or to administer drugs directly into the stomach.

intumescence *n.* a swelling or an increase in the volume of an organ.

intussusception *n.* the telescoping (*invagination*) of one part of the bowel into another: most common in young children under the age of four. As the contents of the intestine are pushed onwards by muscular contraction more and more intestine is dragged into the invaginating portion, resulting in obstruction. Symptoms include intermittent pain, vomiting, and the passing of red jelly with the stools; if the condition does not receive prompt surgical treatment, shock from gangrene of the bowel may result.

inulin *n.* a carbohydrate with a high molecular weight, used in a test of kidney function called *inulin clearance*. Inulin is filtered from the bloodstream by the kidneys. By injecting it into the blood and measuring the amount that appears in the urine over a given period, it is possible to calculate how much filtrate the kidneys are producing in a given time.

inunction *n.* the rubbing in with the fingers of an ointment or liniment.

invagination *n.* **1.** the infolding of the wall of a solid structure to form a cavity. It occurs in some stages of embryonic development. **2.** *see* intussusception.

inversion *n.* **1.** the turning inwards or inside-out of a part or organ: commonly applied to the state of the womb after childbirth when its upper part is pulled through the cervical canal. **2.** a chromosome mutation in which a block of genes within a chromosome are in reverse order, due to that section of the chromosome becoming inverted. The centromere may be included in the inverted segment (*pericentric inversion*) or not (*paracentric inversion*).

invertebrate 1. *n.* an animal without a backbone. The following are invertebrate groups of medical importance: *insects, *ticks, *nematodes, *flukes, *protozoans, and *tapeworms. **2.** *adj.* not possessing a backbone.

in vitro Latin: describing biological phenomena that are made to occur outside the living body (traditionally in a test-tube).

in vitro fertilization *see* test-tube baby.

in vivo Latin: describing biological phenomena that occur or are observed occurring within the bodies of living organisms.

involucrum *n.* a growth of new bone, formed from the *periosteum, that sometimes surrounds a mass of infected and dead bone in osteomyelitis.

involuntary muscle muscle that is not under conscious control, such as the muscle of the gut, stomach, blood vessels, and heart. *See also* cardiac muscle, smooth muscle.

involution *n.* **1.** the shrinking of the womb to its normal size after childbirth. **2.** atrophy of an organ in old age.

involutional melancholia a severe *depression, usually psychotic, appearing for the first time in the involutional period of middle life (approximately 40–55 for women, 50–65 for men). Such an illness classically has characteristic features, including agitation; delusions of ill-health, poverty, sin, and sometimes of the nonexistence of the world; and preoccupations with death and loss. However, the features are not always classical, and many authorities do not regard the condition as a clinical entity separate from depressive psychosis. *See* manic-depressive psychosis.

iodine *n.* an element required in small amounts for healthy growth and development. An adult body contains about 30 mg of iodine, mostly concentrated in the thyroid gland: this gland requires iodine to synthesize *thyroid hormones. A deficiency of iodine leads to *goitre. The daily requirement of iodine in an adult is thought to be about 150 μg per day; dietary sources of iodine are sea food and vegetables grown in soil containing iodide and also iodized table salt. Radioactive isotopes of iodine (usually iodine-131), which are *radioopaque, are used in the diagnosis and treatment of diseases of the thyroid gland. Iodine is also used as an antiseptic.

iodipamide *n.* a *radio-opaque iodine-containing compound used as a *contrast medium in radiography.

iodism *n.* iodine poisoning. The main features are a characteristic staining of the mouth and odour on the breath. Vomited material may be yellowish or bluish. There is pain and burning in the throat, intense thirst, and diarrhoea, with dizziness, weakness, and convulsions. Emergency treatment includes administration of starch or flour in water and lavage with sodium thiosulphate solution.

iontophoresis *n.* the technique of introducing through the skin, by means of an electric current, charged particles of a drug, so that it reaches a deep site. The method has been used to transfer salicylate ions through the skin in the treatment of deep rheumatic pain. *See also* cataphoresis.

iopanoic acid *n.* a *radio-opaque iodine-containing compound used in radiography to outline the gall bladder (*see* cholecystography). Given by intravenous injection, the iopanoic acid is concentrated in the bile by the liver and thus shows up the gall bladder clearly during X-ray examination.

iophendylate *n.* a *radio-opaque iodine-containing compound that is sometimes used in radiography to show up the spinal canal (*see* myelography).

It is injected through a *lumbar puncture needle.

ipecacuanha *n.* a plant extract used in small doses, usually in the form of tinctures and syrups, as an *expectorant to relieve coughing and to induce vomiting. Ipecacuanha irritates the digestive system, and high doses may cause severe digestive upsets.

iprindole *n.* a drug administered by mouth for the treatment of depression (*see* antidepressant). Response may take place gradually, and side-effects, such as dry mouth, blurred vision, constipation, and sweating, may occur. Trade name: **Prondol**.

iproniazid *n.* a drug administered by mouth to treat all types of depression (*see* antidepressant). Side-effects may include constipation, dizziness, difficulty in urination, insomnia, headaches, and impotence. Trade name: **Marsilid**.

ipsilateral (**ipselateral, homolateral**) *adj.* on or affecting the same side of the body: applied particularly to paralysis (or other symptoms) occurring on the same side of the body as the brain lesion that caused them. *Compare* contralateral.

IQ *see* intelligence quotient.

irid- (irido-) *prefix denoting* the iris.

iridectomy *n.* an operation on the eye in which a part of the iris is removed.

iridencleisis *n.* an operation for *glaucoma in which a small incision is made into the eye, beneath the *conjunctiva and close to the cornea, and part of the iris is drawn into it. The iris acts like a wick and keeps the incision open for the drainage of fluid from the front chamber of the eye to the tissue beneath the conjunctiva.

iridocyclitis *n.* inflammation of the iris and ciliary body of the eye. *See* uveitis.

iridodialysis *n.* a tear, caused by injury to the eye, in the attachment of the iris to the ciliary body. Usually a black crescentic gap is seen at the edge of the iris where the tear has occurred, and the pupil is displaced away from the site of the tear.

iridodonesis *n.* tremulousness of the iris when the eye is moved. It is due to absence of support from the lens, against which the iris normally lies, and occurs when the lens is absent or dislocated from its normal position.

iridoplegia *n.* paralysis of the iris, which is usually associated with *cycloplegia and results from injury, inflammation, or the use of drugs in the eye. In the case of injury, the pupil is usually larger than normal and moves little, if at all, in response to light and drugs.

iridotomy *n.* an operation on the eye in which an incision is made in the iris.

iris *n.* the part of the eye that regulates the amount of light that enters. It forms a coloured muscular diaphragm across the front of the lens; light enters through a central opening, the *pupil*. A ring of muscle round the margin contracts in bright light, causing the pupil to become smaller (*see* pupillary reflex). In dim light a set of radiating muscles contract and the constricting muscles relax, increasing the size of the pupil. The outer margin of the iris is attached to the *ciliary body.

iris bombé an abnormal condition of the eye in which the iris bulges forward towards the cornea. It is due to pressure from the aqueous humour behind the iris when its passage through the pupil to the anterior chamber of the eye is obstructed.

iritis *n.* inflammation of the iris. *See* uveitis.

iron *n.* an element essential to life. The body of an adult contains on average 4 g of iron, over half of which is contained in *haemoglobin in the red blood cells, the rest being distributed between myoglobin in muscles, *cytochromes, and iron stores in the form of *ferritin and *haemosiderin. Iron is an essential component in the transfer of oxygen in the body. The absorption and loss of iron is very finely controlled. A good dietary source is meat, particularly liver. The recommended daily intake of iron is 10 mg per day for men and 12 mg per day for women during their reproductive life. A deficiency of iron may lead to *anaemia.

Many preparations of iron are used to treat iron-deficiency anaemia. These include preparations taken by mouth, such as *ferrous sulphate, and those administered by injection, such as *iron dextran.

iron dextran a drug containing *iron and *dextran, administered by intramuscular or intravenous injection to treat iron-deficiency anaemia. Side-effects can include pain at the site of injection, rapid beating of the heart, and allergic reactions. Trade name: **Imferon**.

iron lung *see* respirator.

iron-storage disease *see* haemochromatosis.

irradiation *n.* the therapeutic application of electromagnetic radiation (usually alpha, beta, gamma, or X-rays) to a particular structure. *See* radiotherapy.

irreducible *adj.* unable to be replaced in a normal position: applied particularly to a type of *hernia.

irrigation *n.* the process of washing out a wound or hollow organ with a continuous flow of water or medicated solution.

irritability *n.* (in physiology) the property of certain kinds of tissue that enables them to respond in a specific way to outside stimuli. Irritability is shown by nerve cells, which can gener-

ate and transmit electrical impulses when stimulated appropriately, and by muscle cells, which contract when stimulated by nerve impulses.

irritable bowel syndrome (spastic colon, mucous colitis) a common condition in which recurrent abdominal pain with constipation and/or diarrhoea continues for years without any general deterioration in health. There is no detectable structural disease; the symptoms are caused by abnormal muscular contractions in the colon. The cause is unknown, but the condition is often associated with stress or anxiety and may follow severe infection of the intestine.

irritant *n.* any material that causes irritation of a tissue, ranging from nettles (causing pain and swelling) to tear gas (causing watering of the eyes). Chronic irritation by various chemicals can give rise to *dermatitis.

isch- (ischo-) *prefix denoting* suppression or deficiency.

ischaemia *n.* an inadequate flow of blood to a part of the body, caused by constriction or blockage of the blood vessels supplying it. Ischaemia of heart muscle produces *angina pectoris.

ischi- (ischio-) *prefix denoting* the ischium.

ischiorectal abscess an abscess in the space between the sheet of muscle that assists in control of the rectum (levator ani) and the pelvic bone. It may occur spontaneously, but is often secondary to an anal fissure, thrombosed *haemorrhoids, or other disease of the anus. Symptoms are severe throbbing pain near the anus with swelling and fever. Pus is drained from the abscess by surgical incision.

ischium *n.* a bone forming the lower part of each side of the *hip bone (*see also* pelvis). —**ischiac, ischial** *adj.*

ischuria *n.* retention or suppression of the urine. *See* anuria, retention.

island *n.* (in anatomy) an area of tissue or group of cells clearly differentiated from surrounding tissues.

islet *n.* (in anatomy) a small group of cells that is structurally distinct from the cells surrounding it.

islets of Langerhans small groups of cells, scattered through the material of the *pancreas, that secrete the hormones *insulin and *glucagon. There are three main histological types of cells: alpha (α), beta (β), and D-cells (α_1). The alpha and beta cells produce glucagon and insulin, respectively.

iso- *prefix denoting* equality, uniformity, or similarity.

isoagglutinin (isohaemagglutinin) *n.* one of the antibodies occurring naturally in the plasma that cause *agglutination of red blood cells of a different group.

isoagglutinogen *n.* one of the *antigens naturally occurring on the surface of red blood cells that is attacked by an isoagglutinin in blood plasma of a different group, so causing *agglutination.

isoaminile *n.* a drug administered in capsules and linctuses to suppress coughs (*see* antitussive). Rarely, it may cause dizziness, nausea, constipation, and diarrhoea. Trade name: **Dimyril**.

isoantibody *n.* an *antibody that occurs naturally against the components of foreign tissues from an individual of the same species.

isoantigen *n.* an antigen that forms a natural component of an individual's tissues. Thus the antigens of the *HL-A system are isoantigens, as are the agglutinogens of the different *blood groups.

isodactylism *n.* a congenital defect in which all the fingers are the same length.

isoenzyme (isozyme) *n.* a physically distinct form of a given enzyme. Isoenzymes catalyse the same type of reaction but have slight physical and immunological differences. Isoenzymes of dehydrogenases, oxidases, transaminases, phosphatases, and proteolytic enzymes are known to exist.

isograft (isogenic graft, syngraft) *n.* a *graft of tissue from one identical twin to another or between animals that are genetically identical.

isohaemagglutinin *n.* *see* isoagglutinin.

isoimmunization *n.* the development of antibodies (*isoantibodies*) within an individual against antigens from another individual of the same species.

isolation *n.* **1.** the separation of a person with an infectious disease from noninfected people. *See also* quarantine. **2.** (in surgery) the separation of a structure from surrounding structures by the use of instruments.

isoleucine *n.* an *essential amino acid. *See also* amino acid.

isomerase *n.* any one of a group of enzymes that catalyse the conversion of one isomer of a compound into another.

isometric exercises (isometrics) a system of exercises based on the principle of *isometric contraction* of muscles. This occurs when the fibres are called upon to contract and do work, but despite an increase in tension do not shorten in length. It can be induced in muscles that are used when a limb is made to pull or push against something that does not move. The exercises increase fitness and build muscle.

isometropia *n.* an equal power of *refraction in both eyes.

isomorphism *n.* the condition of two or more objects being alike in shape or structure. It can exist at any structural level, from molecules to whole organisms. —**isomorphic, isomorphous** *adj.*

isoniazid (isonicotinic acid hydrazide, INH) *n.* a drug used in the treatment of tuberculosis, usually taken by mouth. Because tuberculosis bacteria soon become resistant to isoniazid, it is usually given in conjunction with streptomycin or PAS. Occasional side-effects include digestive disturbances and dry mouth; high doses or prolonged treatment may cause inflammation of the nerves, which can be countered by including pyridoxine (vitamin B₆) in the preparation.

isoprenaline *n.* a *sympathomimetic drug used to dilate the air passages in asthma and other bronchial conditions. It also stimulates the heart and is used to treat some heart conditions involving reduced heart activity. It is administered by inhalation, by mouth, by injection, or in suppositories. Side-effects such as increased heart rate, palpitations, chest pain, dizziness, and fainting may occur. Trade names: **Aleudrin, Lomupren, Medihaler-Iso, Prenomiser**.

isopropamide *n.* a *parasympatholytic drug that prevents muscle spasm in the digestive system and helps to reduce acid secretion in the stomach. It is administered by mouth for the treatment of stomach and duodenal ulcers. Side-effects can include dry mouth, disturbed vision, increased heart rate, difficulty in urination, and constipation.

isosthenuria *n.* inability of the kidneys to produce either a concentrated or a dilute urine. This occurs in the final stages of renal failure.

isotonic *adj.* **1.** describing solutions that have the same osmotic pressure. *See* osmosis. **2.** describing muscles that have equal *tonicity.

isotope *n.* any one of the different forms of an element, possessing the same number of protons (positively charged particles) in the nucleus, and thus the same atomic number, but different numbers of neutrons. Isotopes therefore have different atomic weights. Radioactive isotopes decay into other isotopes or elements, emitting alpha, beta, or gamma radiation. Some radioactive isotopes may be produced artificially by bombarding elements with neutrons. These are known as *nuclides* and are used extensively in *radiotherapy for the treatment of cancer.

isoxuprine *n.* a drug that dilates blood vessels and is used to improve blood flow in such conditions as cerebrovascular disease and arteriosclerosis and to inhibit contractions in premature labour. It is administered by mouth or injection and rarely it may cause flushing, increased heart rate, dizziness, and nausea. Trade names: **Duvalidan, Defencin**.

isozyme *n. see* isoenzyme.

isthmus *n.* a constricted or narrowed part of an organ or tissue, such as the band of thyroid tissue connecting the two lobes of the thyroid gland.

itch *n.* **1.** local discomfort or irritation of the skin, prompting the sufferer to scratch or rub the affected area. *See* pruritus. **2.** a rarely used common name for *scabies.

itch mite *see* Sarcoptes.

-itis *suffix denoting* inflammation of an organ, tissue, etc. Examples: *arthritis* (of a joint); *peritonitis* (of the peritoneum).

IUD (intrauterine device) a plastic or metal coil, spiral, or other shape, about 25 mm long, that is inserted into the cavity of the womb to prevent conception. Its exact mode of action is unknown but it is thought to interfere with implantation of the embryo. Early IUDs (such as the *Lippes loop*) were made of plastic; later variants (such as the *Gravigard*) are covered with copper, which slowly dissolves and augments the contraceptive action. Devices such as the *Progestasert* release small amounts of a contraceptive hormone drug. About one-third of women fitted with an IUD find the side-effects (heavy menstrual bleeding or back pain) unacceptable, but most have no complaints. The unwanted pregnancy rate is about 2 per 100 woman-years. If pregnancy should occur there is normally no need to remove the device (it may, however, become detached spontaneously).

IVP *see* intravenous pyelogram.

Ixodes *n.* a genus of widely distributed parasitic ticks. Several species are responsible for transmitting the diseases *tularaemia, Queensland tick typhus, and *Russian spring-summer encephalitis. The bite of a few species can give rise to a serious paralysis, caused by a toxin in the tick's saliva.

ixodiasis *n.* any disease caused by the presence of *ticks.

Ixodidae *n.* a family of *ticks.

J

Jacksonian epilepsy *see* epilepsy.

Jacquemier's sign (Spiegelberg's sign) a bluish or purplish coloration of the membrane lining the vagina: a possible indication of pregnancy.

jactitation *n.* restless tossing and turning of a person suffering from a severe disease, frequently one with a high fever.

jamais vu one of the manifestations of temporal lobe *epilepsy, in which there is a sudden feeling of unfamiliarity with everyday surroundings.

jaundice *n.* a yellowing of the skin or whites of the eyes, indicating excess bilirubin (a bile pigment) in the blood. Jaundice is classified into three types. *Obstructive jaundice* occurs when bile made in the liver fails to reach the intestine due to obstruction of the *bile ducts (e.g. by gallstones) or to *cholestasis. The urine is dark, the faeces pale, and the patient may itch. *Hepatocellular jaundice* is due to disease of the liver cells, such as *hepatitis, when the liver is unable to utilize the bilirubin, which accumulates in the blood. The urine may be dark but the faeces retain their colour. *Haemolytic jaundice* occurs when there is excessive destruction of red cells in the blood (*see* haemolysis). Urine and faeces retain their normal colour. Medical name: **icterus**.

jaw *n.* either the *maxilla (upper jaw) or the *mandible (lower jaw). The jaws form the framework of the mouth and provide attachment for the teeth.

jejun- (jejuno-) *prefix denoting* the jejunum.

jejunal biopsy removal of a piece of the lining (mucosa) of the upper small intestine. This can be done by a surgical operation but is usually performed by a special metal capsule, swallowed by the patient. When the capsule is in the *jejunum a small knife within it is triggered by suction on an attached tube, cutting off a small piece of mucosa. The specimen may be examined microscopically to assist in the diagnosis of *coeliac disease or intestinal infections, or its enzyme content may be measured chemically to detect, for example, *lactase deficiency.

jejunal ulcer *see* peptic ulcer, Zollinger-Ellison syndrome.

jejunectomy *n.* surgical removal of the jejunum or part of the jejunum.

jejunoileostomy *n.* an operation in which the jejunum is joined to the ileum (small intestine), when either the end of the jejunum or the beginning of the ileum has been removed or is to be bypassed. It is usually performed for intestinal disease (e.g. Crohn's disease) but sometimes for the treatment of obesity.

jejunostomy *n.* a surgical operation in which the jejunum is brought through the abdominal wall and opened.

jejunotomy *n.* a surgical incision into the jejunum in order to inspect the interior or remove something from within it.

jejunum *n.* part of the small *intestine. It comprises about two-fifths of the whole small intestine and connects the duodenum to the ileum. —**jejunal** *adj.*

jerk *n.* the sudden contraction of a muscle in response to a nerve impulse. The *knee jerk* (*see* patellar reflex) is the reflex kicking movement produced by contraction of the quadriceps muscle of the thigh after it has been stretched by tapping the tendon below the knee. Eliciting this and other jerks, such as the ankle and elbow jerks, is a means of testing the nerve pathways, via the spinal cord, which are involved in *reflexes.

jigger *n. see* Tunga.

joint *n.* the point at which two or more bones are connected. The opposing surfaces of bone are lined with cartilaginous, fibrous, or soft (synovial) tissue. The three main classes of joint are *diarthrosis (freely movable), *amphiarthrosis (slightly movable), and *synarthrosis (immovable).

joule *n.* the *SI unit of work or energy, equal to the work done when the point of application of a force of 1 newton is displaced through a distance of 1 metre in the direction of the force. In electrical terms the joule is the work done per second when a current of 1 ampere flows through a resistance of 1 ohm. Symbol: J. *See also* calorie.

jugular *adj.* relating to or supplying the neck or throat.

jugular vein any one of several veins in the neck. The *internal jugular* is a very large paired vein running vertically down the side of the neck and draining blood from the brain, face, and neck. It ends behind the sternoclavicular joint, where it joins the subclavian vein. The *external jugular* is a smaller paired vein running superficially down the neck to the subclavian vein and draining blood from the face, scalp, and neck. Its tributary, the *anterior jugular*, runs down the front of the neck.

jugum *n.* (in anatomy) a ridge or furrow that connects two parts of a bone.

junction *n.* (in anatomy) the point at which two different tissues or structures are in contact. *See also* neuromuscular junction.

juxta- *prefix denoting* proximity to. Example: *juxta-articular* (near a joint).

K

Kahn reaction a test for syphilis, in which antibodies specific to the disease are detected in a sample of the patient's blood by means of a *precipitin reaction. The test is not as reliable as the *Wassermann reaction, but is useful as confirmation.

kala-azar (visceral leishmaniasis, Dumdum fever) *n.* a tropical disease caused by the parasitic protozoan *Leishmania donovani*. The parasite, transmitted to man by *sandflies, invades the cells of the lymphatic system, spleen, and bone marrow. Symptoms include enlargement and subsequent lesions of the liver and spleen; anaemia; a low *leucocyte count; weight loss; and irregular fevers. The disease occurs in Asia, South America, the Mediterranean area, and Africa.

Drugs containing antimony are used in the treatment of this potentially fatal disease.

kallidin *n.* a naturally occurring polypeptide consisting of ten amino acids. Kallidin is a powerful vasodilator and causes contraction of smooth muscle; it is formed in the blood under certain conditions. *See* kinin.

kallikrein *n.* one of a group of enzymes found in the blood and body fluids that act on certain plasma globulins to produce bradykinin and kallidin. *See* kinin.

kanamycin *n.* an *antibiotic used to treat a wide range of bacterial infections. It is administered mainly by injection but is given by mouth for infections of the intestine and by inhalation for respiratory infections. Mild side-effects sometimes occur, including skin rashes, fever, headache, nausea, vomiting, and tingling sensations. Trade name: **Kantrex**.

kaolin *n.* a white clay that contains aluminium and silicon and is purified and powdered for use as an adsorbent. It is taken by mouth to treat the diarrhoea and vomiting due to food poisoning and other digestive disorders. Kaolin is also used in dusting powders and poultices.

Kaposi's sarcoma a malignant tumour usually arising in the skin. It is common in Africa but rare in the western world, except in patients with *AIDS. The tumour evolves slowly; radiotherapy is the treatment of choice but chemotherapy may be of value in metastatic disease.

kary- (karyo-) *prefix denoting* a cell nucleus.

karyokinesis *n.* division of the nucleus of a cell, which occurs during cell division before division of the cytoplasm (*cytokinesis*). *See* mitosis.

karyolysis *n.* the breakdown of the cell nucleus in mitosis.

karyoplasm *n. see* nucleoplasm.

karyosome *n.* the dense mass of *chromatin found in the cell nucleus, which is composed mainly of chromosomes.

karyotype *n.* **1.** the *chromosome set of an individual or species described in terms of both the number and structure of the chromosomes. **2.** the representation of the chromosome set in a diagram.

katathermometer *n.* a thermometer used to measure the cooling power of the air surrounding it, having its bulb covered with water-moistened material. The instrument is brought to a steady temperature of 100°F and then exposed to the air. The time taken for the temperature recorded by the thermometer to fall to 95°F gives an index of the air's cooling power.

Kayser-Fleischer ring a brownish-yellow ring in the outer rim of the cornea of the eye. It is a deposit of copper granules and is diagnostic of *Wilson's disease. When well developed it can be seen by unaided observation, but faint Kayser-Fleischer rings may only be detected by specialized ophthalmological examination.

keloid (cheloid) *n.* hard prominent irregular scar tissue in the skin that often increases in size. It often forms where healing injuries, burns, or surgical incisions are under tension; for example, on the back or neck.

kelvin *n.* the *SI unit of temperature, formally defined as the fraction 1/273.16 of the temperature of the triple point of water. A temperature in kelvins is equal to a Celsius temperature plus 273.15°C. Symbol: K.

kerat- (kerato-) *prefix denoting* **1.** the cornea. Example: *keratopathy* (disease of). **2.** horny tissue, especially of the skin.

keratalgia *n*. pain arising from the cornea.

keratectasia *n*. bulging of the cornea at the site of scar tissue (which is thinner than normal corneal tissue).

keratectomy *n*. an operation in which a part of the cornea is removed, usually a superficial layer.

keratin *n*. a fibrous protein that forms the body's horny tissues, such as fingernails. It is also found in the skin and hair.

keratinization (cornification) *n*. the process by which cells become horny due to the deposition of *keratin within them. It occurs in the *epidermis of the skin and associated structures (hair, nails, etc.), where the cells become flattened, lose their nuclei, and are filled with keratin as they approach the surface.

keratitis *n*. inflammation of the *cornea of the eye. The eye waters and is very painful and vision is blurred. It may be due to physical or chemical agents (abrasions, exposure to dust, vapours, ultraviolet light, etc.) or result from infection. Keratitis not due to infection usually responds to keeping the eyes covered until the corneal surface has healed; infections often require specific drug treatment, e.g. with antibiotics.

keratoacanthoma (molluscum sebaceum) *n*. a firm nodule, appearing singly on the skin and growing to around 2 cm across in about six weeks, gradually disappearing during the next few months. Men are affected more often than women, commonly between the ages of 50 and 70. Keratoacanthomas occur on the nose, face, hands and fingers and sometimes on the scalp or neck. The cause is not known. Although the nodules disapppear spontaneously they may leave an unsightly scar, therefore treatment by curettage, cautery, or excision and suture is often carried out.

keratocele (descemetocele) *n*. outward bulging of the base of a deep ulcer of the cornea. The deep layer of the cornea (Descemet's membrane) is elastic and very resistant to ulceration; it therefore bulges when the overlying cornea has been destroyed.

keratoconjunctivitis *n*. combined inflammation of the cornea and conjunctiva of the eye.

keratoconus *n*. conical cornea: an abnormal condition of the eye in which the cornea, instead of having a regular curvature, comes to a rounded apex towards its centre. The 'cone' tends to become sharper with age. It is usually due to a congenital weakness of the centre of the cornea, but may not produce symptoms until later childhood.

keratoglobus (megalocornea) *n*. a congenital disorder of the eye in which the whole cornea bulges forward in a regular curve. *Compare* keratoconus.

keratoma *n*. *see* keratosis.

keratomalacia *n*. a progressive disease of the eye due to vitamin A deficiency. The cornea softens and may become perforated. This condition is very serious and blindness is usually inevitable. *See also* xerophthalmia.

keratome *n*. any instrument designed for cutting the cornea. The simplest type has a flat triangular blade attached at its base to a handle, the other two sides being very sharp and tapering to a point. Power-driven keratomes have oscillating or rotating blades.

keratometer (ophthalmometer) *n*. an instrument for measuring the radius of curvature of the cornea. It is used for assessing the degree of abnormal curvature of the cornea in *astigmatism. Usually the vertical and horizontal curvatures are measured. All keratometers work on the principle that the size of the image of an object reflected from a convex mirror (in this case, the cornea) depends on the curvature of the mirror. The steeper the curve, the smaller the image. —**keratometry** n.

keratoplasty (corneal graft) n. an eye operation in which any diseased parts of the cornea are replaced by clear corneal tissue from a donor. All layers of the cornea may be replaced (*penetrating keratoplasty*) or only some of its layers, the deeper layer remaining (*lamellar keratoplasty*). In the latter case the thickness of the replacement cornea is correspondingly reduced.

keratoscope (Placido's disc) n. an instrument for detecting abnormal curvature of the cornea. It consists of a black disc, about 20 cm in diameter, marked with concentric white rings. The examiner looks through a small lens in the centre at the reflection of the rings in the patient's cornea. A normal cornea will reflect regular concentric images of the rings; a cornea that is abnormally curved (for example in *keratoconus) or scarred reflects distorted rings.

keratosis (keratoma) n. any horny growth of the skin. There are two common types. *Actinic keratosis* is a well-defined red or skin-coloured warty growth, usually occurring in middle or old age, caused by overexposure to the sun. *Seborrhoeic keratosis* (or *warts*) are yellow or brown oval spots with clearly marked perimeters and raised surfaces, developing in middle age.

keratotomy n. an incision into the cornea.

kerion n. a soft inflammatory swelling covered with pustules, caused by a ringworm fungus infection.

kernicterus n. staining and subsequent damage of the brain by bile pigment (bilirubin), which may occur in severe cases of *haemolytic disease of the newborn. Immature brain cells in the *basal ganglia are affected, and as brain development proceeds a pattern of *cerebral palsy emerges at about six months, with uncoordinated movements, deafness, disturbed vision, and feeding and speech difficulties.

Kernig's sign a symptom of *meningitis in which the hamstring muscles in the legs are so stiff that the patient is unable to extend his legs at the knee when the thighs are held at a right angle to the body.

ketogenesis n. the production of *ketone bodies. These are normal products of lipid metabolism and can be used to provide energy. The condition of *ketosis can occur when excess ketone bodies are produced.

ketogenic diet a diet that promotes the formation of *ketone bodies in the tissues. A ketogenic diet is one in which the principal energy source is fat rather than carbohydrate.

ketonaemia n. the presence in the blood of *ketone bodies.

ketone n. any member of a group of organic compounds consisting of a carbonyl group ($=CO$) flanked by two alkyl groups. The ketones acetoacetic acid, acetone, and β-hydroxybutyrate (known as *ketone* (or *acetone*) *bodies*) are produced during the metabolism of fats. *See also* ketosis.

ketonuria (acetonuria) n. the presence in the urine of *ketone (acetone) bodies. This may occur in diabetes mellitus, starvation, or after persistent vomiting and results from the partial oxidation of fats. Ketone bodies may be detected by adding a few drops of 5% sodium nitroprusside solution and a solution of ammonia to the urine; the gradual development of a purplish-red colour indicates their presence.

ketoprofen n. an *analgesic that reduces inflammation, administered by mouth to treat various arthritic and rheumatic diseases. Side-effects are rare, but indigestion sometimes occurs. Trade name: **Orudis**.

ketose *n.* a simple sugar that terminates with a keto group (–C=O); for example, *fructose.

ketosis *n.* raised levels of *ketone bodies in the body tissues. Ketone bodies are normal products of fat metabolism and can be oxidized to produce energy. Elevated levels arise when there is an imbalance in fat metabolism, such as occurs in diabetes mellitus or starvation. Ketosis may result in severe *acidosis. *See also* ketonuria.

kidney *n.* either of the pair of organs responsible for the excretion of nitrogenous wastes, principally urea, from the blood (see illustration). The kidneys are situated at the back of the abdomen, below the diaphragm, one on each side of the spine; they are supplied with blood by the renal arteries. Each kidney is enclosed in a fibrous capsule and is composed of an outer *cortex* and an inner *medulla*. The active units of the kidney are the *nephrons, within the cortex and medulla, which filter the blood under pressure and then reabsorb water and selected substances back into the blood. The *urine thus formed is conducted from the nephrons via the renal tubules into the *renal pelvis* and

from here to the ureter, which leads to the bladder.

kilo- *prefix denoting* a thousand.

kilocalorie *n.* one thousand calories. *See* calorie.

kilogram *n.* the *SI unit of mass equal to 1000 grams and defined in terms of the international prototype (a cylinder of platinum-iridium alloy) kept at Sèvres, near Paris. Symbol: kg.

kin- (kine-) *prefix denoting* movement.

kinaesthesia *n.* the sense that enables the brain to be constantly aware of the position and movement of muscles in different parts of the body. This is achieved by means of *proprioceptors, which send impulses from muscles, joints, and tendons. Without this sense, coordinated movement would be impossible with the eyes closed.

kinaesthesiometer *n.* an instrument for measuring a patient's awareness of the muscular and joint movements of his own body: used during the investigation of nervous and muscular disorders and certain forms of brain damage.

kinanaesthesia *n.* inability to sense the positions and movements of parts of the body, with consequent disordered physical activity.

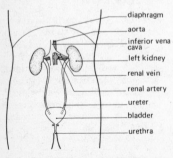

diaphragm
aorta
inferior vena cava
left kidney
renal vein
renal artery
ureter
bladder
urethra

Position of the kidneys

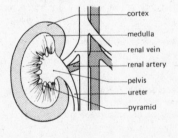

cortex
medulla
renal vein
renal artery
pelvis
ureter
pyramid

Section through a kidney

kinase *n.* **1.** an agent that can convert the inactive form of an enzyme (*see* proenzyme) to the active form. **2.** an enzyme that catalyses the transfer of phosphate groups. An example is *phosphofructokinase.

kinematics *n.* the study of motion and the forces required to produce it. This includes the different forces at work during the movement of a single part of the body, and more complex movements such as running and climbing.

kineplasty *n.* a method of amputation in which the muscles and tendons of the affected limb are arranged so that they can be integrated with a specially made artificial replacement. This enables direct movement of the artificial hand or limb by the muscles.

-kinesis *suffix denoting* movement.

kinetochore *n. see* centromere.

kinin *n.* one of a group of naturally occurring *polypeptides that are powerful *vasodilators, which lower blood pressure, and cause contraction of smooth muscle. The kinins *bradykinin* and *kallidin* are formed in the blood by the action of proteolytic enzymes (*kallikreins*) on certain plasma globulins (*kininogens*). Kinins are not normally present in the blood, but are formed under certain conditions; for example when tissue is damaged or when there are changes in the pH and temperature of the blood. They are thought to play a role in inflammatory response.

kiss of life emergency *artificial respiration, performed mouth-to-mouth, by blowing air into the victim's lungs to inflate them and then allowing exhalation to occur automatically. The operator should aim to produce roughly 20 cycles of respiration per minute, or more for a younger victim.

Klebsiella *n.* a genus of Gram-negative rodlike nonmotile mostly lactose-fermenting bacteria found in the respiratory, intestinal, and urinogenital tracts of animals and man. The species *K. aerogenes* is associated with human urinary infections; *K. pneumoniae* is associated with pneumonia and other respiratory infections. The species *K. rhinoscleromatis* causes *rhinoscleroma, a chronic infection of the nose and pharynx.

Klebs-Loeffler bacillus *see* Corynebacterium.

klepto- *prefix denoting* stealing.

kleptomania *n.* a pathologically strong impulse to steal, often in the absence of any desire for the stolen object(s). It is sometimes associated with *depression.

Klinefelter's syndrome a genetic disorder in which there are three sex chromosomes, XXY, rather than the normal XX or XY. Affected individuals are apparently male, but are tall and thin, with small testes, failure of normal sperm production (azoospermia), enlargement of the breasts (gynaecomastia), and absence of facial and body hair.

Klumpke's paralysis a partial paralysis of the arm caused by injury to a baby's *brachial plexus during birth. This may result from an obstetric manoeuvre in which the arm is raised at the shoulder to an extreme degree, which damages the lower cervical (neck) and upper thoracic (chest) nerve roots of the spinal cord. It results in weakness and wasting of the muscles of the hand.

kneading *n. see* petrissage.

knight's-move thought a form of thought disorder, characteristic of *schizophrenia, in which the *associations of ideas are bizarre and tortuous.

knock-knee *n.* abnormal in-curving of the legs, resulting in a gap between the feet when the knees are in contact. In severe cases there is stress on the knee, ankle, and foot joints, resulting eventually in degenerative arthritis. The condition may be corrected by *osteotomy. Medical name: **genu valgum**.

Koch's bacillus *see* Mycobacterium.

Köhler's disease inflammation of the *navicular bone of the foot (*see* osteochondritis). It occurs in children, causing pain and limping, and is treated by strapping the foot.

koilonychia *n.* the development of thin (brittle) concave (spoon-shaped) nails, a common disorder that can occur with anaemia due to iron deficiency, though the cause is not known. Treatment is by treating any underlying disease.

Koplik's spots small red spots with bluish-white centres that often appear on the mucous membranes of the mouth in *measles.

koro *n.* a state of acute anxiety, seen only in certain cultures (such as that of the Chinese of SE Asia), characterized by a sudden belief that the penis is shrinking into the abdomen and will disappear. Occasionally women have a similar belief that their breasts are disappearing into their body. It is usually treated with tranquillizing drugs and reassurance.

Korsakoff's syndrome (Korsakoff's psychosis) an organic disorder affecting the brain that results in a memory defect in which new information fails to be learnt although events from the past are still recalled; *disorientation for time and place; and a tendency to invent material to fill memory blanks (*see* confabulation). The commonest cause of the condition is alcoholism, especially when this has led to deficiency of thiamin (vitamin B_1). Large doses of thiamin are given as treatment. The condition often becomes chronic.

kraurosis *n.* shrinking of a body part, usually the vulva in elderly women (*kraurosis vulvae*).

Krebs cycle (citric acid cycle) a complex cycle of enzyme-catalysed reactions, occurring within the cells of all living animals, in which acetate, in the presence of oxygen, is broken down to produce energy in the form of *ATP (via the *electron transport chain) and carbon dioxide. The cycle is the final step in the oxidation of carbohydrates, fats, and proteins; some of the intermediary products of the cycle are used in the synthesis of amino acids.

Krukenberg tumour a rapidly developing malignant growth in one or (more often) both ovaries: a type of *fibrosarcoma. The tumour usually arises following the development of a similar growth in the stomach or intestine.

krypton-81m *n.* a radioactive gas that is the shortest-lived isotope in medical use (half-life 13 seconds). It can be used to investigate the function of the lungs. The patient breathes a small quantity of the gas, the arrival of which in different parts of the lungs is recorded by means of a *gamma camera. *See also* rubidium-81.

Kupffer's cells phagocytic cells that line the sinusoids of the *liver (*see* macrophage). They are particularly concerned with the formation of *bile and are often seen to contain fragments of red blood cells and pigment granules derived from the breakdown of haemoglobin.

kuru (trembling disease) *n.* a disease that affects only members of the Fore tribe of New Guinea. It involves a progressive degeneration of the nerve cells of the central nervous system, particularly in the region of the brain that controls movement. Muscular control becomes defective and shiver-like tremors occur in the trunk, limbs, and head. Kuru affects mainly women and children and usually proves fatal within 9–12 months. It is thought to be caused by a virus and transmitted by cannibalism.

kwashiorkor *n.* a form of malnutrition due to a diet deficient in protein and energy-producing foods, common among certain African tribes. Kwashiorkor develops when, after prolonged breast feeding, the child is weaned onto an inadequate traditional family diet. The diet is such that it is physically impossible for the child to consume the required quantity in order to obtain sufficient protein and energy. Kwashiorkor is most common in children between the ages of one and three years. The symptoms are *oedema, loss of appetite, diarrhoea, general discomfort, and apathy; the child fails to thrive and there is usually associated gastrointestinal infection.

Kyasanur Forest disease a tropical disease, common in southern India, caused by a virus transmitted to man through the bite of the forest-dwelling tick *Haemaphysalis spinigera*. Symptoms include fever, headache, muscular pains, vomiting, conjunctivitis, exhaustion, bleeding of nose and gums and, subsequently, internal bleeding and the *necrosis of various tissues. General therapy, in the absence of specific treatment, involves relief of dehydration and loss of blood; analgesics are given to alleviate pain.

kymograph *n.* an instrument for recording the flow and varying pressure of the blood within blood vessels. —**kymography** *n.*

kypho- *prefix denoting* a hump.

kyphos *n.* a sharply localized forward angulation of the spine, resulting in the appearance of a lump (the deformity of the traditional hunchback). The deformity is due to collapse of the anterior part of a vertebra, usually caused by osteoporosis, a secondary malignant deposit, or tuberculosis.

kyphoscoliosis *n.* abnormal curvature of the spine both forwards and sideways: *kyphosis combined with *scoliosis. The deformity may occur during growth for no apparent reason (*idiopathic kyphoscoliosis*) or may result from any of several diseases involving the vertebrae and spinal muscles. Special braces can reduce the extent of the deformity; *osteotomy of the backbone may be required to correct severe deformity.

kyphosis *n.* excessive outward curvature of the spine, causing hunching of the back. A *mobile kyphosis* may be caused by bad posture or muscle weakness or may develop to compensate for another condition, such as hip deformity. A *fixed kyphosis* may result from collapse of the vertebrae (as in senile *osteoporosis), from *osteochondritis in the young, or from ankylosing *spondylitis. Lesser degrees of fixed kyphosis may be balanced by *lordosis (inward curvature) in another part of the spine. Treatment depends on the cause, and may include physiotherapy, bracing, and spinal *osteotomy in severe cases. *See also* kyphos, kyphoscoliosis.

L

labial *adj.* **1.** relating to the lips or to a labium. **2.** designating the surface of a tooth adjacent to the lips.

labio- *prefix denoting* the lip(s).

labiomancy *n.* lip-reading.

labioplasty (cheiloplasty) *n.* surgical repair of injury or deformity of the lips.

labium *n.* (*pl.* **labia**) a lip-shaped structure, especially either of the two pairs of skin folds that enclose the *vulva. The larger outer pair are known as the *labia* *majora* and the smaller inner pair the *labia minora*.

labour *n.* the sequence of actions by which a baby and the afterbirth are expelled from the womb at childbirth. The process usually starts spontaneously about 280 days after conception, but it may be started by artificial means (*see* induction). In the first stage the muscular wall of the womb begins contracting while the muscle fibres of the cervix (neck of the womb) relax so that the cervix expands. A portion of the membranous sac (amnion) surrounding the baby is pushed into the opening and bursts under the pressure, releasing *amniotic fluid to the exterior. In the second stage the baby's head appears at the cervix and the contractions of the womb strengthen. The passage of the infant through the vagina is assisted by contractions of the abdominal muscles and conscious pushing by the mother. When the top of the baby's head appears at the vaginal opening the whole infant is eased clear of the vagina, and the umbilical cord is cut. If the emergence of the head is impeded a cut may be made in the surrounding tissue (*see* episiotomy). In the final stage the placenta and membranes are pushed out by the continuing contraction of the womb, which eventually returns to its unexpanded state. The average duration of labour is about 13 hours in first pregnancies and about 8 hours in subsequent pregnancies. Labour pains can be lessened by previous training of the abdominal muscles and by the use of drugs. *See also* Caesarean section.

labrum *n.* (*pl.* **labra**) a lip or liplike structure; occurring, for example, around the margins of the articulating socket (acetabulum) of the hip bone.

labyrinth (inner ear) *n.* a convoluted system of cavities and ducts comprising the organs of hearing and balance. The *membranous labyrinth* is a series of interconnected membranous canals and chambers consisting of the *semicircular canals, *utricle, and *saccule (concerned with balance) and the central cavity of the *cochlea (concerned with hearing). (See illustration.) It is filled with a fluid – *endolymph*. The *bony labyrinth* is the system of the bony canals and chambers that surround the membranous labyrinth. It is embedded in the petrous part of the *temporal bone and is filled with fluid (*perilymph*).

superior semicircular canal

ampulla of semicircular canal

lateral semicircular canal

endolymphatic duct

cochlear nerve

posterior semicircular canal

cochlea

utricle

spiral ganglion

saccule

Membranous labyrinth of the right ear

labyrinthitis (otitis interna) *n.* inflammation of the inner ear (labyrinth). *See* otitis.

laceration *n.* a tear in the flesh producing a wound with irregular edges.

lacertus *n.* a band of fibres or a tendon-like structure.

lacrimal apparatus the structures that produce and drain away fluid from the eye (see illustration). The *lacrimal gland* secretes *tears, which drain away through small openings (*puncta*) at the inner corner of the eye into two *lacrimal canaliculi*. From there the tears pass into the nasal cavity via the *lacrimal sac* and the *nasolacrimal duct.

lacrimal bone the smallest bone of the face: either of a pair of rectangular bones that contribute to the orbits. *See* skull.

lacrimal gland

lacrimal canaliculus

lacrimal sac

nasal cavity

excretory ducts of lacrimal glands

punctum

nasolacrimal duct

The lacrimal apparatus

lacrimation *n.* the production of excess tears; crying. *See also* lacrimal apparatus.

lacrimator *n.* an agent that irritates the eyes, causing excessive secretion of tears.

lact- (lacti-, lacto-) *prefix denoting* **1.** milk. **2.** lactic acid.

lactalbumin *n.* a milk protein present in milk at a lower concentration than *casein. Unlike casein, it is not precipitated from milk under acid conditions; it is therefore a constituent of cheese made from whey rather than curd.

lactase *n.* an enzyme, secreted by the glands of the small intestine, that converts lactose (milk sugar) into glucose and galactose during digestion.

lactation *n.* the secretion of milk by the *mammary glands of the breasts, which usually begins at the end of pregnancy. A fluid called *colostrum is secreted before the milk is produced; both secretions are released in response to the sucking action of the infant on the nipple. Lactation is controlled by hormones (*see* prolactin, oxytocin); it stops when the baby is no longer fed at the breast.

lacteal *n.* a blind-ended lymphatic vessel that extends into a villus of the small *intestine. Digested fats are absorbed into the lacteals.

lactic acid a compound that forms in the cells as the end-product of glucose metabolism in the absence of oxygen (*see* glycolysis). During strenuous exercise pyruvic acid is reduced to lactic acid, which may accumulate in the muscles and cause cramp. Lactic acid (owing to its low pH) is an important food preservative. The lactic acid produced by the fermentation of milk is responsible for the preservation and flavour of cheese, yoghurt, and other fermented milk products.

lactiferous *adj.* transporting or secreting milk, as the *lactiferous ducts* of the breast.

lactifuge *n.* a drug that reduces the secretion of milk. Oestrogenic drugs, such as *chlorotrianisene and *dienoestrol, have this effect and are used to suppress milk production in mothers not breast feeding.

Lactobacillus *n.* a genus of Gram-positive nonmotile rodlike bacteria capable of growth in acid media and of producing lactic acid from the fermentation of carbohydrates. They are found in fermenting animal and plant products, especially dairy products, and in the alimentary tract and vagina. They are responsible for the souring of milk. The species *L. acidophilus* is found in milk and is associated with dental caries. It occurs in very high numbers in the faeces of breast- or bottle-fed infants.

lactogenic hormone *see* prolactin.

lactose *n.* a sugar, consisting of one molecule of glucose and one of galactose, found only in milk. Lactose is split into its constituent sugars by the enzyme *lactase, which is secreted in the small intestine. This enzyme is missing or is of low activity in certain people of some Eastern and African races. This leads to the inability to absorb lactose, known as *lactose intolerance*.

lactosuria *n.* the presence of milk sugar (*lactose) in the urine. This often occurs during pregnancy and breastfeeding or if the milk flow is suppressed.

lacuna *n.* (*pl.* **lacunae**) (in anatomy) a small cavity or depression; for example, one of the spaces in compact bone in which a bone cell lies.

laetrile *n.* a cyanide-containing compound extracted from peach stones. It has been used, despite the lack of evidence for its therapeutic value, in the treatment of various forms of cancer.

laevo- *prefix. see* levo-.

laevocardia *n.* the normal position of the heart, in which its apex is directed towards the left. *Compare* dextrocardia.

lagaena (lagena) *n.* the closed end of the spiral *cochlea. This term is more commonly used to describe the structure homologous to the cochlea in primitive vertebrates.

lagophthalmos *n.* any condition in which the eye does not close completely. It may lead to corneal damage from undue exposure.

laking *n.* the physical or chemical treatment of blood to abolish the structure of the red cells and thus form a homogeneous solution. Laking is an important preliminary step in the analysis of haemoglobin or enzymes present in red cells.

-lalia *suffix denoting* a condition involving speech.

lallation (lalling) *n.* **1.** unintelligible speech-like babbling, as heard from infants. **2.** the immature substitution of one consonant for another (e.g. *l* for *r*).

lambda *n.* the point on the skull at which the lambdoidal and sagittal *sutures meet.

lambdoidal suture *see* suture (def. 1).

lambliasis *n. see* giardiasis.

lamella *n.* (*pl.* **lamellae**) **1.** a thin layer, membrane, scale, or plate-like tissue or part. In *bone tissue, lamellae are thin bands of calcified matrix arranged concentrically around a Haversian canal. **2.** a thin gelatinous medicated disc used to apply drugs to the eye. The disc is placed on the eyeball; the gelatinous material dissolves and the drug is absorbed.

lamina *n.* (*pl.* **laminae**) a thin membrane or layer of tissue.

laminectomy (rachiotomy) *n.* surgical cutting into the backbone to obtain access to the spinal cord. The surgeon excises the rear part (the posterior arch) of one or more vertebrae. The operation is performed to remove tumours, to treat injuries to the spine, such as prolapsed intervertebral (slipped) disc (in which the affected disc is removed), or to relieve pressure on a spinal nerve.

lanatoside *n.* a drug similar to *digitalis, used in the treatment of heart failure. It is administered by mouth or injection. High doses may cause loss of appetite, nausea, vomiting, headache, disturbed vision, and abnormal heart activity. Trade name: **Cedilanid**.

Lancefield classification a classification of the *Streptococcus bacteria based on the presence or absence of antigenic carbohydrate on the cell surface. Species are classified into the groups A–P. Most species causing disease in man belong to group A.

lancet *n.* a broad two-edged surgical knife with a sharp point.

lancinating *adj.* describing a sharp stabbing or cutting pain.

Landry's paralysis a rapidly progressive form of the *Guillain-Barré syndrome.

Lange curve a method of detecting excess globulins in the protein of the cerebrospinal fluid. It is useful in the diagnosis of neurosyphilis and multiple sclerosis.

lanugo *n.* fine hair covering the body and limbs of the human fetus. It is most profuse at about the seventh month of gestation and is shed in the ninth month.

laparo- *prefix denoting* the loins or abdomen.

laparoscope (peritoneoscope) *n.* a surgical instrument (a type of *endoscope) comprising an illuminated viewing tube that is inserted through the abdominal wall to enable the surgeon to view the organs in the abdomen (*see* laparoscopy).

laparoscopy (peritoneoscopy, abdominoscopy) *n.* examination of the abdominal structures (which are contained within the peritoneum) by means of an illuminated tubular instrument (*laparoscope) passed through a small incision in the wall of the abdomen. Laparoscopy is often used for examining the ovaries and Fallopian tubes as well as for performing one method of sterilization.

laparotomy *n.* a surgical incision into the abdominal cavity. The operation is done to examine the abdominal organs as a help to diagnosis; for example, to establish the spread of a growth (*exploratory laparotomy*) or as a prelude to major surgery.

lardaceous *adj.* resembling lard: often applied to tissue infiltrated with the starchlike substance amyloid (*see* amyloidosis).

larva *n.* (*pl.* **larvae**) the preadult or immature stage hatching from the egg of some animal groups, e.g. insects and nematodes, which may be markedly different from the sexually mature adult and have a totally different way of life. For example, the larvae of some flies are parasites of animals and cause disease whereas the adults are free-living. —**larval** *adj.*

larva migrans *see* creeping eruption.

laryng- (laryngo-) *prefix denoting* the larynx.

laryngeal reflex a cough produced by irritating the larynx.

laryngectomy *n.* surgical removal of the whole or a part of the larynx, as in the treatment of laryngeal carcinoma.

laryngismus *n.* closure of the vocal cords by sudden contraction of the laryngeal muscles, followed by a noisy indrawing of breath. It occurs in young children and was in the past associated with low-calcium rickets. Now it occurs when the larynx has been irritated following administration of anaesthetic, when a foreign body has lodged in the larynx, or in *croup.

laryngitis *n.* inflammation of the larynx and vocal cords, due to infection by bacteria or viruses or irritation by gases, chemicals, etc. The cords lose their vibrance (owing to swelling) and the voice becomes husky or is lost completely; breathing is harsh and difficult (*see* stridor); and the cough is painful and honking. Obstruction of the airways may occasionally be serious, especially in children (*see* croup). The patient should rest his voice and remain in a warm moisture-laden atmosphere; steam inhalations for 15–20 minutes every 2–3 hours are traditionally beneficial. The patient should avoid cold air or fog and smoking.

laryngocele *n.* a developmental defect in which an air sac communicates with the larynx. The sac forms a swelling in the neck that dilates on coughing or straining.

laryngofissure *n.* *see* laryngotomy.

laryngology *n.* the study of diseases of the larynx and vocal cords.

laryngopharynx *n.* the part of the pharynx that lies below the hyoid bone.

laryngoscope *n.* an instrument for examining the larynx. There are several types, the simplest consisting of a curved blunt metal blade, used to press the tongue out of the line of vision, and a small light to illuminate the field.

laryngospasm *n.* closure of the larynx, obstructing the flow of air to the lungs. It usually occurs as part of an allergic reaction, such as *angioneurotic oedema.

laryngotomy (laryngofissure) *n.* surgical incision of the larynx. *Inferior laryngotomy*, in which an incision is made in the cricothyroid membrane beneath the larynx, is a life-saving operation when there is obstruction to breathing at or above the larynx. *See* tracheostomy.

laryngotracheobronchitis *n.* a severe infection of the respiratory tract, especially of young children, in whom there may be a dangerous degree of obstruction either at the larynx (*see* croup) or main air passages (bronchi) due to the thickness and stickiness of the fluid (exudate) produced by the inflamed tissues. Treatment: as for *laryngitis, with *tracheostomy if necessary and bronchoscopy in addition, during which it may be possible to clear the obstructing exudate by bronchial lavage and suction.

larynx *n.* the organ responsible for the production of vocal sounds, also serving as an air passage conveying air from the pharynx to the lungs. It is situated in the front of the neck, above the trachea. It is made up of a framework of nine cartilages (see illustration) – the epiglottis, thyroid, cricoid, arytenoid (two), corniculate (two), and cuneiform (two) – bound together by ligaments and muscles and lined with mucous membrane. Within are a pair of *vocal cords, which function in the production of voice. —**laryngeal** *adj.*

epiglottis

hyoid bone

thyroid cartilage

arytenoid cartilage

cricoid cartilage

trachea

Cartilages of the larynx

laser *n.* a device that produces a very thin beam of light in which high energies are concentrated. In surgery lasers can be used to operate on small areas of abnormality (for example, in the retina of the eye) without damaging delicate surrounding tissue.

Lasix *n. see* frusemide.

Lassa fever a serious virus disease confined to Central West Africa. After an incubation period of 3–21 days, headache, high fever, and severe muscular pains develop; difficulty in swallowing often arises. Death from kidney or heart failure occurs in over 50% of cases. Treatment with plasma from recovered patients is the best therapy.

latah *n.* a pattern of behaviour seen only in certain cultures, such as that of Malaysia. After a psychological shock the affected individual becomes very anxious and very suggestible and shows excessive obedience and pathological imitation of the actions of another person (echopraxia).

latent period (in neurology) the pause of a few milliseconds between the time that a nerve impulse reaches a muscle fibre and the time that the fibre starts to contract.

lateral *adj.* **1.** situated at or relating to the side of an organ or organism. **2.** (in anatomy) relating to the region or parts of the body that are furthest from the *median plane. **3.** (in radiology) in the *sagittal plane.

lateroversion *n.* a turning or displacement of an organ, for example the womb (*uterine lateroversion*) to one side.

lathyrism *n.* a disease, characterized by muscular weakness and paralysis, found among people whose staple diet consists mostly of large quantites of *Lathyrus sativus*, a kind of chick pea, and/or vetches and pulses related it. Except in mild cases complete recovery does not occur, despite administration of an adequate diet and physiotherapy.

laudanum *n.* a hydroalcoholic solution containing 1% morphine, prepared from macerated raw opium. It was formerly widely used as a narcotic analgesic, taken by mouth.

laughing gas *see* nitrous oxide.

lavage *n.* washing out a body cavity, such as the colon or stomach, with water or a medicated solution.

laxative (cathartic, purgative) *n.* a drug used to stimulate or increase the frequency of bowel evacuation, or to encourage a softer or bulkier stool. The common laxatives are the irritants castor oil and jalop; senna and its derivatives; magnesium sulphate and other mineral salts; and methylcellulose and other bulking agents.

LD$_{50}$ the dose of a toxic compound that causes death in 50% of a group of experimental animals to which it is administered: used as a measure of the toxicity of drugs.

L-dopa *n. see* levodopa.

lead^1 *n.* a soft bluish-grey metallic element that forms several poisonous compounds. Acute lead poisoning, which may follow inhalation of lead fumes or dust, causes abdominal pains, vomiting, and diarrhoea, with paralysis and convulsions and sometimes *encephalitis. In chronic poisoning a characteristic bluish marking of the gums ('lead line') is seen and the peripheral nerves are affected; there is also anaemia. Treatment is with *EDTA. The use of lead in paints is now strictly controlled. Symbol: Pb.

lead^2 *n.* a portion of an electrocardiographic record that is obtained from a single electrode or a combination of electrodes placed on a particular part of the body (*see* electrocardiogram, electrocardiography). In the conventional ECG, 12 leads are recorded. Each lead represents the electrical activity of the heart as 'viewed' from a different position on the body surface and may help to localize myocardial damage.

lecithin *n.* one of a group of *phospholipids that are important constituents of cell membranes and are involved in the metabolism of fat by the liver. An example is *phosphatidylcholine*.

lecithinase *n.* an enzyme from the small intestine that breaks *lecithin down into its constituents (i.e. glycerol, fatty acids, phosphoric acid, and choline).

Ledermycin *n. see* demethylchlortetracycline.

leech *n.* a type of worm that possesses suckers at both ends of its body. Leeches occur in tropical forests and grasslands and in water. Certain parasitic species suck blood from animals and man, and their bites cause irritation and, occasionally, infection. Rarely, leeches are taken in with foul drinking water and pass from the mouth to the nose, where they provoke headache and nose bleeds. A leech can be detached from its host either by applying salt or by touching it with a lighted cigarette. Calamine lotion eases the irritation of the bites. Leeches were formerly used in bloodletting.

Legg-Calvé-Perthes disease (Perthes disease, pseudocoxalgia) inflammation of the heads of the femurs (thighbones), resulting in loss of the blood supply and death of the outer layer of bone (avascular necrosis) (*see* osteochondritis). It occurs most commonly in boys between the ages of 5 and 10, and causes aching and a limp. Unless early and effective treatment by bed rest and calipers is carried out, deformity, shortening, and secondary osteoarthritis of the bones result.

legionnaires' disease a bacterial infection of the lungs, named after an outbreak of 182 cases at the American Legion convention in Pennsylvania in 1976. Symptoms appear after an incubation period of about seven days: malaise and muscle pain are succeeded by a fever, dry cough, chest pain, and breathlessness. There is loss of protein in the urine and impaired kidney function. X-ray of the lungs shows patchy consolidation. Erythromycin provides the most effective therapy.

leio- *prefix denoting* smoothness. Example: *leiodermia* (abnormal smoothness of the skin).

leiomyoma *n.* a benign tumour of smooth muscle. Such tumours occur most commonly in the uterus (*see* fibroid) but can also arise in the digestive tract, walls of blood vessels, etc. They may undergo malignant change (*see* leiomyosarcoma).

leiomyosarcoma *n.* a malignant tumour of smooth muscle, most commonly found in the womb, stomach, small bowel, and at the base of the bladder. It is the second most common *sarcoma of soft tissues. This tumour is rare in children, occurring most com-

monly in the bladder, prostate, and stomach.

Leishman-Donovan body *see* Leishmania.

Leishmania *n.* a genus of parasitic flagellate protozoans, several species of which cause disease in man (*see* leishmaniasis). The parasite assumes a different form in each of its two hosts. In man, especially in *kala-azar patients, it is a small rounded structure, with no flagellum, called a *Leishman-Donovan body*, which is found within the cells of the lymphatic system, spleen, and bone marrow. In the insect carrier it is long and flagellated.

leishmaniasis *n.* a disease, common in the tropics and subtropics, caused by parasitic protozoans of the genus *Leishmania*, which are transmitted by the bite of sandflies. There are two principal forms of the disease: *visceral leishmaniasis*, in which the cells of various internal organs are affected (*see* kala-azar); and *cutaneous leishmaniasis*, which affects the tissues of the skin. Cutaneous leishmaniasis itself has several different forms, depending on the region in which it occurs and the species of *Leishmania* involved. In Asia it is common in the form of *oriental sore. In America there are several forms of leishmaniasis (*see* chiclero's ulcer, espundia). Leishmaniasis is treated with drugs containing antimony.

lemniscus *n.* a ribbon-like tract of nerve tissue conveying information from the spinal cord and brainstem upwards through the midbrain to the higher centres. On each side a *medial lemniscus* acts as a pathway from the spinal cord, while an outer *lateral lemniscus* commences higher up and is mainly concerned with hearing.

lens *n.* **1.** (in anatomy) the transparent crystalline structure situated behind the pupil of the eye and enclosed in a thin transparent *capsule*. It helps to refract incoming light and focus it onto the *retina. *See also* accommodation. **2.** (in optics) a piece of glass shaped to refract rays of light in a particular direction. *Convex lenses* converge the light, and *concave lenses* diverge it; they are worn to correct faulty eyesight. *See also* bifocal lenses, contact lenses, trifocal lenses.

lenticonus *n.* a condition in which the central part of the front surface of the lens of the eye (or sometimes, the back) has a much steeper curvature than normal and bulges forwards in a blunted cone. It is usually congenital.

lenticular nucleus (lentiform nucleus) *see* basal ganglia.

lentigo *n.* a brown roundish flat spot on the skin caused by excess development of melanin. Commoner in old people, lentigo sometimes turns into a slow-growing skin cancer.

leontiasis *n.* overgrowth of the skull bones, said to resemble the appearance of a lion's head: a rare feature of untreated *Paget's disease. Medical name: **leontiasis ossea**.

lepidosis *n.* any skin eruption that causes scaling.

lepra reaction an aggravation of lumps on the skin caused by *leprosy, accompanied by fever and malaise.

leproma *n.* a lump on the skin characteristic of *leprosy.

lepromin *n.* a chemical prepared from lumps on the skin caused by lepromatous *leprosy.

leprosy (Hansen's disease) *n.* a chronic disease, caused by the bacterium *Mycobacterium leprae*, that affects the skin, mucous membranes, and nerves. It is confined mainly to the tropics and is transmitted by direct contact. After an incubation period of 1–30 years, symptoms develop gradually and mainly involve the skin and nerves. *Lepromatous leprosy* is a contagious steadily progressive form of the disease characterized by the development of widely distributed lumps on the skin, thickening of the skin and nerves, and in serious cases by severe numbness of the skin, muscle weakness, and paralysis leading to disfigurement and deformity. Tuberculosis is a common complication. *Tuberculoid leprosy* is a benign, often self-limiting, form of leprosy causing discoloration and disfiguration of patches of skin (sparsely distributed) associated with localized numbness. *Indeterminate leprosy* is a form of the disease in which skin manifestations represent a combination of the two main types. Leprosy can be controlled, but not cured, by prolonged treatment with *sulphone drugs.

lept- (lepto-) *prefix denoting* **1.** slender; thin. **2.** small. **3.** mild; slight.

leptocyte *n.* a red blood cell (*erythrocyte) that is abnormally thin. Leptocytes are seen in certain types of anaemia.

leptomeninges *pl. n.* the inner two *meninges: the arachnoid and pia mater.

leptomeningitis *n.* inflammation of the inner membranes (the *pia mater and *arachnoid) of the brain and spinal cord. *See also* meningitis.

leptophonia *n.* weakness of the voice.

Leptospira *n.* a genus of spirochaete bacteria, commonly bearing hooked ends. They are not visible with ordinary light microscopy and are best seen using dark-ground microscopy. The parasitic species *L. icterohaemorrhagiae* is the main causative agent of *leptospirosis (Weil's disease), but many closely related species cause similar symptoms.

leptospirosis (Weil's disease) *n.* an infectious disease, caused by bacteria of the genus *Leptospira*, that occurs in rodents, dogs, and other mammals and may be transmitted to people whose work brings them into contact with these animals. The disease begins with a fever and may affect the liver (causing jaundice) or meninges (resulting in meningitis); in some cases the kidneys are involved.

leptotene *n.* the first stage in the first prophase of *meiosis, in which the chromosomes become visible as single long threads.

leresis *n.* rambling speech, immature both in syntax and pronunciation. It is a feature of dementia.

lesbianism *n.* the condition in which a woman is sexually attracted to, or engages in sexual behaviour with, another woman (*see also* homosexuality). Treatment for lesbianism varies: many therapists prefer to reduce the anxiety and guilt associated with the condition rather than try to change it directly. —**lesbian** *adj., n.*

lesion *n.* a zone of tissue with impaired function as a result of damage by disease or wounding. Apart from direct physical injury, examples of primary lesions include abscesses, ulcers, tumours; secondary lesions (such as crusts and scars) are derived from primary ones.

lethal gene a gene that, under certain conditions, causes the death of the individual carrying it. Lethal genes are usually *recessive: an individual will die only if both his parents carry the gene. If only one parent is affected, the lethal effects of the gene will be masked by the dominant *allele inherited from the normal parent.

lethargy *n.* mental and physical sluggishness: a degree of inactivity and unresponsiveness approaching or verging on the unconscious. The condition results from disease (such as sleeping sickness) or hypnosis.

Letterer-Siwe disease *see* reticuloendotheliosis.

leuc- (leuco-, leuk-, leuko-) *prefix denoting* 1. lack of colour; white. 2. leucocytes.

leucine *n.* an *essential amino acid. *See also* amino acid.

leucocidin *n.* a bacterial *exotoxin that selectively destroys white blood cells (leucocytes).

leucocyte (white blood cell) *n.* any blood cell that contains a nucleus. In health there are three major subdivisions: *granulocytes, *lymphocytes and *monocytes, which are involved in protecting the body against foreign substances and in antibody production. In disease, a variety of other types may appear in the blood, most notably immature forms of the normal red or white blood cells.

leucocytosis *n.* an increase in the number of white blood cells (leucocytes) in the blood. *See* basophilia, eosinophilia, lymphocytosis, monocytosis.

leucoderma *n. see* vitiligo.

leucolysin *n. see* lysin.

leucoma *n.* a white opacity in the cornea. Most leucomas result from scarring after corneal inflammation or ulceration. Congenital types may be associated with other abnormalities of the eye.

leuconychia *n.* white discoloration of the nails, which may be total or partial. The cause is unknown.

leucopenia *n.* a reduction in the number of white blood cells (leucocytes) in the blood. *See* eosinopenia, lymphopenia, neutropenia.

leucoplakia (leukoplakia) *n.* thickened white patches on mucous membranes, such as the mouth lining or vulva, due to an overgrowth of the tissues. Some leucoplakia may be caused by excessive smoking or alcohol or by certain infections; occasionally it can become malignant.

leucopoiesis *n.* the process of the production of white blood cells (leucocytes), which normally occurs in the blood-forming tissue of the *bone marrow. *See also* granulopoiesis, haemopoiesis, lymphopoiesis, monoblast.

leucorrhoea (whites) *n.* a whitish or yellowish discharge of mucus from the vaginal opening. It may occur normally at all times, the quantity increasing before and after menstruation. An abnormally large discharge may indicate infection of the lower reproductive tract, e.g. by the protozoan *Trichomonas vaginalis* (*see* vaginitis).

leucotomy *n.* the surgical operation of interrupting the pathways of white nerve fibres within the brain: it is the most common procedure in *psychosurgery. In the original form, *prefrontal leucotomy* (*lobotomy*), the operation involved cutting through the nerve fibres connecting the *frontal lobe with the *thalamus and the association fibres of the frontal lobe. This was often successful in reducing severe emotional tension but had serious side-effects, including epilepsy and changes in the personality towards apathy and irresponsibility.

Modern procedures use *stereotaxy and make selective lesions in smaller areas of the brain. Side-effects are uncommon and the operation is used for intractable pain, severe depression, obsessional neurosis, and chronic anxiety, where very severe emotional tension has not been relieved by other treatments.

leukaemia *n.* any of a group of malignant diseases in which the bone marrow and other blood-forming organs produce increased numbers of certain types of white blood cells (*leucocytes). Overproduction of these white cells, which are immature or abnormal forms, suppresses the production of normal white cells, red cells, and platelets. This leads to increased susceptibility to infection (due to *neutropenia), *anaemia, and bleeding (due to *thrombocytopenia). Other symptoms include enlargement of the spleen, liver, and lymph nodes.

Leukaemias are classified into *acute* or *chronic* varieties depending on the rate of progression of the disease. They are also classified according to the type of white cell that is proliferating abnormally; for example *lymphoblastic leukaemia* (*see* lymphoblast) and *acute myeloblastic leukaemia* (*see* myeloblast). (*See also* myeloid leukaemia.) Leukaemias are treated with radiotherapy or *cytotoxic drugs, which are aimed at suppressing the reproduction of the abnormal cells.

leukoplakia *n.* *see* leucoplakia.

leukotaxine *n.* a chemical, present in inflammatory exudates, that attracts white blood cells (leucocytes) and increases the permeability of blood capillaries. It is probably produced by injured cells.

levallorphan *n.* a drug that counteracts the depression in breathing caused by narcotic analgesics such as morphine without affecting their pain-relieving effects. It is administered by injection, usually before or at the same time as the analgesic. Trade name: **Lorfan**.

levator *n.* **1.** a surgical instrument used for levering up displaced bone fragments in a depressed fracture of the skull. **2.** any muscle that lifts the structure into which it is inserted; for example, the *levator scapulis* helps to lift the shoulder blade.

levo- (laevo-) *prefix denoting* **1.** the left side. **2.** (in chemistry) levorotation.

levodopa (L-dopa) *n.* a naturally occurring amino acid administered by mouth to treat *parkinsonism. Com-

levorphanol

mon side-effects are nausea, vomiting, loss of appetite, and involuntary facial movements; high doses may cause weakness, faintness, and dizziness. Trade names: **Berkdopa**, **Brocadopa**, **Larodopa**, **Veldopa**.

levorphanol *n.* a narcotic analgesic, similar to *morphine, used to relieve severe pain. It is administered by mouth or injection and may cause nausea, vomiting, loss of appetite, constipation, and confusion. Dependence may develop. Trade name: **Dromoran**.

levulosuria *n. see* fructosuria.

Leydig cells *see* interstitial cells.

LH *see* luteinizing hormone.

Lhermitte's sign a tingling shocklike sensation passing down the arms or trunk when the neck is flexed. It is a nonspecific indication of disease in the cervical (neck) region of the spinal cord.

libido *n.* the sexual drive: the term is often used to refer to the intensity of sexual desires. In psychoanalytic theory, the libido (like the death instinct) is one of the fundamental sources of energy for all mental life. The normal course of development (*see* psychosexual development) can be altered by fixation at one level and by regression.

Librium *n. see* chlordiazepoxide.

lice *pl. n. see* louse.

lichen *n.* any of several types of skin disease in which small round hard lesions occur close together. For example, *lichen planus* is an inflammatory condition in which wide flat mauve pimples are found mainly on the forearms, neck, and between the thighs. It may occur in the mouth and often causes symptomless white patches; occasionally it forms painful erosions.

lichenification *n.* the thickening of certain cell layers in the epidermis causing brown or violet patches in the

skin with exaggeration of the normal creases. A criss-cross appearance results, containing lozenge-shaped flat-topped shiny areas. The cause is abnormal scratching or rubbing of the skin.

lichenoid *adj.* describing any skin disease that resembles *lichen.

Lieberkuhn's glands (crypts of Lieberkuhn) simple tubular glands in the mucous membrane of the *intestine. In the small intestine they lie between the villi. They are lined with columnar *epithelium in which various types of secretory cells are found. In the large intestine Lieberkuhn's glands are longer and contain more mucus-secreting cells.

lien *n. see* spleen.

lien- (lieno-) *prefix denoting* the spleen. Example: *lienopathy* (disease of).

lientery *n.* diarrhoea with the passage of undigested food in the faeces. This may indicate simply rapid transit of food through the digestive tract or some form of *malabsorption.

life table an actuarial presentation of the ages at which a group of males and/or females will die and from which mean *life expectancy* at any age can be estimated, based on the assumption that mortality patterns current at the time of preparation of the table will continue to apply.

ligament *n.* **1.** a tough band of white fibrous connective tissue that links two bones together at a joint. Ligaments are inelastic but flexible; they strengthen the joint and limit its movements to certain directions. **2.** a sheet of peritoneum that supports or links together abdominal organs.

ligation *n.* the application of a *ligature.

ligature *n.* any material – for example, nylon, silk, catgut, or wire – that is tied firmly round a blood vessel to stop it bleeding or around the base of a structure (such as the *pedicle of a growth) to constrict it.

light adaptation reflex changes in the eye to enable vision either in normal light after being in darkness or in very bright light after being in normal light. The pupil contracts (*see* pupillary reflex) and the pigment in the *rods is bleached. *Compare* dark adaptation.

lightening *n.* the descent of the womb into the pelvic cavity at a late stage of pregnancy, usually two to three weeks before labour begins but sometimes, in women who have given birth previously, not until the onset of labour. Lightening occurs when the head of the fetus turns down towards the vagina.

light reflex *see* pupillary reflex.

lignocaine *n.* a widely used local *anaesthetic administered by injection for minor surgery and dental procedures. It can also be applied directly to the eye, throat, and mouth as it is absorbed through mucous membranes. Lignocaine is also injected to treat conditions involving abnormal heart rhythm, particularly myocardial infarction. When used as a local anaesthetic, side-effects are rare. Trade names: **Xylocaine, Xylotox.**

limbic system a complex system of nerve pathways and networks in the brain, involving several different nuclei, that is involved in the expression of instinct and mood in activities of the endocrine and motor systems of the body. Among the brain regions involved are the *amygdala, *hippocampal formation, and *hypothalamus. The activities of the body that are governed are those concerned with self-preservation (e.g. searching for food, fighting) and preservation of the species (e.g. reproduction and the care of offspring), the expression of fear, rage, and pleasure, and the establishment of

memory patterns. *See also* reticular activating system.

limbus *n.* (in anatomy) an edge or border; for example, the *limbus sclerae* is the junction of the cornea and sclera of the eye.

limen *n.* (in anatomy) a border or boundary. The *limen nasi* is the boundary between the bony and cartilaginous parts of the nasal cavity.

liminal *adj.* (in physiology) relating to the threshold of perception.

limosis *n.* abnormal hunger or an excessive desire for food.

lincomycin *n.* an *antibiotic used to treat infections caused by a narrow range of bacteria, including osteomyelitis. It is administered by mouth or injection and occasionally causes diarrhoea, nausea, and stomach pains. Trade names: **Lincocin, Mycivin.**

linctus *n.* a syrupy liquid medicine, particularly one used in the treatment of irritating coughs.

Lindau's tumour *see* haemangioblastoma.

linea *n.* (*pl.* **lineae**) (in anatomy) a line, narrow streak, or stripe. The *linea alba* is a tendinous line, extending from the xiphoid process to the pubic symphysis, where the flat abdominal muscles are attached.

linear accelerator (linac) a machine that accelerates particles to produce high-energy radiation, used in the treatment of malignant disease.

lingual *adj.* relating to, situated close to, or resembling the tongue (lingua). The lingual surface of a tooth is the surface adjacent to the tongue.

lingula *n.* **1.** the thin forward-projecting portion of the anterior lobe of the cerebellum, in the midline. **2.** a small section of the upper lobe of the left lung, extending downwards in front of the heart. **3.** a bony spur on the inside of the mandible, above the angle of the jaw. **4.** a small backward-pointing projection on each side of the sphenoid bone.

liniment *n.* a medicinal preparation that is rubbed onto the skin or applied on a surgical dressing. Liniments often contain camphor and alcohol.

linin *n.* the lightly staining material surrounding the much more deeply staining *chromatin in the nucleus of a cell not undergoing division.

lining *n.* (in dentistry) a protective layer placed in a prepared tooth cavity before a restoration is inserted.

linkage *n.* the situation in which two or more genes lie close to each other on a chromosome and are therefore very likely to be inherited together. The further two genes are apart the more likely they are to be separated by *crossing over during meiosis and to come to lie on different homologous chromosomes.

linoleic acid *see* essential fatty acid.

linolenic acid *see* essential fatty acid.

lint *n.* a material used in surgical dressings, made of scraped linen or a cotton substitute. It is usually fluffy one side and smooth the other.

liothyronine *n.* a hormone produced by the thyroid gland that is similar to *thyroxine and used to treat conditions of thyroid deficiency. It is administered by mouth or injection and has a rapid but short-lived effect.

lip- (lipo-) *prefix denoting* **1.** fat. **2.** lipid.

lipaemia *n.* the presence in the blood of an abnormally large amount of fat, such as *cholesterol.

lipase (steapsin) *n.* an enzyme, produced by the pancreas and the glands of the small intestine, that breaks down fats into glycerol and fatty acids during digestion.

lipid *n.* one of a group of naturally occurring compounds that are soluble in solvents such as chloroform or alcohol, but insoluble in water. Lipids are important dietary constituents, not only because of their high energy value but also because certain vitamins and essential fatty acids are associated with them. The group includes *fats, *steroids, *phospholipids, and *glycolipids.

lipidosis (lipoidosis) *n.* (*pl.* **-ses**) any disorder of lipid metabolism within the cells of the body. The *brain lipidoses* (*see* Gaucher's disease, Hurler's syndrome, Tay-Sachs disease) are inborn defects causing the accumulation of lipids within the brain.

lipochondrodystrophy *n.* multiple congenital defects affecting lipid (fat) metabolism, cartilage and bone, skin, and the major internal organs, leading to mental retardation, dwarfism, and deformities of the bones.

lipochrome *n.* a pigment that is soluble in fat and therefore gives colour to fatty materials. An example is *carotene, the pigment responsible for the colour of egg yolks and butter.

lipodystrophy *n.* any disturbance of fat metabolism or of the distribution of fat in the body. In *inferior lipodystrophy* fat is absent from the legs; in *insulin lipodystrophy*, sometimes occurring in diabetics, it disappears from the areas at which insulin is injected.

lipofuscin *n.* a brownish pigment staining with certain fat stains. It is most common in the cells of heart muscle, nerves, and liver and is normally contained within the *lysosomes.

lipogenesis *n.* the process by which glucose and other substances, derived from carbohydrate in the diet, are converted to *fatty acids in the body.

lipogranulomatosis *n.* an abnormality of lipid metabolism causing deposition of yellowish nodules in the skin.

lipoic acid a sulphur-containing compound that can be readily interconverted to and from its reduced form, *dihydrolipoic acid*. Lipoic acid functions in carbohydrate metabolism as one of the *coenzymes in the oxidative decarboxylation of pyruvate and other α-keto acids.

lipoid factor one of the substances involved in the clotting of blood, important for the activation of plasma *thromboplastin.

lipoidosis *n. see* lipidosis.

lipolysis *n.* the process by which lipids, particularly triglycerides in fat, are broken down into their constituent fatty acids in the body by the enzyme *lipase. —**lipolytic** *adj.*

lipoma *n.* a common benign tumour composed of well-differentiated fat cells. It is doubtful whether malignant change ever occurs.

lipomatosis *n.* **1.** the presence of an abnormally large amount of fat in the tissues. **2.** the presence of multiple *lipomas.

lipopolysaccharide *n.* a complex molecule containing both a lipid and a polysaccharide component. Lipopolysaccharides are constituents of the cell walls of Gram-negative bacteria and are important in determining the antigenic properties of these bacteria.

lipoprotein *n.* one of a group of proteins, found in blood plasma and lymph, that are combined with fats or other lipids (such as cholesterol). Lipoproteins are important for the transport of lipids in the blood and lymph.

liposarcoma *n.* a malignant tumour of fat cells. It is most commonly found in the thigh and is rare under the age of 30 years. There are four main histological types: *well-differentiated, myxoid, pleomorphic,* and *round-cell liposarcomas,* the first two of which are the most sensitive to treatment.

liposome *n.* a microscopic spherical membrane-enclosed vesicle or sac (20–30 nm in diameter) made artificially in the laboratory by the addition of an aqueous solution to a phospholipid gel. The membrane resembles a cell membrane and the whole vesicle is similar to a cell organelle. Liposomes can be incorporated into living cells and are used to transport relatively toxic drugs into diseased cells, where they can exert their maximum effects. For example, liposomes containing *methotrexate can be injected into the patient's blood. The cancerous organ is heated to a temperature higher than body temperature, so that when the liposome passes through its blood vessels the membrane melts and the drug is released.

lipotrophin *n.* a hormone-like substance from the anterior pituitary gland that stimulates the transfer of fat from the body stores to the bloodstream.

lipotropic *adj.* describing a substance that promotes the transport of fatty acids from the liver to the tissues or accelerates the utilization of fat in the liver itself. An example of such a substance is the amino acid methionine.

lipping *n.* overgrowth of bone as seen in X-rays near a joint margin. This is a characteristic sign of degenerative or inflammatory joint disease and occurs most frequently and prominently in osteoarthrosis. *See also* osteophyte.

lipuria *n.* the presence of fat or oil droplets in the urine.

liquor *n.* (in pharmacy) any solution, usually an aqueous solution.

Listeria *n.* a genus of Gram-positive aerobic motile rodlike bacteria that are parasites of warm-blooded animals.

lith-

The single species, *L. monocytogenes*, infects many domestic and wild animals and, on transmission to man, causes *meningoencephalitis and occasionally infection of the womb.

lith- (litho-) *prefix denoting* a calculus (stone). Example: *lithogenesis* (formation of).

-lith *suffix denoting* a calculus (stone). Example: *faecalith* (a stony mass of faeces).

lithaemia *n. see* hyperuricaemia.

lithagogue *n.* an agent that promotes the removal of stones (calculi), such as kidney stones in the urine or gallstones from the gall bladder.

lithiasis *n.* formation of stones (*see* calculus) in an internal organ, such as the gall bladder (*see* gallstone), urinary system, pancreas, or appendix.

lithium (lithium carbonate) *n.* a drug given by mouth to prevent manic-depressive psychosis or to treat mania. Side-effects include tremor, weakness, nausea, thirst, and excessive urination. Thyroid function can be interfered with, and changes in the kidney can appear after long-term treatment. Excessive doses can cause an *encephalopathy and even death. The levels of lithium in the blood are therefore usually checked during long-term therapy. Trade names: **Camcolit, Priadel**.

litholapaxy (lithotripsy) *n.* the operation of crushing a stone in the bladder, using an instrument called a *lithotrite*. The small fragments of stone can then be removed by irrigation and suction.

lithonephrotomy *n.* surgical removal of a stone from the kidney. *See* nephrolithotomy, pyelolithotomy.

lithopaedion *n.* a fetus that has died in the womb or abdominal cavity and has become calcified (stony).

lithotomy *n.* the surgical removal of a stone (calculus) from the urinary tract. *See* nephrolithotomy, pyelolithotomy, ureterolithotomy.

lithotripsy *n. see* litholapaxy.

lithotrite *n.* a surgical instrument used for crushing a stone in the bladder. *See* litholapaxy.

lithotrophic *adj. see* autotrophic.

lithuresis *n.* the passage of small stones or *gravel in the urine.

lithuria *n. see* hyperuricuria.

litre *n.* a unit of volume equal to the volume occupied by 1 kilogram of pure water at 4°C and 760 mmHg pressure. In *SI units the litre is treated as a special name for the cubic decimetre, but is not used when a high degree of accuracy is required (1 litre = 1.0000028 dm^3). For approximate purposes 1 litre is assumed to be equal to 1000 cubic centimetres (cm^3), therefore 1 millilitre (ml) is often taken to be equal to 1 cm^3. This practice is now deprecated.

Little's disease a form of *cerebral palsy involving both sides of the body and affecting the legs more severely than the arms.

livedo *n.* a discoloured area or spot on the skin, often caused by local congestion of the circulation.

liver *n.* the largest gland of the body, weighing 1200–1600 g. Situated in the top right portion of the abdominal cavity, the liver is divided by fissures (*fossae*) into four lobes: the *right* (the largest lobe), *left*, *quadrate*, and *caudate lobes*. It is connected to the diaphragm and abdominal walls by five ligaments: the membranous *falciform* (which separates the right and left lobes), *coronary*, and *right* and *left triangular ligaments* and the fibrous *round ligament*, which is derived from the embryonic umbilical vein. Venous blood containing digested food is brought to the liver in the *hepatic portal vein* (*see* portal system).

Branches of this vein pass in between the lobules and terminate in the *sinusoids* (see illustration). Oxygenated blood is supplied in the *hepatic artery*. The blood leaves the liver via a central vein in each lobule, which drains into the *hepatic vein. The liver is supplied by parasympathetic nerve fibres from the vagus nerve, and by sympathetic fibres from the solar plexus. The liver has a number of important functions. It synthesizes *bile, which drains into the *gall bladder before being released into the duodenum. The liver is an important site of metabolism of carbohydrates, proteins, and fats. It regulates the amount of blood sugar, converting excess glucose to *glycogen; it removes excess amino acids by breaking them down into ammonia and finally *urea; and it stores and metabolizes fats. The liver also synthesizes *fibrinogen and *prothrombin (essential blood-clotting substances) and *heparin, an anticoagulant. It forms red blood cells in the fetus and is the site of production of plasma proteins. It has an important role in the detoxification of poisonous substances and it breaks down worn out red cells and other unwanted substances, such as excess oestrogen in the male (*see also* Kupffer's cells). The liver is also the site of *vitamin A synthesis; this vitamin is stored in the liver, together with vitamins B_{12}, D, and K.

liver spot a local brown discoloration on the skin known medically as senile *lentigo. The term is sometimes also used for *chloasma and some medical sources also apply the term to *pityriasis versicolor* – a mild chronic infection of the skin, caused by the fungus *Malassezia furfur*, that produces discrete depigmented areas on the body.

livid *adj.* denoting a bluish colour of the skin, such as that produced locally by a bruise or of the general complexion in *cyanosis.

The microscopic structure of the liver

Loa *n.* a genus of parasitic nematode worms (*see* filaria). The adult eye worm, *L. loa*, lives within the tissues beneath the skin, where it causes inflammation and swelling (*see* loiasis). The motile embryos, present in the blood during the day, may be taken up by bloodsucking *Chrysops* flies. Here they develop into infective larvae, ready for transmission to a new human host.

lobe *n.* a major division of an organ or part of an organ, especially one having a rounded form and often separated from other lobes by fissures or bands of connective tissue. For example, the brain, liver, and lung are divided into lobes. **—lobar** *adj.*

lobectomy *n.* the surgical removal of a lobe of an organ or gland, such as the lung, thyroid, or brain. Lobectomy of the lung may be performed for cancer or other disease of the lung.

lobeline *n.* a drug administered by injection to stimulate breathing or given by mouth as a smoking deterrent. Side-effects can include nausea, vomiting, coughing, headache, tremors, and dizziness.

lobotomy (prefrontal leucotomy) *see* leucotomy.

lobule *n.* a subdivision of a part or organ that can be distinguished from the whole by boundaries, such as septa, that are visible with or without a microscope. For example, the *lobule of the liver* is a structural and functional unit seen in cross-section under a microscope as a column of cells drained by a central vein and bounded by a branch of the portal vein. The *lung lobule* is a practical subdivision of the lung tissue seen macroscopically in lung slices as outlined by incomplete septa of fibrous tissue. It is made up of three to five lung *acini.

lochia *n.* the material eliminated from the womb through the vagina after the completion of labour. The first discharge, *lochia rubra* (*lochia cruenta*), consists largely of blood. This is followed by *lochia serosa*, a brownish mixture of blood and mucus, and finally *lochia alba* (*lochia purulenta*), a yellowish or whitish discharge containing microbes and cell fragments. Each stage may last for several days. —**lochial** *adj.*

lockjaw *n. see* tetanus.

locomotor ataxia *see* tabes dorsalis.

loculus *n.* (in anatomy) a small space or cavity.

locum tenens a doctor who stands in temporarily for a colleague who is absent or ill and looks after the patients in his practice. Often shortened to **locum**.

locus *n.* **1.** (in anatomy) a region or site. The *locus ceruleus* is a small pigmented region in the floor of the fourth ventricle in the brain. **2.** (in

genetics) the region of a chromosome occupied by a particular gene.

log- (logo-) *prefix denoting* words; speech.

logopaedics *n.* the scientific study of defects and disabilities of speech and of the methods used to treat them; speech therapy.

logorrhoea *n.* a rapid flow of voluble speech, often with incoherence, such as is encountered in *mania.

-logy (-ology) *suffix denoting* field of study. Example: *cytology* (study of cells).

loiasis *n.* a disease, occurring in West and Central Africa, caused by the eye worm *Loa loa*. The adult worms live and migrate within the skin tissues, causing the appearance of transitory *calabar* swellings. These are probably an allergic reaction to the worms' waste products, and they sometimes lead to fever and itching. Worms often migrate across the eyeball just beneath the conjunctiva, where they cause irritation and congestion. Loiasis is treated with *diethylcarbamazine, which kills both the adults and larval forms.

loin *n.* the region of the back and side of the body between the lowest rib and the pelvis.

long-sightedness *n. see* hypermetropia.

loop *n.* **1.** a bend in a tubular organ, e.g. *Henle's loop in a kidney tubule. **2.** one of the patterns of dermal ridges in *fingerprints.

lorazepam *n.* a *tranquillizer used to relieve moderate or severe anxiety and tension and to treat insomnia. It is administered by mouth and may cause drowsiness, dizziness, blurred vision, and nausea. Trade name: **Ativan**.

lordosis *n.* inward curvature of the spine. A certain degree of lordosis is normal in the lumbar and cervical regions of the spine: loss of this is a sign of ankylosing *spondylitis. Exaggerated lordosis may occur in adolescence, through faulty posture or as a result of disease affecting the vertebrae and spinal muscles. *Compare* kyphosis.

lotion *n.* a medicinal solution for washing or bathing the external parts of the body. Lotions usually have a cooling, soothing, or antiseptic action.

loupe *n.* a small magnifying hand lens used for examining the front part of the eye. It is usually used with a pocket torch to provide illumination.

louse *n.* (*pl.* **lice**) a small wingless insect that is an external parasite of man. Lice attach themselves to hair and clothing using their well-developed legs and claws. Their flattened leathery bodies are resistant to crushing and their mouthparts are adapted for sucking blood. Lice thrive in overcrowded and unhygienic conditions and they may transmit disease. *See also* Pediculus, Phthirus.

lozenge *n.* a medicated tablet containing sugar. Lozenges should dissolve slowly in the mouth so that the medication is applied to the mouth and throat.

LSD *see* lysergic acid diethylamide.

lubb-dupp *n.* a representation of the normal heart sounds as heard through the stethoscope. Lubb (the first heart sound) coincides with closure of the mitral and tricuspid valves; dupp (the second heart sound) is due to closure of the aortic and pulmonary valves.

Ludwig's angina severe inflammation caused by infection of both sides of the floor of the mouth, resulting in massive swelling of the neck. If untreated, it may obstruct the airways, necessitating tracheostomy.

lues *n.* a serious infectious disease such as syphilis.

lumbago *n.* low backache, of any cause or description. Severe lumbago, of sudden onset while bending or lifting, can be due either to a slipped disc or to a strained muscle or ligament. When associated with *sciatica it is probably due to a slipped disc.

lumbar *adj.* relating to the loin.

lumbar puncture a procedure in which cerebrospinal fluid is withdrawn by means of a hollow needle inserted into the *subarachnoid space in the region of the lower back (usually between the third and fourth lumbar vertebrae). The fluid thus obtained is examined for diagnostic purposes. The procedure is usually without risk to the patient, but in patients with raised intracranial pressure it may be hazardous and the optic fundi must be examined for the presence of *papilloedema. *See also* Queckenstedt test.

lumbar vertebrae the five bones of the *backbone that are situated between the thoracic vertebrae and the sacrum, in the lower part of the back. They are the largest of the unfused vertebrae and have stout processes for attachment of the strong muscles of the lower back. *See also* vertebra.

lumbo- *prefix denoting* the loin; lumbar region.

lumbosacral *adj.* relating to part of the spine composed of the lumbar vertebrae and the sacrum.

lumen *n.* **1.** the space within a tubular or sac-like part, such as a blood vessel, the intestine, or the stomach. **2.** the *SI unit of luminous flux, equal to the amount of light emitted per second in unit solid angle of 1 steradian by a point source of 1 candela. Symbol: lm.

lunate bone a bone of the wrist (*see* carpus). It articulates with the capitate bone in front and with the radius and ulna behind.

lung

lung *n.* one of the pair of organs of
*respiration, situated in the chest cavity
on either side of the heart and enclosed
by a serous membrane (*see* pleura). The
lungs are fibrous elastic sacs that are
expanded and compressed by movements of the rib cage and diaphragm
during *breathing. They communicate
with the atmosphere through the *trachea, which opens into the pharynx.
The trachea divides into two bronchi
(*see* bronchus), which enter the lungs
and branch into *bronchioles. These
divide further and terminate in minute
air sacs (*see* alveolus), the sites of
gaseous exchange. (See illustration.)
Atmospheric oxygen is absorbed and
carbon dioxide from the blood of the
pulmonary capillaries is released into
the lungs; in each case down a concentration gradient (*see* pulmonary circulation). The total capacity of the lungs in
an adult male is about 5.5 litres, but
during normal breathing only about
500 ml of air is exchanged (*see also*
residual volume). Other functions of
the lung include water evaporation: an
important factor in the fluid balance
and heat regulation of the body.

lung cancer cancer arising in the
epithelium of the air passages (*bronchial cancer*) or lung. It is a very
common form of cancer, particularly in
Britain, and is strongly associated with
cigarette smoking and exposure to industrial air pollutants (including asbestos). There are often no symptoms in
the early stages of the disease, when
diagnosis is made on X-ray examination. Treatment includes surgical removal of the affected lobe or lung (20%
of cases are suitable for surgery), radiotherapy, and chemotherapy.

lunula *n.* the whitish crescent-shaped
area at the base of a *nail.

lupus *n.* any of several chronic skin
diseases. Used alone, lupus generally
refers to tuberculosis of the skin (*lupus
vulgaris). *See also* lupus erythematosus,
lupus verrucosus.

lupus erythematosus (LE) a chronic
inflammatory disease of connective tissue, affecting the skin and various

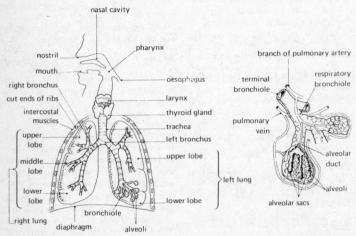

The lungs and main air passages, with details of the alveoli internal organs. Typically, there is a red scaly rash on the face, affecting the nose and cheeks; arthritis; and progressive damage to the kidneys. Often the heart, lungs, and brain are also affected by progressive attacks of inflammation followed by the formation of scar tissue (fibrosis). In a milder form of the disease only the skin is affected. LE is regarded as an *autoimmune disease and can be diagnosed by the presence of abnormal antibodies in the bloodstream, most easily detected by a test that reveals characteristic white blood cells (*LE cells*). The disease is treated with corticosteroids.

lupus verrucosus a tuberculous infection of the skin – commonly the arm or hand – typified by warty lesions. It occurs in those who have been reinfected with tuberculosis.

lupus vulgaris tuberculous infection of the skin, usually due to direct inoculation of the tuberculosis bacillus into the skin. This type of lupus often starts in childhood, with dark red patches on the nose or cheek. Unless treated lupus vulgaris spreads, ulcerates, and causes extensive scarring. Treatment is with antituberculous drugs.

lute *n.* (in dentistry) a thin layer of cement inserted into the minute space between a prepared tooth and a crown or inlay to hold it permanently in place.

lutein *n.* **1.** *see* xanthophyll. **2.** the yellow pigment of the corpus luteum.

luteinizing hormone (LH) a hormone (*see* gonadotrophin), synthesized and released by the anterior pituitary gland, that stimulates ovulation, *corpus luteum formation, progesterone synthesis by the ovary (*see also* menstrual cycle), and androgen synthesis by the interstitial cells of the testes. Also called: **interstitial cell stimulating hormone (ICSH)**.

luteo- *prefix denoting* **1.** yellow. **2.** the corpus luteum.

luteotrophic hormone (luteotrophin) *see* prolactin.

lux *n.* the *SI unit of intensity of illumination, equal to 1 lumen per square metre. This unit was formerly called the metre candle. Symbol: lx.

luxation *n. see* dislocation.

lyase *n.* one of a group of enzymes that catalyse the linking of groups by double bonds.

lycanthropy *n.* a very rare symptom of mental disorder in which an individual believes that he can change into a wolf.

lymph *n.* the fluid present within the vessels of the *lymphatic system. It consists of the fluid that bathes the tissues, which is derived from the blood and is drained by the lymphatic vessels. Lymph passes through a series of filters (*lymph nodes) and is ultimately returned to the bloodstream via the *thoracic duct. It is similar in composition to plasma, but contains less protein and some cells, mainly *lymphocytes.

lymphaden- (lymphadeno-) *prefix denoting* lymph node(s).

lymphadenectomy *n.* surgical removal of lymph nodes, an operation commonly performed when a cancer has invaded nodes in the drainage area of an organ infiltrated by a malignant growth.

lymphadenitis *n.* inflammation of lymph nodes, which become swollen, painful, and tender. Some cases may be chronic (e.g. tuberculous lymphadenitis) but most are acute and localized adjacent to an area of infection. The most commonly affected lymph nodes are those in the neck, in association with tonsillitis. The lymph nodes help to contain and combat the infection. Occasionally generalized lymphadenitis occurs as a result of virus infections. The treatment is that of the cause.

lymphadenoma *n.* an obsolete term for *lymphoma.

lymphagogue *n.* an agent that stimulates the secretion of lymph.

lymphangi- (lymphangio-) *prefix denoting* a lymphatic vessel.

lymphangiectasis *n.* dilatation of the lymphatic vessels, which is usually congenital and produces enlargement of various parts of the body (e.g. the leg in Milroy's disease). It may also be caused by obstruction of the lymphatic vessels (*see* lymphoedema).

lymphangiography *n.* X-ray examination of the lymphatic vessels and lymph nodes after a contrast medium has been injected into them (*see* angiography). Its main uses are in the investigation of the extent and spread of cancer of the lymphatic system and in the investigation of lymphoedema.

lymphangioma *n.* a localized collection of distended lymphatic vessels, which may result in a large cyst in the neck or armpit (*cystic hygroma*). This can be removed surgically.

lymphangiosarcoma *n.* a malignant tumour of the lymphatic vessels. It is most commonly seen in the chronically swollen (oedematous) arms of women who have had a mastectomy for breast cancer.

lymphangitis *n.* inflammation of the lymphatic vessels, which can be seen most commonly as red streaks in the skin adjacent to a focus of streptococcal infection. Occasionally a more chronic form results in *lymphoedema. The infected part is rested and the infection can be eliminated by an antibiotic (e.g. penicillin).

lymphatic 1. *n.* a lymphatic vessel. *See* lymphatic system. **2.** *adj.* relating to or transporting lymph.

lymphatic system a network of vessels that conveys electrolytes, water, pro-

teins, etc. – in the form of *lymph – from the tissue fluids to the bloodstream (see illustration). It consists of fine blind-ended lymphatic capillaries, which unite to form lymphatic vessels. At various points along the lymphatic vessels are *lymph nodes. Lymph drains into the capillaries and passes into the lymphatic vessels, which have valves to prevent backflow of lymph. The lymphatics lead to two large channels – the *thoracic duct* and the *right lymphatic duct* – which return the lymph to the bloodstream via the innominate veins.

The lymphatic system

lymph node one of a number of small swellings found at intervals along the lymphatic system. Groups of nodes are found in many parts of the body; for example, in the groin and armpit and behind the ear. They are composed of lymphoid tissue and act as filters for the lymph, preventing foreign particles from entering the bloodstream; they also produce lymphocytes.

lympho- *prefix denoting* lymph or the lymphatic system.

lymphoblast *n.* an abnormal cell present in the blood and blood-forming organs in a type of leukaemia (*lymphoblastic leukaemia*). It has a large nucleus with very scanty cytoplasm and was once thought to be the precursor of the lymphocyte. —**lymphoblastic** *adj.*

lymphocyte *n.* a variety of white blood cell (leucocyte), present also in the lymph nodes, spleen, thymus gland, gut wall, and bone marrow. With *Romanowsky stains, lymphocytes are seen to have dense nuclei with clear pale-blue cytoplasm. Lymphocytes with scanty cytoplasm are *small lymphocytes*; those with abundant cytoplasm are *large lymphocytes*. There are normally $1.5–4.0 \times 10^9$ lymphocytes per litre of blood. They are involved in *immunity and can be subdivided into *B-lymphocytes*, which produce antibodies, and *T-lymphocytes*, which are involved in graft rejection, etc. —**lymphocytic** *adj.*

lymphocytopenia *n. see* lymphopenia.

lymphocytosis *n.* an increase in the number of *lymphocytes in the blood. Lymphocytosis may occur in a wide variety of diseases, including chronic lymphocytic *leukaemia and infections due to viruses.

lymphoedema *n.* an accumulation of lymph in the tissues, producing swelling. It may be due to a congenital abnormality of the lymphatic vessels or result from obstruction of the lymphatic vessels by a tumour, parasites, in-

flammation, or injury. The legs are most often affected. Treatment consists of elastic support, by stockings or bandages, and diuretic drugs. A variety of surgical procedures have been devised but with little success.

lymphogranuloma venereum a venereal disease that is caused by a virus and is most common in tropical regions. An initial lesion on the genitals is followed by swelling and inflammation of the lymph nodes in the groin; the lymph vessels in the genital region may become blocked, causing thickening of the skin of that area. Early treatment with sulphonamides or tetracyclines is usually effective.

lymphography *n.* the technique of injecting *radio-opaque material into the lymphatic system in a particular region of the body so that X-ray photographs may be taken of the lymph vessels and nodes. Lymphography can indicate the presence of tumours in the lymphatic system.

lymphoid tissue a tissue responsible for the production of lymphocytes and antibodies. It occurs as discrete organs, in the form of the lymph nodes, tonsils, thymus, and spleen, and also as diffuse groups of cells not separated from surrounding tissue.

lymphoma *n.* any malignant tumour of lymph nodes, excluding Hodgkin's disease. There is a broad spectrum of malignancy, with prognosis ranging from a few months to many years. The patient usually shows evidence of multiple enlarged lymph nodes and may have constitutional symptoms such as weight loss, fever, and sweating. Disease is usually widespread, but in some cases is confined to a single area, such as the tonsil. Treatment is with drugs such as chlorambucil or combinations of cyclophosphamide, vincristine and prednisone, sometimes with the addition of doxorubicin and/or bleomycin; response to these drugs is often dramatic. Localized disease may be treated with radiotherapy followed by drugs.

lymphopenia (lymphocytopenia) *n.* a decrease in the number of *lymphocytes in the blood, which may occur in a wide variety of diseases.

lymphopoiesis *n.* the process of the production of *lymphocytes, which occurs in the *bone marrow as well as in the lymph nodes, spleen, thymus gland, and gut wall. The precursor cell from which lymphocytes are derived has not yet been identified.

lymphorrhagia *n.* the escape of the lymph from lymphatic vessels that have been injured.

lymphosarcoma *n.* an old term for certain types of *lymphoma. On the whole these tend to be the types with a better prognosis, and some may not need treatment for months or years after the patient has first been examined.

lymphuria *n.* the presence in the urine of lymph.

lynoestrenol *n.* a synthetic female sex hormone (*see* progestogen) used mainly in *oral contraceptives, together with an oestrogen. It is also used to treat menstrual disorders.

lys- (lysi-, lyso-) *prefix denoting* lysis; dissolution.

lysergic acid diethylamide (LSD) a *psychedelic drug that is also a *hallucinogen. It has been used to aid treatment of psychological disorders. Side-effects include digestive upsets, dizziness, tingling, anxiety, sweating, dilated pupils, muscle incoordination and tremor. Alterations in sight, hearing and other senses occur, psychotic effects, depression, and confusion are common, and tolerance to the drug develops rapidly. Because of these toxic effects, LSD is used only to treat severe cases.

lysin *n.* a protein component in the blood that is capable of bringing about the destruction (lysis) of whole cells. Names are given to varieties of lysin with different targets; for example, *haemolysin* attacks red blood cells; *leucolysin* white cells; and a *bacteriolysin* bacterial cells.

lysine *n.* an *essential amino acid. *See also* amino acid.

lysis *n.* the destruction of cells through damage or rupture of the plasma membrane, allowing escape of the cell contents. *See also* autolysis, lysozyme.

-lysis *suffix denoting* **1.** lysis; dissolution. **2.** remission of symptoms.

lysogenic *adj.* producing *lysis.

lysogeny *n.* an interaction between a *bacteriophage and its host in which a latent form of the phage (*prophage*) exists within the bacterial cell, which is not destroyed. Under certain conditions (e.g. irradiation of the bacterium) the phage can develop into an active form, which reproduces itself and eventually destroys the bacterial cell.

lysosome *n.* a particle in the cytoplasm of cells that contains enzymes responsible for breaking down substances in the cell and is bounded by a single membrane. Lysosomes are especially abundant in liver and kidney cells. Foreign particles (e.g. bacteria) taken into the cell are broken down by the enzymes of the lysosomes. When the cell dies, these enzymes are released to break down the cell's components.

lysozyme *n.* an enzyme found in tears and egg white. It catalyses the destruction of the cell walls of certain bacteria. Bacterial cells that are attacked by lysozyme are said to have been *lysed*.

M

maceration *n.* **1.** the softening of a solid by leaving it immersed in a liquid. **2.** (in obstetrics) the natural breakdown of a dead fetus within the womb.

macr- (macro-) *prefix denoting* large size. Example: *macrencephaly* (abnormally enlarged brain).

macrocephaly (megalocephaly) *n.* abnormal largeness of the head in relation to the rest of the body. *Compare* microcephaly.

macrocheilia *n.* hypertrophy of the lips: a congenital condition in which the lips are abnormally large. *Compare* microcheilia.

macrocyte (megalocyte) *n.* an abnormally large red blood cell (*erythrocyte). *See also* macrocytosis. —**macrocytic** *adj.*

macrocytosis *n.* the presence of abnormally large red cells (*macrocytes*) in the blood. Macrocytosis is a feature of certain anaemias (*macrocytic anaemias*), including those due to deficiency of vitamin B_{12} or folic acid, and also of anaemias in which there is an increase in the rate of red cell production.

macrodactyly *n.* abnormally large size of one or more of the fingers or toes.

macrodontia *n.* a condition in which the teeth are unusually large.

macrogamete *n.* the nonmotile female sex cell of the malarial parasite (*Plasmodium*) and other single-celled animals (*see* Protozoa). The macrogamete is similar to the ovum of higher animal groups and larger than the male sex cell (*see* microgamete).

macrogametocyte *n.* a cell that undergoes meiosis to form mature female sex cells (macrogametes) of the malarial parasite (*Plasmodium*). Macrogametocytes are found in the blood of man but must be ingested by a mosquito before developing into macrogametes.

macrogenitosoma *n.* excessive bodily growth with marked enlargement of the genitalia. *Macrogenitosoma praecox* is a variant occurring in early childhood.

macroglia *n.* one of the two basic classes of *glia (the non-nervous cells of the central nervous system), divided into *astrocytes and *oligodendrocytes. *Compare* microglia.

macroglobulin (immunoglobulin M) *n.* a protein of the globulin series that is present in the blood and functions as an antibody, forming an effective first-line defence against bacteria in the bloodstream. *See also* immunoglobulin.

macroglobulinaemia *n.* the presence in the blood of an abnormal form of immunoglobulin-M (*see* macroglobulin), produced by a tumour of the lymphocytes.

macroglossia *n.* an abnormally large tongue. It may be due to a congenital defect, such as thyroid deficiency (cretinism); to infiltration of the tongue with *amyloid or a tumour; or to obstruction of the lymph vessels.

macrognathia *n.* marked overgrowth of one jaw relative to the growth of the other.

macromastia *n.* abnormally large size of the breasts.

macromelia *n.* abnormally large size of the arms or legs. *Compare* micromelia.

macronormoblast *n.* an abnormal form of any of the cells (*normoblasts) that form a series of precursors of red blood cells. Macronormoblasts are un-

macrophage

usually large but have normal nuclei (*compare* megaloblast); they are seen in certain anaemias in which red cell production is impaired.

macrophage (clasmocyte) *n.* a large scavenger cell (a *phagocyte) present in connective tissue and many major organs and tissues, including the bone marrow, spleen, *lymph nodes, liver (*see* Kuppfer's cells), and the central nervous system (*see* microglia). They are closely related to *monocytes. *Fixed macrophages* (*histiocytes*) are stationary within connective tissue; *free macrophages* wander between cells and aggregate at focal sites of infection, where they remove bacteria or other foreign bodies from blood or tissues. *See also* reticuloendothelial system.

macropolycyte *n.* an abnormal form of *neutrophil (a type of white blood cell) the nucleus of which has an excessively large number of lobes. Macropolycytes are seen in vitamin B_{12} or folic acid deficiency.

macropsia *n.* a condition in which objects appear larger than they really are. It is usually due to disease of the retina affecting the *macula but may also occur in spasm of *accommodation and in some brain disorders.

macroscopic *adj.* visible to the naked eye. *Compare* microscopic.

macula *n.* (*pl.* **maculae**) **1.** a small anatomical area that is distinguishable from the surrounding tissue. The *macula lutea* is the yellow spot on the retina at the back of the eye, which surrounds the greatest concentration of cones (*see* fovea). Maculae occur in the saccule and utricle of the inner ear (see illustration). Tilting of the head causes the otoliths to bend the hair cells, which send impulses to the brain via the vestibular nerve. *See also* labyrinth. **2.** *see* macule.

A macula of the inner ear

macule (macula) *n.* a spot, discoloration, or thickening of the skin that forms a distinct area from the surrounding normal surface. *Compare* papule.

maculopapular *adj.* describing a rash that consists of both *macules and *papules.

madarosis *n.* **1.** a congenital deficiency of the eyelashes and eyebrows, which are sometimes absent altogether. **2.** a deficiency of the eyelashes alone, caused by chronic ulcerative *blepharitis.

Madura foot an infection of the tissues and bones of the foot producing chronic inflammation (mycetoma), occurring in the tropics. It is caused by various filamentous fungi (e.g. *Madurella*) and certain bacteria of the genera *Nocardia* and *Streptomyces*. Medical name: **maduromycosis**.

Madurella *n.* a genus of widely distributed fungi. The species *M. grisea* and *M. mycetomi* cause the tropical infection *Madura foot.

maduromycosis *n. see* Madura foot.

magenta *n. see* fuchsin.

maggot *n.* the wormlike larva of a fly, which occasionally infests human tissues (*see* myiasis). Formerly maggots were, in some cases, allowed to feed on dead and rotting tissues and so assist in the cleaning and healing of serious wounds.

magnesium *n.* a metallic element essential to life. The body of an average adult contains about 25 g of magnesium, concentrated mostly in the bones. Magnesium is necessary for the proper functioning of muscle and nervous tissue. It is required as a *cofactor for approximately 90 enzymes. A good source of magnesium is green leafy vegetables.

magnesium carbonate a weak *antacid used to relieve indigestion and also pain due to stomach and duodenal ulcers; it is also used as a mild laxative. It is usually given with other compounds in mixtures, powders, and tablets.

magnesium hydroxide a magnesium salt with effects and uses similar to those of *magnesium carbonate. Trade name: **Milk of Magnesia**.

magnesium sulphate a magnesium salt given in mixtures or enemas to treat constipation (*see* laxative). It is also administered by injection to treat magnesium deficiency.

magnesium trisilicate a compound of magnesium with antacid and absorbent properties, used in the treatment of peptic ulcers and other digestive disorders.

mal *n.* illness or disease. *See also* grand mal, petit mal.

mal- *prefix denoting* disease, disorder, or abnormality.

malabsorption *n.* a state in which absorption of one or more substances by the small intestine is reduced. It commonly affects fat (causing *steatorrhoea), vitamins (such as B_{12}, folic acid, vitamin D, and vitamin K), *electrolytes (such as calcium, potassium), iron, and amino acids. Symptoms (depending on the substances involved) include weight loss, diarrhoea, anaemia, swelling (oedema), and vitamin deficiencies. The commonest causes are *coeliac disease, *pancreatitis, *cystic fibrosis, *stagnant-loop syndrome, or surgical removal of a length of small intestine.

malacia *n.* abnormal softening of a part, organ, or tissue, such as bone (*see* osteomalacia).

-malacia *suffix denoting* abnormal softening of a tissue. Example: *keratomalacia* (of the cornea).

malaise *n.* a general feeling of being unwell. The feeling may be accompanied by identifiable physical discomfort and may indicate the presence of disease.

malar bone *see* zygomatic bone.

malaria (ague, marsh fever, periodic fever, paludism) *n.* an infectious disease due to the presence of parasitic protozoa of the genus *Plasmodium* (*P. falciparum*, *P. malariae*, *P. ovale*, or *P. vivax*) within the red blood cells. The disease is transmitted by the *Anopheles* mosquito and is confined mainly to tropical and subtropical areas.
Parasites in the blood of an infected person are taken into the stomach of the mosquito as it feeds. Here they multiply and then invade the salivary glands. When the mosquito bites an individual, parasites are injected into the bloodstream and migrate to the liver and other organs, where they multiply. After an incubation period varying from 12 days (*P. falciparum*) to 10 months (some varieties of *P. vivax*), parasites return to the bloodstream and invade the red blood cells. Rapid multiplication of the parasites results in destruction of the red cells and the release of more parasites capable of infecting other red cells. This causes a short bout of shivering, fever, and sweating, and the loss of healthy red cells results in anaemia. When the next batch of parasites is released symptoms reappear. The interval between fever

attacks varies in different types of malaria: in *quartan malaria* (or *fever*), caused by *P. malariae*, it is three days; in *tertian malaria* (*P. ovale* or *P. vivax*) two days; and in *malignant tertian* (or *quotidian*) *malaria* (*P. falciparum*) – the most severe kind – from a few hours to two days (*see also* blackwater fever). Preventative and curative treatment relies on such drugs as *chloroquine, *mepacrine, and *proguanil.

Malassezia *n.* a genus of fungi producing superficial infections of the skin. The species *M. furfur* is the causative organism of a form of ringworm.

malformation *n.* any variation from the normal physical structure, due either to congenital or developmental defects or to disease or injury.

malignant *adj.* **1.** describing a tumour that invades and destroys the tissue in which it originates and can spread to other sites in the body via the bloodstream and lymphatic system. If untreated such tumours cause progressive deterioration and death. *See* cancer. **2.** describing any disorder that becomes progressively worse if untreated. *Compare* benign.

malingering *n.* pretending to be ill, usually in order to avoid work or gain attention. It may be a sign of mental disorder (*see* Munchhausen's syndrome).

malleolus *n.* either of the two protuberances on each side of the ankle: the *lateral malleolus* at the lower end of the *fibula or the *medial malleolus* at the lower end of the *tibia.

malleus *n.* a hammer-shaped bone in the middle *ear that articulates with the incus and is attached to the eardrum. *See* ossicle.

Mallory's triple stain a histological stain consisting of water-soluble aniline blue or methyl blue, orange G, and oxalic acid. Before the stain is applied the tissue is mordanted, then treated with acid fuchsin and phosphomolybdic acid. Nuclei stain red, muscle red to orange, nervous tissue lilac, collagen dark blue, and mucus and connective tissue become blue.

malnutrition *n.* the condition caused by an improper balance between what an individual eats and what he requires to maintain health. This can result from eating too little (*subnutrition* or *starvation*) but may also imply dietary excess or an incorrect balance of basic foodstuffs such as protein, fat, and carbohydrate. A deficiency (or excess) of one or more minerals, vitamins, or other essential ingredients may arise from *malabsorption of digested food or metabolic malfunction of one or more parts of the body as well as from an unbalanced diet.

malocclusion *n.* the condition in which the upper and lower teeth are abnormally related.

Malpighian body the part of a *nephron comprising the blood capillaries of the glomerulus and its surrounding Bowman's capsule.

Malpighian layer the stratum germinativum: one of the layers of the *epidermis.

malposition *n.* abnormal location of any part of the body.

malpractice *n.* professional misconduct: treatment falling short of the standards of skill and care that can reasonably be expected from a qualified medical practitioner.

malpresentation *n.* arrival of the fetus at the opening from the womb other than in the normal head-first position (*see* presentation). Malpresentation is likely to make birth difficult and may necessitate delivery by *Caesarean section.

malt *n.* a mixture of carbohydrates, predominantly maltose, produced by the breakdown of starch contained in barley or wheat grains. The cereal grain is allowed to germinate and the malt is extracted with hot water. Malt is used for brewing and distilling; it has been used as a source of nutrients in wasting diseases.

Malta fever *see* brucellosis.

maltase *n.* an enzyme, present in saliva and pancreatic juice, that converts maltose into glucose during digestion.

maltose *n.* a sugar consisting of two molecules of glucose. Maltose is formed from the digestion of starch and glycogen and is found in germinating cereal seeds. .

malunion *n.* deformity of a bone resulting from *union of a fracture in which the bone ends are poorly aligned. Arthritis of adjoining joints may develop as a complication later. *Osteotomy may be needed to correct the deformity and prevent the complication.

mamilla *n. see* nipple.

mamillary bodies two paired rounded swellings in the floor of the *hypothalamus, immediately behind the pituitary gland.

mamma *n. see* breast.

mammary gland the milk-producing gland of female mammals. *See* breast.

mammography *n.* the making of X-ray or infra-red ray photographs of the breast: used for the early detection of abnormal growths. *See also* radiography, thermography.

mammoplasty *n.* plastic surgery of the breasts, in order to alter their shape or increase or decrease their size. In the case of sagging breasts skin and glandular tissue are removed and the remaining breast tissue is fixed in the normal position. When the breasts are too small, a *prosthesis may be inserted to improve the contour.

mammothermography *n.* the technique of examining the breasts for the presence of tumours or other abnormalities by *thermography.

M-AMSA (amsacrine) *n.* a *cytotoxic drug undergoing evaluation in the treatment of malignant disease. Side-effects include marrow suppression.

mancinism *n.* the condition of being left-handed.

mandelic acid a drug that prevents bacterial growth and was formerly used to treat infections of the urinary system (it has now largely been replaced by antibiotics). Mandelic acid is administered by mouth.

mandible *n.* the lower jawbone. It consists of a horseshoe-shaped *body*, the upper surface of which bears the lower teeth (*see* alveolus (def. 2)), and two vertical parts (*rami*). Each ramus divides into a *condyle* and a *coronoid process. The condyle articulates with the temporal bone of the cranium to form the *temporomandibular joint* (a hinge joint). *See also* maxilla, skull. —**mandibular** *adj.*

manganese *n.* a greyish metallic element, the oxide of which, when inhaled by miners in under-ventilated mines, causes brain damage and symptoms very similar to those of *parkinsonism.

mania *n.* a state of mind characterized by excessive cheerfulness and increased activity. The mood is euphoric and changes rapidly to irritability. Thought and speech are rapid to the point of incoherence and the connections between ideas may be impossible to follow. Behaviour is overactive, extravagant, overbearing, and sometimes violent. Judgment is impaired, and therefore the sufferer may damage his own interests. There may be grandiose delusions. Treatment is usually with drugs such as lithium or phenothiazines. Hospital admission is frequently necessary. Lithium can also be taken to prevent relapses. *See* manic-depressive psychosis. —**manic** *adj.*

-mania *suffix denoting* obsession, compulsion, or exaggerated feeling for. Example: *pyromania* (for starting fires).

manic-depressive psychosis a severe mental illness causing repeated episodes of *depression, *mania, or both. These episodes can be precipitated by upsetting events but are out of proportion to these causes. Sometimes chronic depression or chronic mania can result. There is a genetically inherited predisposition to the illness. Treatment is with *phenothiazine drugs for mania and with *antidepressant drugs or *electroconvulsive therapy for depression. *Lithium can prevent or reduce the frequency and severity of attacks, and the sufferer is usually well in the intervals between them.

manikin *n. see* homunculus.

manipulation *n.* the use of the hands to produce a desired movement or therapeutic effect in part of the body. Physiotherapists and osteopaths use manipulation to restore normal working to stiff joints.

mannitol *n.* a *diuretic administered by injection to supplement other diuretics in the treatment of fluid retention (oedema), to treat some kidney disorders, and to relieve pressure in brain injuries. Headache, chest pain, and dry mouth may occur following injection.

mannomustine *n.* a drug that prevents the growth of cancer cells and is used in the treatment of some types of leukaemia and other cancers. It is administered by injection or by mouth and often causes nausea and vomiting. Trade name: **Degranol**.

Mann-Whitney U test *see* significance.

manometer *n.* a device for measuring pressure in a gas. A manometer often consists of a U-tube containing mer-

cury, water, or other liquid, open at one end and exposed to the gas under pressure at the other end. The pressure can be read directly from a graduated scale. *See also* sphygmomanometer.

manpower committee (in Britain) a special committee established regionally (*Regional Manpower Committee*) and centrally (*Central Manpower Committee*) by the Department of Health and Social Security to advise on medical staffing by specialty and to consider the relative numbers of consultants and training grades of doctors in the National Health Service.

Manpower Services Commission *see* Employment Service Division.

Mantoux test *see* tuberculin.

manubrium *n.* (*pl.* **manubria**) **1.** the upper section of the breastbone (*see* sternum). It articulates with the clavicles and the first costal cartilage; the second costal cartilage articulates at the junction between the manubrium and body of the sternum. **2.** the handle-like part of the *malleus (an ear ossicle), attached to the eardrum. —**manubrial** *adj.*

MAO *see* monoamine oxidase.

MAO inhibitor a drug that prevents the activity of the enzyme *monoamine oxidase (MAO) in brain tissue and therefore affects mood. MAO inhibitors include *iproniazid, isocarboxacid, *phenelzine, and *tranylcypromine. They are *antidepressants, whose use is now restricted because of the severity of their side-effects. These include interactions with other drugs (e.g. ephedrine, amphetamine) and foods containing *tyramine (e.g. cheese) to produce a sudden increase in blood pressure.

maple syrup urine disease an inborn defect of amino acid metabolism causing an excess of valine, leucine, isoleucine, and alloisoleucine in the urine, which has an odour like maple syrup.

Untreated it leads to mental retardation and death in infancy.

maprotiline *n.* a drug used to treat all types of depression, including that associated with anxiety (*see* antidepressant). It is administered by mouth and may cause drowsiness, dizziness, and tremor. Trade name: **Ludiomil**.

marasmus *n.* severe wasting in infants, when body weight is below 75% of that expected for age. The infant looks 'old', pallid, apathetic, lacks skin fat, and has subnormal temperature. The condition may be due to *malabsorption, wrong feeding, metabolic disorders, repeated vomiting, diarrhoea, severe disease of the heart, lungs, kidneys, or urinary tract, or chronic bacterial or parasitic disease (especially in tropical climates). Maternal rejection of an infant may cause marasmus through undereating. Acute infection may precipitate death. Treatment depends on the underlying cause, but initially very gentle nursing and the provision of nourishment and fluids by gradual steps is appropriate for all.

marble-bone disease *see* osteopetrosis.

Marburg disease (green monkey disease) a virus disease of vervet (green) monkeys transmitted to man by contact (usually in laboratories) with blood or tissues from an infected animal. Symptoms include fever, malaise, severe headache, vomiting, diarrhoea and bleeding from mucous membranes in the mouth and elsewhere. Treatment with antiserum and measures to reduce the bleeding are sometimes effective.

Marfan's syndrome an inherited disorder of connective tissue characterized by excessive height, abnormally long and slender fingers and toes (*arachnodactyly*), heart defects, and partial dislocation of the lenses of the eyes.

marihuana *n. see* cannabis.

marrow *n. see* bone marrow.

marsupialization *n.* an operative technique for curing a cyst. The cyst is opened, its contents removed, and the edges then stitched to the skin incision. The wound is kept open until it has healed by *granulation.

Marzine *n. see* cyclizine.

masculinization *n.* development of excess body and facial hair, deepening of the voice, and increase in muscle bulk (secondary male sexual characteristics) in a female due to a hormone disorder or to hormone therapy. *See also* virilism, virilization.

masochism *n.* sexual pleasure derived from the experience of pain. The word is sometimes used loosely for all forms of behaviour that lead to pain or humiliation. *See* perversion. —**masochist** *n.* —**masochistic** *adj.*

massage *n.* manipulation of the soft tissues of the body with the hands. Massage is used to improve circulation, reduce oedema where present, prevent *adhesions in tissues after injury, reduce muscular spasm, and improve the tone of muscles. *See also* effleurage, petrissage, tapotement.

masseter *n.* a thick muscle in the cheek extending from the zygomatic arch to the outer corner of the mandible. It is important for mastication and acts by closing the jaws.

mast- (masto-) *prefix denoting* the breast.

mastalgia *n.* pain in the breast.

mastatrophy (mastatrophia) *n.* reduction in size (atrophy) of the breasts.

mast cell a large cell in *connective tissue with many coarse cytoplasmic granules. These granules contain the chemicals *heparin, *histamine, and *serotonin, which are released during inflammation and allergic responses.

mastectomy

mastectomy *n.* surgical removal of a breast. If the operation is to combat cancer a *radical mastectomy* is performed: as well as the breast itself, the lymph nodes in the nearest armpit and the muscles linking the upper part of the chest with the shoulder are also removed, in case the cancer has spread to them.

mastication *n.* the process of chewing food.

mastitis *n.* inflammation of the breast, usually caused by bacterial infection through damaged nipples. It most often occurs as acute *puerperal mastitis*, which develops during the period of breast-feeding, about a month after childbirth, and sometimes involves the discharge of pus. Chronic *cystic mastitis* has a different cause and does not involve inflammation. The breast feels lumpy due to the presence of cysts, and the condition is thought to be caused by hormone imbalance.

mastoid *n.* the *mastoid process of the temporal bone. *See also* mastoiditis.

mastoidectomy *n.* an operation to remove some or all of the air cells in the bone behind the ear (the *mastoid process of the temporal bone) when they have become infected (*see* mastoiditis).

mastoiditis *n.* inflammation of the *mastoid process behind the ear and of the air space (*mastoid antrum*) connecting it to the cavity of the middle ear. It is usually caused by bacterial infection that spreads from the middle ear (*see* otitis (media)). Usually the infection responds to antibiotics, but surgery (*see* mastoidectomy) may be required in severe cases.

mastoidotomy *n.* surgical incision of the mastoid bone, usually done to treat infection (*see* mastoidectomy).

mastoid process a nipple-shaped process on the *temporal bone that extends downward and forward behind the ear canal and is the point of attachment of several neck muscles. It contains many air spaces (*mastoid cells*), which communicate with the cavity of the middle ear via an air-filled channel, the *mastoid antrum*. This provides a possible route for the spread of infection from the middle ear (*see* mastoiditis).

mastoplasia (mazoplasia) *n.* increase in the size of the breasts because of multiplication and growth (*hyperplasia) of normal mammary gland cells.

mastoptosis *n.* sagging of the breasts.

masturbation *n.* physical stimulation of the male or female external genital organs in order to produce sexual pleasure, which may result in orgasm.

matched pair study *see* case control study.

materia medica the study of drugs used in medicine, including *pharmacognosy, *pharmacy, *pharmacology, and therapeutics.

maternal mortality rate the number of deaths due to complications of pregnancy, childbirth, and the puerperium expressed as a proportion of all births (i.e. including *stillbirths). Formerly the rate was expressed per 1000 births but with the low levels currently reported it is customary to use a base of a 100,000 births. Concern with maternal mortality resulted in Britain in a special confidential enquiry being held into every such death to try and pinpoint the possible shortfall in resources or care.

matrix *n.* the substance of a tissue or organ in which more specialized structures are embedded; for example, the ground substance of connective tissue.

matrix band a flexible strip that is placed round a tooth to restore a wall, thus simplifying insertion of a dental filling.

maturation *n.* the process of attaining full development. The term is applied particularly to the development of mature germ cells (ova and sperm).

maxilla *n.* (*pl.* **maxillae** or **maxillas**) loosely, the upper jaw, which bears the upper teeth. Strictly, the maxilla is one of a pair of bones that partly form the upper jaw, the outer walls of the maxillary sinus, and the floor of the orbit. *See also* mandible, skull. —**maxillary** *adj.*

maxillary sinus (maxillary antrum) *see* paranasal sinuses.

maxillofacial *adj.* describing or relating to the region of the face, jaws, and related structures.

maxwell *n.* a unit of magnetic flux equal to a flux of 1 gauss per square centimetre.

mazindol *n.* a drug that reduces the appetite and is used in the treatment of obesity. It is administered by mouth and may cause constipation, dry mouth, and insomnia. Trade name: **Teronac**.

McBurney's point the point on the abdomen that overlies the anatomical position of the appendix and is the site of maximum tenderness in acute appendicitis. It lies one-third of the way along a line drawn from the anterior superior iliac spine (the projecting part of the hipbone) to the umbilicus.

meals on wheels *see* social services.

mean (arithmetic mean) *n.* the average of a group of observations calculated by adding their values and dividing by the number in the group. When one or more observations are substantially different from the rest, which can influence the arithmetic mean unduly, it is preferable to use the *geometric mean* (a similar calculation based on the logarithmic values of the observations) or – more commonly – the *median* (the middle observation of the series arranged in ascending order). A further method of obtaining an average value of a group is to identify the *mode* – the observation (or group of observations when these occur as a continuous quantitative *variable) that occurs most often in the series.

measles *n.* a highly infectious virus disease that tends to appear in epidemics every 2–3 years and mainly affects children. After an incubation period of 8–15 days, symptoms resembling those of a cold develop accompanied by a high fever. Small red spots with white centres (*Koplik's spots*) may appear on the inside of the cheeks. On the third to fifth day a blotchy slightly elevated pink rash develops, first behind the ears then on the face and elsewhere; it lasts 3–5 days. The patient is infectious throughout this period. In most cases the symptoms soon subside but patients are susceptible to pneumonia and middle ear infections. Complete recovery may take 2–4 weeks. Vaccination against measles provides effective immunity. Medical names: **rubeola**, **morbilli**.

meat- (meato-) *prefix denoting* a meatus. Example: *meatotomy* (incision into the urethral meatus).

meatus *n.* (in anatomy) a passage or opening. The *external auditory meatus* is the passage leading from the pinna of the outer *ear to the eardrum. A *nasal meatus* is one of three groovelike parts of the nasal cavity beneath each of the nasal conchae. The *urethral meatus* is the external opening of the urethra.

mecamylamine *n.* a drug used to lower high blood pressure. It is administered by mouth and may cause dizziness, blurred vision, digestive upsets, and dry mouth. Trade name: **Inversine**.

mechanoreceptor *n.* a group of cells that respond to mechanical distortion, such as that caused by stretching or compressing a tissue, by generating a nerve impulse in a sensory nerve (*see* receptor). Touch receptors, *proprioceptors, and the receptors for hearing and balance all belong to this class.

mechanotherapy *n.* the use of mechanical equipment during physiotherapy to produce regularly repeated movements in part of the body. This is done to improve the functioning of muscles and joints.

Meckel's cartilage a cartilaginous bar in the fetus around which the *mandible develops. Part of Meckel's cartilage develops into the malleus (an ear ossicle) in the adult.

Meckel's diverticulum *see* diverticulum.

meclozine *n.* an *antihistamine drug used mainly to prevent and treat nausea and vomiting, particularly in travel sickness, and also to relieve allergic reactions. It is administered by mouth.

meconism *n.* poisoning from the effects of eating or smoking *opium or the products derived from it, especially *morphine.

meconium *n.* the first stools of a newborn baby, which are sticky and dark green and composed of cellular debris, mucus, and bile pigments. The presence of meconium in the amniotic fluid during labour indicates fetal distress. *See also* (meconium) ileus.

media (tunica media) *n.* **1.** the middle layer of the wall of a *vein or *artery. It is the thickest of the three layers, being composed of elastic fibres and smooth muscle fibres in alternating layers. **2.** the middle layer of various other organs or parts.

medial *adj.* relating to or situated in the central region of an organ, tissue, or the body.

median *adj.* **1.** (in anatomy) situated in or towards the plane that divides the

body into right and left halves. **2.** (in statistics) *see* mean.

mediastinitis *n.* inflammation of the midline partition of the chest cavity (mediastinum), usually complicating a rupture of the oesophagus (gullet).

mediastinum *n.* the space in the thorax (chest cavity) between the two pleural sacs. The mediastinum contains the heart, aorta, trachea, oesophagus, and thymus gland and is divided into anterior, middle, posterior, and superior regions.

medical *adj.* **1.** of or relating to medicine, the diagnosis, treatment and prevention of disease. **2.** of or relating to conditions that require the attention of a physician rather than a surgeon. For example, a *medical ward* accommodates patients with such conditions.

medical certificate a certificate stating a doctor's diagnosis of a patient's medical condition, disability, or fitness to work.

medical committee 1. (in a hospital) a group of doctors of consultant grade (some or all of the consultants on the hospital staff) who give medical viewpoints on affairs concerned with overall policies on patient care, resource allocation, and the running of the hospital. Representatives of other hospital professions (nursing, administration, planning, and junior doctors) are usually in attendance. It is generally subdivided into specialist subgroups known colloquially as the *Cogwheel divisions*, representing the broad divisions of hospital practice (medical, surgical, paediatric, etc.). Usually the chairmen of each Cogwheel division form an executive committee for day-to-day decisions that are ratified at less frequent (quarterly) meetings of the medical committee. **2.** (local) (in Britain) a group of representatives of the general practitioners under contract with a single *Family Practitioner Committee. The members act as spokesmen for the local practitioners, by whom they are elected. Similar arrangements and responsibilities apply for the *local dental committee*, *local pharmaceutical committee*, and the *local optical committee*. **3.** (in Britain) a group of representative specialists and general practitioners who serve as medical advisors and spokesmen to a District or Regional Health Authority (*District Medical Committee* or *Regional Medical Committee*). *See also* National Health Service.

medical jurisprudence the study or practice of the legal aspects of medicine. *See* forensic medicine.

Medical Officer of Health formerly, the chief health executive of local government. *See* community physician.

medical social worker a person with some medical training, employed to assist patients with domestic problems that may arise through illness.

medicated *adj.* containing a medicinal drug: applied to lotions, soaps, sweets, etc.

medication *n.* **1.** a substance administered by mouth, applied to the body, or introduced into the body for the purpose of treatment. Medicated dressings are applied to wounds to prevent infection and allow normal healing. *See also* premedication. **2.** treatment of a patient using drugs.

medicine *n.* **1.** the science or practice of the diagnosis, treatment, and prevention of disease. **2.** the science or practice of nonsurgical methods of treating disease. **3.** any drug or preparation used for the treatment or prevention of disease, particularly a preparation that is taken by mouth.

medicochirurgical *adj.* of or describing matters that are related to both medicine and surgery. A medicochirurgical disorder is one that calls for treatment by both a physician and a surgeon.

Mediterranean fever 1. *see* brucellosis. **2.** *see* polyserositis.

medium *n.* **1.** any substance, usually a broth, agar, or gelatin, used for the *culture of microorganisms or tissue cells. An *assay medium* is used to determine the concentration of a growth factor or chemical by measuring the amount of growth it produces in a particular microorganism; all other nutrients are present in amounts adequate for growth. **2.** *see* contrast medium.

medroxyprogesterone *n.* a synthetic female sex hormone (*see* progestogen) used to treat menstrual disorders, including amenorrhoea, to prevent miscarriage, and (in combination with an oestrogen) in *oral contraceptives. It is administered by mouth or injection. Trade name: **Provera**.

medulla *n.* **1.** the inner region of any organ or tissue when it is distinguishable from the outer region (the cortex), particularly the inner part of the kidney, adrenal glands, or lymph nodes. **2.** *see* medulla oblongata. **3.** the *myelin layer of certain nerve fibres. —**medullary** *adj.*

medulla oblongata (myelencephalon) the extension within the skull of the upper end of the spinal cord, forming the lowest part of the *brainstem. Besides forming the major pathway for nerve impulses entering and leaving the skull, the medulla contains centres that are responsible for the regulation of the heart and blood vessels, respiration, salivation, and swallowing. *Cranial nerves VI–XII leave the brain in this region.

medullated (myelinated) nerve fibre any nerve fibre that has a sheath of *myelin surrounding and insulating its axon.

medulloblastoma *n.* a *cerebral tumour that occurs during childhood. It is derived from cells that have the apparent potential to mature into neurones. The medulloblastoma usually develops adjacent to the fourth ventricle. It causes an unsteady gait and shaky limb movements. Obstruction to the flow of cerebrospinal fluid causes *hydrocephalus. The tumour is sensitive to radiotherapy.

mefenamic acid an *analgesic that also reduces inflammation and fever and is used to treat headache, toothache, rheumatic pain, and similar conditions. It is administered by mouth; side-effects include digestive upsets, drowsiness, and skin rashes. Trade name: **Ponstan**.

mega- *prefix denoting* 1. large size, or abnormal enlargement or distention. Example: *megacaecum* (of the caecum). 2. a million. Example: *megavolt* (a million volts).

megacolon *n.* dilatation, and sometimes lengthening, of the colon. It is caused by obstruction of the colon, *Hirschsprung's disease, or longstanding constipation, or it may occur as a complication of ulcerative *colitis (*toxic megacolon*).

megakaryoblast *n.* a cell that gives rise to the platelet-forming cell *megakaryocyte, found in the blood-forming tissue of the bone marrow. It is derived from a *haemopoietic stem cell and matures via an intermediate stage (*promegakaryocyte*) into a megakaryocyte.

megakaryocyte *n.* a cell in the bone marrow that produces *platelets. It is large (35–160 μm in diameter), with an irregularly lobed nucleus, and with *Romanowsky stains its abundant cytoplasm appears pale blue with fine reddish granules. *See also* thrombopoiesis.

megal- (megalo-) *prefix denoting* abnormal enlargement. Example: *megalomelia* (of limbs).

megaloblast *n.* an abnormal form of any of the cells that are precursors of red blood cells (*see* erythroblast). Megaloblasts are unusually large and their nuclei fail to mature in the normal way; they are seen in the bone marrow in certain anaemias (*megaloblastic anaemias*) due to deficiency of vitamin B_{12} or folic acid. —**megaloblastic** *adj.*

megalocephaly *n.* 1. *see* macrocephaly. 2. overgrowth and distortion of skull bones (*see* leontiasis).

megalocyte *n. see* macrocyte.

megalomania *n.* delusions of grandeur, such as being God, royalty, etc. It may be a feature of a schizophrenic or manic illness or of cerebral syphilis.

-megaly *suffix denoting* abnormal enlargement. Example: *splenomegaly* (of spleen).

megaureter *n.* gross dilatation of the *ureter. This occurs above the site of a long-standing obstruction in the ureter, which blocks the free flow of urine from the kidney. A common cause of megaureter is reflux of urine from the bladder into the ureters (*see* vesicoureteric reflux), but some of the most striking examples are found in so-called *idiopathic megaureter*. In this condition, which may affect one or both ureters, there is a segment of normal ureter of varying length at the extreme lower end of the bladder, above which the ureter is enormously dilated. Both reflux and idiopathic megaureter progress to urinary infection and/or renal impairment. Treatment is by corrective surgery.

megestrol *n.* a synthetic female sex hormone (*see* progestogen) that is used in combination with an oestrogen in *oral contraceptives.

meibomian cyst *n. see* chalazion.

meibomian glands (tarsal glands) small sebaceous glands that lie under the conjunctiva of the eyelids.

meiosis (reduction division) *n.* a type of cell division that produces four daughter cells, each having half the number of chromosomes of the original cell. It occurs before the formation of sperm and ova and the normal (*diploid) number of chromosomes is restored after fertilization. Meiosis also produces genetic variation in the daughter cells, brought about by the process of *crossing over. Meiosis consists of two successive divisions, each divided into four stages (*see* prophase, metaphase, anaphase, telophase). (See illustration.) *Compare* mitosis. —**meiotic** *adj.*

Meissner's plexus (submucous plexus) a fine network of parasympathetic nerve fibres in the wall of the alimentary canal, supplying the muscles and mucous membrane.

melaena *n.* black tarry faeces due to the presence of partly digested blood from higher up the digestive tract. Melaena is not apparent unless at least 500 ml of blood has entered the gut. It often occurs after vomiting blood (*see* haematemesis) and the causes are the same.

melan- (melano-) *prefix denoting* **1.** black coloration. **2.** melanin. Example: *melanaemia* (presence in the blood).

melancholia *n. see* depression, involutional melancholia.

melanin *n.* a dark-brown to black pigment occurring in the hair, the skin, and in the iris and choroid layer of the eyes. Melanin is contained within special cells (*chromatophores*); in the skin these are found in the *dermis. Production of melanin in the skin is increased by the action of sunlight (producing tanning), which protects the underlying skin layers from the sun's radiation.

Stages in meiosis

melanism (melanosis) *n.* an unusually pronounced darkening of body tissues caused by excessive production of the pigment *melanin. For example, melanism may affect the hair, the skin (after sunburn, during pregnancy, or in *Addison's disease), or the eye.

melanocyte (melanophore) *n.* a cell within the epidermis of skin that produces the dark brown pigment *melanin.

melanocyte-stimulating hormone (MSH) a hormone synthesized and released by the pituitary gland. In amphibians MSH brings about colour changes in the skin but its physiological role in man is uncertain.

melanoderma *n.* an abnormal increase in the skin pigment (*melanin).

melanoma *n.* a highly malignant tumour of melanin-forming cells, the *melanocytes. Such tumours usually occur in the skin but are also found in the eye and the mucous membranes. They may contain melanin (*melanotic melanomas*) or be free of pigment (*amelanotic melanomas*). Spread of this cancer to other parts of the body, especially to the lymph nodes and liver, is common. In these cases melanin or its precursors (*melanogens*) may be excreted in the urine and the whole of the skin may be deeply pigmented.

melanonychia *n.* blackening of the nails with the pigment *melanin.

melanophore *n. see* melanocyte.

melanoplakia *n.* pigmented areas of *melanin in the mucous membrane lining the inside of the cheeks.

melanosis *n.* **1.** *see* melanism. **2.** a disorder in the body's production of the pigment melanin. **3.** *cachexia associated with the spread of the skin cancer *melanoma. —**melanotic** *adj.*

melanuria *n.* the presence of dark pigment in the urine. This may be caused by the presence of melanin or its precursors, in some cases of *melanoma; it may alternatively be caused by metabolic disease, such as *porphyria.

melasma *n. see* chloasma.

melioidosis *n.* a disease of wild rodents caused by the bacterium *Pseudomonas pseudomallei*. It can be transmitted to man, possibly by rat fleas, causing pneumonia, multiple abscesses, and septicaemia. It is often fatal.

melomelus *n.* a fetus with one or more pairs of supernumery limbs.

melphalan *n.* a drug used to treat various types of cancer, including malignant melanoma, tumours of the breast and ovaries, and Hodgkin's disease. It is administered by mouth or injection. Side-effects include digestive upsets, mouth ulcers, and temporary hair loss. Trade name: **Alkeran**.

membrane *n.* **1.** a thin layer of tissue surrounding the whole or part of an organ or tissue lining a cavity, or separating adjacent structures or cavities. *See also* basement membrane, mucous membrane, serous membrane. **2.** the lipoprotein envelope surrounding a cell (*plasma* or *cell membrane*). —**membranous** *adj.*

membrane bone a bone that develops in connective tissue by direct *ossification, without cartilage being formed first. The bones of the face and skull are membrane bones.

membranous labyrinth *see* labyrinth.

men- (meno-) *prefix denoting* menstruation.

menarche *n.* the start of the menstrual periods. This may happen at any age between about 10 and 17 years.

mendelism *n.* the theory of inheritance based on *Mendel's laws.

Mendel's laws rules of inheritance based on the breeding experiments of

Gregor Mendel, which showed that the inheritance of characteristics is controlled by particles now known as *genes. In modern terms they are as follows. (1) Each body (somatic) cell of an individual carries two factors (genes) for every characteristic and each gamete carries only one. It is now known that the genes are arranged on chromosomes, which are present in pairs in somatic cells and separate during gamete formation by the process of *meiosis. (2) Each pair of factors segregates independently of all other pairs at meiosis, so that the gametes show all possible combinations of factors. This law applies only to genes on different chromosomes; those on the same chromosome are affected by *linkage. *See also* dominant, recessive.

menidrosis (menhidrosis) *n.* the production of sweat, sometimes containing blood, instead of the normal menstrual flow.

Ménière's disease (Ménière's syndrome) a disease affecting the inner ear in which deafness is associated with buzzing in the ears (tinnitus) and vertigo; its cause is not known. Typically, the attacks of vertigo are sudden and explosive and associated with pallor, nausea, and vomiting. Between attacks there may be months without symptoms, but as the disease progresses the deafness becomes more marked. Neither medical nor surgical treatment is uniformly successful.

mening- (meningo-) *prefix denoting* the meninges.

meninges *pl. n.* (*sing.* **meninx**) the three connective tissue membranes that line the skull and vertebral canal and enclose the brain and spinal cord (see illustration). The outermost layer – the *dura mater (pachymeninx) – is inelastic, tough, and thicker than the middle layer (the *arachnoid mater) and the innermost layer (the *pia mater). The inner two membranes are together

called the *leptomeninges*; between them circulates the *cerebrospinal fluid.

Section through the skull and brain to show meninges

meningioma *n.* a tumour arising from the fibrous coverings of the brain and spinal cord (*meninges). It is usually slow-growing and produces symptoms by pressure on the underlying nervous tissue. In the brain the tumour is a cause of focal *epilepsy and gradually progressive neurological disability. In the spinal cord it causes paraplegia and the *Brown-Séquard syndrome. Some meningiomas (known as *meningeal sarcomas*) are malignant and invade neighbouring tissues. Treatment of the majority of cases is by surgical removal if the tumour is accessible. The more malignant varieties may also require additional radiotherapy. Some patients have been known to have symptoms for as long as 30 years before the tumour has been discovered.

meningism *n.* stiffness of the neck mimicking that found in meningitis. It is most common in childhood and is usually a symptom of chest infection or inflammation in the upper respiratory tract. Examination of the *cerebrospinal fluid reveals no abnormalities.

meningitis *n.* an inflammation of the *meninges due to infection by viruses or by the bacteria responsible for pneumonia, syphilis, or tuberculosis. Meningitis causes an intense headache, fever, loss of appetite, intolerance to light and sound, rigidity of muscles, especially those in the neck (*see also* Kernig's sign), and in severe cases convulsions, vomiting, and delirium leading to death. Bacterial meningitis can be effectively treated with antibiotics or sulphonamides. Viral meningitis does not respond to drugs; prolonged bed rest, darkness, and quiet is the only treatment. *See also* cerebrospinal fever, leptomeningitis, pachymeningitis.

meningocele *n. see* neural tube defects.

meningococcaemia *n.* the presence of meningococci (bacteria of the species *Neisseria meningitidis*) in the bloodstream. *See* meningitis.

meningococcus *n.* (*pl.* **meningococci**) one of the bacteria causing meningitis: *Neisseria meningitidis*. —**meningococcal** *adj.*

meningoencephalitis *n.* inflammation of the brain and its membranous coverings (the meninges) caused by infection, as with the mumps virus or *Brucella* (the bacterium causing brucellosis). *Brucellosis may also involve the spinal cord, producing *myelitis with paralysis of both legs, sometimes called *meningomyelitis*.

meningoencephalocele *n. see* neural tube defects.

meningomyelitis *n. see* meningoencephalitis.

meningomyelocele *n. see* neural tube defects.

meningovascular *adj.* relating to or affecting the meninges covering the brain and spinal cord and the blood vessels that penetrate them to supply the underlying neural tissues. The term is usually used to describe secondary syphilitic infection of the nervous system.

meninx *n.* the thin layer of mesoderm that surrounds the brain of the embryo. It gives rise to most of the skull and the membranes that surround the brain. *See also* chondrocranium.

meniscectomy *n.* surgical removal of a cartilage (meniscus) in the knee. This is carried out when the meniscus has been torn or is diseased, to relieve pain and 'locking' of the knee joint.

meniscus *n.* (in anatomy) a crescent-shaped structure, such as the fibrocartilaginous disc that divides the cavity of a synovial joint.

menopause (climacteric) *n.* the time in a woman's life when the ovaries cease to produce an egg cell every four weeks and therefore menstruation ceases and the woman is no longer able to bear children. The menopause can occur at any age between the middle thirties and the late fifties. Menstruation may decrease gradually in successive periods or the intervals between periods may lengthen; alternatively there may be a sudden and complete stoppage of the monthly periods. At the time of the menopause there is a change in the balance of sex hormones in the body, which sometimes leads to hot flushes, palpitations, and dryness of the mucous membrane lining the vagina. Some women may also experience emotional disturbances. —**menopausal** *adj.*

menorrhagia (epimenorrhagia) *n.* abnormally heavy bleeding at menstruation, which may or may not be associated with abnormally long periods. Menorrhagia may be associated with high blood pressure, hormonal disturbances, inflammation or tumours (e.g.

fibroids) in the pelvic cavity, anaemia, sugar diabetes, kidney disease, and many other conditions.

menses *n.* the blood and other materials discharged from the womb at menstruation.

menstrual cycle the periodic sequence of events in sexually mature nonpregnant women by which an egg cell (ovum) is released from the ovary at four-weekly intervals until the change of life (*see* menopause). The stages of the menstrual cycle are shown in the diagram. An ovum develops within a *Graafian follicle in the ovary. When mature, it bursts from the follicle and travels along the Fallopian tube to the womb. A temporary endocrine gland – the corpus luteum – develops in the ruptured follicle and secretes the hormone *progesterone, which causes the lining of the womb to become thicker and richly supplied with blood in preparation for pregnancy. If the ovum is not fertilized the cycle continues: the corpus luteum shrinks and the womb lining is shed at *menstruation. If fertilization does take place the fertilized ovum becomes attached to the womb lining and the corpus luteum continues to secrete progesterone, i.e. pregnancy begins.

menstruation (catamenia) *n.* the discharge of blood and fragments of womb lining from the vagina at intervals of about one month in women of child-bearing age (*see* menarche, menopause). Menstruation is that stage of the *menstrual cycle during which the womb lining, which is thickened in readiness to receive a fertilized egg cell (ovum), is cast off if fertilization does not occur within a limited period of time. The normal duration of discharge varies from three to seven days. In *anovular menstruation*, discharge takes place without previous release of an egg cell from the ovary. *Vicarious menstruation* is bleeding from a mucous membrane other than the womb lining when normal menstruation is due. *See also* amenorrhoea, dysmenorrhoea, epimenorrhoea, hypomenorrhoea, menorrhagia, oligomenorrhoea.

mental[1] *adj.* relating to or affecting the mind.

mental[2] *adj.* relating to the chin.

mental age a measure of an individual's level of intellectual functioning; for example, someone described as having a mental age of 6 years would be functioning at the level of an average 6-year-old child. This measure has largely been replaced by a comparison

The menstrual cycle

of the functioning of persons of the same age group (*see* intelligence quotient, intelligence test).

mental deficiency *see* subnormality.

Mental Health Acts the Acts of Parliament governing the care of the mentally disordered. The Mental Health Act 1959 provided the framework for England and Wales; similar Acts in 1960 and 1961 provided for Scotland and Northern Ireland. They abolished the old system of certification and established a legal framework for voluntary treatment of the mentally ill on the same basis as other patients. The Act also provides for *compulsory admission when the mentally disordered put themselves or other people into danger. It also enjoined local authorities to provide for the community treatment of mental disorder. The Mental Health (Amendment) Act of 1982 made further provisions for the protection of the civil rights of patients, the restriction of grounds for detention and compulsory treatment, and for a commission to regulate aspects of the practice of psychiatry (*see* Mental Health Act Commission).

Mental Health Act Commission a regulating body set up by the Mental Health (Amendment) Act of 1982. Its members comprise some 90 psychiatrists, nurses, lawyers, members of other clinical professions, and lay people. They have the responsibilities of regularly visiting psychiatric hospitals (yearly for ordinary hospitals; more frequently for *special hospitals), reviewing psychiatric care, giving second opinions on the need for certain psychiatric treatments, and acting as a forum for the discussion of psychiatric issues.

mental illness a disorder of one or more of the functions of the mind (such as emotion, perception, memory, or thought), which causes suffering to the patient or others. If the sole problem is that the individual's behaviour as a whole is out of line with society's expectations, then the term 'illness' is not appropriate.

Mental illness should be distinguished from *subnormality, in which an individual has a general failure of development of the normal intellectual capacities. It is broadly divided into *psychosis, in which the capacity for appreciating reality is lost, and *neurosis, in which insight is retained.

mental impairment the presence of seriously antisocial or irresponsible behaviour in a person with mental *subnormality.

mental welfare officer (in Britain) an employee of a local authority with special training in and responsibility for people with mental illness. He obtains court orders for *compulsory admission where necessary and provides surveillance and support for those being treated at home or in designated hostel accommodation, including those discharged from hospital. *See also* after care.

mento- *prefix denoting* the chin.

mentum *n.* the chin.

mepacrine *n.* a drug used to treat various infections and infestations, particularly malaria, giardiasis, and taeniasis. It is administered by mouth. Digestive upsets and headache may occur and the skin often turns yellow. Trade names: **Atebrin, Quinacrine.**

mephenesin *n.* a *muscle-relaxant drug used to relieve muscular spasm and abnormal movements in such diseases as parkinsonism, chorea, and athetosis. It is administered by mouth or injection. Side-effects usually include digestive upsets. Trade name: **Myanesin.**

meprobamate *n.* a mild *tranquillizer used to relieve anxiety and nervous tension. It is administered by mouth or injection; side-effects include digestive upsets, headache, and drowsiness. Trade names: **Equanil**, **Mepavlon**, **Miltown**.

mepyramine *n.* an *antihistamine drug administered by mouth or injection to treat allergies and sensitivity reactions and applied as a cream to treat skin allergies and itching. Drowsiness is a common side-effect and digestive upsets may occur. Trade name: **Anthisan**.

meralgia paraesthetica painful tingling and numbness felt over the outer surface of the thigh when the lateral cutaneous nerve is trapped as it passes through the fibrous and muscular tissues of the thigh.

mercaptopurine *n.* a drug that prevents the growth of cancer cells and is administered by mouth, chiefly in the treatment of some types of leukaemia (*see* antimetabolite). It commonly reduces the numbers of white blood cells; mouth ulcers and digestive upsets may also occur. Trade name: **Puri-Nethol**.

mercurialism (hydrargyria) *n.* mercury poisoning. Metallic mercury is absorbed through the skin and alimentary canal, and its vapour is taken in through the lungs. Acute poisoning causes vomiting, severe abdominal pains, bloody diarrhoea, and kidney damage, with failure to produce urine. Treatment is with *dimercaprol. Chronic poisoning causes mouth ulceration, loose teeth, loss of appetite, and intestinal and renal disturbances, with anaemia and nervous irritability. Treatment is removing the patient from further exposure.

mercury *n.* a silvery metallic element that is liquid at room temperature. Its toxicity has caused a decline in the use of its compounds in medicine during this century, but mercurial compounds in the form of ointments were formerly used in the treatment of syphilis. The main uses of mercury salts today are in antiseptics, fungicides, and antiparasitic agents. Symbol: Hg. *See also* mercurialism.

merocrine (eccrine) *adj.* describing a type of *secretion in which the glandular cells remain intact during the process of secretion.

merozoite *n.* a stage in the life cycle of the malaria parasite (*Plasmodium*). Many merozoites are formed during the asexual division of the schizont (*see* schizogony). The released merozoites may invade new red blood cells or new liver cells, and continue the asexual phase with the production of yet more merozoites, effectively spreading the infection. Alternatively, merozoites invade red blood cells and begin the sexual cycle with the formation of male and female sex cells (*see* microgametocyte, macrogametocyte).

mes- (meso-) *prefix denoting* middle or medial.

mesaortitis *n.* inflammation of the middle layer (media) of the wall of the aorta, generally the result of late syphilis. Aneurysm formation may result. The infection can be eradicated with penicillin.

mesarteritis *n.* inflammation of the middle layer (media) of an artery, which is often combined with inflammation in all layers of the artery wall. It is seen in syphilis, polyarteritis, temporal arteritis, and Buerger's disease.

mescaline *n.* an alkaloid present in *mescal buttons* (the dried tops of the Mexican cactus *Lophophora williamsii*) that produces inebriation and vivid colourful hallucinations when ingested.

mesencephalon *n. see* midbrain.

mesenchyme *n.* the undifferentiated tissue of the early embryo that forms almost entirely from *mesoderm. It is loosely organized and the individual cells migrate to different parts of the body where they form most of the skeletal and connective tissue, the blood and blood system, and the visceral (smooth) muscles.

mesentery *n.* a double layer of *peritoneum attaching the stomach, small intestine, pancreas, spleen, and other abdominal organs to the posterior wall of the abdomen. It contains blood and lymph vessels and nerves supplying these organs. —**mesenteric** *adj.*

mesial *adj.* **1.** medial. **2.** relating to or situated in the *median line or plane. **3.** designating the surface of a tooth towards the midline of the jaw.

mesiodens *n.* an extra tooth that may occur in the midline of the palate, between the central incisors, and may interfere with their eruption.

mesmerism *n.* *hypnosis based on the ideas of the 18th-century physician Franz Mesmer, sometimes employing magnets and a variety of other equipment.

mesna *n.* a drug administered intravenously by injection or infusion to prevent the toxic effect of *ifosfamide and *cyclophosphamide on the bladder. It binds with the toxic metabolite acrolein in the urine.

mesoappendix *n.* the *mesentery of the appendix.

mesocolon *n.* the fold of peritoneum by which the colon is fixed to the posterior abdominal wall. Usually only the *transverse* and *sigmoid mesocolons* persist in the adult, attached to the transverse and sigmoid colon, respectively.

mesoderm *n.* the middle *germ layer of the early embryo. It gives rise to cartilage, muscle, bone, blood, kidneys, gonads and their ducts, and connective tissue. It separates into two layers – an outer *somatic* and an inner *splanchnic mesoderm*, separated by a cavity (*coelom*) that becomes the body cavity. The

dorsal somatic mesoderm becomes segmented into a number of *somites. *See also* mesenchyme. —**mesodermal** *adj.*

mesometrium *n.* the broad ligament of the uterus (womb): a sheet of connective tissue that carries blood vessels to the uterus (womb) and attaches it to the abdominal wall.

mesomorphic *adj.* describing a *body type that has a well developed skeletal and muscular structure and a sturdy upright posture. —**mesomorph** *n.* —**mesomorphy** *n.*

mesonephros (Wolffian body) *n.* the second area of kidney tissue to develop in the embryo. Its excretory function only lasts for a very brief period before it degenerates. However, parts of it become incorporated into the male reproductive structures. Its duct – the *mesonephric* (or *Wolffian*) *duct* – persists in males as the epididymis and vas deferens, which conduct sperm from the testis. —**mesonephric** *adj.*

mesophilic *adj.* describing organisms, especially bacteria, that grow best at temperatures of about 25–45°C. *Compare* psychrophilic, thermophilic.

mesosalpinx *n.* a fold of peritoneum that surrounds the Fallopian tubes. It is the upper part of the broad ligament, which surrounds the womb.

mesosome *n.* a structure occurring in some bacterial cells, formed by infolding of the cell membrane. Mesosomes are associated with the DNA and play a part in cell division.

mesotendon *n.* the delicate connective tissue membrane that surrounds a tendon.

mesothelioma *n.* a tumour of the epithelium making up the pleura, peritoneum, or pericardium. The occurrence of pleural mesothelioma has a strong association with exposure to asbestos dust (*see* asbestosis), and workers in the asbestos industry who develop such tumours are entitled to industrial compensation. In other cases, however, there is no history of asbestos exposure. Some tumours can be surgically removed but most are inoperable; for these cases chemotherapy with *doxorubicin may be tried.

mesothelium *n.* the single layer of cells that lines *serous membranes. It is derived from embryonic mesoderm. *Compare* epithelium.

mesovarium *n.* the *mesentery of the ovaries.

messenger RNA a type of RNA that carries the information of the *genetic code of the DNA from the cell nucleus to the ribosomes, where the code is translated into protein. *See* transcription, translation.

mestranol *n.* a synthetic female sex hormone that is one of the most commonly used oestrogens in *oral contraceptive pills.

met- (meta-) *prefix denoting* **1.** distal to; beyond; behind. **2.** change; transformation.

metabolism *n.* **1.** the sum of all the chemical and physical changes that take place within the body and enable its continued growth and functioning. Metabolism involves the breakdown of complex organic constituents of the body with the liberation of energy, which is required for other processes (*see* catabolism) and the building up of complex substances, which form the material of the tissues and organs, from simple ones (*see* anabolism). *See also* basal metabolism. **2.** the sum of the biochemical changes undergone by a particular constituent of the body; for example, protein metabolism. —**metabolic** *adj.*

metabolite *n.* a substance that takes part in the process of *metabolism. Metabolites are either produced during metabolism or are constituents of food taken into the body.

metacarpal 1. *adj.* relating to the bones of the hand (*metacarpus). **2.** *n.* any of the bones forming the metacarpus.

metacarpus *n.* the five bones of the hand that connect the *carpus (wrist) to the *phalanges (digits).

metacentric *n.* a chromosome in which the centromere is at or near the centre of the chromosome. —**metacentric** *adj.*

metacercaria *n.* (*pl.* **metacercariae**) a mature form of the *cercaria larva of a fluke. Liver fluke metacercariae are enveloped by thin cysts and develop on various kinds of vegetation.

metachromasia (metachromatism) *n.* **1.** the property of a dye of staining certain tissues or cells a colour that is different from that of the stain itself. **2.** the variation in colour produced in certain tissue elements that are stained with the same dye. **3.** abnormal coloration of a tissue produced by a particular stain. —**metachromatic** *adj.*

Metagonimus *n.* a genus of small flukes, usually less than 3 mm in length, common as parasites of dogs and cats in the Far East, N. Siberia, and the Balkan States. Adult flukes of *M. yokogawai* occasionally infect the duodenum of man if undercooked fish (the intermediate host) is eaten. They may cause inflammation and some ulceration of the intestinal lining, which produces a mild diarrhoea. Flukes can be easily removed with tetrachlorethylene.

metamorphopsia *n.* a condition in which objects appear distorted. It is usually due to a disorder of the retina affecting the *macula (the most sensitive part).

metamyelocyte *n.* an immature *granulocyte (a type of white blood cell), having a kidney-shaped nucleus (*compare* myelocyte) and cytoplasm containing neutrophil, eosinophil, or basophil granules. It is normally found in the blood-forming tissue of the bone marrow but may appear in the blood in a wide variety of diseases, including acute infections. *See also* granulopoiesis.

metanephros *n.* the excretory organ of the fetus, which develops into the kidney and is formed from the rear portion of the *nephrogenic cord. It does not become functional until birth, since urea is transferred across the placenta to the mother.

metaphase *n.* the second stage of *mitosis and of each division of *meiosis, in which the chromosomes line up at the centre of the *spindle, with their centromeres attached to the spindle fibres.

metaphysis *n.* the growing portion of a long bone that lies between the *epiphyses (the ends) and the *diaphysis (the shaft).

metaplasia *n.* an abnormal change in the nature of a tissue. For instance, columnar epithelium lining the bronchi may be converted to squamous epithelium (*squamous metaplasia*): this may be an early sign of malignant change. *Myeloid metaplasia* is the development of bone marrow elements, normally found only within the marrow cavities of the bones, in organs such as the spleen and liver. This may occur after bone marrow failure.

metastasis *n.* the distant spread of malignant tumour from its site of origin. This occurs by three main routes: (1) through the bloodstream; (2) through the lymphatic system; (3) across body cavities, e.g. through the peritoneum. Highly malignant tumours have a greater potential for metastasis. Individual tumours may spread by one or all of the above routes, although

*carcinoma is said classically to metastasize via the lymphatics and *sarcoma via the bloodstream. —**metastatic** *adj.*

metastasize *vb.* (of a malignant tumour) to spread by *metastasis.

metatarsal 1. *adj.* relating to the bones of the foot (*metatarsus). **2.** *n.* any of the bones forming the metatarsus.

metatarsalgia *n.* aching pain in the metatarsal bones of the foot. Repeated injury and deformities of the foot are common causes, and corrective footwear may be prescribed.

metatarsus *n.* the five bones of the foot that connect the *tarsus (ankle) to the *phalanges (toes).

metathalamus *n.* a part of the *thalamus consisting of two nuclei through which impulses pass from the eyes and ears to be distributed to the cerebral cortex.

metencephalon *n.* part of the hindbrain, formed by the pons and the cerebellum and continuous below with the medulla oblongata. *See* brain.

meteorism *n. see* tympanites.

-meter *suffix denoting* an instrument for measuring. Example: *perimeter* (instrument for measuring the field of vision).

metformin *n.* a drug that reduces blood sugar levels and is used to treat *diabetes. It is administered by mouth and may cause loss of appetite and minor digestive upsets. Trade name: **Glucophage**.

methadone *n.* a potent narcotic *analgesic drug administered by mouth or injection to relieve severe pain and as a linctus to suppress coughs. It is also used to treat heroin addiction. Digestive upsets, drowsiness, and dizziness may occur, and prolonged use may lead to dependence. Trade name: **Physopeptone**.

methaemalbumin *n.* a chemical complex of the pigment portion of haemoglobin (*haem*) with the plasma protein *albumin. It is formed in the blood in anaemias in which red blood cells are destroyed and free haemoglobin is released into the plasma. In such conditions methaemalbumin can be detected in both the blood and urine.

methaemoglobin *n.* a substance formed when the iron atoms of the blood pigment *haemoglobin have been oxidized from the ferrous to the ferric form (*compare* oxyhaemoglobin). Methaemoglobin cannot bind molecular oxygen and therefore cannot transport oxygen round the body. The presence of methaemoglobin in the blood (*methaemoglobinaemia*) may result from ingestion of oxidizing drugs or from an inherited abnormality of the haemoglobin molecule. Symptoms are fatigue, headache, dizziness and *cyanosis.

methandienone *n.* a synthetic male sex hormone with *anabolic properties, used to build up tissues in wasting diseases, such as osteoporosis, and during convalescence. Methandienone is administered by mouth; side-effects are uncommon, but nausea, menstrual abnormalities, and fluid retention may occur. Trade name: **Dianabol**.

methandriol *n.* a synthetic male sex hormone (*see* androgen) with the same actions and uses as *methandienone. Side-effects may include symptoms of virilization in women, such as growth of body hair and voice changes.

methanol *n. see* methyl alcohol.

methapyrilene *n.* an *antihistamine used to relieve *hay fever and other allergic reactions. It is administered by mouth and may cause drowsiness.

methaqualone *n.* a hypnotic and *sedative drug used to treat insomnia. It is administered by mouth; side-effects include headache, drowsiness,

and digestive upsets. Trade name: **Revonal**.

methenamine *n. see* hexamine.

methenolone *n.* a synthetic male sex hormone with body-building actions (*see* anabolic). It is administered by mouth or injection and may cause symptoms of virilization in women, such as growth of body hair and voice changes.

methimazole *n.* a drug that reduces thyroid activity, used to treat *thyrotoxicosis and to prepare patients for surgical removal of the thyroid gland. It is administered by mouth or injection; side-effects include rashes, digestive upsets, and headache.

methionine *n.* a sulphur-containing *essential amino acid. *See also* amino acid.

methixene *n.* a drug with effects similar to those of *atropine, used to control the tremors and other symptoms in parkinsonism and to relieve spasm of smooth muscle in digestive disorders. It is administered by mouth; side-effects can include dry mouth, disturbed vision, flushing, and dizziness. Trade name: **Tremonil**.

methoin *n.* an *anticonvulsant drug used to prevent or reduce the severity of grand mal fits in *epilepsy. It is administered by mouth; common side-effects are drowsiness, dizziness, and nausea. Trade name: **Mesontoin**.

methoserpidine *n.* a drug that lowers the blood pressure. It is administered by mouth; common side-effects include lethargy, drowsiness, and digestive upsets. Trade name: **Decaserpyl**.

methotrexate *n.* a drug that interferes with cell growth and is used to treat various types of cancer, including leukaemia (*see* antimetabolite). It is administered by mouth or injection; common side-effects include mouth sores, digestive upsets, skin rashes, and hair loss.

methotrimeprazine *n.* a tranquillizing, sedative, and analgesic drug used to treat anxiety, tension, and agitation and to relieve moderate or severe pain. It is administered by mouth or injection; common side-effects are drowsiness and weakness. Trade name: **Veractil**.

methoxamine *n.* a *sympathomimetic drug that causes blood vessels to constrict and thus raises blood pressure. It is administered by injection to maintain the blood pressure during surgical operations. High doses may cause headache and vomiting. Trade name: **Vasoxine**.

methoxyphenamine *n.* a *sympathomimetic drug used to treat asthma and other allergic conditions, such as rhinitis, and added to cough mixtures. It is administered by mouth and may cause nausea, dizziness, and dry mouth. Trade name: **Orthoxine**.

methyl alcohol (methanol) wood alcohol: an alcohol that is oxidized in the body much more slowly than ethyl alcohol and forms poisonous products. As little as 10 ml of pure methyl alcohol can produce permanent blindness, and 100 ml is likely to be fatal. The breakdown product formaldehyde is responsible for damage to the eyes; it is itself converted to formic acid, which causes acidosis and death from respiratory failure. *See also* methylated spirits.

methylamphetamine *n.* a drug with actions and side-effects similar to those of *amphetamine. It is administered by mouth to treat narcolepsy and parkinsonism and some depressive states, and to reduce appetite. It is also administered by injection in psychiatry, to restore the blood pressure in surgical procedures, and to treat drug overdosage. Its use is restricted to hospitals.

methylated spirits a mixture consisting mainly of ethyl alcohol with *methyl alcohol and petroleum hydrocarbons. The addition of pyridine gives it an objectionable smell, and the dye methyl violet is added to make it recognizable as unfit to drink. It is used as a solvent, cleaning fluid, and fuel.

methylcellulose *n.* a compound that absorbs water and is used as a bulk *laxative to treat constipation, to control diarrhoea, and in patients with a *colostomy. It is administered by mouth and usually has no side-effects. Trade names: **Celevac**, **Cellucon**, **Cologel**.

methyldopa *n.* a drug that reduces blood pressure (*see* sympatholytic). It is administered by mouth or injection, and drowsiness commonly occurs during the first days of treatment. Trade names: **Aldomet**, **Dopamet**, **Hydromet**, **Medomet**.

methylene blue a blue antiseptic dye that has been used to treat infections of the urinary system, methaemoglobinaemia, and in a test for kidney function. It is also used to stain bacterial cells for microscopic examination.

methylergometrine *n.* a drug that stimulates contractions of the womb. It is used in childbirth to control bleeding following delivery and to help the womb return to normal. It is administered by mouth or injection and may cause headache and vertigo.

methyl green a basic dye used for colouring the stainable part of the cell nucleus (chromatin) and – with pyronin – for the differential staining of RNA and DNA, which give a red and a green colour respectively.

methylphenidate *n.* a *sympathomimetic drug that also stimulates the central nervous system. It is used to improve mental activity in convalescence and some depressive states and to overcome lethargy associated with drug treatment. It is administered by mouth or injection; side-effects such as nervousness and insomnia may occur. Trade name: **Ritalin**.

methyl salicylate oil of wintergreen: a liquid with *counterirritant and *analgesic properties, applied to the skin to relieve pain in lumbago, sciatica, and rheumatic conditions.

methyltestosterone *n.* a synthetic male sex hormone (*see* androgen) administered by mouth to treat sexual underdevelopment in men. It is also used to suppress lactation, to treat menstrual and menopausal disorders, and to treat breast cancer in women. Side-effects are those of *testosterone.

methylthiouracil *n.* a drug that inhibits thyroid activity, used to treat overactivity of the thyroid gland (*see* thyrotoxicosis). It is administered by mouth; side-effects may include rashes, digestive upsets, and headache.

methyl violet (gentian violet) a dye used mainly for staining Protozoa.

methyprylone *n.* a hypnotic and *sedative drug used to treat insomnia and to relieve anxiety and tension. It is administered by mouth; side-effects such as headache and drowsiness may occur. Trade name: **Noludar**.

methysergide *n.* a drug used to prevent severe migraine attacks and to control diarrhoea associated with tumours in the digestive system. It is administered by mouth; common side-effects are digestive upsets, dizziness, and drowsiness. Trade name: **Deseril**.

metoclopramide *n.* a drug that speeds up digestion. It is used to treat nausea, vomiting, indigestion, heartburn, and flatulence. It is administered by mouth or injection; high doses may cause drowsiness and muscle spasms. Trade names: **Maxolon, Primperan**.

metolazone *n.* a *diuretic used to treat fluid retention (oedema) and high blood pressure. It is administered by mouth; side-effects include headache,

loss of appetite, and digestive upsets, and blood potassium levels may be reduced. Trade name: **Zoroxolyn**.

metoprolol *n.* a drug that controls the activity of the heart (*see* beta blocker) and is used to treat high blood pressure and angina. It is administered by mouth; the commonest side-effects are tiredness and digestive upsets. Trade names: **Betaloc, Lopressor**.

metr- (metro-) *prefix denoting* the womb.

metralgia *n.* pain in the womb.

metre *n.* the *SI unit of length that is equal to 39.37 inches. It is formally defined as the length of the path travelled by light in vacuum during a time interval of 1/299,792,458 of a second. Symbol: m.

metritis *n.* inflammation of the womb. *See also* endometritis, myometritis.

metrocolpocele *n.* protrusion of the womb into the vagina, which consequently becomes displaced downwards.

metronidazole *n.* a drug used to treat infections of the urinary, genital, and digestive systems, such as trichomoniasis, amoebiasis, and giardiasis, and acute ulcerative gingivitis. It is administered by mouth or in suppositories; side-effects are rare but may include digestive upsets, drowsiness, and headache. Trade name: **Flagyl**.

metropathia haemorrhagica (essential uterine haemorrhage) abnormal loss of blood in the womb, resulting from disease. The lining membrane of the womb usually thickens and there may be fluid-filled sacs in the ovary.

metroptosis (uterine prolapse) *n.* the downward displacement of the womb. The neck (cervix) of the womb sometimes protrudes from the vaginal opening. The womb usually drops under the influence of gravity because the supporting tissues are weak or damaged, especially in women who have given birth. A surgical operation may be required in order to correct the condition. *Compare* metrocolpocele.

metrorrhagia *n.* bleeding from the womb when menstruation is not due. Metrorrhagia may indicate the presence of cancer of the cervix (neck of the womb) or some other disease of the womb.

metrostaxis *n.* a slight but incessant loss of blood from the womb.

-metry *suffix denoting* measuring or measurement.

mianserin *n.* a drug used to relieve moderate or severe depression and anxiety. It is administered by mouth; side-effects are usually milder than with other potent antidepressants, the commonest being drowsiness. Trade name: **Bolvidon**.

micelle *n.* one of the microscopic particles into which the products of fat digestion (i.e. fatty acids and monoglycerides), present in the gut, are dispersed by the action of *bile salts. Fatty material in this finely dispersed form is more easily absorbed by the small intestine.

micr- (micro-) *prefix denoting* 1. small size. 2. one millionth part.

microaerophilic *adj.* describing microorganisms that grow best at very low oxygen concentrations (i.e. below the atmospheric level).

microaneurysm *n.* a minute localized swelling of a capillary wall, which is found in the retina of patients with diabetic *retinopathy. It is recognized as a small red dot when the interior of the eye is examined with an *ophthalmoscope.

microangiopathy *n.* damage to the walls of the smallest blood vessels. It may result from a variety of diseases, including diabetes mellitus, collagen diseases, infections, and cancer. Common manifestations of microangiopathy are kidney failure, haemolysis (damage to red blood cells), and purpura (bleeding into the skin). The treatment is that of the underlying cause.

microbe *n. see* microorganism.

microbiology *n.* the science of *microorganisms. Microbiology in relation to medicine is concerned mainly with the isolation and identification of the microorganisms that cause disease. —**microbiological** *adj.* —**microbiologist** *n.*

microblepharon (microblepharism) *n.* the condition of having abnormally small eyelids.

microcephaly *n.* abnormal smallness of the head in relation to the size of the rest of the body: a congenital condition in which the brain is not fully developed. *Compare* macrocephaly.

microcheilia *n.* abnormally small size of the lips. *Compare* macrocheilia.

Micrococcus *n.* a genus of spherical Gram-positive bacteria occurring in colonies. They are saprophytes or parasites. The species *M. tetragenus* (formerly *Gaffkya tetragena*) is normally a harmless parasite in man but it can become pathogenic, causing arthritis, endocarditis, meningitis, or abscesses in tissues. It occurs in groups of four.

microcyte *n.* an abnormally small red blood cell (*erythrocyte). *See also* microcytosis. —**microcytic** *adj.*

microcytosis *n.* the presence of abnormally small red cells (*microcytes*) in the blood. Microcytosis is a feature of certain anaemias (*microcytic anaemias*), including iron-deficiency anaemias, certain *haemoglobinopathies, anaemias associated with chronic infections, etc.

microdactyly *n.* abnormal smallness or shortness of the fingers.

microdissection *n.* the process of dissecting minute structures under the microscope. Miniature surgical instruments, such as knives made of glass, are manipulated by means of geared connections that reduce the relatively coarse movements of the operator's fingers into microscopic movements. Using this technique it is possible to dissect the nuclei of cells and even to separate individual chromosomes. *See also* microsurgery.

microdontia *n.* a condition in which the teeth are unusually small.

microelectrode *n.* an extremely fine wire used as an electrode to measure the electrical activity in small areas of tissue. Microelectrodes can be used for recording the electrical changes that occur in the membranes of cells, such as those of nerve and muscle.

microfilaria *n.* (*pl.* **microfilariae**) the motile embryo of certain nematodes (*see* filaria). The slender microfilariae, 150–300 μm in length, are commonly found in the circulating blood or lymph of patients suffering an infection with any of the filarial worms, e.g. *Wuchereria*. They mature into larvae, which are infective, within the body of a bloodsucking insect, such as a mosquito.

microgamete *n.* the motile flagellate male sex cell of the malarial parasite (*Plasmodium*) and other single-celled animals (*see* Protozoa). The microgamete is similar to the sperm cell of higher animal groups and smaller than the female sex cell (*see* macrogamete).

microgametocyte *n.* a cell that undergoes meiosis to form 6–8 mature male sex cells (microgametes) of the malarial parasite (*Plasmodium*). Microgametocytes are found in the blood of man but must be ingested by a mosquito before developing into microgametes.

microglia *n.* one of the two basic classes of *glia (the non-nervous cells of the central nervous system), having a mainly scavenging function (*see* macrophage). *Compare* macroglia.

microglossia *n.* abnormally small size of the tongue.

micrognathia *n.* a condition in which one jaw is unusually small.

microgram *n.* one millionth of a gram. Symbol: μg.

micrograph (photomicrograph) *n.* a photograph of an object viewed through a microscope. An *electron micrograph* is photographed through an electron microscope; a *light micrograph* through a light microscope.

microgyria *n.* a developmental disorder of the brain in which the folds (convolutions) in its surface are small and its surface layer (cortex) is structurally abnormal. It is associated with mental and physical retardation.

microhaematocrit *n.* a measurement of the proportion of red blood cells in a volume of circulating blood. It is determined by taking a sample of the patient's blood in a fine tube and spinning it in a centrifuge until settling is complete. *See* packed cell volume.

micromanipulation *n.* the manipulation of extremely small structures under the microscope, as in *microdissection, or *microsurgery.

micromastia (micromazia) *n.* the condition of having abnormally small breasts.

micromelia *n.* abnormally small size of the arms or legs. *Compare* macromelia.

micrometer *n.* an instrument for making extremely fine measurements of thickness or length, often relying upon the movement of a screw thread and the principle of the *vernier.

micrometre *n.* one millionth of a metre (10^{-6} m). Symbol: μm.

microorganism (microbe) *n.* any organism too small to be visible to the naked eye. Microorganisms include *bacteria, some *fungi, *mycoplasmas, *protozoa, *rickettsiae, and *viruses.

microphotograph *n.* **1.** a photograph reduced to microscopic proportions. **2.** (loosely) a *photomicrograph.

micropipette *n.* an extremely fine tube from which minute volumes of liquid can be delivered. It can also be used to draw up minute quantities of liquid for examination. Using a micropipette it is possible to add or take away material from individual cells under the microscope.

micropsia *n.* a condition in which objects appear smaller than they really are. It is usually due to disease of the retina affecting the *macula but may occur in paralysis of *accommodation and in some brain disorders.

microscope *n.* an instrument for producing a greatly magnified image of an object, which may be so small as to be invisible to the naked eye. *Light* or *optical microscopes* use light as a radiation source for viewing the specimen and combinations of lenses to magnify the image, usually an *objective and an *eyepiece. *See also* electron microscope, operating microscope, ultramicroscope. **—microscopical** *adj.* **—microscopy** *n.*

microscopic *adj.* **1.** too small to be seen clearly without the use of a microscope. **2.** of, relating to, or using a microscope.

microsome *n.* a small particle consisting of a piece of *endoplasmic reticulum with ribosomes attached. Microsomes are formed when homogenized cells are centrifuged. **—microsomal** *adj.*

microsonation *n.* the use of ultrasound waves generated inside the body

from an extremely small source, such as the tip of a needle or a bubble within the tissues. This technique is used to obtain a picture of the fine structure of the neighbouring tissues. It is a specialized form of *ultrasonography.

Microsporum *n.* a genus of fungi causing *ringworm of the skin, hair, and nails. The species *M. audouini* causes ringworm of the scalp (tinea capitis).

microsurgery *n.* the branch of surgery in which extremely intricate operations are performed through highly refined *operating microscopes using miniaturized precision instruments (forceps, scissors, needles, etc.). The technique enables surgery of previously inaccessible parts of the eye, inner ear, spinal cord, and brain (e.g. for the removal of tumours and repair of cerebral aneurysms), as well as the reattachment of amputated fingers (necessitating the suturing of minute nerves and blood vessels) and the reversal of vasectomies.

microtome *n.* an instrument for cutting extremely thin slices of material that can be examined under a microscope. The material is usually embedded in a suitable medium, such as paraffin wax. A common type of microtome is a steel knife.

microvillus *n.* (*pl.* **microvilli**) one of a number of microscopic hairlike structures (about 5 μm long) projecting from the surface of epithelial cells (*see* epithelium). They serve to increase the surface area of the cell and are seen on absorptive and secretory cells. In some regions (particularly the intestinal tract) microvilli form a dense covering on the free surface of the cells: this is called a *brush border*.

microwave therapy a form of *diathermy using electromagnetic waves of extremely short wavelength. In modern apparatus the electric currents induced in the tissues have frequencies of up to 25,000 million cycles per second.

micturition *n. see* urination.

midbrain (mesencephalon) *n.* the small portion of the *brainstem, excluding the pons and the medulla, that joins the hindbrain to the forebrain.

middle ear (tympanic cavity) the part of the *ear that consists of an air-filled space within the petrous part of the temporal bone. It is lined with mucous membrane and is connected to the pharynx by the *Eustachian tube and to the outer ear by the eardrum (*tympanic membrane). Within the middle ear are three bones – the auditory *ossicles – which transmit sound vibrations from the outer ear to the inner ear (*see* labyrinth).

midgut *n.* the middle portion of the embryonic gut, which gives rise to most of the small intestine and part of the large intestine. Early in development it is connected with the *yolk sac outside the embryo via the *umbilicus.

midwifery *n.* the profession of providing assistance and medical care to women undergoing labour and childbirth. *See also* domiciliary midwife, obstetrics. —**midwife** *n.*

migraine *n.* a recurrent throbbing headache that characteristically affects one side of the head. There is sometimes forewarning of an attack (an *aura*) consisting of flickering bright lights or blurring of vision, which clears up as the headache develops. It is often accompanied by prostration and vomiting.

miliaria *n. see* prickly heat.

miliary *adj.* describing or characterized by very small nodules or lesions, resembling millet seed.

miliary tuberculosis acute generalized *tuberculosis characterized by le-

sions in affected organs, which resemble millet seeds.

milium *n.* (*pl.* **milia**) a white nodule in the skin, particularly on the face. Up to 4 mm in diameter, milia are round masses of *keratin occurring just beneath the outer layer (epidermis) of the skin.

milk *n.* the liquid food secreted by female mammals from the mammary gland. It is the sole source of food for the young of most mammals at the start of life. Milk is a complete food in that it has most of the nutrients necessary for life: protein, carbohydrate, fat, minerals, and vitamins. The composition of milk varies very much from mammal to mammal. Cows' milk contains nearly all the essential nutrients but is comparatively deficient in vitamins C and D. Human milk contains more sugar (lactose) and less protein than cows' milk.

milk leg *see* white leg.

milk teeth *Colloquial.* the deciduous teeth of young children. *See* dentition.

milli- *prefix denoting* one thousandth part.

milliampere *n.* one thousandth of an ampere (10^{-3} A). Symbol: mA.

milligram *n.* one thousandth of a gram. Symbol: mg.

millilitre *n.* one thousandth of a litre. Symbol: ml. *See* litre.

millimetre *n.* one thousandth of a metre (10^{-3} m). Symbol: mm.

Miltown *n. see* meprobamate.

MIND the National Association for Mental Health. It is a voluntary association, registered as a charity, that promotes the welfare of those with *mental illness through advice, education, campaigning, and the provision of resources.

mineralocorticoid *n. see* corticosteroid.

minim *n.* a unit of volume used in pharmacy, equivalent to one sixtieth part of a fluid *drachm.

Minimata disease a form of mercury poisoning (from ingesting methyl mercury in contaminated fish) that caused 43 deaths in the Japanese coastal town of Minimata during 1953–56. The source of mercury was traced to an effluent containing mercuric sulphate from a local PVC factory. Symptoms include numbness, difficulty in controlling the limbs, and impaired speech and hearing.

mio- *prefix denoting* **1.** reduction or diminution. **2.** rudimentary.

miosis (myosis) *n.* constriction of the pupil. This occurs normally in bright light, but persistent miosis is most commonly due to drug therapy for glaucoma. *See also* miotic. *Compare* mydriasis.

miotic *n.* a drug that causes the pupil of the eye to contract. Miotics, such as *physostigmine and *pilocarpine, are used to counteract the dilation of the pupil caused by drugs such as ephedrine and phenylephrine and to reduce the pressure in the eye in the treatment of glaucoma.

miracidium *n.* (*pl.* **miracidia**) the first-stage larva of a parasitic *fluke. Miracidia hatch from eggs released into water with the host's excreta. They have *cilia and swim about until they reach a snail. The miracidia then bore into the snail's soft tissues and there continue their development as *sporocysts.

miscarriage *n. see* abortion.

miso- *prefix denoting* hatred. Example: *misopedia* (of children).

missed case a person suffering from an infection in whom the symptoms and signs are so minimal that either there is no request for medical assistance or the doctor fails to make the diagnosis. The patient usually has partial immunity to the disease, but since the infecting organisms (pathogens) are of normal virulence, nonimmune contacts can be affected with the full manifestations of the illness. The period of infectivity is confined to the shortened duration of the illness (in contrast to a *carrier, in whom the pathogen is present without necessarily causing any ill effect). Alternatively the subject has had the disease but retains some of the pathogens (e.g. in the throat or bowel) and so acts as a continuing reservoir of infection.

Misuse of Drugs Act (1971) (in the UK) an Act of Parliament restricting the use of dangerous drugs. These controlled drugs include the natural *opiates and their synthetic substitutes, many stimulants (including amphetamine, cocaine, and pemoline), hallucinogens such as LSD and cannabis, and the sedative methaqualone. The Act specifies certain requirements for writing prescriptions for these drugs.

mite *n.* a free-living or parasitic arthropod belonging to a group (Acarina) that also includes the *ticks. Most mites are small, averaging 1 mm or less in length. A mite has no antennae or wings, and its body is not divided into a distinct head, thorax, and abdomen. Medically important mites include the many species causing dermatitis (e.g. *Dermatophagoides*) and the harvest mite (*see* Trombicula), which transmits scrub typhus.

mithramycin *n.* an *antibiotic that prevents the growth of cancer cells. It is used mainly to treat cancer of the testis and is administered by injection. Common side-effects are digestive upsets and mouth ulcers and, more seriously, nosebleeds and vomiting of blood.

mitobronitol *n.* a drug that prevents growth of cancer cells, used to treat leukaemia. It is administered by mouth; common side-effects are digestive upsets, hair loss, skin disorders, menstrual abnormalities, and reduction in the numbers of normal blood cells. Trade name: **Myelobromol**.

mitochondrion (chondriosome) *n.* (*pl.* **mitochondria**) a structure, occurring in varying numbers in the cytoplasm of every cell, that is the site of the cell's energy production. Mitochondria contain *ATP and the enzymes involved in the cell's metabolic activities; each is bounded by a double membrane, the inner being folded inwards to form projections (*cristae*). —**mitochondrial** *adj.*

mitogen *n.* any substance that can cause cells to begin division (*mitosis).

mitomycin C an antibiotic that inhibits the growth of cancer cells. It causes severe marrow suppression but is of use in the treatment of stomach and breast cancers.

mitosis *n.* a type of cell division in which a single cell produces two genetically identical daughter cells. It is the way in which new body cells are produced for both growth and repair. Division of the nucleus (*karyokinesis*) takes place in four stages (*see* prophase, metaphase, anaphase, telophase) and is followed by division of the cytoplasm (*cytokinesis*) to form two daughter cells (see illustration). *Compare* meiosis. —**mitotic** *adj.*

mitral incompetence failure of the *mitral valve to close, allowing a reflux of blood from the left ventricle of the heart to the left atrium. It most often results from scarring of the mitral valve by rheumatic fever, but it can also develop as a complication of myocardial infarction or cardiomyopathies. It may occur as a congenital defect. Its manifestations include breathlessness, atrial *fibrillation, embolism, enlargement of the left ventricle, and a systolic *murmur. Mild cases are symptomless and require no treatment, but in severe cases the affected valve should be

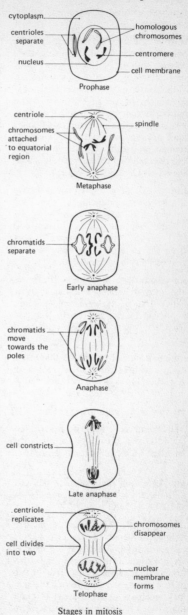

Stages in mitosis

mitral stenosis

replaced with an artificial one (*mitral prosthesis*).

mitral stenosis narrowing of the opening of the mitral valve: a result of chronic scarring that follows rheumatic fever. It may be seen alone or combined with *mitral incompetence. The symptoms are similar to those of mitral incompetence except that the patient has a diastolic *murmur. Mild cases need no treatment, but severe cases are treated surgically by reopening the stenosis (*mitral valvotomy*) or by inserting an artificial valve (*mitral prosthesis*).

mitral valve (bicuspid valve) a valve in the heart consisting of two flaps (cusps) attached to the walls at the opening between the left atrium and left ventricle. It allows blood to pass from the atrium to the ventricle, but prevents any backward flow.

mittelschmerz *n.* pain in the lower abdomen experienced about midway between successive menstrual periods, i.e. when the egg cell is being released from the ovary. *See also* menstrual cycle.

mixed connective tissue disease a disease with features in common with systemic *lupus erythematosus, *polymyositis, and *scleroderma.

ml *abbrev. for* millilitre. *See* litre.

MLD minimal lethal dose: the smallest quantity of a toxic compound that is recorded as having caused death. *See also* LD_{50}.

mmHg a unit of pressure equal to 1 millimetre of mercury. 1 mmHg = 133.3224 pascals.

modality *n.* **1.** a form of sensation, such as smell, hearing, tasting, or detecting temperature. Differences in modality are not due to differences in the structure of the nerves concerned, but to differences in the working of the sensory receptors and the areas of brain that receive the messages. **2.** one form

of therapy as opposed to another, such as the modality of physiotherapy contrasted with that of radiotherapy.

mode *n. see* mean.

modelling *n.* a technique used in *behaviour modification, whereby an individual learns a behaviour by observing someone else doing it. Together with *prompting, it is useful for introducing new behaviours to the individual.

modiolus *n.* the conical central pillar of the *cochlea in the inner ear.

Mogadon *n. see* nitrazepam.

molar *n.* in the permanent *dentition, the sixth, seventh, or eighth tooth from the midline on each side in each jaw (*see also* wisdom tooth). In the deciduous dentition, molars are the fourth and fifth teeth from the midline on each side in each jaw.

molarity *n.* the strength of a solution, expressed as the weight of dissolved substance in grams per litre divided by its molecular weight, i.e. the number of moles per litre. Molarity is indicated as 0.1 M, 1 M, 2 M, etc.

molar solution a solution in which the number of grams of dissolved substance per litre equals its molecular weight, i.e. a solution of molarity 1 M.

mole[1] *n.* the *SI unit of amount of substance, equal to the amount of substance that contains as many elementary units as there are atoms in 0.012 kilograms of carbon-12. The elementary units, which must be specified, may be atoms, molecules, ions, electrons, etc., or a specified group of such entities. One mole of a compound has a mass equal to its molecular weight expressed in grams. Symbol: mol.

mole[2] *n.* an area of pigment, usually brown, in the skin. Some moles are flat; others are raised and occasionally have hairs growing from them. Certain types of mole can become malignant.

molecular biology the study of the molecules that are associated with living organisms, especially proteins and nucleic acids.

molluscum n. any of several skin diseases typified by the development of soft rounded tumours. Commonly, the term is used for *molluscum contagiosum*, a virus disease that produces small rounded pearl-like swellings with craters containing broken-down matter. The condition is chronic and treatment is by removal with a *curette, *electrocautery, or by instilling carbolic acid locally. *See also* keratoacanthoma (molluscum sebaceum).

mon- (mono-) *prefix denoting* one, single, or alone.

mongolism n. *see* Down's syndrome.

Monilia n. the former name of the genus of fungi now known as *Candida*.

moniliasis n. *see* candidiasis.

monoamine oxidase (MAO) an enzyme that catalyses the oxidation of a large variety of monoamines, including adrenaline, noradrenaline, and serotonin. Monoamine oxidase is found in most tissues, particularly the liver and nervous system. Drugs that act as inhibitors of this enzyme are widely used in the treatment of depression (*see* MAO inhibitor).

monoarthritis n. *see* arthritis.

monoblast n. the earliest identifiable cell that gives rise to a *monocyte. It is probably identical with the *myeloblast and matures via an intermediate stage (*promonocyte*). It is normally found in the blood-forming tissue of the *bone marrow but may appear in the blood in certain diseases, most notably in acute monoblastic *leukaemia.

monochromat n. a person who is completely colour-blind. There are two types. The *rod monochromat* appears to have totally defective *cones: he has very poor visual acuity as well as the inability to discriminate colours. The *cone monochromat* has normal visual acuity: his cones appear to respond normally to light but to be completely unable to discriminate colours. It is possible in this case that the defect does not lie in the cones themselves but in the integration of the nerve impulses as they pass from the cones to the brain. Both types of colour blindness are probably inherited.

monoclonal antibody an antibody produced artificially from a cell *clone and therefore consisting of a single type of immunoglobulin. Monoclonal antibodies are produced by fusing antibody-forming lymphocytes from mouse spleen with mouse myeloma cells. The resulting hybrid cells multiply rapidly (like cancer cells) and produce the same antibody as their parent lymphocytes.

monocular *adj.* relating to or used by one eye only. *Compare* binocular.

monocyte n. a variety of white blood cell, 16–20 μm in diameter, with a kidney-shaped nucleus and greyish-blue cytoplasm (when treated with *Romanowsky stains). Its function is the ingestion of foreign particles, such as bacteria and tissue debris. There are normally 0.2–0.8 × 10^9 monocytes per litre of blood. —**monocytic** *adj.*

monocytosis n. an increase in the number of *monocytes in the blood. Monocytosis occurs in a variety of diseases, including certain leukaemias (*monocytic leukaemias*) and infections due to some bacteria and protozoa.

monodactylism n. the congenital absence of all but one digit on each hand and foot.

monoiodotyrosine n. an iodine-containing substance produced in the thyroid gland from which the *thyroid hormones are derived.

monomania *n.* the state in which a particular delusion or set of delusions is present in an otherwise normally functioning person. *See also* paranoia.

mononeuritis *n.* disease affecting a single peripheral nerve. Entrapment of the nerve or interference with its blood supply are the commonest causes. *Mononeuritis multiplex* is the separate involvement of two or more nerves. *Compare* polyneuropathy.

mononucleosis *n.* the condition in which the blood contains an abnormally high number of mononuclear leucocytes (*monocytes). *See* glandular fever (infectious mononucleosis).

monophobia *n.* an extreme fear of being alone.

monophyletic *adj.* describing a number of individuals, species, etc., that have evolved from a single ancestral group. *Compare* polyphyletic.

monoplegia *n.* paralysis of one limb. —**monoplegic** *adj.*

monoploid *adj.* *see* haploid.

monorchism *n.* absence of one testis. This is usually due to failure of one testicle to descend into the scrotum before birth. The term is sometimes used for the condition in which one testicle has been removed surgically or destroyed by injury or disease. If the single testis is normal, no adverse effects result from the absence of the other.

monosaccharide *n.* a simple sugar having the general formula $(CH_2O)_n$. Monosaccharides may have between three and nine carbon atoms, but the most common number is five or six. Monosaccharides are classified according to the number of carbon atoms they possess. Thus *trioses* have three carbon atoms, *tetroses* four, *pentoses* five, and *hexoses* six. The most abundant monosaccharide is glucose (a hexose).

monosomy *n.* a condition in which there is one chromosome missing from the normal (*diploid) set. *Compare* trisomy. —**monosomic** *adj.*

monozygotic twins *see* twins.

mons *n.* (in anatomy) a rounded eminence. The *mons pubis* is the mound of fatty tissue lying over the pubic symphysis.

Moraxella *n.* a genus of short rodlike Gram-negative aerobic bacteria, usually occurring in pairs. They exist as parasites in many warm-blooded animals. The species *M. lacunata* causes conjunctivitis.

morbid *adj.* diseased or abnormal; pathological.

morbidity *n.* the state of being diseased. The *morbidity rate* is the number of cases of a disease found to occur in a stated number of the population, usually given as cases per 100,000 or per million. Annual figures for morbidity rate give the incidence of the disease, which is the number of new cases reported in the year. *See also* incidence rate, prevalence rate.

morbilli *n.* *see* measles.

morbilliform *adj.* describing a skin rash resembling that of measles.

morbus *n.* disease. The term is usually used as part of the medical name of a specific disease.

mordant *n.* (in microscopy) a substance, such as alum or phenol, used to fix a *stain in a tissue.

moribund *adj.* dying.

morning sickness nausea and vomiting during early pregnancy. In some women the symptoms disappear if a small amount of food is eaten before rising in the morning. *Compare* hyperemesis. Medical name: **nausea gravidarum**.

moron *n. Obsolete.* a person afflicted by a mild degree of mental subnormality. *See* feeblemindedness.

morphine *n.* a potent analgesic and *narcotic drug used mainly to relieve severe and persistent pain. It is administered by mouth or injection; common side-effects are loss of appetite, nausea, constipation, and confusion. Morphine causes feelings of euphoria; *tolerance develops rapidly and *dependence may occur.

morpho- *prefix denoting* form or structure.

morphoea *n.* a localized form of *scleroderma in which the skin and sometimes the underlying tissues are replaced with connective tissue, forming areas or bands of infiltrating tissue. These bands may follow the course of nerves. The sweat glands and hair follicles disappear in the affected area.

morphogenesis *n.* the development of form and structure of the body and its parts.

morphology *n. see* anatomy.

-morphous *suffix denoting* form or structure (of a specified kind).

Morquio-Brailsford disease *see* chondrodysplasia.

mortality (mortality rate) *n.* the incidence of death in the population in a given period. The *annual mortality rate* is the number of registered deaths in a year, multiplied by 1000 and divided by the population at the middle of the year. *See also* infant mortality rate, maternal mortality rate.

mortification *n. see* necrosis.

morula *n.* an early stage of embryonic development formed by *cleavage of the fertilized ovum. It consists of a solid ball of cells and is an intermediate stage between the zygote and *blastocyst.

mosaicism *n.* a condition in which the cells of an individual do not all contain identical chromosomes; there may be two or more genetically different populations of cells. Often one of the cell populations is normal and the other one carries a chromosome defect such as *Down's syndrome or *Turner's syndrome. In affected individuals the chromosome defect is usually not fully expressed. —**mosaic** *adj.*

mosquito *n.* a small winged bloodsucking insect belonging to a large group – the *Diptera (two-winged flies). Its mouthparts are formed into a long proboscis for piercing the skin and sucking blood. Female mosquitoes transmit the parasites responsible for several major infectious diseases, such as *malaria. *See* Anopheles, Aëdes, Culex.

motile *adj.* being able to move spontaneously, without external aid: usually applied to a *microorganism or a cell (e.g. a sperm cell).

motion sickness *see* travel sickness.

motor cortex the region of the *cerebral cortex that is responsible for initiating nerve impulses that bring about voluntary activity in the muscles of the body. It is possible to map out the cortex to show which of its areas is responsible for which particular part of the body. The motor cortex of the left cerebral hemisphere is responsible for muscular activity in the right side of the body.

motor nerve one of the nerves that carry impulses outwards from the central nervous system to bring about activity in a muscle or gland. *Compare* sensory nerve.

motor neurone one of the units (*neurones) that goes to make up the nerve pathway between the brain and an effector organ, such as a skeletal muscle. An *upper motor neurone* has a cell body in the brain and an axon that extends into the spinal cord, where it ends in synapses. It is thus entirely within the central nervous system. A *lower motor neurone*, on the other hand, has a cell body in the spinal cord or brainstem and an axon that extends outwards in a cranial or spinal motor nerve to reach an effector.

motor neurone disease a progressive degenerative disease of the motor system occurring in middle age and causing muscle weakness and wasting. It primarily affects the cells of the anterior horn of the spinal cord, the motor nuclei in the brainstem, and the corticospinal fibres. There are three clinically distinct forms: *amyotrophic lateral sclerosis* (*ALS*), *progressive muscular atrophy*, and *progressive bulbar palsy*.

mould *n.* any multicellular filamentous fungus that commonly forms a rough furry coating on decaying matter.

moulding *n.* the changing of the shape of an infant's head during labour, brought about by the pressures to which it is subjected when passing through the birth passage.

mountain sickness *see* altitude sickness.

mouthwash *n.* an aqueous solution with antiseptic, astringent, or deodorizing properties used for daily rinsing of the mouth and teeth. Mouthwashes are used to prevent dental *caries (*see also* chlorhexidine) and to treat mild throat infections.

moxibustion *n.* a form of treatment favoured in Japan, in which cones of sunflower pith or down from the leaves of the plant *Artemisia moxa* are stuck to the skin and ignited. The heat produced by the smouldering cones acts as a counterirritant and is reputed to cure a variety of disorders.

MSH *see* melanocyte-stimulating hormone.

mucilage *n.* (in pharmacy) a thick aqueous solution of a gum used as a lubricant in skin preparations (*see also* glycerin), for the production of pills, and for the suspension of insoluble substances. The most important mucilages are of acacia, tragacanth, and starch.

mucin *n.* the principal constituent of *mucus. Mucin is a *glycoprotein.

muco- *prefix denoting* **1.** mucus. **2.** mucous membrane.

mucocele *n.* a space or organ distended with mucus. For example, it may occur in the gall bladder when the exit duct becomes obstructed so that the mucus secretions are retained and dilate the cavity of the organ. A mucocele in the soft tissues arising from a salivary gland occurs when the duct is blocked or ruptured.

mucolytic *n.* an agent, such as carbocysteine or tyloxapol, that dissolves or breaks down mucus. Mucolytics are used to treat chest conditions involving excessive or thickened mucus secretions.

mucopolysaccharide *n.* one of a group of complex carbohydrates functioning mainly as structural components in connective tissue. Mucopolysaccharide molecules are usually built up of two repeating sugar units, one of which is an amino sugar. An example of a mucopolysaccharide is *chondroitin, occurring in cartilage.

mucoprotein *n.* one of a group of proteins found in the *globulin fraction of blood plasma. Mucoproteins are globulins combined with a carbohydrate group (an amino sugar). They are similar to *glycoproteins but contain a greater proportion of carbohydrate.

mucopurulent *adj.* containing mucus and pus. *See* mucopus.

mucopus *n.* a mixture of *mucus and *pus.

Mucor *n.* a genus of mould fungi commonly seen on dead and decaying organic matter. They can be pathogenic in man (*see* mucormycosis).

mucormycosis *n.* a disease caused by a fungus of the genus *Mucor*, affecting the external ear, skin, and respiratory passages.

mucosa *n. see* mucous membrane. —**mucosal** *adj.*

mucous membrane (mucosa) the moist membrane lining many tubular structures and cavities, including the nasal sinuses, respiratory tract, gastrointestinal tract, biliary, and pancreatic systems. The surface of the mouth is lined by mucous membrane, the nature of which varies according to its site. The mucous membrane consists of a surface layer of *epithelium, which contains glands secreting *mucus, with underlying layers of connective tissue (lamina propria) and muscularis mucosae, which forms the inner boundary of the mucous membrane.

mucoviscidosis *n. see* cystic fibrosis.

mucus *n.* a viscous fluid secreted by *mucous membranes. Mucus acts as a protective barrier over the membranes, a lubricant, and a carrier of enzymes. It consists chiefly of *glycoproteins, particularly *mucin*. —**mucous** *adj.*

MUGA scan (multiple-gated arteriography) a method of studying left-ventricular function and wall motion of the heart by injecting the patient's red cells with radioactive technetium-99 to form an image of the blood pool within the heart at specific points in the cardiac cycle, using an ECG, gamma camera, and computer.

Müllerian duct *see* paramesonephric duct.

multifactorial *adj.* describing a condition that is believed to have resulted from the interaction of genetic factors, usually polygenes, with an environmental factor or factors. Many disorders, e.g. spina bifida and anencephaly, are thought to be multifactorial.

multifocal lenses lenses in which the power (*see* dioptre) of the lower part gradually increases towards the lower edge. There is no dividing line on the lens as there is between the upper and lower segments of *bifocal lenses. The wearer can see clearly at any distance by lowering or raising his eyes.

multigravida *n.* a woman who has been pregnant at least twice.

multipara *n.* a woman who has given birth to a live child after each of at least two pregnancies.

multiple sclerosis (disseminated sclerosis) a chronic disease of the nervous system affecting young and middle-aged adults. The *myelin sheaths surrounding nerves in the brain and spinal cord are damaged, which affects the function of the nerves involved. The course of the illness is characterized by recurrent relapses followed by remissions. The disease affects different parts of the brain and spinal cord, resulting in typically scattered symptoms. These include unsteady gait and shaky movements of the limbs (ataxia), rapid involuntary movements of the eyes (*nystagmus), defects in speech pronunciation (dysarthria), spastic weakness, and *retrobulbar neuritis. The underlying cause of the nerve damage remains unknown.

multivariate analysis *see* correlation.

mummification *n.* **1.** the conversion of dead tissue into a hard shrunken mass, chiefly by dehydration. **2.** (in dentistry) the application of a fixative to the dental pulp to prevent decomposition.

mumps *n.* a common virus infection mainly affecting children between the ages of five and 15. Symptoms appear 2–3 weeks after exposure: fever, headache, and vomiting may precede a

Munchhausen's syndrome

typical swelling of the *parotid salivary glands. The gland on one side of the face often swells up days before the other but sometimes only one side is affected. The symptoms usually vanish within three days, the patient remaining infectious until the swelling has completely disappeared, but the infection may spread to other salivary glands and to the pancreas, brain, and testicles. In adult men, mumps can cause sterility. Most people acquire immunity through a childhood infection. Medical name: **infectious parotitis**.

Munchhausen's syndrome a mental disorder in which the patient persistently tries to obtain hospital treatment for an illness that is nonexistent: an extreme form of malingering. The disease may be described in vivid detail, and in some cases injury may be deliberately self-inflicted in an attempt to give the appearance of authenticity to the claims being made.

murmur (bruit) *n.* a noise, heard with the aid of a stethoscope, that is generated by turbulent blood flow within the heart or blood vessels. Turbulent flow is produced by damaged valves, *septal defects, narrowed arteries, or arteriovenous communications. Heart murmurs can also be heard in normal individuals, especially those who have hyperac-

tive circulation, and frequently in normal children (*innocent murmurs*). Murmurs are classified as *systolic* or *diastolic* (heard in ventricular *systole or *diastole respectively); *continuous murmurs* are heard throughout systole and diastole.

muscae volitantes *pl. n.* black spots seen floating before the eyes usually due to the presence of opaque specks in the vitreous humour.

muscle *n.* a tissue whose cells have the ability to contract, producing movement or force (see illustration). Muscles possess mechanisms for converting energy derived from chemical reactions into mechanical energy. The major functions of muscles are to produce movements of the body, to maintain the position of the body against the force of gravity, to produce movements of structures inside the body, and to alter pressures or tensions of structures in the body. There are three types of muscle: *striated muscle, attached to the skeleton; *smooth muscle, which is found in such tissues as the stomach, gut, and blood vessels; and *cardiac muscle, which forms the walls of the heart.

muscle relaxant an agent that reduces tension in muscles. Drugs such as *chlormezanone, *diazepam, and *mephensin are used to relieve skeletal muscular spasms in various spastic

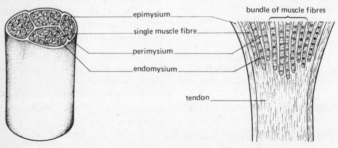

A voluntary muscle in transverse section (left) and in longitudinal section at its junction with a tendon (right)

conditions, parkinsonism, and tetanus. Other drugs, e.g. *gallamine, *suxamethonium, and *tubocurarine, paralyse voluntary muscles and are used in addition to anaesthetics to relax the muscles during surgical operations.

muscle spindle a specialized receptor, sensitive to stretch, that is embedded between and parallel to the fibres of striated muscles. These receptors are important for coordinated muscular movement. *See also* stretch receptor.

muscular dystrophy any one of a group of muscle diseases in which there is a recognizable pattern of inheritance. They are marked by weakness and wasting of selected muscles: the affected muscle fibres degenerate and are replaced by fatty tissue. The muscular dystrophies are classified according to the patient's age at onset, distribution of the weakness, the progression of the disease, and the mode of inheritance. Confirmation of the diagnosis is based upon *electromyography and muscle biopsy.

The most common form is *Duchenne dystrophy*, which is inherited as a sex-linked recessive character and is nearly always restricted to boys. It usually begins before the age of four, with selective weakness and wasting of the muscles of the pelvic girdle and back. The child has a waddling gait and *lordosis of the lumbar spine. The calf muscles – and later the shoulders and upper limbs – often become firm and bulky. Although the disease cannot be cured, physiotherapy and orthopaedic measures can relieve the disability. *See also* dystrophia myotonica.

muscularis *n.* a muscular layer of the wall of a hollow organ (such as the stomach) or a tubular structure (such as the intestine or ureter). The *muscularis mucosae* is the muscular layer of a mucous membrane complex, especially that of the stomach or intestine.

muscular rheumatism any aching pain in the muscles and joints. Commonly the symptoms are due to *fibrositis; wear and tear of the joints (*osteoarthritis); or to inflammation of the muscles associated with abnormal immune reactions (*polymyalgia rheumatica).

musculo- *prefix denoting* muscle.

musculocutaneous nerve a nerve of the *brachial plexus that supplies some muscles of the arm and the skin of the lateral part of the forearm.

mushroom *n.* the aerial fruiting (spore-producing) body of various fungi. Edible mushrooms include the field and cultivated mushrooms (*Agaricus campestris* and *A. bisporus*), the chanterelle (*Cantherellus cibarius*), and the parasol (*Lepiota procera*). However, great care must be taken in identifying edible fungi. Many species are poisonous, especially the death cap and panther cap (*see* Amanita).

mustine (nitrogen mustard) *n.* a drug used to treat various types of cancer, including Hodgkin's disease and some types of leukaemia. It is administered by injection; common side-effects include nausea and vomiting, and the drug may damage the bone marrow, causing serious blood disorders.

mutagen *n.* an external agent that, when applied to cells or organisms, can increase the rate of *mutation. Mutagens usually only increase the number of mutants formed and do not cause mutations not found under natural conditions. Several kinds of radiation, many chemicals, and some viruses can act as mutagens. *Compare* antimutagen.

mutant *n.* **1.** an individual in which a mutation has occurred, especially when the effect of the mutation is visible. **2.** a characteristic showing the effects of a mutation. —**mutant** *adj.*

mutation *n.* a change in the genetic material (*DNA) of a cell, or the change this causes in a characteristic of the individual, which is not caused by normal genetic processes. In a *point* (or *gene*) *mutation* there is a change in a single gene; in a *chromosome mutation* there is a change in the structure or number of the chromosomes. All mutations are rare events and may occur spontaneously or be caused by external agents (*mutagens). If a mutation occurs in developing sex cells (gametes) it may be inherited. Mutations in any other cells (*somatic mutations*) are not inherited.

mutism *n.* inability or refusal to speak; dumbness. Innate speechlessness most commonly occurs in those who have been totally deaf since birth (*deaf-mutism*). Inability to speak may result from brain damage (*see* aphasia). It may also be caused by depression or psychological trauma, in which case the patient either does not speak at all or speaks only to particular persons or in particular situations. This latter condition is called *elective mutism*.
Treatment of mutism due to psychological causes is increasingly by behavioural means, such as *prompting: people that the patient does not address are slowly introduced into the situation where the patient does speak. This may be done either alone or in combination with more traditional psychotherapy. —**mute** *adj., n.*

mutualism *n.* the intimate but not necessarily obligatory association between two different species of organism in which there is mutual aid and benefit. *Compare* symbiosis.

my- (myo-) *prefix denoting* muscle.

myalgia *n.* pain in the muscles.

myasthenia gravis a chronic disease marked by abnormal fatiguability and weakness of selected muscles, which is relieved by rest or *anticholinesterase drugs. The degree of fatigue is so extreme that these muscles are temporarily paralysed. Other symptoms include drooping of the upper eyelid (ptosis), double vision, and *dysarthria. The cause is uncertain, but appears to be associated with impaired ability of the neurotransmitter acetylcholine to induce muscular contraction. It chiefly affects adolescents and young adults (usually women) and adults over 40. Drug treatment and surgical removal of the thymus lessen the severity of the symptoms.

myc- (myco-, mycet(o)-) *prefix denoting* a fungus.

mycelium *n.* (*pl.* **mycelia**) the tangled mass of fine branching threads that make up the feeding and growing part of a *fungus.

mycetoma *n.* a chronic inflammation of tissues caused by a fungus. *See* Madura foot.

Mycobacterium *n.* a genus of rodlike Gram-positive aerobic bacteria that can form filamentous branching structures. Some species are pathogenic to animals and man: *M. leprae* (*Hansen's bacillus*) causes *leprosy; *M. tuberculosis* (*Koch's bacillus*) causes *tuberculosis. *M. bovis* causes tuberculosis in cattle but can also infect the lungs, joints, and intestines of man.

mycology *n.* the science of fungi. *See also* microbiology. —**mycologist** *n.*

mycoplasma *n.* one of a group of minute nonmotile microorganisms that lack a rigid cell wall and hence display a variety of forms. They are regarded by some authorities as primitive bacteria. The group includes some species that cause severe respiratory disease in cattle, sheep, and goats; one of these, *Mycoplasma pneumoniae*, causes a pneumonia-like disease in man. The group also includes the *pleuropneumonia-like organisms* (*PPLO*).

mycosis *n.* any disease caused by a fungus, including actinomycosis, aspergillosis, cryptococcosis, rhinosporidiosis, ringworm, and sporotrichosis.

mycosis fungoides a disease that is a variety of *reticulosis usually confined to the skin. Chronic irritating eruptions occur, resembling eczema or psoriasis. Purplish tumours develop and then ulcerate. The disease is fatal, though partial remission may be effected with anti-cancer drugs.

Mycota *n. see* undecenoic acid.

mydriasis *n.* widening of the pupil, which occurs normally in dim light. The commonest cause of prolonged mydriasis is drug therapy (*see* mydriatic) or injury to the eye. *See also* cycloplegia. *Compare* miosis.

mydriatic *n.* a drug that causes the pupil of the eye to dilate. Examples are *atropine, *cyclopentolate, and *phenylephrine. Mydriatics are used to aid examination of the eye and to treat some eye inflammations such as iritis and cyclitis.

myectomy *n.* a surgical operation to remove part of a muscle.

myel- (myelo-) *prefix denoting* **1.** the spinal cord. **2.** bone marrow. **3.** myelin.

myelencephalon *n. see* medulla oblongata.

myelin *n.* a complex material formed of protein and *phospholipid that is laid down as a sheath around the *axons of certain neurones, known as *myelinated* (or *medullated*) *nerve fibres*. The material is produced and laid down in concentric layers by *Schwann cells at regular intervals along the nerve fibre (see illustrations). Myelinated nerves conduct impulses more rapidly than nonmyelinated nerves.

Formation of a myelin sheath by a Schwann cell

Longitudinal section through a myelinated nerve fibre

myelination *n.* the process in which *myelin is laid down as an insulating layer around the axons of certain nerves. Myelination of nerve tracts in the central nervous system is completed by the second year of life.

myelitis *n.* **1.** an inflammatory disease of the spinal cord. The most usual kind (*transverse myelitis*) most often occurs during the development of multiple sclerosis, but it is sometimes a manifestation of *encephalomyelitis, when it can occur as an isolated attack. The inflammation spreads more or less completely across the tissue of the spinal cord, resulting in a loss of its normal function to transmit nerve impulses up and down. It is as though the spinal cord had been severed: paralysis and numbness affects the legs and trunk below the level of the diseased tissue. **2.** inflammation of the bone marrow. *See* osteomyelitis.

myeloblast *n.* the earliest identifiable cell that gives rise to a *granulocyte, having a large nucleus and scanty cytoplasm. It is normally found in the blood-forming tissue of the bone marrow, but may appear in the blood in a variety of diseases, most notably in acute myeloblastic *leukaemia. *See also* granulopoiesis. —**myeloblastic** *adj.*

myelocele *n. see* neural tube defects.

myelocyte *n.* an immature form of *granulocyte having a round nucleus (*compare* metamyelocyte) and neutrophil, eosinophil, or basophil granules in its cytoplasm (*compare* promyelocyte). It is normally found in the blood-forming tissue of the bone marrow, but may appear in the blood in a variety of diseases, including infections, infiltrations of the bone marrow, and certain leukaemias. *See also* granulopoiesis.

myelofibrosis *n.* a chronic but progressive disease characterized by *fibrosis of the bone marrow, which leads to anaemia and the presence of immature red and white blood cells in the circulation. Other features include enlargement of the spleen and the presence of blood-forming (myeloid) tissue in abnormal sites, such as the spleen and liver. Its cause is unknown.

myelography *n.* a specialized method of X-ray examination to demonstrate the spinal canal that involves injection of a radio-opaque contrast medium into the subarachnoid space. The X-rays obtained are called *myelograms*. It is of importance in the recognition of tumours of the spinal cord and other conditions compressing the cord or the nerve roots.

myeloid *adj.* **1.** like, derived from, or relating to bone marrow. **2.** resembling a *myelocyte. **3.** relating to the spinal cord.

myeloid leukaemia a variety of *leukaemia in which the type of blood cell that proliferates abnormally originates in the blood-forming (myeloid) tissue of the bone marrow. Myeloid leukaemias may be acute or chronic and may involve any one of the cells produced by the marrow.

myeloid tissue a tissue in the *bone marrow in which the various classes of blood cells are produced. *See also* haemopoiesis.

myeloma (multiple myeloma, myelomatosis) *n.* a malignant disease of the bone marrow, characterized by two or more of the following criteria: (1) the presence of an excess of abnormal malignant plasma cells in the bone marrow; (2) typical deposits in the bones on X-ray, giving the appearance of holes; (3) the presence in the serum of an abnormal gamma globulin, usually IgG (an immunoglobulin; *see* paraprotein). *Bence-Jones protein may also be found in the serum or urine. The patient may complain of tiredness due to anaemia and of bone pain and may develop pathological fractures. Treatment is usually with such drugs as melphalan or cyclophosphamide, with local radiotherapy to particular areas of pain. Radiotherapy of the whole body is also used in the primary treatment of myeloma. *See also* plasmacytoma.

myelomalacia *n.* softening of the tissues of the spinal cord, most often caused by an impaired blood supply.

myelomatosis *n. see* myeloma.

myelomeningocele *n. see* neural tube defects.

myenteric reflex a reflex action of the intestine in which a physical stimulus causes the intestine to contract above and relax below the point of stimulation.

myenteron *n.* the muscular layer of the *intestine, consisting of a layer of circular muscle inside a layer of longitudinal muscle. These muscles are used in *peristalsis. —**myenteric** *adj.*

myiasis *n.* an infestation of a living organ or tissue by maggots. The flies normally breed in decaying animal and vegetable matter; myiasis therefore generally occurs only in regions of poor hygiene, and in most cases the infestations are accidental. Various genera may infect man. *Gasterophilus, *Hypoderma, *Dermatobia,* and *Cordylobia* affect the skin; *Fannia* invades the alimentary canal and the urinary system; *Phormia* and *Wohlfahrtia* infest open wounds and ulcers; *Oestrus* attacks the eyes; and *Cochliomyia* invades the nasal passages. Treatment of external myiases involves the destruction and removal of maggots followed by the application of antibiotics to wounds and lesions.

mylohyoid *n.* a muscle in the floor of the mouth, attached at one end to the mandible and at the other to the hyoid bone.

myo- *prefix. see* my-.

myoblast *n.* a cell that develops into a muscle fibre. —**myoblastic** *adj.*

myocardial infarction death of a segment of heart muscle, which follows interruption of its blood supply (*see* coronary thrombosis). Myocardial infarction is usually confined to the left ventricle. The patient experiences a 'heart attack': sudden severe chest pain, which may spread to the arms and throat. The main danger is that of ventricular *fibrillation, which accounts for most of the fatalities. Other *arrhythmias are also frequent; *ectopic beats in the ventricle are especially important as they predispose to ventricular fibrillation. Other complications include heart failure, rupture of the heart, phlebothrombosis, pulmonary embolism, pericarditis, shock, mitral incompetence, and perforation of the septum between the ventricles.
The best results from the management of patients with myocardial infarction follow mobile and hospital-based coronary care with facilities for the early detection, prevention, and treatment of arrhythmias and *cardiac arrest. Most survivors of myocardial infarction are able to return to a full and active life, including those who have been successfully resuscitated from cardiac arrest.

myocarditis *n.* acute or chronic inflammation of the heart muscle. It may be seen alone or as part of pancarditis (*see* endomyocarditis).

myocardium *n.* the middle of the three layers forming the wall of the heart (*see also* endocardium, epicardium). It is composed of *cardiac muscle and forms the greater part of the heart wall, being thicker in the ventricles than in the atria. —**myocardial** *adj.*

myoclonus *n.* a sudden spasm of the muscles typically lifting and flexing the arms. Occasional *myoclonic jerks* occur between fits in patients with idiopathic *epilepsy, and myoclonus is a major feature of some progressive neurological illnesses with extensive degeneration of brain cells. —**myoclonic** *adj.*

myocyte *n.* a muscle cell.

myodynia *n.* pain in the muscles.

myoepithelium *n.* a tissue consisting of cells of epithelial origin having a contractile cytoplasm. Myoepithelial cells play an important role in encouraging the secretion of substances into ducts.

myofibril *n.* one of numerous contractile filaments found within the cytoplasm of *striated muscle cells. When viewed under a microscope myofibrils show alternating bands of high and low refractive index, which give striated muscle its characteristic appearance.

myogenic *adj.* originating in muscle: applied to the inherent rhythmicity of contraction of some muscles (e.g. cardiac muscle), which does not depend on neural influences.

myoglobin *n.* an iron-containing pigment, resembling *haemoglobin, found in muscle cells. It acts as an oxygen reservoir within the muscle fibres.

myoglobinuria *n.* the presence in the urine of the pigment myoglobin.

myogram *n.* a recording of the activity of a muscle. *See* electromyography.

myograph *n.* an instrument for recording the activity of muscular tissues. *See* electromyography.

myokymia *n.* prominent quivering of a few muscle fibres, not associated with any other abnormal features. It is a benign condition. *See also* fasciculation.

myology *n.* the study of the structure, function, and diseases of the muscles.

myoma *n.* a benign tumour of muscle. It may originate in smooth muscle (*see* leiomyoma) or in striated muscle (*see* rhabdomyoma).

myomectomy *n.* an operation in which benign tumours (fibromyomas or fibroids) are removed from the muscular wall of the womb. It is performed instead of hysterectomy when the patient wishes for further pregnancies.

myometritis *n.* inflammation of the muscular wall (myometrium) of the womb.

myometrium *n.* the muscular tissue of the uterus (womb), which surrounds the *endometrium. It is composed of smooth muscle that undergoes small regular spontaneous contractions. The frequency and amplitude of these contractions alter in response to the hormones *oestrogen, *progesterone, and *oxytocin, which are present at particular stages of the menstrual cycle and pregnancy.

myoneural junction *see* neuromuscular junction.

myopathy *n.* any disease of the muscles. The myopathies are usually subdivided into those that are inherited (*see* muscular dystrophy) and those that are acquired. The acquired myopathies include *polymyositis and muscular diseases complicating endocrine disorders or carcinoma. All are typified by weakness and wasting of the muscles in the upper parts of the arms and legs.

myopia (short-sightedness) *n.* the condition in which parallel light rays are brought to a focus in front of the retina (see illustration). Objects further than six metres from the eye are blurred and cannot be made sharp by *accommodation. The condition is corrected by wearing spectacles with concave lenses. *Compare* emmetropia, hypermetropia. —**myopic** *adj.*

focusing point falls short of retina

Uncorrected

Corrected

concave lens diverges light rays falling on the eye

Myopia (short-sightedness)

myoplasm *n.* *see* sarcoplasm.

myoplasty *n.* the plastic surgery of muscle, in which part of a muscle is partly detached and used to repair tissue defects or deformities in the vicinity of the muscle.

myosarcoma *n.* a malignant tumour of muscle. *See also* leiomyosarcoma, rhabdomyosarcoma.

myosin *n.* the most abundant protein in muscle fibrils, having the important properties of elasticity and contractility. With actin, it comprises the principal contractile element of muscles. *See* striated muscle.

myosis *n. see* miosis.

myositis *n.* any of a group of muscle diseases in which inflammation and degenerative changes occur. *Polymyositis is the most commonly occurring example, but myositis may be found in relation to systemic *collagen disorders and a minority are caused by bacterial or parasitic infections.

myotactic *adj.* relating to the sense of touch in muscles.

myotatic reflex *see* stretch reflex.

myotome *n.* that part of the segmented mesoderm in the early embryo that gives rise to all the skeletal muscle of the body. Visceral (smooth) muscles develop from unsegmented mesoderm (*see* mesenchyme). *See also* somite.

myotomy *n.* the dissection or surgical division of a muscle.

myotonia *n.* a disorder of the muscle fibres that results in abnormally prolonged contractions. The patient has difficulty in relaxing a movement (e.g. his grip) after any vigorous effort. It is a feature of a hereditary condition starting in infancy or early childhood (*myotonia congenita*) and of a form of muscular dystrophy (*dystrophia myotonica*).

myotonic *adj.* relating to muscle tone.

myotonus *n.* **1.** a tonic muscular spasm. **2.** muscle tone.

myringa *n.* the eardrum (*see* tympanic membrane).

myringitis *n.* inflammation of the eardrum. *See* otitis (media).

myringoplasty (tympanoplasty) *n.* surgical reconstruction of an eardrum damaged by infection (*otitis media) or injury.

myringotomy (tympanotomy) *n.* incision of the eardrum to create an artificial opening, which relieves pressure and allows drainage of fluid from an inflamed middle ear (*otitis media).

myx- (myxo-) *prefix denoting* mucus.

myxoedema *n.* **1.** a dry firm waxy swelling of the skin and subcutaneous tissues found in patients with underactive thyroid glands (*see* hypothyroidism). **2.** the clinical syndrome due to hypothyroidism in adult life, including coarsening of the skin, intolerance to cold, weight gain, and mental dullness. The symptoms are abolished with thyroxine treatment.

myxofibroma *n.* a benign tumour of fibrous tissue that contains myxomatous elements (*see* myxoma) or has undergone mucoid degeneration.

myxoma *n.* a benign gelatinous tumour of connective tissue. *Atrial myxoma* is a tumour of the heart, usually of the left side, arising from the septum dividing the two upper chambers. Symptoms may include fever, lassitude, joint pains, and sudden loss of consciousness due to obstruction of the bloodflow. The tumour may be wrongly diagnosed as stenosis of the mitral valve as it can produce a similar murmur. Treatment is by surgical removal. —**myxomatous** *adj.*

myxosarcoma *n.* a *sarcoma containing mucoid material. It is doubtful whether this represents a true entity and it may be simply a variant of other sarcomas, such as a *liposarcoma or a *fibrosarcoma.

myxovirus *n.* one of a group of RNA-containing viruses that includes those causing influenza in animals and man. The related *paramyxoviruses* include the *respiratory syncytial virus (RSV) and the agents causing measles, mumps, and parainfluenza.

N

nabothian follicle (nabothian cyst, nabothian gland) one of a number of cysts on the neck (cervix) of the womb, near its opening to the vagina. The sacs, which contain a thick liquid, form when the ducts of the glands in the cervix are blocked by a new growth of surface cells (epithelium) over an area damaged through infection.

NAD (nicotinamide adenine dinucleotide) a *coenzyme that acts as a hydrogen acceptor in oxidation-reduction reactions, particularly in the *electron transport chain in cellular respiration. NAD and the closely related coenzyme *NADP* (*nicotinamide adenine dinucleotide phosphate*) are derived from nicotinic acid; they are reduced to *NADH* and *NADPH*, respectively.

NADP (nicotinamide adenine dinucleotide phosphate) *see* NAD.

Naegleria *n.* a genus of *amoebae that normally live in damp soil or mud. *Naegleria* species can, however, live as parasites in man and are believed to have caused some rare, but fatal, infections of the brain.

naevus *n.* (*pl.* **naevi**) a birthmark: a clearly defined malformation of the skin, present at birth. There are many different types of naevi. Some are composed of small blood vessels (*see* haemangioma). These blood-vessel birthmarks include the *strawberry mark*, which usually disappears in early life, and the *port-wine stain*, which does not disappear and is best left untreated. Another kind of naevus is the *mole.

Naga sore *see* tropical ulcer.

nail *n.* a horny structure, composed of keratin, formed from the epidermis on the dorsal surface of each finger and toe (see illustration). The exposed part of the nail is the *body*, behind which is the *root*. The whitish crescent-shaped area at the base of the body is called the *lunula*. Growth of the nail occurs at the end of the nail root by division of the germinative layer of the underlying *epidermis (which forms part of the *matrix*). The growing nail slides forward over the *nail bed*. The fold of skin that lies above the root is the *nail fold*;

Longitudinal section through the fingertip and nail

folds of skin on either side of the nail are the *nail walls*. The epidermis of the nail fold that lies next to the nail root is called the *eponychium* (forming the 'cuticle' at the base of the nail). Anatomical name: **unguis**.

nalidixic acid a drug active against various bacteria and used to treat infections of the urinary and digestive systems. It is administered by mouth; common side-effects are nausea, vomiting, and skin reactions. Trade name: **Negram**.

nalorphine *n.* a drug that reduces the effects of morphine and similar narcotic drugs and is used to stimulate breathing and restore consciousness after an overdose of these drugs. It is administered by injection and, given alone, may depress breathing and cause drowsiness or restlessness. Trade name: **Lethidrone**.

nandrolone *n.* a synthetic male sex hormone with effects and uses similar to those of *methandienone. It is administered by injection and high doses may cause signs of *virilization in women. Trade name: **Durabolin**.

nano- *prefix denoting* **1.** extremely small size. **2.** one thousand-millionth part (10^{-9}).

nanometre *n.* one thousand-millionth of a metre (10^{-9} m). One nanometre is equal to 10 angstrom. Symbol: nm.

naphazoline *n.* a drug that constricts small blood vessels and is used to relieve congestion in rhinitis and sinusitis. It is administered as nasal drops and may cause slight irritation.

napkin rash 1. a painful raw area of skin around the anus and buttocks due to contact with frequent irritant stools. It is common between birth and six months of age. **2.** reddening over the genitals and napkin area due to the formation of ammonia in urine-soaked

napkins. A neglected rash will become ulcerated. It is common from six to 16 months. **3.** red raised areas of skin in the napkin region due to candidiasis. It has some resemblance to *psoriasis, hence its alternative name *napkin psoriasis*.

naprapathy *n.* a system of medicine based on the belief that a great many diseases are attributable to displacement of ligaments, tendons, and other connective tissues and that cure can be brought about only by manipulation to correct these displacements.

naproxen *n.* an analgesic drug that also reduces inflammation and fever. It is used to treat rheumatoid arthritis, ankylosing spondylitis, and gout. It is administered by mouth; side-effects may include digestive upsets and rashes. Trade name: **Naprosyn**.

narcissism *n.* excessive self-regard, with or without some rational basis. In Freudian terms it is a state in which the *ego has taken itself as a love object. Some degree of narcissism is present in most individuals, but when it is shown to an extreme degree it may be a symptom of schizophrenia, personality disorder, and other conditions. —**narcissistic** *adj.*

narco- *prefix denoting* narcosis; stupor.

narcolepsy *n.* an extreme tendency to fall asleep in quiet surroundings or when engaged in monotonous activities. The patient can be woken easily and is immediately alert. It is often associated with *cataplexy, and when falling asleep the patient may experience auditory hallucinations or transient attacks of muscular paralysis. —**narcoleptic** *adj., n.*

narcosis *n.* a state of diminished consciousness or complete unconsciousness caused by the use of *narcotic drugs, which have a depressant action on the nervous system. The body's normal reactions to stimuli are diminished and the body may become sedated or completely anaesthetized.

narcotic *n.* a drug that induces stupor and insensibility and relieves pain. The term is used particularly for *morphine and other derivatives of opium (*see* opiate) but is also applied to other drugs that depress brain function (e.g. general anaesthetics and hypnotics). In legal terms a narcotic is any addictive drug subject to illegal use. Narcotics (i.e. morphine and morphine-like drugs) have been largely replaced as sleeping drugs because of their ability to cause *dependence and tolerance; they are still used for relief of severe pain (*see* analgesic).

nares *pl. n.* (*sing.* **naris**) openings of the nose. The two *external* (or *anterior*) *nares* are the nostrils, leading from the nasal cavity to the outside. The two *internal* (or *posterior*) *nares* (*choanae*) are the openings leading from the nasal cavity into the pharynx.

nasal bone either of a pair of narrow oblong bones that together form the bridge and root of the nose. *See* skull.

nasal cavity the space inside the nose that lies between the floor of the cranium and the roof of the mouth. It is divided into two halves by a septum: each half communicates with the outside via the nostrils and with the nasopharynx through the posterior nares.

nasal concha (turbinate bone) any of three thin scroll-like bones that form the sides of the *nasal cavity. The *superior* and *middle nasal conchae* are part of the *ethmoid bone; the *inferior nasal conchae* are a separate pair of bones of the face. *See* skull.

nasion *n.* the point on the bridge of the nose at the centre of the suture between the nasal and frontal bones.

naso- *prefix denoting* the nose.

nasolacrimal *adj.* relating to the nose and the lacrimal (tear-producing) apparatus.

nasolacrimal duct the duct that passes through the hole (*nasolacrimal canal*) in the palatine bone of the skull. It drains the tears away from the *lacrimal apparatus into the inferior meatus of the nose.

nasopharynx (rhinopharynx) *n.* the part of the *pharynx that lies above the soft palate.

nates *pl. n.* the buttocks. —**natal** *adj.*

National Assistance Act (1945) an Act of Parliament providing for the needs of those who, through age, infirmity, or lack of qualifying contributions, are ineligible for benefit under the terms of the National Insurance Act. Cash payments (*supplementary benefit*) may be made from exchequer funds providing the applicants qualify in a means test. Under the terms of Part III of the Act local authorities are required to provide accommodation for those in need of care and attention that is not otherwise available to them (*Part III accommodation*). Such accommodation has replaced the workhouse, but the associated stigma – and dislike of the means test – deter many who are eligible from applying for help to which they are entitled.

national census *see* Office of Population Censuses and Surveys.

National Health Service (in Britain) a comprehensive service offering therapeutic and preventive medical and surgical care, including the prescription and dispensing of medicines, spectacles, and medical and dental appliances. Exchequer funds pay for the services of doctors, nurses, and other professionals and meet a substantial part of the cost of the medicines and appliances. Legislation enacted in 1946 was implemented in 1948 and the services were subjected to substantial reorganization in 1974 and again in 1982. In England overall responsibility is vested in the Secretary of State for Health and Social Security assisted by a comprehensive department (*see* Department of Health and Social Security). Administration is based on a system of delegation downwards and accountability upwards through a hierarchy of 15 regions, each subdivided into a number of districts. In general, *Regional Health Authorities* (*RHA*), whose members are all appointed by the Secretary of State, are responsible for overall planning and monitoring and for allocating funds to the *District Health Authorities* (*DHA*). DHA, whose chairmen are appointed by the Secretary of State and the majority of their members by the RHA, are responsible for local planning, some of which may be delegated to districts. Each tier has a team of officers consisting of a medical officer (*see* community physician), administrator, treasurer, and *nursing officer. The team has executive powers, and decisions are made on the basis of consensus with ultimate accountability to the appropriate authority.

Health authorities are expected to provide all the normal health services from their own resources except the salaries and fees for general practitioners, pharmacists, opticians, and dentists, which come from a separate fund through the *Family Practitioner Committee. Some of the special resources for patients with rarer complaints are shared on a regional or supraregional basis. Wherever possible, districts have common boundaries with local authorities in order to try and ensure liaison with the Social Service Department, which provides many important services to support the sick and aged (*see* social services). However, many districts include part of more than one local authority since the division tends to be made on the basis of the catchment area of a district general hospital. Executive power is vested in the *District Management Team* (*DMT*), which has equivalent composition to the District Team of Officers with the addition of a general practitioner and a hospital consultant.

Different arrangements apply in Northern Ireland and Wales, where the appropriate Secretary of State is responsible and the regional tier is omitted. In Scotland (for which there is a separate Act) the Secretary of State is also responsible and there is an intermediate tier by which districts are grouped into areas (*see* Chief Administrative Medical Officer).

natriuresis *n.* the excretion of sodium in the urine: a normal phenomenon.

natriuretic *n.* an agent that promotes the excretion of sodium salts in the urine. Most *diuretics are natriuretics.

naturopathy *n.* a system of medicine that relies upon the use of only 'natural' substances for the treatment of disease, rather than drugs. Herbs, food grown without artificial fertilizers and prepared without the use of preservatives or colouring material, pure water, sunlight, and fresh air are all employed in an effort to rid the body of 'unnatural' substances, which are said to be at the root of most illnesses.

nausea *n.* the feeling that one is about to vomit, as experienced in seasickness and in morning sickness of early pregnancy. Actual vomiting often occurs subsequently.

navel *n.* see umbilicus.

navicular bone a boat-shaped bone of the ankle (*see* tarsus) that articulates with the three cuneiform bones in front and with the talus behind.

nearthrosis *n. see* pseudarthrosis.

nebula *n.* a faint opacity of the cornea that remains after an ulcer has healed.

nebulizer *n.* an instrument used for applying a liquid in the form of a fine spray.

Necator *n.* a genus of *hookworms that live in the small intestine. The human hookworm, *N. americanus*, occurs in tropical Africa, Central and South America, India, and the Pacific Islands. The worm possesses two pairs of sharp cutting plates inside its mouth cavity, which enable it to feed on the blood and tissues of the gut wall. *Compare* Ancylostoma.

necatoriasis *n.* an infestation of the small intestine by the parasitic hookworm *Necator americanus*. *See also* hookworm disease.

necro- *prefix denoting* death or dissolution.

necrobiosis *n.* a gradual process by which cells lose their function and die. *Necrobiosis lipoidica* is patchy degeneration of the skin causing areas of white scarring and thinning. It is most commonly seen in diabetics but is found occasionally in nondiabetics.

necrology *n.* the study of the phenomena of death, involving determination of the moment of death and the different changes that occur in the tissues of the body after death.

necromania *n.* morbid desire for a dead body or bodies. This may be necrophilism, but the attraction is sometimes not sexual. A bereaved person, for instance, who is not grieving normally, may occasionally treasure the body of a loved one.

necrophilism (necrophilia) *n.* sexual attraction to corpses. *See also* perversion. —**necrophile** *n.*

necropsy *n. see* autopsy.

necrosis (mortification) *n.* the death of some or all of the cells in an organ or tissue, caused by disease, physical or chemical injury, or interference with the blood supply (*see* gangrene). *Caseous necrosis* occurs in pulmonary tuberculosis, the lung tissue becoming soft, dry, and cheeselike.

necrospermia *n.* the presence of either dead or motionless spermatozoa in the semen. *See* infertility.

necrotomy *n.* **1.** the removal of a dead piece of bone (*see* sequestrum). **2.** dissection of a dead body.

needle *n.* a slender sharp-pointed instrument used for a variety of purposes. Needles used for sewing up tissue during surgical operation are of various designs, for specific operations, and are equipped with an eye for threading suture material. Hollow needles are used to inject substances into the body (in hypodermic syringes), to obtain specimens of tissue (*see* biopsy), or to withdraw fluid from a cavity (*see* aspiration). *See also* stop needle.

needling *n.* a form of *capsulotomy in which a sharp needle is used to make a hole in the capsule surrounding the lens of the eye.

negativism *n.* behaviour that is the opposite of that suggested by others. In *active negativism* the individual does the opposite of what he is asked (for example, he screws his eyes up when asked to open them). This is uncommon in adult life and is usually associated with other features of *catatonia. In *passive negativism* the person fails to cooperate (for example, he does not eat). This occurs in *schizophrenia and *depression.

Neisseria *n.* a genus of spherical Gram-negative aerobic nonmotile bacteria characteristically grouped in pairs. They are parasites of animals, and some species are normal inhabitants of the respiratory tract of man. The species *N. gonorrhoeae* (the *gonococcus*) causes *gonorrhoea. Gonococci are found within pus cells of urethral and vaginal discharge; they can be cultured only on serum or blood agar. *N. meningitidis* (the *meningococcus*) causes *cerebrospinal fever and *meningitis. Meningococci are found within pus cells of infected cerebrospinal fluid and blood or in the nasal passages of carriers. They too can only be cultured on serum or blood agar.

nematode (roundworm) *n.* any one of a large group of worms having an unsegmented cylindrical body, tapering at both ends. This distinguishes nematodes from other *helminths. Nematodes occur either as free-living forms in the sea, fresh water, and soil or as parasites of plants, animals, and man. *Hookworms and *pinworms infest the alimentary canal. *Filariae are found in the lymphatic tissues. The *guinea worm and *Onchocerca affect connective tissue. Some nematodes (e.g. pinworms) are transmitted from host to host by the ingestion of eggs; others (e.g. *Wuchereria) by the bite of a bloodsucking insect.

Nembutal *n. see* pentobarbitone.

neo- *prefix denoting* new or newly formed.

neocerebellum *n.* the middle lobe of the *cerebellum, excluding the pyramid and uvula. In evolutionary terms it is the newest part, occurring only in mammals.

neologism *n.* (in psychiatry) the invention of words to which meanings are attached. It is common in childhood, but when it occurs in an adult it may be a symptom of a psychotic illness, such as *schizophrenia. It should be distinguished from *paraphasia, in which new meanings are attached to ordinary words.

neomycin *n.* an antibiotic used to treat infections caused by a wide range of bacteria, mainly those affecting the skin and eyes. It is usually applied in creams or drops with other antibiotics, but can also be given by mouth.

neonatal death rate *see* infant mortality rate.

neonate *n.* an infant at any time during the first four weeks of life. The word is particularly applied to infants just born or in the first week of life. —**neonatal** *adj.*

neopallium *n.* an enlargement of the wall of each cerebral hemisphere. In evolutionary terms it is the newest part of the cerebrum, formed by the development of new pathways for sight and hearing in mammals.

neoplasm *n.* a new and abnormal growth: any *benign or *malignant tumour.

neostigmine *n.* a *parasympathomimetic drug that acts by inhibiting the enzyme cholinesterase (*see also* anticholinesterase). It is used mainly to diagnose and treat *myasthenia gravis and as an antidote to some *muscle-relaxant drugs, such as tubocurarine. It is also used to treat some intestinal disorders and glaucoma. Neostigmine is administered by mouth, injection, or in eye-drops; side-effects include digestive upsets and increased saliva flow. Trade name: **Prostigmin.**

nephr- (nephro-) *prefix denoting* the kidney(s).

nephralgia *n.* pain in the kidney. The pain is felt in the loin and can be caused by a variety of kidney complaints.

nephrectomy *n.* surgical removal of a kidney. When performed for cancer of the kidney, the entire organ is removed together with its surrounding fat and the adjacent adrenal gland (*radical nephrectomy*). Removal of either the upper or lower pole of the kidney is termed *partial nephrectomy.*

nephritis (Bright's disease) *n.* inflammation of the kidney. Nephritis is a nonspecific term used to describe a condition resulting from a variety of causes. *See* glomerulonephritis.

nephroblastoma (Wilms' tumour) *n.* a malignant tumour of the kidney found in children (*see* cancer). It is rare over the age of eight years and the most obvious symptom is an abdominal swelling. Treatment is by *nephrectomy followed by radiotherapy and *cytotoxic drugs. Considerable improvement in the results of treatment has occurred in recent years since the use of cytotoxic drugs as a routine.

nephrocalcinosis *n.* the presence of calcium deposits in the kidneys. This can be caused by excess calcium in the blood, as caused by overactivity of the parathyroid glands, or it may result from an underlying abnormality of the kidney. The cause of nephrocalcinosis must be detected by full biochemical, radiological, and urological investigation so that appropriate treatment can be undertaken.

nephrogenic cord either of the paired ridges of tissue that run along the dorsal surface of the abdominal cavity of the embryo. Parts of it develop into the kidney, ovary, or testis and their associated ducts. Intermediate stages of these developments are the *pronephros, *mesonephros, and *metanephros.

nephrolithiasis *n.* the presence of stones in the kidney (*see* calculus). Such stones can cause pain and blood in the urine, but they may produce no symptoms. Full investigation is undertaken to determine the underlying cause of stone formation. When stones are associated with urinary obstruction and infection they usually require surgical removal (*see* nephrolithotomy, pyelolithotomy).

nephrolithotomy *n.* the surgical removal of a stone from the kidney by an incision into the kidney substance. It is normally performed in combination with an incision into the renal pelvis (*see* pyelolithotomy). *See also* percutaneous nephrolithotomy.

nephrology *n.* the branch of medicine concerned with the study, investigation, and management of diseases of the kidney. *See also* urology. —**nephrologist** *n.*

nephron *n.* the active unit of excretion in the kidney (see illustration). Blood, supplied by branches of the renal artery, is filtered through a knot of capillaries (*glomerulus*) into the cup-shaped *Bowman's capsule* so that water, nitrogenous waste, and many other substances (excluding colloids) pass into the *renal tubule*. Here most of the substances are reabsorbed back into the blood, the remaining fluid (*urine) passing into the collecting duct, which drains into the *ureter.

nephropexy *n.* an operation to fix a mobile kidney. The kidney is fixed to the twelfth rib and adjacent posterior abdominal wall to prevent descent of the kidney on standing (*see* nephroptosis).

nephroptosis *n.* abnormal descent of a kidney into the pelvis on standing, which may occur if it is excessively mobile (for example, in thin women). If this is accompanied by pain and obstruction to free drainage of urine by the kidney, *nephropexy may be advised.

nephrosclerosis *n.* hardening of the arteries and arterioles of the kidneys. *Arteriolar nephrosclerosis* is associated with *hypertension.

nephroscope *n.* an instrument used for examining the inside of the kidney (*nephroscopy*) at open operation, usually in an attempt to locate small fragments of calculi in the calyces.

nephrosis *n.* (in pathology) degenerative changes in the epithelium of the kidney tubules. The term is sometimes used loosely for the *nephrotic syndrome.

distal convoluted tubule

efferent arteriole

afferent arteriole

Bowman's capsule

glomerulus

proximal convoluted tubule

collecting duct

loop of Henle

A single nephron

nephrostomy *n.* drainage of urine from the kidney by a tube (catheter) passing through the kidney via the skin surface. This is commonly used as a temporary procedure after operations on the kidney. Long-term urine drainage by nephrostomy may be complicated by the attendant problems of infection and obstruction of the catheter by debris.

nephrotic syndrome a condition in which there is great loss of protein in the urine, reduced levels of albumin in the blood, and generalized swelling of the tissues due to *oedema. It can be caused by a variety of disorders, most usually *glomerulonephritis.

nephrotomy *n.* surgical incision into the substance of the kidney. This is usually undertaken to remove a kidney stone (*see* nephrolithotomy).

nephroureterectomy (ureteronephrectomy) *n.* surgical removal of a kidney together with its ureter. This operation is performed of cancer of the kidney pelvis or ureter. It is also undertaken when the kidney has been destroyed by *vesicoureteric reflux, to prevent subsequent continuing reflux into the stump of the ureter that would occur if the kidney alone were removed.

nerve *n.* a bundle of conducting *nerve fibres (see illustration) that transmit impulses from the brain or spinal cord to the muscles and glands (*motor nerves*) or inwards from the sense organs to the brain and spinal cord (*sensory nerves*). Most large nerves are *mixed nerves*, containing both motor and sensory nerve fibres running to and from a particular region of the body.

nerve fibre

myelin sheath

neurilemma

endoneurium

epineurium

perineurium

fascicle (a group of fibres)

Transverse section through a nerve

nerve block a method of producing *anaesthesia in part of the body by blocking the passage of pain impulses in the sensory nerves supplying it. A local anaesthetic, such as lignocaine, is injected into the tissues in the region of

nerve cell

a nerve. In this way anaesthesia can be localized, so that minor operations can be performed without the necessity of giving a general anaesthetic.

nerve cell *see* neurone.

nerve ending the final part (terminal) of one of the branches of a nerve fibre, where a *neurone makes contact either with another neurone at a synapse or with a muscle or gland cell at a neuromuscular or neuroglandular junction.

nerve fibre the long fine process that extends from the cell body of a *neurone and carries nerve impulses. Bundles of nerve fibres running together form a *nerve. Each fibre has a sheath, which in medullated nerve fibres is a relatively thick layer containing the fatty insulating material *myelin.

nerve gas any gas that disrupts the normal functioning of nerves and thus of the muscles they supply. There are two groups, the *G agents* and the *V agents*. The latter are more than 300 times as deadly as mustard gas: one inhalation can kill by paralysing the respiratory muscles. V agents also act through the skin, therefore gas masks are ineffective protection against them.

nerve impulse the electrical activity in the membrane of a *neurone that – by its rapid spread from one region to the next – is the means by which information is transmitted within the nervous system along the axons of the neurones. The membrane of a resting nerve is charged (*polarized*) because of the different concentrations of ions inside and outside the cell. When a nerve impulse is triggered, a wave of *depolarization spreads, and ions flow across the membrane (*see* action potential). Until the nerve has undergone *repolarization no further nerve impulses can pass.

nervous system the vast network of cells specialized to carry information (in the form of *nerve impulses) to and from all parts of the body in order to bring about bodily activity. The brain and spinal cord together form the *central nervous system; the remaining nervous tissue is known as the *peripheral nervous system and includes the *autonomic nervous system, which is itself divided into the sympathetic and parasympathetic nervous systems. The basic functional unit of the nervous system is the *neurone (nerve cell).

nettle rash an allergic skin reaction causing blisters and wheals, resembling those caused by nettle stings. *See* urticaria.

neur- (neuro-) *prefix denoting* nerves or the nervous system.

neural arch *see* vertebra.

neural crest the two bands of ectodermal tissue that flank the *neural plate of the early embryo. Cells of the neural crest migrate throughout the embryo and develop into sensory nerve cells and peripheral nerve cells of the autonomic nervous system.

neuralgia *n.* a severe burning or stabbing pain often following the course of a nerve. *Postherpetic neuralgia* is an intense debilitating pain felt at the site of a previous attack of shingles. In *trigeminal neuralgia* (*tic douloureux*) there are brief paroxysms of searing pain felt in the distribution of one or more branches of the *trigeminal nerve in the face. The facial pain of *migrainous neuralgia* lasts for 30–60 minutes and occurs at roughly the same time on successive days.

neural plate the strip of ectoderm lying along the central axis of the early embryo that forms the *neural tube and subsequently the central nervous system.

neural spine the spinous process situated on the neural arch of a *vertebra.

neural tube the embryological structure from which the brain and spinal cord develop. It is a hollow tube of ectodermal tissue formed when two edges of a groove in a plate of primitive neural tissue (*neural plate*) come together and fuse. Failure of normal fusion results in a number of congenital defects (*see* neural tube defects).

neural tube defects a group of congenital abnormalities caused by failure of the *neural tube to close. In *spina bifida the bony arches of the spine, which protect the spinal cord and its coverings (the meninges), fail to close. More severe defects of fusion of these bones result in increasingly serious neurological conditions. A *meningocele* is the protrusion of the meninges through the gap in the spine, the skin covering being vestigial. There is a constant risk of damage to the meninges, with resulting infection. Urgent surgical treatment to protect the meninges is required. In a *meningomyelocele* (*myelomeningocele*, *myelocele*) the spinal cord and the nerve roots are exposed, often adhering to the fine membrane that overlies them. There is a constant risk of infection and this condition is accompanied by paralysis and numbness of the legs and urinary incontinence. *Hydrocephalus and the *Arnold-Chiari malformation are usually present. A failure of fusion at the cranial end of the neural tube (*cranium bifidum*) gives rise to comparable disorders. The bone defect is most often in the occipital region of the skull but it may occur in the frontal or basal regions. A protrusion of the meninges alone is called a *cranial meningocele*. The terms *meningoencephalocele*, *encephalocele*, and *cephalocele* are used to indicate the protrusion of brain tissue through the skull defect. This is accompanied by severe mental and physical disorders.

neurapraxia *n.* temporary loss of nerve function resulting in tingling, numbness, and weakness. It is usually caused by compression of the nerve and there is no structural damage involved. Complete recovery occurs.

neurasthenia *n.* a set of psychological and physical symptoms, including fatigue, irritability, headache, dizziness, anxiety, and intolerance of noise. It can be caused by organic damage, such as a head injury, or it can be due to neurosis. —**neurasthenic** *adj., n.*

neurectasis *n.* the surgical procedure for stretching a peripheral nerve.

neurectomy *n.* the surgical removal of the whole or part of a nerve.

neurilemma (neurolemma) *n.* the sheath of the *axon of a nerve fibre. The neurilemma of a medullated fibre contains *myelin laid down by Schwann cells. —**neurilemmal** *adj.*

neurilemmoma *n. see* neurofibroma.

neurinoma *n. see* neurofibroma.

neuritis *n.* a disease of the peripheral nerves showing the pathological changes of inflammation. The term is also used in a less precise sense as an alternative to *neuropathy. *See also* retrobulbar neuritis.

neuroanatomy *n.* the study of the structure of the nervous system, from the gross anatomy of the brain down to the microscopic details of neurones.

neurobiotaxis *n.* the predisposition of a nerve cell to move towards the source of its stimuli during development.

neuroblast *n.* any of the nerve cells of the embryo that give rise to functional nerve cells (neurones).

neuroblastoma *n.* a malignant tumour composed of embryonic nerve cells. It may originate in any part of the sympathetic nervous system, most commonly in the medulla of the adrenal gland, and secondary growths are often widespread in other organs and in bones.

neurocranium *n*. the part of the skull that encloses the brain.

neurodermatitis (neurodermatosis) *n*. a skin disease in which localized areas itch persistently and, because of constant scratching, become thickened (*see* lichenification). Women suffer more than men and the cause is uncertain, though psychological factors probably play a part. Common sites are the back of the neck, forearm, upper inner thighs, inner side of knees, and outer side of ankle.

neuroendocrine system the system of dual control of certain activities of the body by means of both nerves and circulating hormones. The functioning of the autonomic nervous system is particularly closely linked to that of the pituitary and adrenal glands. *See* neurohormone, neurosecretion.

neuroepithelioma *n*. a malignant tumour of the retina of the eye. It is a form of *glioma and commonly spreads into the brain.

neuroepithelium *n*. a type of epithelium associated with organs of special sense. It contains sensory nerve endings and is found in the retina, the membranous labyrinth of the inner ear, the mucous membrane lining the nasal cavity, and the taste buds. —**neuroepithelial** *adj*.

neurofibril *n*. one of the microscopic threads of cytoplasm found in the cell body of a *neurone and also in the *axoplasm of peripheral nerves.

neurofibroma (neurilemmoma, neurinoma, neuroma, Schwannoma) *n*. a benign tumour growing from the fibrous coverings of a peripheral nerve: it is usually symptomless. When it develops from the sheath of a nerve root, it causes pain and may compress the spinal cord.

neurofibromatosis (von Recklinghausen's disease) *n*. a congenital disease, typified by numerous benign tumours growing from the fibrous coverings of nerves (*see* neurofibroma). Tumours may occur in the spinal canal, where they may press on the spinal cord. The tumours can be felt beneath the skin along the course of the nerves; they sometimes become malignant, giving rise to *neurofibrosarcomas*. Pigmented patches on the skin (*café au lait spots*) are commonly found. This condition is often associated with the adrenal tumour *phaeochromocytoma.

neurogenesis *n*. the growth and development of nerve cells.

neurogenic *adj*. **1.** caused by disease or dysfunction of the nervous system. **2.** arising in nervous tissue. **3.** caused by nerve stimulation.

neuroglia *n*. *see* glia.

neurohormone *n*. a hormone that is produced within specialized nerve cells and is secreted from the nerve endings into the circulation. Examples are the hormones oxytocin and vasopressin, produced within the nerve cells of the hypothalamus and released into the circulation in the posterior pituitary gland, and noradrenaline, released from *chromaffin tissue in the adrenal medulla.

neurohumour *n*. a *neurohormone or a *neurotransmitter.

neurohypophysis *n*. the posterior lobe of the *pituitary gland.

neurolemma *n*. *see* neurilemma.

neurology *n*. the study of the structure, functioning, and diseases of the nervous system (including the brain, spinal cord, and all the peripheral nerves). —**neurological** *adj*. —**neurologist** *n*.

neuroma *n*. *see* neurofibroma.

neuromuscular junction (myoneural junction) the meeting point of a nerve fibre and the muscle fibre that it supplies. Between the enlarged end of the nerve fibre (*motor end-plate*) and the membrane of the muscle is a gap across which a *neurotransmitter must diffuse from the nerve to trigger contraction of the muscle.

neuromyelitis optica (Devic's disease) a condition that is closely related to multiple sclerosis. Typically there is a transverse *myelitis, producing paralysis and numbness of the legs and trunk below the inflamed spinal cord, and *retrobulbar (optic) neuritis affecting both optic nerves. The attacks of myelitis and optic neuritis may coincide or they may be separated by days or weeks. Recovery from the initial attack is often incomplete, but relapses appear to be less common than in conventional multiple sclerosis.

neurone (nerve cell) *n.* one of the basic functional units of the nervous system: a cell specialized to transmit electrical *nerve impulses and so carry information from one part of the body to another (see illustration). Each neurone has an enlarged portion, the *cell body* (*perikaryon*), containing the nucleus; from the body extend several processes (*dendrites*) through which impulses enter from their branches. A longer process, the nerve fibre (*see* axon), extends outwards and carries impulses away from the cell body. This is normally unbranched except at the *nerve ending. The point of contact of one neurone with another is known as a *synapse.

neuronophagia *n.* the process whereby damaged or degenerating nerve cells finally disintegrate and are removed by scavenger cells (*phagocytes).

neuronoplasty *n.* reconstructive surgery for damaged or severed peripheral nerves.

neuropathy *n.* any disease of the peripheral nerves, usually causing weakness and numbness. In a *mononeu-*

Types of neurone: motor (left) and sensory (right)

ropathy a single nerve is affected and the extent of the symptoms depends upon the distribution of that nerve. In a *polyneuropathy* many or all of the nerves are involved and the symptoms are most profound at the extremities of the limbs.

neurophysiology *n.* the study of the complex chemical and physical changes that are associated with the activity of the nervous system.

neuropil *n.* nerve tissue that is visible microscopically as a mass of interwoven and interconnected nerve endings, dendrites, and other neurone components, rather than an ordered array of axons.

neuroretinitis *n.* combined inflammation of the optic nerve and the retina.

neurosecretion *n.* any substance produced within, and secreted by, a nerve cell. Important examples are the hormone-releasing factors produced by the cells of the *hypothalamus and released into blood vessels of the pituitary gland, on which they act.

neurosis *n.* (*pl.* **neuroses**) a mental illness in which insight is retained but there is a maladaptive way of behaving or thinking that causes suffering (*compare* psychosis). The classification of neuroses is based on the symptoms, which may be a pathologically severe emotional state, as in *anxiety state or *depression; distressing behaviour and thoughts, as in *phobias or *obsessions; or physical complaints, as in *hysteria or *hypochondria. In practice the distinction between neurosis and psychosis is often blurred, as the amount of insight retained is very variable. Neurotic symptoms are occasionally the result of overwhelming stress (e.g. in soldiers in battle), but usually represent a complex interaction between stresses and a vulnerable personality.
Treatment for neurosis can include chemotherapy (often with *tranquillizers), *psychotherapy, or *behaviour therapy. The little evidence there is favours the use of behavioural techniques, such as *desensitization and *flooding. —**neurotic** *adj.*

neurosurgery *n.* the surgical or operative treatment of diseases of the brain and spinal cord. This includes the management of head injuries, the relief of raised intracranial pressure and compression of the spinal cord, the eradication of infection, the control of intracranial haemorrhage, and the diagnosis and treatment of tumours. The development of neurosurgery has been sup-ported by advances in anaesthetics, radiology, and antiseptics.

neurosyphilis *n.* *syphilis affecting the nervous system.

neuroticism *n.* a dimension of personality derived from questionnaires and psychological tests. People with high scores in neuroticism are anxious and intense and more prone to develop neurosis.

neurotomy *n.* the surgical procedure of severing a nerve.

neurotoxic *adj.* poisonous or harmful to nerve cells.

neurotransmitter *n.* a chemical substance released from nerve endings to transmit impulses across *synapses to other nerves and across the minute gaps between the nerves and the muscles or glands that they supply. Outside the central nervous system the chief neurotransmitter is *acetylcholine; *noradrenaline is released by nerve endings of the sympathetic system. In the central nervous system, besides acetylcholine and noradrenaline, *dopamine, *serotonin, *gamma-aminobutyric acid and several other substances are thought to act as transmitters.

neurotrophic *adj.* relating to the growth and nutrition of neural tissue in the body.

neurotropic *adj.* growing towards or having an affinity for neural tissue. The term may be applied to viruses, chemicals, or toxins.

neutropenia *n.* a decrease in the number of *neutrophils in the blood. Neutropenia may occur in a wide variety of diseases, including certain hereditary defects, aplastic *anaemias, tumours of the bone marrow, *agranulocytosis, and acute leukaemias. It results in an increased susceptibility to infections.

neutrophil (polymorph) *n.* a variety of *granulocyte (a type of white blood cell) distinguished by a lobed nucleus and the presence in its cytoplasm of fine granules that stain purple with *Romanowsky stains. It is capable of ingesting and killing bacteria and provides an important defence against infection. There are normally 2.0–7.5 × 10⁹ neutrophils per litre of blood.

newton *n.* the *SI unit of force, equal to the force required to impart to 1 kilogram an acceleration of 1 metre per second per second. Symbol: N.

nexus *n.* (in anatomy) a connection or link.

niacin *n. see* nicotinic acid.

nialamide *n.* a drug with effects similar to *phenelzine, used to treat all types of depression. It is administered by mouth; headache, nausea, dizziness, and giddiness are common side-effects. Trade name: **Niamid**.

niche *n.* (in anatomy) a recess or depression in a smooth surface.

nicotinamide *n.* a B vitamin: the amide of *nicotinic acid.

nicotinamide adenine dinucleotide *see* NAD.

nicotine *n.* a poisonous alkaloid derived from *tobacco, responsible for the dependence of regular smokers on cigarettes. In small doses nicotine has a stimulating effect on the autonomic nervous system, causing in regular smokers such effects as raised blood pressure and pulse rate and impaired appetite. Large doses cause paralysis of the autonomic ganglia.

nicotinic acid (niacin) a B vitamin. Nicotinic acid is a derivative of pyridine and is interchangeable with its amide, *nicotinamide*. Both forms of the vitamin are equally active. Nicotinamide is a component of the coenzymes *NAD (nicotinamide adenine dinucleotide) and NADP, its phosphate. Nicotinic acid is required in the diet but can

also be formed in small amounts in the body from the essential amino acid tryptophan. A deficiency of the vitamin leads to *pellagra. Good sources of nicotinic acid are meat, yeast extracts, and some cereals. Nicotinic acid is present in some cereals (e.g. maize) in a bound unavailable form. The adult recommended intake is 18 mg equivalent per day (1 mg equivalent is equal to 1 mg of available nicotinic acid or 60 mg tryptophan).

nicotinyl *n.* a drug that dilates blood vessels. It is similar to *nicotinic acid and is used to treat disorders due to poor circulation, such as chilblains and Raynaud's disease. It is administered by mouth; side-effects are rare, but temporary flushing of the face may occur. Trade name: **Ronicol**.

nictitation *n.* exaggerated and frequent blinking or winking of the eyes.

nidation *n. see* implantation.

nidus *n.* a place in which bacteria have settled and multiplied because of particularly suitable conditions: a focus of infection.

nifuratel *n.* a drug active against various microorganisms, used mainly to treat fungus infections of the genital and urinary systems (such as candidiasis of the vagina). It is administered by mouth and in pessaries; side-effects are rare, but some digestive discomfort may occur. Trade name: **Magmilor**.

night blindness the inability to see in dim light or at night. It is due to a disorder of the cells in the retina that are responsible for vision in dim light (*see* rod), and can result from dietary deficiency of *vitamin A. If the vitamin deficiency is allowed to continue night blindness may progress to *xerophthalmia and *keratomalacia. Medical name: *nyctalopia*. *Compare* day blindness.

night sweat copious sweating during sleep. Night sweats may be an early indication of tuberculosis or other disease.

night terror the condition in which a child (usually aged 2–4 years), soon after falling asleep, starts screaming and appears terrified. The child cannot be comforted because he remains mentally inaccessible; the attack ceases when he wakes up fully and is never remembered. Attacks sometimes follow a stressful experience.

Nile blue an oxazine chloride, used for staining lipids and lipid pigments. *Nile blue A* (*Nile blue sulphate*), which stains fatty acids, changes from blue to purplish at pH 10–11.

ninhydrin reaction a histochemical test for proteins, in which ninhydrin (triketohydrindene hydrate) is boiled with the test solution and gives a blue colour in the presence of amino acids and proteins.

nipple (mamilla, papilla) *n.* the protuberance at the centre of the *breast. In females the milk ducts open at the nipple.

niridazole *n.* an anthelmintic drug used particularly in the treatment of schistosomiasis. It is administered by mouth and side-effects may include agitation and confusion, abdominal discomfort, digestive upsets, and headache. Niridazole should not be used in patients with impaired liver function.

Nissl granules collections of darkstaining material, containing RNA, seen in the cell bodies of neurones on microscopic examination.

nit *n.* the egg of a *louse. The eggs of head lice are firmly cemented to the hair, usually at the back of the head; those of body lice are fixed to the clothing. Nits, 0.8×0.3 mm, are visible as light white specks.

nitrazepam *n.* a *hypnotic drug administered by mouth to treat insomnia and sleep disturbances. It is often preferred to other hypnotics since side-effects are not severe, though morning drowsiness sometimes occurs. Trade names: **Mogadon, Remnos**.

nitric acid a strong corrosive mineral acid, HNO_3, the concentrated form of which is capable of producing severe burns of the skin. Swallowing the acid leads to intense burning pain and ulceration of the mouth and throat. Treatment is by immediate administration of alkaline solutions, followed by milk or olive oil.

nitrofurantoin *n.* a drug used to treat bacterial infections of the urinary system. It is administered by mouth and may cause nausea, vomiting, and skin rashes. Trade names: **Berkfurin, Furadantin, Furan, Macrodantin**.

nitrogen *n.* a gaseous element and a major constituent of air (79 per cent). Nitrogen is an essential constituent of proteins and nucleic acids and is obtained by man in the form of proteincontaining foods (atmospheric nitrogen cannot be utilized directly). Nitrogenous waste is excreted as *urea. Symbol: N.

nitrogen mustard *see* mustine.

nitroglycerin *n. see* glyceryl trinitrate.

nitrous oxide a colourless gas used as an *anaesthetic with good *analgesic properties. It is administered by inhalation, in conjunction with oxygen, and is used as a vehicle for potent anaesthetic vapours, such as halothane. A mixture of oxygen and nitrous oxide provides effective analgesia for some dental procedures and in childbirth; such a state is known as *relative analgesia. Nitrous oxide was formerly referred to as *laughing gas* because of its tendency to excite the patient when used alone.

nm *abbrev. for* nanometre.

NMR *see* nuclear magnetic resonance.

Nocardia *n.* a genus of rodlike or filamentous Gram-positive nonmotile bacteria found in the soil. As cultures age, filaments form branches, but these soon break up into rodlike or spherical cells. Three or more spores may form in each cell; these germinate to form filaments. Some species are pathogenic: *N. asteroides* causes *nocardiosis and *N. madurae* is associated with the disease *Madura foot.

nocardiosis *n.* a disease caused by bacteria of the genus *Nocardia*, primarily affecting the lungs, skin, and brain, resulting in the formation of abscesses. Treatment involves antibiotics and sulphonamides.

noci- *prefix denoting* pain or injury.

nociceptive *adj.* describing nerve fibres, endings, or pathways that are concerned with the condition of pain.

noct- (nocti-) *prefix denoting* night.

noctambulation *n.* *see* somnambulism.

nocturia *n.* the passage of urine at night. In the absence of a high fluid intake, sleep is not normally interrupted by the need to pass urine. Nocturia usually occurs in elderly men with enlarged prostate glands, and is a common reason for patients to request *prostatectomy.

node *n.* a small swelling or knot of tissue. *See* atrioventricular node, sinoatrial node.

node of Ranvier one of the gaps that occur at regular intervals in the *myelin sheath of medullated nerve fibres, between adjacent *Schwann cells.

nodule *n.* a small swelling or aggregation of cells.

noma *n.* a gangrenous infection of the mouth that spreads to involve the face. It is rare in civilized communities and is usually found in debilitated or malnourished individuals. Noma is a severe form of *ulcerative gingivitis.

nondisjunction *n.* a condition in which pairs of homologous chromosomes fail to separate during meiosis or a chromosome fails to divide at *anaphase of mitosis or meiosis. It results in a cell with an abnormal number of chromosomes (*see* monosomy, trisomy).

nonigravida *n.* a woman who has been pregnant nine times.

nonipara *n.* a woman who has been pregnant at least nine times and has given birth to an infant capable of survival after each of nine pregnancies.

nonsecretor *n.* a person in whose body fluids it is not possible to detect soluble forms of the A, B, or O agglutinogens that determine blood group. *Compare* secretor.

noradrenaline (norepinephrine) *n.* a hormone, closely related to *adrenaline and with similar actions, secreted by the medulla of the *adrenal gland and also released as a *neurotransmitter by sympathetic nerve endings. Among its many actions are constriction of small blood vessels leading to an increase in blood pressure, increased blood flow through the coronary arteries and a slowing of the heart rate, increase in the rate and depth of breathing, and relaxation of the smooth muscle in intestinal walls.

norepinephrine *n.* *see* noradrenaline.

norethandrolone *n.* a synthetic male sex hormone with body-building action. It has the same effects and uses as *methandienone and is administered by mouth or injection.

norethisterone *n.* a synthetic female sex hormone (*see* progestogen) administered by mouth to treat menstrual disorders, including amenorrhoea. It is also used in oral contraceptives, often in combination with an oestrogen.

norma *n.* a view of the skull from one of several positions, from which it can be described or measured. For example the *norma lateralis* is a side view of the skull; the *norma verticalis* is the view of the top of the skull.

normalization *n.* (in psychiatry) the process of making the living conditions of people with mental *subnormality as similar as possible to those of people who are not handicapped. This includes moves to living outside institutions and encouragement to cope with work, pay, social life, and civil rights.

normo- *prefix denoting* normality.

normoblast *n.* a nucleated cell that forms part of the series giving rise to the red blood cells and is normally found in the blood-forming tissue of the bone marrow. Normoblasts pass through three stages of maturation: *early* (or *basophilic*), *intermediate* (or *polychromatic*), and *late* (or *orthochromatic*) forms. *See also* erythroblast, erythropoiesis.

normocyte *n.* a red blood cell of normal size. A *normocytic anaemia* is one characterized by the presence of such cells. —**normocytic** *adj.*

normotensive *adj.* describing the state in which the arterial blood pressure is within the normal range. *Compare* hypertension, hypotension.

nortriptyline *n.* a tricyclic *antidepressant drug used to relieve all types of depression. It is administered by mouth; side-effects may include dry mouth and drowsiness. Trade names: **Allegron, Aventyl.**

nose *n.* the organ of olfaction, which also acts as an air passage that warms, moistens, and filters the air on its way to the lungs. The *external nose* is a triangular projection in the front of the face that is composed of cartilage and

covered with skin. It leads to the *nasal cavity* (*internal nose*), which is lined with mucous membrane containing olfactory cells and is divided into two chambers (*fossae*) by the *nasal septum*. The lateral wall of each chamber is formed by the three scroll-shaped *nasal conchae, below each of which is a groovelike passage (*meatus*). The *paranasal sinuses open into these meatuses.

nosebleed *n.* bleeding from the nose, which may be caused by physical injury or may be associated with fever, high blood pressure, or blood disorders. The blood often comes from a vessel just inside the nostril, in which case the flow may be stopped by applying pressure on the side of the nose. Otherwise gauze packing may be effective in controlling the loss of blood. Medical name: **epistaxis.**

noso- *prefix denoting* disease.

nosocomial infection an infection originating in a hospital. It may develop in a hospitalized patient without having been present or incubating at the time of admission, or it may be acquired in hospital but only appears after discharge. The term also includes infections developing among hospital staff.

nosology *n.* the naming and classification of diseases.

Nosopsyllus *n.* a genus of fleas. The common rat flea of temperate regions, *N. fasciatus*, will, in the absence of rats, bite man and may therefore transmit plague or murine typhus from an infected rat population. The rat flea is also an intermediate host for the larval stage of two tapeworms, *Hymenolepis diminuta* and *H. nana*.

nostrils *n. see* nares.

notch *n.* (in anatomy) an indentation, especially one in a bone.

notifiable disease a disease that must be reported to the health authorities in order that speedy control and preventive action may be undertaken if necessary. In Great Britain such diseases must be notified to the Proper Officer for the control of communicable diseases (formerly to the Medical Officer of Health). They include cholera, diphtheria, dysentery, food poisoning, infective jaundice, malaria, measles, poliomyelitis, smallpox, tuberculosis, typhoid, and whooping cough. The list varies for different countries.

notochord *n.* a strip of mesodermal tissue that develops along the dorsal surface of the early embryo, beneath the *neural tube. It becomes almost entirely obliterated by the development of the vertebrae, persisting only as part of the intervertebral discs.

novobiocin *n.* an antibiotic administered by mouth or injection to treat certain infections resistant to other antibiotics. Side-effects, including digestive upsets and rashes, occur frequently and for this reason other antibiotics are usually preferred.

nucha *n.* the nape of the neck. —**nuchal** *adj.*

nuclear cardiology the study and diagnosis of heart disease by the intravenous injection of a radionuclide. The radionuclide emits gamma rays, enabling a gamma camera and computer to form an image of the heart. *See* MUGA scan, thallium scan.

nuclear magnetic resonance (NMR) a technique of chemical analysis used in the diagnosis of brain abnormalities, vascular disease, and cancer. Based on the absorption of specific radio frequencies by atomic nuclei, it enables the imaging of parts of the body in any plane.

nuclease *n.* an enzyme that catalyses the breakdown of nucleic acids by cleaving the bonds between adjacent nucleotides. Examples are *ribonuclease*, which acts on RNA, and *deoxyribonuclease*, which acts on DNA.

nucleic acid either of two organic acids, *DNA or *RNA, present in the nucleus and in some cases the cytoplasm of all living cells. Their main functions are in heredity and protein synthesis.

nucleolus *n.* (*pl.* **nucleoli**) a dense spherical structure within the cell *nucleus that disappears during cell division. The nucleolus contains *RNA for the synthesis of *ribosomes and plays an important part in RNA and protein synthesis.

nucleoplasm (karyoplasm) *n.* the protoplasm making up the nucleus of a cell.

nucleoprotein *n.* a compound that occurs in cells and consists of nucleic acid and protein tightly bound together. *Ribosomes are nucleoproteins containing RNA; *chromosomes are nucleoproteins containing DNA.

nucleoside *n.* a compound consisting of a nitrogen-containing base (a *purine or *pyrimidine) linked to a sugar. Examples are *adenosine, *guanosine, *cytidine, *thymidine, and *uracil.

nucleotide *n.* a compound consisting of a nitrogen-containing base (a *purine or *pyrimidine) linked to a sugar and a phosphate group. Nucleic acids (DNA and RNA) are long chains of linked nucleotides (*polynucleotide* chains), which in DNA contain the purine bases adenine and guanine and the pyrimidines thymine and cytosine; in RNA, thymine is replaced by uracil.

nucleus *n.* **1.** the part of a *cell that contains the genetic material, *DNA. The DNA, which is combined with protein, is normally dispersed throughout the nucleus as *chromatin. During cell division the chromatin becomes visible as the *chromosomes. The nucleus also contains *RNA, most of which is located in the *nucleolus. The nucleus is separated from the cytoplasm by a double membrane, the *nuclear envelope*. **2.** an anatomically and functionally distinct mass of nerve cells within the brain or spinal cord.

nuclide *n.* an artificially produced isotope that emits radioactive waves and may be used in radiotherapy for the treatment of tumours. *See* caesium-137, cobalt, yttrium-90.

nuisance *n.* any noxious substance, accumulating in refuse or as dust or effluent, that is deemed by British law to be injurious to health or offensive. It can also include dwellings, work premises, or animals.

null hypothesis *see* significance.

nullipara *n.* a woman who has never given birth to an infant capable of survival.

nurse *n.* a person trained and experienced in medical matters and entrusted with the care of the sick and the carrying out of medical and surgical routines under the supervision of a doctor. In Britain student nurses must receive a specified period of training in a hospital approved by the General Nursing Council and pass an examination before qualifying for the State Roll of Assistant Nurses (*State Enrolled Nurse*) or State Register of Nurses (*State Registered Nurse*). *See also* domiciliary midwife, health visitor, home nurse, nursing officer, school nurse.

nursing officer a higher grade of nurse concerned with administration and management in either tier of the British *National Health Service (*Regional* or *District Nursing Officer*). There are in addition the grades of *Principal Nursing Officer*, who has responsibility for part of the nursing organization within a hospital or in community nursing, and *Senior Nursing Officer*, who is respon-

sible for a group of nurses caring for a designated specialty (e.g. surgical).

nutation *n.* the act of nodding the head.

nutrient *n.* a substance that must be consumed as part of the diet to provide a source of energy, material for growth, or substances to regulate growth or energy production. Nutrients include carbohydrates, fats, proteins, minerals, and vitamins.

nutrition *n.* the study of food in relation to the physiological processes that depend on its absorption by the body (growth, energy production, repair of body tissues, etc.). The science of nutrition includes the study of diets and deficiency diseases.

nux vomica the seed of the tree *Strychnos nux-vomica*, which contains the poisonous alkaloid *strychnine.

nyct- (nycto-) *prefix denoting* night or darkness.

nyctalopia *n. see* night blindness.

nyctophilia *n.* an intense preference for the darkness and an avoidance of activity in daylight hours. This is sometimes a form of social *phobia.

nyctophobia *n.* extreme fear of the dark. It is common in children and not unusual in normal adults.

nyctophonia *n.* speaking in the night but not in the daytime: a form of elective *mutism.

nymph *n.* **1.** an immature stage in the life history of certain insects, such as grasshoppers and *reduviid bugs. On emerging from the eggs, nymphs resemble the adult insects except that they are smaller, do not have fully developed wings, and are not sexually mature. **2.** the late larval stage of a tick.

nympho- *prefix denoting* **1.** the labia minora. **2.** female sexuality.

nymphomania *n.* an extreme degree of sexual promiscuity in a woman. *Compare* satyriasis. —**nymphomaniac** *adj., n.*

nystagmus *n.* rapid involuntary movements of the eyes that may be from side to side, up and down, or rotatory. Nystagmus may be congenital and associated with poor sight; it also occurs in disorders of the part of the brain responsible for eye movements and their coordination and in disorders of the organ of balance in the ear or the associated parts of the brain. *Optokinetic nystagmus* occurs in normal people when they try to look at a succession of objects moving quickly across their line of sight. Jerking movements sometimes occur in normal people when tired, on exaggerated movement of the eyes. These are called *nystagmoid jerks* and they do not imply disease.

nystatin *n.* an antibiotic active against fungi. It is applied as a cream for skin infections, by mouth for intestinal infections, as pessaries or suppositories for vaginal or anal infections, or as eye-drops for eye infections. Side-effects include mild digestive upsets. Trade name: **Nystan**.

O

oat cell a cell type of carcinoma of the bronchus. Oat cells are small round or oval cells with darkly staining nuclei and scanty indistinct cytoplasm. Oat-cell carcinoma is usually related to smoking and accounts for about one quarter of bronchial carcinomas.

obesity *n.* the condition in which excess fat has accumulated in the body, mostly in the subcutaneous tissues. Obesity is usually considered to be present when a person is 20% above the recommended weight for his/her height and build. The accumulation of fat is caused by the consumption of more food than is required for producing enough energy for daily activities. Obesity is the most common nutritional disorder of recent years. —**obese** *adj.*

obex *n.* the curved lower margin of the fourth *ventricle of the brain, between the medulla oblongata and the cerebellum.

objective *n.* (in microscopy) the arrangement of lenses in a light microscope that is nearest to the object under examination and furthest from the *eyepiece. In many microscopes interchangeable objectives with different powers of magnification are provided.

obligate *adj.* describing an organism that is restricted to one particular way of life; for example, an *obligate parasite* cannot exist without a host. *Compare* facultative.

observer error *see* validity.

obsession *n.* a recurrent thought, feeling, or action that is unpleasant and provokes anxiety but cannot be got rid of. Although an obsession dominates the person, he (or she) realizes its senselessness and struggles to expel it. The obsession may be a vivid image, a thought, a fear (for example, of contamination), or an impulse (for example, to wash the hands repetitively). It is a feature of obsessional neurosis and sometimes of depression and of organic states, such as encephalitis. It can be treated with behaviour therapy and also with psychotherapy and tranquillizers. *See also* anankastic. —**obsessional** *adj.*

obstetrics *n.* the branch of medical science concerned with the care of women during pregnancy, childbirth, and the period of about six weeks following the birth, when the reproductive organs are recovering. *Compare* gynaecology. —**obstetrical** *adj.* —**obstetrician** *n.*

obstipation *n. Chiefly US.* severe or complete constipation.

obstructive lung disease *see* bronchospasm.

obtund *vb.* to blunt or deaden sensitivity; for example, by the application of a local anaesthetic, which reduces or causes complete loss of sensation in nearby nerves.

obturator *n.* **1.** *see* obturator muscle. **2.** a wire or rod within a cannula or hollow needle for piercing tissues or fitting aspirating needles. **3.** a removable form of denture that both closes a defect in the palate and also bears artificial teeth for cosmetic purposes. The defect may be congenital, as in a cleft palate, or result from the removal of a tumour.

obturator foramen a large opening in the *hip bone, below and slightly in front of the acetabulum. *See also* pelvis.

obturator muscle either of two muscles that cover the outer surface of the anterior wall of the pelvis (the *obturator externus* and *obturator internus*) and are responsible for lateral rotation of the thigh and movements of the hip.

obtusion *n.* the weakening or blunting of normal sensations. This may be associated with disease.

occipital bone a saucer-shaped bone of the *skull that forms the back and part of the base of the cranium. At the base of the occipital are two *occipital condyles*: rounded surfaces that articulate with the first (atlas) vertebra of the backbone. Between the condyles is the *foramen magnum*, the cavity through which the spinal cord passes.

occiput *n.* the back of the head. —**occipital** *adj.*

occlusal *adj.* (in dental anatomy) denoting or relating to the biting surface of a premolar or molar tooth.

occlusal rim the occlusal extension of a denture base to allow the recording of jaw relations in the construction of *dentures.

occlusion *n.* **1.** the closing or obstruction of a hollow organ or part. **2.** (in dentistry) the relation of the upper and lower teeth when they are in contact. Maximum contact between the teeth is known as *centric occlusion. See also* malocclusion.

occult *adj.* not apparent to the naked eye; not easily determined or detected. For example *occult blood* is blood present in such small quantities, for example in the faeces, that it can only be detected microscopically or by chemical testing.

occupational disease any one of various specific diseases to which workers in certain occupations are particularly prone. *Industrial diseases*, associated with a particular industry or group of industries, fall within this category. Examples of such diseases include the various forms of *pneumoconiosis, which affect the lungs of workers continually exposed to dusty atmospheres; cataracts in glassblowers; decompression sickness in divers; poisoning from toxic metals in factory and other workers; and infectious diseases contracted from animals by farm workers. *See also* prescribed disease, sickness benefit.

occupational mortality rates and causes of death in relation to different jobs, occupational and socioeconomic groups, or *social class. Because some occupations have older incumbents than others (e.g. judges) allowance for age bias is made by comparing either *standardized mortality ratios* for those aged 15–64 years or related but less familiar indices, such as *comparative mortality figure* or *proportional mortality ratio*.

occupational therapy the treatment of physical and psychiatric conditions by encouraging patients to undertake specific selected activities that will help them to reach their maximum level of function and independence in all aspects of daily life. These activities are designed to make the best use of the patient's capabilities and are based on individual requirements. They range from woodwork, metalwork, and printing to pottery and other artistic activities, household management, social skills (for psychiatric patients), and leisure activities (for geriatic patients). Occupational therapy also includes assessment for mechanical aids and adaptations in the home.

ochronosis n. the presence of brown-black pigment in the skin, cartilage, and other tissues due to the abnormal accumulation of homogentisic acid that occurs in the metabolic disease *alcaptonuria.

oct- (octa-, octi-, octo-) prefix denoting eight.

octigravida n. a woman who has been pregnant eight times.

octipara n. a woman who has been pregnant at least eight times and has given birth to an infant capable of survival after each of eight pregnancies.

ocular adj. of or concerned with the eye or vision.

oculist n. a North American term for an *ophthalmologist.

oculo- prefix denoting the eye(s).

oculogyric adj. causing or concerned with movements of the eye.

oculomotor adj. concerned with eye movements.

oculomotor nerve the third *cranial nerve (III), which is composed of motor fibres distributed to muscles in and around the eye. Fibres of the parasympathetic system are responsible for altering the size of the pupil and the lens of the eye. Fibres outside the eye run to the upper eyelid and to muscles that turn the eyeball in different directions.

oculonasal adj. concerned with the eye and nose.

odont- (odonto-) prefix denoting a tooth. Example: odontalgia (toothache).

odontoblast n. a cell that forms dentine. Odontoblasts line the pulp and have small processes that extend into the dentine.

odontoid process a toothlike process from the upper surface of the axis vertebra. See cervical vertebrae.

odontology n. the study of the teeth.

odontome n. an abnormal mass of calcified dental tissue.

-odynia suffix denoting pain in (a specified part).

odynophagia n. a sensation of pain behind the sternum as food or fluid is swallowed; particularly, the burning sensation experienced by patients with reflux *oesophagitis when hot, spicy, or alcoholic liquid is swallowed.

oedema n. excessive accumulation of fluid in the body tissues: popularly known as dropsy. The resultant swelling may be local, as with an injury or inflammation, or more general, as in heart or kidney failure. In generalized oedema there may be collections of fluid within the chest cavity (pleural effusions), abdomen (see ascites), or within the air spaces of the lung (pulmonary oedema). It may result from heart or kidney failure, cirrhosis of the liver, acute nephritis, the nephrotic syndrome, starvation, allergy, or drugs (e.g. phenylbutazone or cortisone derivatives). In such cases the kidneys can usually be stimulated to get rid of the excess fluid by the administration of *diuretic drugs. Subcutaneous oedema commonly occurs in the legs and ankles due to the influence of gravity and (in women) before menstruation; the swelling subsides with rest and elevation of the legs. —**oedematous** *adj.*

Oedipus complex repressed sexual feelings of a child for its opposite-sexed parent, combined with rivalry towards the same-sexed parent: a normal stage of development, first described by Freud. The end of the Oedipus complex in children is marked by a loss of sexual feelings towards the opposite-sexed parent and an increase in identification with the same-sexed parent. Arrest of development at the Oedipal stage is said to be responsible for sexual deviations and other neurotic behaviour.

oesophag- (oesophago-) *prefix denoting* the oesophagus. Example: *oesophagectomy* (surgical removal of).

oesophageal ulcer *see* peptic ulcer, oesophagitis.

oesophagitis *n.* inflammation of the oesophagus (gullet). Frequent regurgitation of acid and peptic juices from the stomach causes *reflux oesophagitis*, the commonest form, which may be associated with a hiatus *hernia. The main symptoms are heartburn, regurgitation of bitter fluid, and sometimes difficulty in swallowing; complications include bleeding, narrowing (*stricture) of the oesophageal canal, and ulceration. It is treated by antacid medicines, weight reduction, and avoidance of bending; in severe cases surgery may be required. *Corrosive oesophagitis* is caused by the ingestion of caustic acid or alkali. It is often severe and may lead to perforation of the oesophagus or to extensive stricture formation. Treatment includes avoidance of food and administration of antibiotics and corticosteroids; later dilatation of the stricture may be needed. *Infective oesophagitis* is most commonly due to a fungus (*Candida*) infection in debilitated patients, especially those being treated with antibiotics, corticosteroids, and immunosuppressive drugs, but is occasionally due

to viruses (such as cytomegalovirus or herpes virus).

oesophagocele *n.* protrusion of the lining (mucosa) of the oesophagus (gullet) through a tear in its muscular wall.

oesophagoscope *n.* an illuminated optical instrument used to inspect the interior of the oesophagus (gullet), dilate its canal (in cases of stricture), obtain material for biopsy, or remove a foreign body. It may be a rigid metal tube or a flexible fibreoptic instrument (*see* gastroscope). —**oesophagoscopy** *n.*

Oesophagostomum *n.* a genus of parasitic nematodes occurring in Brazil, Africa, and Indonesia. It is a rare intestinal parasite of man, producing symptoms of dysentery in cases of heavy infection. The worms may also invade the tissues of the gut wall, giving rise to abscesses. The worms can be eliminated with *tetrachloroethylene.

oesophagostomy *n.* a surgical operation in which the oesophagus (gullet) is opened onto the neck. It is usually performed after operations on the throat as a temporary measure to allow feeding.

oesophagotomy *n.* surgical opening of the oesophagus (gullet) in order to inspect its interior or to remove or insert something.

oesophagus *n.* the gullet: a muscular tube, about 23 cm long, that extends from the pharynx to the stomach. It is lined with mucous membrane, whose secretions lubricate food as it passes from the mouth to the stomach. Waves of *peristalsis assist the passage of food.

oestradiol *n.* the major female sex hormone produced by the ovary. *See* oestrogen.

oestriol *n.* one of the female sex hormones produced by the ovary. *See* oestrogen.

oestrogen *n.* one of a group of steroid hormones (including oestriol, oestrone, and oestradiol) that control female sexual development, promoting the growth and function of the female sex organs (*see* menstrual cycle) and female secondary sexual characteristics (such as breast development). Oestrogens are synthesized mainly by the ovary; small amounts are also produced by the adrenal cortex, testes, and placenta. In men excessive production of oestrogen gives rise to *feminization.

Naturally occurring and synthetic oestrogens, given by mouth or injection, are used to treat *amenorrhoea, menopausal disorders, androgen-dependent cancers (e.g. cancer of the prostate), and to inhibit lactation. Synthetic oestrogens are a major constituent of *oral contraceptives. Side-effects of oestrogen therapy may include nausea and vomiting, headache and dizziness, irregular vaginal bleeding, fluid and salt retention, and feminization in men. Oestrogens should not be used in patients with a history of cancer of the breast, womb, or genital tract. —**oestrogenic** *adj.*

oestrone *n.* one of the female sex hormones produced by the ovary. *See* oestrogen.

Oestrus *n.* a genus of widely distributed nonbloodsucking flies, occurring wherever sheep and goats are raised. The parasitic larvae of *O. ovis*, the sheep nostril fly, may occasionally and accidentally infect man. By means of large mouth hooks, it attaches itself to the conjunctiva of the eye, causing a painful *myiasis that may result in loss of sight. This is an occupational disease of shepherds. Larvae can be removed with forceps following anaesthesia.

Office of Population Censuses and Surveys (in Britain) a department of central government responsible for the compilation and publication of statistics relating to national and local population and the demographic patterns of births, marriages, and deaths (including the medical cause of death). It organizes a *national census* at ten-yearly intervals based n the actual presence of individuals in a house or institution on a designated night as distinct from their official address.

ohm *n.* the *SI unit of electrical resistance, equal to the resistance between two points on a conductor when a constant potential difference of 1 volt applied between these points produces a current of 1 ampere. Symbol: Ω.

-oid *suffix denoting* like; resembling. Example: *pemphigoid* (condition resembling pemphigus).

ointment *n.* a greasy material, usually containing a medicament, applied to the skin or mucous membranes.

oleandomycin *n.* an antibiotic used to treat infections caused by a wide range of bacteria. It is administered by mouth or injection and is usually without side-effects.

olecranon process the large process of the *ulna that projects behind the elbow joint.

oleic acid *see* fatty acid.

oleo- *prefix denoting* oil.

oleothorax *n.* the procedure of introducing a light oil into the *pleural cavity so that the lung is allowed to collapse. This was sometimes formerly undertaken to allow healing in a lung damaged by tuberculosis.

oleum *n.* (in pharmacy) an oil.

olfaction *n.* **1.** the sense of smell. **2.** the process of smelling. Sensory cells in the mucous membrane that lines the nasal cavity are stimulated by the presence of chemical particles dissolved in the mucus. *See* nose. —**olfactory** *adj.*

olfactory nerve the first *cranial nerve (I): the special sensory nerve of smell.

Fibres of the nerve run upwards from smell receptors in the nasal mucosa high in the roof of the nose, through minute holes in the skull, join to form the olfactory tract, and pass back to reach the brain.

olig- (oligo-) *prefix denoting* **1.** few. **2.** a deficiency.

oligaemia *n. see* hypovolaemia.

oligoarthritis *n. see* arthritis.

oligodactylism *n.* the congenital absence of some of the fingers and toes.

oligodendrocyte *n.* one of the cells of the *glia, responsible for producing the *myelin sheaths of the neurones of the central nervous system and therefore equivalent to the *Schwann cells of the peripheral nerves.

oligodendroglioma *n.* a tumour of the central nervous system derived from a type of *glia (the supporting tissue) rather than from the nerve cells themselves. *See also* glioma.

oligodipsia *n.* a condition in which thirst is diminished or absent.

oligodontia *n.* the congenital absence of some of the teeth.

oligohydramnios *n.* a condition in which the amount of amniotic fluid bathing a fetus during pregnancy is abnormally small. The developing infant may consequently be vulnerable, for example if the mother falls.

oligomenorrhoea *n.* sparse or infrequent menstruation.

oligophrenia *n. Obsolete.* mental *subnormality.

oligospermia *n.* the presence of less than the normal number of spermatozoa in the semen. Normal semen produced on ejaculation usually contains more than 60 million sperm/ml, of which about 80% are motile and morphologically normal. In oligospermia, the sperm usually have poor motility

and often include many bizarre and immature forms. Treatment is directed to any underlying cause (such as *varicocele). *See also* infertility.

oliguria *n.* the production of an abnormally small volume of urine. This may be a result of copious sweating associated with intense physical activity and/or hot weather. It can also be due to kidney disease, retention of water in the tissues (*see* oedema), loss of blood, diarrhoea, or poisoning.

olive *n.* a smooth oval swelling in the upper part of the medulla oblongata on each side. It contains a mass of nerve cells, mainly grey matter (*olivary nucleus*). —**olivary** *adj.*

-ology *suffix. see* -logy.

om- (omo-) *prefix denoting* the shoulder.

-oma *suffix denoting* a tumour. Examples: *hepatoma* (of the liver); *lymphoma* (of the lymph nodes).

omentectomy *n.* the removal of all or part of the omentum (the fold of peritoneum between the stomach and other abdominal organs).

omentopexy *n.* an operation in which the *omentum is attached to some other tissue, usually the abdominal wall (in order to improve blood flow through the liver) or the heart (to increase the blood supply to the heart).

omentum (epiploon) *n.* a double layer of *peritoneum attached to the stomach and linking it with other abdominal organs, such as the liver, spleen, and intestine. The *great omentum* is a highly folded portion of the omentum, rich in fatty tissue, that covers the intestines in an apron-like fashion. It acts as a heat insulator and prevents friction between abdominal organs. The *lesser omentum* links the stomach with the liver. —**omental** *adj.*

Ommaya reservoir a device inserted into the ventricles of the brain to enable the repeated injection of drugs into the cerebrospinal fluid. It is used, for example, in the treatment of malignant meningitis, particularly in children with leukaemia.

omphal- (omphalo-) *prefix denoting* the navel or umbilical cord.

omphalitis *n.* inflammation of the navel, especially in newborn infants.

omphalocele *n.* an umbilical *hernia.

omphalus *n. see* umbilicus.

Onchocerca *n.* a genus of parasitic worms (*see* filaria) occurring in central Africa and central America. The adult worms are found in fibrous nodules within the connective tissues beneath the skin and their presence causes disease (*see* onchocerciasis). Various species of black fly, in which *Onchocerca* undergoes part of its development, transmit the infective larvae to man.

onchocerciasis *n.* a tropical disease of the skin and underlying connective tissue caused by the parasitic worm *Onchocerca volvulus*. Fibrous nodular tumours grow around the adult worms in the skin; these may take several months to appear, and if secondary bacterial infection occurs they may degenerate into abscesses. The skin also becomes inflamed and itches. The migration of the larvae into the eye can cause total or partial blindness – the *river blindness* of Africa. Onchocerciasis occurs in Central Africa and Central America. The drugs *suramin and *diethylcarbamazine are used in treatment; if possible, the nodules are removed as and when they appear.

onco- *prefix denoting* 1. a tumour. 2. volume.

oncogene *n.* a gene in viruses and mammalian cells that can cause cancer. It probably produces proteins regulating cell division that, under certain conditions, become uncontrolled.

oncogenesis *n.* the development of a new abnormal growth (a benign or malignant tumour).

oncogenic *adj.* describing a substance, organism, or environment that is known to be a causal factor in the production of a tumour. Some animal viruses are known to be oncogenic; others are suspected of being so in man, including some papovaviruses, adenoviruses, and herpesviruses. *See also* carcinogen.

oncology *n.* the study and practice of treating tumours.

oncolysis *n.* the destruction of tumours and tumour cells. This may occur spontaneously or, more usually, in response to treatment with drugs or radiotherapy.

oncometer *n.* an instrument for measuring the volume of blood circulating in one of the limbs. *See* plethysmography.

oncosphere (hexacanth) *n.* the six-hooked larva of a *tapeworm. If ingested by a suitable intermediate host, such as a pig or an ox, the larva will use its hooks to penetrate the wall of the intestine. The larva subsequently migrates to the muscles, where it develops into a *cysticercus.

oncotic *adj.* 1. characterized by a tumour or swelling. 2. relating to an increase in volume or pressure.

oncotic pressure a pressure represented by the pressure difference that exists between the osmotic pressure of blood and that of the lymph or tissue fluid. Oncotic pressure is important for regulating the flow of water between blood and tissue fluid. *See also* osmosis.

oneir- (oneiro-) *prefix denoting* dreams or dreaming.

oneirism n. day-dreaming. Obviously this is a normal phenomenon, but in excess it may impair the ability to cope with life. This is a feature of *schizoid and *asthenic personalities.

onomatomania n. the repeated intrusion of a specific word or a name into a person's thoughts: a form of *obsession.

onomatopoiesis n. inventing words that reflect the sound made by the object or event to be described. It is one of the principles that guide some schizophrenics in the production of *neologisms.

ontogeny n. the history of the development of an individual from the fertilized egg to maturity.

onych- (onycho-) prefix denoting the nail(s).

onychauxis n. thickening or overgrowth of the nails.

onychia n. inflammation of the matrix of the *nail, which results in loss of the nail.

onychogryphosis n. gross thickening and hardening of the nail, which becomes elongated and deformed. The cause is unknown.

onycholysis n. separation or loosening of part or all of a nail from its bed, often due to a poor blood supply. The condition may occur in *psoriasis and in fungus infection of the skin and nail bed.

onychomadesis n. loss of the nails.

onychomycosis n. fungus infection of the nails, usually caused by *Epidermophyton or *Candida. The nails become white, opaque, thickened, and brittle. See also ringworm.

onychosis n. any disease or deformity of the nails.

O'nyong nyong fever (joint-breaker fever) an East African disease caused by an *arbovirus and transmitted to man by mosquitoes of the genus *Anopheles. The disease is similar to *dengue and symptoms include rigor, severe headache, an irritating rash, fever, and pains in the joints. The patient is given drugs to relieve the pain and fever.

oo- prefix denoting an egg; ovum.

oocyesis (ovariocyesis) n. the development of an embryo in the ovary: ovarian pregnancy. See also ectopic pregnancy.

oocyst n. a spherical structure, 50–60 μm in diameter, that develops from the zygote (see ookinete) of the malarial parasite (Plasmodium) on the outer wall of the mosquito's stomach. The oocyst steadily grows in size and its contents divide repeatedly to form *sporozoites, which are released into the body cavity of the mosquito when the oocyst bursts.

oocyte n. a cell in the ovary that undergoes *meiosis to form an ovum. Primary oocytes develop from *oogonia in the fetal ovary as they enter the early stages of meiosis. Only a fraction of the primary oocytes survive until puberty, and even fewer will be ovulated. At ovulation the first meiotic division is completed and a secondary oocyte and a polar body are formed. Fertilization stimulates the completion of the second meiotic division, which produces a second polar body and an ovum.

oogenesis n. the process by which mature ova (egg cells) are produced in the ovary (see illustration). Primordial germ cells multiply to form *oogonia, which start their first meiotic division to become *oocytes in the fetus. This division is not completed until each oocyte is ovulated. The second division is only completed on fertilization. Each meiotic division is unequal, so that one large ovum is produced with a much smaller polar body.

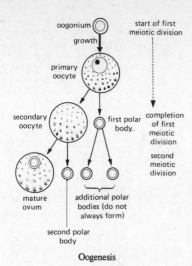

oogonium ◯   start of first meiotic division

growth

primary oocyte

secondary oocyte   first polar body   completion of first meiotic division

second meiotic division

mature ovum   additional polar bodies (do not always form)

second polar body

Oogenesis

oogonium *n.* (*pl.* **oogonia**) a cell produced at an early stage in the formation of an ovum (egg cell). Primordial germ cells that have migrated to the embryonic ovary multiply to form numerous small oogonia. After the fifth month of pregnancy they enter the early stages of the first meiotic division to form *oocytes. *See also* oogenesis.

ookinete *n.* the motile elongated *zygote of the malarial parasite (*Plasmodium*), formed after fertilization of the *macrogamete. The ookinete bores through the lining of the mosquito's stomach and attaches itself to the outer wall, where it later forms an *oocyst.

oophor- (oophoro-) *prefix denoting* the ovary.

oophoralgia (ovarialgia, ovaralgia) *n.* pain in the ovary.

oophorectomy (ovariectomy) *n.* surgical removal of an ovary, performed, for example, when the ovary contains tumours or cysts or is otherwise diseased. *Compare* ovariotomy.

oophoritis (ovaritis) *n.* inflammation of an ovary, either on the surface or within the organ. Oophoritis sometimes results from infection of the Fallopian tubes (*see* salpingitis) or the lower part of the abdominal cavity. *Follicular oophoritis* is inflammation of the ovarian (Graafian) follicles. A bacterial infection usually responds to antibiotics.

oophorocystosis *n.* the formation of an *ovarian cyst.

oophoroma *n.* a rapidly developing cancerous growth in the ovary. *Compare* ovarian cyst.

oophoropexy (oophoropeliopexy, oophorrhaphy) *n.* the stitching of a displaced ovary to the wall of the pelvic cavity.

operant *adj.* describing a unit of behaviour that is defined by its effect on the environment. *See* conditioning.

operating microscope a binocular microscope used in surgery, e.g. in operations to remove a blood clot from an artery (*see* endarterectomy). The field of operation is illuminated through the objective lens by a light source within the microscope (see illustration). Many models incorporate a beam splitter and a second set of eyepieces, to enable the surgeon's assistant to view the operation.

operculum *n.* (*pl.* **opercula**) **1.** a plug of mucus that blocks the cervical canal of the womb in a pregnant woman. **2.** (in embryology) a plug of fibrin and blood cells that develops over the site at which a developing fertilized ovum has become embedded in the wall of the womb. **3.** (in neurology) one of the folded and overlapping regions of cerebral cortex that conceal the *insula on each side of the brain.

operon *n.* a group of closely linked genes that regulate the production of enzymes. An operon is composed of

An operating microscope

one or more *structural genes*, which determine the nature of the enzymes made, and an *operator gene*, which controls the working of the structural genes and is itself controlled by a *regulator gene*, which is not part of the operon.

OPG *see* orthopantomogram.

ophthalm- (ophthalmo-) *prefix denoting* the eye.

ophthalmectomy *n.* an operation in which the eye is removed. *See* enucleation.

ophthalmia *n. Obsolete.* inflammation of the eye, particularly the conjunctiva (*see* conjunctivitis).

ophthalmia neonatorum a form of conjunctivitis occurring in newborn infants, who contract the disease as they pass through an infected birth canal. The most serious condition occurs if the mother has a gonorrhoeal infection: blindness will result unless antibiotic treatment or silver nitrate eyedrops are given promptly.

ophthalmic *adj.* concerned with the eye.

ophthalmic nerve the smallest of the three branches of the *trigeminal nerve. It supplies sensory fibres to the eyeball, conjunctiva, and lacrimal gland, to a small region of the nasal mucous membrane, and to the skin of the nose, brows, and scalp.

ophthalmitis *n.* inflammation of the eye. *See* conjunctivitis, uveitis.

ophthalmodynamometry *n.* measurement of the blood pressure in the vessels of the retina of the eye. A small instrument is pressed against the eye until the vessels are seen (through an *ophthalmoscope) to collapse. The pressure recorded by the instrument reflects the pressure within the vessels of the retina. In certain disorders of the blood circulation to the eye, the pressure in the vessels is reduced and the vessels can be made to collapse by a pressure that is lower than normal.

ophthalmologist *n.* a doctor who specializes in the diagnosis and treatment of eye diseases.

ophthalmology *n.* the branch of medicine that is devoted to the study and treatment of eye diseases. —**ophthalmological** *adj.*

ophthalmometer *n. see* keratometer.

ophthalmoplegia *n.* paralysis of the muscles of the eye. *Internal ophthalmoplegia* affects the muscles inside the eye: the iris (which controls the size of the pupil) and the ciliary muscle (which is responsible for *accommodation). *External ophthalmoplegia* affects the muscles that move the eye.

ophthalmorrhexis *n.* rupture of the eyeball. This is usually due to a severe blow to the eye.

ophthalmoscope *n.* an instrument for examining the interior of the eye (see illustration). There are two types. The *direct ophthalmoscope* enables a fine beam of light to be directed into the eye and at the same time allows the examiner to see the spot where the beam falls inside the eye. Examiner and subject are very close together. In the *indirect ophthalmoscope* an image of the inside of the eye is formed between the subject and the examiner; it is this image that the examiner sees. The examiner and subject are almost at arm's length apart. —**ophthalmoscopy** *n.*

disc for changing lenses

An ophthalmoscope

ophthalmotomy *n.* the operation of making an incision in the eyeball.

ophthalmotonometer (tonometer) *n.* a small instrument for measuring the pressure inside the eye. There are two types, both applied to the cornea after a drop of local anaesthetic has been put in the eye. The *indentation* (*Schiotz*) *tonometer* uses a small plunger that indents the cornea by an amount corresponding to the softness (determined by pressure) of the eye. The *applanation tonometer* measures the pressure required to flatten a constant area of the cornea. A high pressure is required when the pressure inside the eye is increased, and vice versa.

-opia *suffix denoting* a defect of the eye or of vision. Example: *asthenopia* (eyestrain).

opiate *n.* one of a group of drugs derived from opium, including *apomorphine, *codeine, *morphine, and *papaverine. Opiates depress the central nervous system: they relieve pain, suppress coughing, and stimulate vomiting. The most important opiate – morphine – and its synthetic derivative heroin are *narcotics, producing feelings of euphoria before inducing stupor. They are only used for severe pain since they cause *dependence.

opisth- (opistho-) *prefix denoting* **1.** dorsal; posterior. **2.** backwards.

opisthorchiasis *n.* a condition caused by the presence of the parasitic fluke *Opisthorchis* in the bile ducts. The infection is acquired through eating raw or undercooked fish that contains the larval stage of the parasite. Heavy infections can lead to considerable damage of the tissues of the bile duct and liver, progressing in advanced cases to *cirrhosis. Symptoms may include loss of weight, abdominal pain, indigestion, and sometimes diarrhoea. The disease, occurring in E Europe and the Far East, is treated with *chloroquine.

Opisthorchis *n.* a genus of parasitic flukes occurring in E Europe and parts of SE Asia. *O. felineus* is normally a parasite of fish-eating mammals but accidental infections of man have occurred. The adult flukes, which live in the bile ducts, can cause *opisthorchiasis.

opisthotonos *n.* the position of the body in which the head, neck, and spine are arched backwards. It is assumed involuntarily by patients with tetanus and strychnine poisoning.

opium *n.* an extract from the poppy *Papaver somniferum*, which has analgesic and narcotic action due to its content of *morphine. It has the same uses and side-effects as morphine and prolonged use may lead to *dependence. *See also* opiate.

opponens *n.* one of a group of muscles in the hand that bring the digits opposite to other digits. For example, the *opponens pollicis* is the principal muscle causing opposition of the thumb.

opposition *n.* (in anatomy) the position of the thumb in relation to the other fingers when it is moved towards the palm of the hand.

-opsia *suffix denoting* a condition of vision. Example: *erythropsia* (red vision).

opsonic index a numerical measurement of the power of a person's serum to attack invading bacteria and prepare them for destruction by *phagocytes. It is measured by dividing the average number of bacteria in the blood per phagocyte in the presence of immune serum by the corresponding number in the presence of normal serum. A vaccine increases the opsonic index.

opsonin *n.* a serum component that attaches itself to invading bacteria and apparently makes them more attractive to *phagocytes and thus more likely to be engulfed and destroyed.

opsonization *n.* the process by which opsonins render bacteria more attractive to *phagocytes by attaching themselves to their outer surfaces and changing their physical and chemical composition.

opt- (opto-) *prefix denoting* vision or the eye.

optic *adj.* concerned with the eye or vision.

optical activity the property possessed by some substances of rotating the plane of polarization of polarized light. A compound that rotates the plane to the left is described as *laevorotatory* (or l-); one that rotates the plane to the right is described as *dextrorotatory* (or d-).

optical committee (local) *see* medical committee (local).

optic atrophy degeneration of the optic nerve. It may be secondary to disease within the eye or it may follow damage to the nerve itself resulting from injury or inflammation.

optic chiasma (optic commissure) the X-shaped structure formed by the two optic nerves, which pass backwards from the eyeballs to meet in the midline beneath the brain, near the pituitary gland (see illustration). Nerve fibres from the nasal side of the retina of each eye cross over to join fibres from the lateral side of the retina of the opposite eye. The optic tracts resulting from the junction pass backwards to the occipital lobes.

The optic chiasma

optic cup either of the paired cup-shaped outgrowths of the embryonic brain that form the retina and iris of the eyes.

optic disc (optic papilla) the start of the optic nerve, where nerve fibres from the rods and cones leave the eyeball. *See* blind spot.

optic foramen the groove in the top of the *orbit that contains the optic nerve and the ophthalmic artery.

optician *n.* a person who either makes and fits glasses (*dispensing optician*) or who both tests people for glasses and also makes and fits them (*ophthalmic optician* or *optometrist*).

optic nerve the second *cranial nerve (II), which is responsible for vision. Each nerve contains about one million fibres that receive information from the rod and cone cells of the retina. It passes into the skull behind the eyeball to reach the *optic chiasma, after which the visual pathway continues to the cortex of the occipital lobe of the brain on each side.

optic neuritis *see* retrobulbar neuritis.

optometer (refractometer) *n.* an instrument for measuring the *refraction of the eye. Because the design and use of optometers is very complex, errors of refraction are usually determined using a *retinoscope.

optometrist *n. see* optician.

oral *adj.* **1.** relating to the mouth. **2.** taken by mouth: applied to medicines, etc.

oral cavity the mouth.

oral contraceptive the Pill: a preparation, consisting of one or more synthetic female sex hormones, taken by women to prevent conception. Most oral contraceptives are combined pills, consisting of an *oestrogen, which blocks the normal process of ovulation, and a *progestogen, which acts on the pituitary gland to block the normal control of the menstrual cycle. Progestogens also alter the lining of the womb and the viscosity of mucus in its outlet, the cervix, so that conception is less likely should ovulation occur. These pills are taken every day for three weeks and then stopped for a week, during which time menstruation occurs. Side-effects may include headache, weight gain, nausea, skin changes, and depression. There is also a small risk that blood clots may form in the veins, especially those of the legs (which may lead to *pulmonary embolism), or that prolonged use of hormonal contraceptives may reduce fertility. The unwanted pregnancy rate is less than 1 per 100 woman-years.

Other hormonal contraceptives include *minipills*, which rely on a progestogen alone, and injections of progestogen, which need be given only every three months. The unwanted pregnancy rate is slightly higher with these preparations: 1–2 per 100 woman-years.

oral rehabilitation the procedure of rebuilding a dentition that has been mutilated as a result of disease, wear, or trauma.

Orbenin *n. see* cloxacillin sodium.

orbicularis *n.* either of two circular muscles of the face. The *orbicularis oris*, around the mouth, closes and compresses the lips. The *orbicularis oculi*, around each orbit, is responsible for closing the eye.

orbit *n.* the cavity in the skull that contains the eye. It is formed from parts of the frontal, sphenoid, zygomatic, lacrimal, ethmoid, palatine, and maxillary bones. —**orbital** *adj.*

orbitotomy *n.* a surgical incision into the bony orbit containing the eye.

orchi- (orchido-, orchio-) *prefix denoting* the testis or testicle. Example: *orchioplasty* (plastic surgery of).

orchidalgia *n.* pain in the testicle. The pain may not be due to a primary condition of the testicle itself: it may be caused by a hernia in the groin, the presence of a stone in the lower ureter, or the presence of a *varicocele.

orchidectomy *n.* surgical removal of a testis, usually to treat such diseases as *seminoma (a malignant tumour of the testis). Removal of both testes (*castration) causes sterility.

orchidopexy *n.* the operation of mobilizing an undescended testis in the groin and fixing it in the scrotum. The operation should be performed well before puberty to allow the testis every chance of normal development (*see* cryptorchidism).

orchidotomy *n.* an incision into the testis, usually done to obtain *biopsy material for histological examination, particularly in men with few or no sperm in their semen (*see* azoospermia, oligospermia).

orchitis *n.* inflammation of the testis. This causes pain, redness, and swelling of the scrotum, and may be associated with inflammation of the epididymis (*epididymo-orchitis*). The condition may affect one or both testes; it is usually caused by infection spreading down the vas deferens but can develop in mumps. Mumps orchitis affecting both testes may result in sterility. Treatment of epididymo-orchitis is by local support and administration of analgesics and antibiotics; mumps orchitis often responds to *corticosteroids.

orciprenaline *n.* a drug used to relieve bronchitis and asthma. It has the same actions and side-effects as *isoprenaline. Trade name: **Alupent**.

orf *n.* a virus infection of sheep and goats that can be transmitted to man, causing a mild skin eruption on the fingers, hands, and forearms.

organ *n.* a part of the body, composed of more than one tissue, that forms a structural unit responsible for a particular function (or functions). Examples are the heart, lungs, and liver.

organelle *n.* a structure within a cell that is specialized for a particular function. Examples of organelles are the nucleus, endoplasmic reticulum, Golgi apparatus, lysosomes, and mitochondria.

organic *adj.* **1.** relating to any or all of the organs of the body. **2.** describing chemical compounds containing carbon, found in all living systems.

organic disorder a disorder associated with changes in the structure of an organ or tissue. *Compare* functional disorder.

organism *n.* any living thing, which may consist of a single cell (*see* microorganism) or a group of differentiated but interdependent cells.

organo- *prefix denoting* organ or organic. Examples: *organogenesis* (formation of); *organopathy* (disease of).

organ of Corti (spiral organ) the sense organ of the *cochlea of the inner ear, which converts sound signals into nerve impulses that are transmitted to the brain via the cochlear nerve.

organ of Jacobson (vomeronasal organ) a small blind sac in the wall of the nasal cavity. In man it never develops properly and has no function, but in lower animals (e.g. snakes) it is one of the major organs of olfaction.

organotrophic *adj. see* heterotrophic.

orgasm *n.* the climax of sexual excitement, which – in men – occurs simultaneously with *ejaculation. In women its occurrence is much more variable, being dependent upon a number of physiological and psychological factors.

oriental sore (Baghdad boil, Delhi boil, Aleppo boil) a skin disease, occurring in tropical and subtropical Africa and Asia, caused by the parasitic protozoan *Leishmania tropica* (*see* leishmaniasis). The disease commonly affects children and takes the form of a slow-healing open sore or ulcer, which sometimes becomes secondarily infected with bacteria. Antibiotics are administered to combat the infection.

orientation *n.* (in psychology) awareness of oneself in time, space, and place. Orientation may be disturbed in such conditions as organic brain disease, toxic drug states, and concussion.

origin *n.* (in anatomy) **1.** the point of attachment of a muscle that remains relatively fixed during contraction of the muscle. *Compare* insertion. **2.** the point at which a nerve or blood vessel branches from a main nerve or blood vessel.

ornithine *n.* an *amino acid produced in the liver as a by-product during the conversion of ammonia to *urea.

Ornithodoros (Ornithodorus) *n.* a genus of soft *ticks, a number of species of which are important in various parts of the world in the transmission of *relapsing fever.

ornithosis *n.* an infectious disease of birds, primarily pigeons, due to a viruslike organism of the genus *Chlamydia*; it can be transmitted to man and causes symptoms resembling those of pneumonia. *Compare* parrot disease.

oro- *prefix denoting* the mouth.

oro-antral fistula a connection between the mouth and the maxillary sinus (antrum) as a sequel to tooth extraction. It may resolve or require surgical closure.

oropharynx *n.* the part of the *pharynx that lies between the soft palate and the hyoid bone (which is situated near the upper portion of the epiglottis).

Oroya fever *see* bartonellosis.

orphenadrine *n.* a drug that relieves spasm in muscle, used to treat all types of parkinsonism. It is administered by mouth or injection; side-effects may include dry mouth, sight disturbances, and difficulty in urination. Trade name: **Disipal**.

ortho- *prefix denoting* **1.** straight. Example: *orthograde* (having straight posture). **2.** normal. Example: *orthocrasia* (normal reaction to drugs).

orthochromatic *adj.* describing or relating to a tissue specimen that stains normally.

orthodiagraph *n.* an X-ray photograph designed to give an undistorted picture of part of the body so that accurate measurements may be made from it.

orthodontic appliance an appliance used to move teeth as part of orthodontic treatment. A *fixed appliance* is fitted to the teeth and used to perform complex tooth movements; it is used by dentists with specialist training. A *removable appliance* is a dental plate with appropriate retainers and springs to perform simple tooth movements; it is removed from the mouth for cleaning by the patient.

orthodontics *n.* the branch of dentistry concerned with the growth and development of the dentition and the treatment of irregularities. *See* orthodontic appliance. —**orthodontic** *adj.*

orthopaedics *n.* the science or practice of correcting deformities caused by disease of or damage to the bones and joints of the skeleton. This specialized branch of medicine may require the use of surgery, manipulation, traction, or special apparatus. —**orthopaedic** *adj.*

orthopantomogram (OPG) *n.* a special form of tomogram (*see* tomography) that provides a picture of all the teeth of both jaws on one film.

orthophoria *n.* the condition of complete balance between the movements of the two eyes, such that perfect alignment is maintained even when one eye is covered. This theoretically normal state is in fact rarely seen, since most people have a slight tendency to squint (*see* heterophoria).

orthopnoea *n.* breathlessness that prevents the patient from lying down, so that he has to sleep propped up in bed or sitting in a chair. —**orthopnoeic** *adj.*

orthoptics *n.* the practice of using nonsurgical methods, particularly eye exercises, to treat abnormalities of vision and of coordination of eye movements (most commonly strabismus (squint) and amblyopia). Orthoptics also includes the detection and measurement of the degree of such abnormalities. —**orthoptist** *n.*

orthoptoscope *n. see* amblyoscope.

orthostatic *adj.* relating to the upright position of the body: used when describing this posture or a condition caused by it. *Orthostatic hypotension*, for example, is low blood pressure found in some patients when they stand upright.

os[1] *n.* (*pl.* **ossa**) a bone.

os[2] *n.* (*pl.* **ora**) the mouth or a mouth-like part.

osche- (oscheo-) *prefix denoting* the scrotum. Example: *oscheocele* (a scrotal hernia).

oscilloscope *n.* a cathode-ray tube designed to display electronically a wave form corresponding to the electrical data fed into it. Oscilloscopes are used to provide a continuous record of many different measurements, such as the activity of the heart and brain. *See* electrocardiography, electroencephalography.

osculum *n.* (in anatomy) a small aperture.

-osis *suffix denoting* **1.** a diseased condition. Examples: *nephrosis* (of the kidney); *leptospirosis* (caused by *Leptospira* species). **2.** any condition. Example: *narcosis* (of stupor). **3.** an increase or excess. Example: *leucocytosis* (of leucocytes).

osm- (osmo-) *prefix denoting* **1.** smell or odour. **2.** osmosis or osmotic pressure.

osmic acid *see* osmium tetroxide.

osmiophilic *adj.* describing a tissue that stains readily with osmium tetroxide.

osmium tetroxide (osmic acid) a colourless or faintly yellowish compound used to stain fats or as a *fixative in the preparation of tissues for microscopical study. Osmium tetroxide evaporates readily, the vapour having a toxic action on the eyes, skin, and respiratory tract.

osmole *n.* a unit of osmotic pressure equal to the molecular weight of a solute in grams divided by the number of ions or other particles into which it dissociates in solution.

osmoreceptor *n.* a group of cells in the *hypothalamus that monitor blood concentration. Should this increase abnormally, as in dehydration, the osmoreceptors send nerve impulses to the hypothalamus, which then increases the rate of release of *vasopressin from the posterior pituitary gland. Loss of water from the body in the urine is thus restricted until the blood concentration returns to normal.

osmosis *n.* the passage of a solvent from a less concentrated to a more concentrated solution through a *semipermeable membrane. This tends to equalize the concentrations of the two solutions. In living organisms the solvent is water and cell membranes function as semipermeable membranes, and the process of osmosis plays an impor-

tant role in controlling the distribution of water. The *osmotic pressure* of a solution is the pressure by which water is drawn into it through the semipermeable membrane; the more concentrated the solution (i.e. the more solute molecules it contains), the greater its osmotic pressure. —**osmotic** *adj.*

osseous *adj.* bony: applied to the bony parts of the inner ear (cochlea, semicircular canals, labyrinth).

ossicle *n.* a small bone. The *auditory ossicles* are three small bones (the incus, malleus, and stapes) in the middle *ear. They transmit sound from the outer ear to the labyrinth (inner ear).

ossification (osteogenesis) *n.* the formation of *bone, which takes place in three stages by the action of special cells (osteoblasts). A meshwork of collagen fibres is deposited in connective tissue, followed by the production of a cementing polysaccharide. Finally the cement is impregnated with minute crystals of calcium salts. The osteoblasts become enclosed within the matrix as *osteocytes* (*bone cells*). In *intracartilaginous* (or *endochondral*) *ossification* the bone replaces cartilage. This process starts to occur soon after the end of the second month of embryonic life. *Intramembranous ossification* is the formation of a *membrane bone (e.g. a bone of the skull). This starts in the early embryo and is not complete at birth (*see* fontanelle).

ost- (oste-, osteo-) *prefix denoting* bone. Examples: *ostalgia* (pain in); *osteocarcinoma* (carcinoma of); *osteonecrosis* (death of); *osteoplasty* (plastic surgery of).

ostectomy *n.* the surgical removal of a bone or a piece of bone. *See also* osteotomy.

osteitis *n.* inflammation of bone, due to infection, damage, or metabolic disorder. *Osteitis fibrosa cystica* refers to the characteristic cystic changes that occur in bones during long-standing *hyperparathyroidism. *See also* Paget's disease (of bone) (osteitis deformans).

osteo- *prefix. see* ost-.

osteoarthritis (osteoarthrosis) *n.* a disease of joint cartilage, associated with secondary changes in the underlying bone, which may ultimately cause pain and impair the function of the affected joint (usually the hip, knee, and thumb joints). The condition may result from overuse and is most common in those past middle life; it may also complicate many other diseases involving joints, such as *rheumatoid arthritis (*secondary osteoarthritis*). Osteoarthritis is recognized on X-ray by narrowing of the joint space (due to loss of cartilage) and the presence of *osteophytes and irregularity at the bone margins. Treatment consists of aspirin and other analgesics, reduction of pressure across the joint (by weight loss and the use of a walking stick in osteoarthritis of the hip), and corrective and prosthetic surgery.

osteoarthropathy *n.* any disease of the bone and cartilage adjoining a joint. *Hypertrophic osteoarthropathy* is characterized by the formation of new bony tissue and occurs as a complication of chronic diseases of the chest, including pulmonary abscess, mesothelioma, and lung cancer.

osteoarthrosis *n. see* osteoarthritis.

osteoarthrotomy *n.* surgical excision of the bone adjoining a joint.

osteoblast *n.* a cell, originating in the mesoderm of the embryo, that is responsible for the formation of *bone. *See also* ossification.

osteochondritis *n.* inflammation of a bone associated with pain: the deposition of abnormal bony tissue seen on X-ray (*see* osteosclerosis). The cause is not known and the condition is frequently self-limiting, though permanent deformity of the affected bone may result. Treatment is with analgesics. *See also* Köhler's disease, Legg-Calvé-Perthes disease.

This condition was formerly known as *osteochondrosis.*

osteochondritis dissecans release of a small fragment (or fragments) of bone and cartilage into a joint, most frequently the knee, with resulting pain, swelling, and limitation of movement. If the condition persists, or relapses frequently, *arthrotomy, followed by extraction of the bone fragments, may be required.

osteochondroma *n.* (*pl.* **osteochondromata**) a bone tumour composed of cartilage-forming cells. It appears as a painless mass, usually at the end of a long bone, and is most common between the ages of 10 and 25. As a small proportion of these tumours become malignant if untreated, they are excised.

osteochondrosis *n. see* osteochondritis.

osteoclasia (osteoclasis) *n.* **1.** the deliberate breaking of a malformed or malunited bone, carried out by a surgeon to correct deformity. Also called: **osteoclasty. 2.** dissolution of bone through disease (*see* osteolysis).

osteoclasis *n.* **1.** remodelling of bone by *osteoclasts, during growth or the healing of a fracture. **2.** *see* osteoclasia.

osteoclast *n.* **1.** a large multinucleate cell that resorbs calcified bone. Osteoclasts are only found when bone is being resorbed and may be seen in small depressions on the bone surface. **2.** a device for fracturing bone for therapeutic purposes.

osteoclastoma *n.* a rare tumour of bone, caused by proliferation of *osteoclast cells.

osteocyte *n.* a bone cell: an *osteoblast that has ceased activity and has become embedded in the bone matrix.

osteodystrophy *n.* any generalized bone disease resulting from a metabolic disorder. *Renal osteodystrophy* is the characteristic change in bones occurring in chronic kidney failure.

osteogenesis *n. see* ossification.

osteogenesis imperfecta (fragilitas ossium) a congenital disorder in which the bones are unusually brittle and fragile. No treatment is available, but the tendency to fracture sometimes diminishes at adolescence.

osteology *n.* the study of the structure and function of bones and related structures.

osteolysis (osteoclasia) *n.* dissolution of bone through disease, commonly by infection or loss of the blood supply (ischaemia) to the bone. In *acro-osteolysis* the terminal bones of the fingers or toes are affected: a common feature of some disorders involving blood vessels (including *Raynaud's disease), *scleroderma, and systemic *lupus erythematosus.

osteoma *n.* a benign bone tumour. A *cancellous osteoma* (*exostosis*) is an outgrowth from the end of a long bone, usually rising to a point. A *compact osteoma* (*ivory tumour*) is usually harmless but may rarely compress surrounding structures, as within the skull. An *osteoid osteoma* is an overgrowth of bone-forming cells, usually causing pain in the middle of a long bone. Compact and osteoid osteomas are treated by surgical excision.

osteomalacia *n.* softening of the bones caused by a deficiency of *vitamin D, either from a poor diet or lack of sunshine or both. It is the adult counterpart of *rickets. Vitamin D is necessary for the uptake of calcium from food; the deficiency therefore leads to progressive decalcification of bony tissues, often causing bone pain. The condition may become irreversible if treatment with vitamin D is not given. Osteomalacia is most common in the Middle and Far East, particularly in women of child-bearing age in whom calcium is lost from the skeleton during pregnancy.

osteomyelitis *n.* inflammation of the bone marrow due to infection. This is a hazard following compound fractures and must be rigorously guarded against whenever the marrow is exposed during bone or joint surgery. It may also be caused by blood-borne microorganisms. In *acute osteomyelitis*, most common in children, there is severe pain, swelling, and redness at the site, often in the shaft of a long bone, accompanied by general illness and high fever. *Chronic osteomyelitis* may follow the acute form or develop insidiously; tuberculosis and syphilis are occasional causes. Both forms are treated by antibiotics in high dosage, and in some cases drainage by surgery may be necessary. Delay in eradicating the infection may lead to bone shortening and deformity.

osteopathy *n.* a system of healing based on the theory that most diseases are caused by displacement of bones from their correct positions. Treatment, by manipulation and massage, provides relief for many disorders of bones and joints. —**osteopath** *n.* —**osteopathic** *adj.*

osteopetrosis (Albers-Schönberg disease, marble-bone disease) *n.* a congenital abnormality in which bones become abnormally dense and brittle and tend to fracture. Affected bones appear unusually opaque to X-rays. *See also* osteosclerosis.

osteophyte *n.* a projection of bone, usually shaped like a rose thorn, that occurs at sites of cartilage degeneration or destruction near joints and intervertebral discs. Osteophyte formation is an X-ray sign of *osteoarthritis but is not a cause of symptoms in itself.

osteoporosis *n.* loss of bony tissue, resulting in bones that are brittle and liable to fracture. Infection, injury, and *synovitis can cause localized osteoporosis of adjacent bone. Generalized osteoporosis is common in the elderly, and in women often follows the menopause. It is also a feature of *Cushing's disease and prolonged steroid therapy. The condition may be prevented by oestrogen therapy in the menopause (this use of oestrogens is controversial).

osteosarcoma *n.* a malignant bone tumour. It is usually seen in children and adolescents but can occur in adults of all ages, often in association with *Paget's disease of bone. Osteosarcomas can also occur in soft tissue in elderly patients. In children the usual site for the tumour is the leg, particularly the femur. Secondary growths (metastases) are common, most frequently in the lungs (though other sites, such as the liver, may also be involved). The symptoms are usually pain and swelling at the site of the tumour and there is often a history of preceding trauma, although it is doubtful whether this contributes to the cause. Treatment of disease localized to the primary site is by amputation of the limb. Many centres also give postoperative drug therapy in an attempt to kill any residual microscopic tumour that might have already spread. Drugs used include doxorubicin, vincristine, cyclophosphamide, and methotrexate.

osteosclerosis *n.* an abnormal increase in the density of bone, as a result of poor blood supply, chronic infection, or tumour. The affected bone is more opaque to X-rays than normal bone. *See also* osteopetrosis.

osteotome *n.* a surgical chisel designed to cut bone (see illustration).

An osteotome

osteotomy *n.* a surgical operation to cut a bone into two parts, followed by realignment of the ends to allow healing. The operation is performed to reduce pain and disability in an arthritic joint, for cases in which conservative treatment has failed. Osteotomy of the jaws is performed to improve severe discrepancies in jaw relation.

ostium *n.* (*pl.* **ostia**) (in anatomy) an opening. The *ostium abdominale* is the opening of the Fallopian tube into the abdominal cavity.

-ostomy *suffix. see* -stomy.

ot- (oto-) *prefix denoting* the ear. Example: *ototomy* (surgical incision of).

otalgia *n.* pain in the ear. Apart from local causes it may be due to a lesion of the geniculate ganglion of the facial nerve (*geniculate otalgia*) or to *herpes zoster affecting the facial nerve (Ramsay Hunt syndrome).

otic *adj.* relating to the ear.

otic capsule the cup-shaped cartilage in the head of an embryo that later develops into the bony *labyrinth of the ear.

otitis *n.* inflammation of the ear. *Otitis externa* is inflammation of the canal between the eardrum and the external opening of the ear (the external auditory meatus) and is often found in swimmers (*swimmer's ear*). *Otitis media* is inflammation, usually due to viral or bacterial infection, of the middle ear (the chamber lying behind the eardrum and containing the three bony ossicles that conduct sound to the inner ear). Symptoms include severe pain and a high fever; unless treated (with antibiotics), it may lead to conductive *deafness. *Secretory otitis media* (glue ear) is a chronic accumulation of fluid in the tympanic cavity, causing deafness (*see* grommet). *Otitis interna* (*labyrinthitis*) is inflammation of the inner ear, causing the sudden onset of vomiting, vertigo, and loss of balance.

otoconium *n. see* otolith.

otocyst *n.* a small cavity in the mesoderm of the head of an embryo that later develops into the membranous *labyrinth of the ear.

otolaryngology *n.* the study of diseases of the ears and larynx.

otolith (otoconium) *n.* one of the small particles of calcium carbonate associated with a macula in the *saccule or *utricle of the inner ear.

otology *n.* the study of diseases of the ear.

-otomy *suffix. see* -tomy.

otomycosis *n.* a fungus infection of the ear, causing irritation and inflammation of the canal between the eardrum and the external opening of the ear (external auditory meatus). It is one of the causes of *otitis externa.

otoplasty *n.* surgical repair or reconstruction of the ears after injury or in the correction of a congenital defect (such as 'bat ears').

otorhinolaryngology *n.* the study of ear, nose, and throat diseases (i.e. ENT disorders).

otorrhagia *n.* bleeding from the ear.

otorrhoea *n.* any discharge from the ear, commonly a purulent discharge in chronic middle ear infection (*otitis media).

otosclerosis *n.* a hereditary disorder causing deafness in adult life. An overgrowth of the bone of the inner ear leads to the third ear ossicle (the stapes) becoming fixed to the fenestra ovalis, which separates the middle and inner ears, so that sounds cannot be con-

ducted to the inner ear. *Deafness is progressive and may become very severe, but surgical treatment is highly effective (*see* fenestration, stapedectomy).

otoscope *n. see* auriscope.

ouabain *n.* a drug that stimulates the heart and is used to treat heart failure and other heart conditions. It is administered by mouth or injection and has the same actions and side-effects as *digitalis.

outbreeding *n.* the production of offspring by parents who are not closely related. *Compare* inbreeding.

outer ear the pinna and the external auditory meatus of the *ear.

out-patient *n.* a patient who receives treatment at a hospital, either at a single attendance or at a series of attendances, but is not admitted to a bed in a hospital ward. Large hospitals have *clinics at which out-patients with various complaints can be given specialist treatment. *Compare* in-patient.

oval window *see* fenestra (ovalis).

ovari- (ovario-) *prefix denoting* the ovary.

ovarian cyst a fluid-filled sac, one or more of which may develop in the ovary. Although most ovarian cysts are not malignant, they may reach a very large size or become twisted on their stalks, producing pain and vomiting. In such cases the cysts are usually surgically removed.

ovariectomy *n. see* oophorectomy.

ovariocele *n.* hernia of an ovary.

ovariocyesis *n. see* oocyesis.

ovariotomy *n.* **1.** incision into or surgical removal of an ovary. **2.** surgical removal of a tumour of the ovary.

ovaritis *n. see* oophoritis.

ovary *n.* the main female reproductive organ, which produces ova (egg cells) and steroid hormones in a regular cycle (*see* menstrual cycle) in response to hormones (*gonadotrophins) from the anterior pituitary gland. There are two ovaries, situated in the lower abdomen, one on each side of the womb (*see* reproductive system). Each ovary contains numerous *follicles*, within which the ova develop (see illustration), but only a small proportion of them reach maturity (*see* Graafian follicle, oogenesis). The follicles secrete *oestrogen and small amounts of androgen. After ovulation a *corpus luteum forms at the site of the ruptured follicle and secretes progesterone. Oestrogen and progesterone regulate the changes in the womb throughout the menstrual cycle and pregnancy. —**ovarian** *adj.*

germinal epithelium
developing primary follicle
corpus albicans
maturing follicle
mature Graafian follicle
ovum
released ovum
ruptured follicle
young corpus luteum
connective tissue
fully formed corpus luteum
degenerating follicle

Section of the ovary showing ova in various stages of maturation

overbite *n.* the vertical overlap of the upper incisor teeth over the lower ones.

overcompensation *n.* (in psychology) the situation in which a person tries to overcome a disability by making greater efforts than are required. This may result in the person becoming extremely efficient in what he (or she) is trying to achieve; alternatively, excessive overcompensation may be harmful to the person.

overjet *n.* the horizontal overlap of the upper incisor teeth in front of the lower ones.

overt *adj.* plainly to be seen or detected: applied to diseases with observable signs and symptoms, as opposed to those whose presence may not be suspected for years despite the fact that they cause insidious damage. An infectious disease becomes overt only at the end of an incubation period.

ovi- (ovo-) *prefix denoting* an egg; ovum.

oviduct *n. see* Fallopian tube.

ovulation *n.* the process by which an ovum is released from a mature *Graafian follicle. The fluid-filled follicle distends the surface of the ovary until a thin spot breaks down and the ovum floats out surrounded by a cluster of follicle cells (the cumulus oophoricus) and starts to travel down the Fallopian tube to the womb. Ovulation is stimulated by the secretion of *luteinizing hormone by the anterior pituitary gland.

ovum (egg cell, vitellus) *n.* the mature female sex cell (*see* gamete). The term is often applied to the secondary *oocyte although this is technically incorrect. The final stage of meiosis occurs only when the oocyte has been activated by fertilization.

oxacillin *n.* an antibiotic used to treat infections caused by a wide variety of bacteria. It is administered by mouth or injection; side-effects include allergic reactions and digestive upsets.

oxalic acid an extremely poisonous acid, $C_2H_2O_4$. It is a component of some bleaching powders and is found in many plants, including sorrel and the

perivitelline space

centrosome with two centrioles

nucleus

corona radiata

zona pellucida

ooplasm

A mature ovum (magnification about x 600)

leaves of rhubarb. Oxalic acid is a powerful local irritant; when swallowed it produces burning sensations in the mouth and throat, vomiting of blood, breathing difficulties, and circulatory collapse. Treatment is with calcium lactate or other calcium salts, lime water, or milk.

oxalosis *n.* an inborn defect of metabolism causing deposition of oxalate in the kidneys and elsewhere and eventually leading to renal failure.

oxaluria *n.* the presence in the urine of oxalic acid or oxalates, especially calcium oxalate. Excessive amounts of oxalates are excreted in *oxalosis.

oxazepam *n.* a tranquillizing drug used to relieve anxiety and tension and for the treatment of alcoholism. It is administered by mouth and commonly causes drowsiness. Trade name: **Serenid**. *See also* tranquillizer.

oxethazaine *n.* a local anaesthetic of skin and mucous membranes, used in indigestion mixtures to relieve heartburn and pain due to inflammation of the digestive system. Mild side-effects, including dry mouth and nausea, may occur.

oxidase *n. see* oxidoreductase.

oxidoreductase *n.* one of a group of enzymes that catalyse oxidation-reduction reactions. This class includes the enzymes formerly known either as *dehydrogenases* or as *oxidases*.

oximeter *n.* an instrument for measuring the proportion of oxygenated haemoglobin (oxyhaemoglobin) in the blood.

oxolinic acid an antibacterial drug used to treat infections of the urinary system. It is administered by mouth; side-effects may include digestive upsets and disturbances of vision. Trade name: **Prodoxol**.

oxprenolol *n.* a drug that controls the activity of the heart (*see* beta blocker), used to treat angina, high blood pressure, and abnormal heart rhythm. It is administered by mouth or injection; side-effects may include dizziness, drowsiness, headache, and digestive upsets. Trade name: **Trasicor**.

oxycephaly (turricephaly) *n.* a deformity of the bones of the skull giving the head a pointed appearance. —**oxycephalic** *adj.*

oxygen *n.* an odourless colourless gas that makes up one-fifth of the atmosphere. Oxygen is essential to most forms of life in that it combines chemically with glucose (or some other fuel) to provide energy for metabolic processes. In man oxygen is absorbed into the blood from air breathed into the lungs. Oxygen is administered therapeutically in various conditions in which the tissues are unable to obtain an adequate supply through the lungs (*see* oxygenator, (oxygen) tent). Symbol: O.

oxygenator *n.* a machine that oxygenates blood outside the body. It is used together with pumps to maintain the patient's circulation while he is undergoing open heart surgery (*see* heart-lung machine) or to improve the circulation of a patient with heart or lung disorders that lower the amount of blood oxygen.

oxygen deficit a physiological condition that exists in cells during periods of temporary oxygen shortage. During periods of violent exertion the body requires extra energy, which is obtained by the breakdown of glucose in the absence of oxygen, after the available oxygen has been used up. The breakdown products are acidic and cause muscle pain. The oxygen required to get rid of the breakdown products (called the oxygen deficit) must be made available after the exertion stops.

oxygen tent see tent.

oxyhaemoglobin n. the bright-red substance formed when the pigment *haemoglobin in red blood cells combines reversibly with oxygen. Oxyhaemoglobin is the form in which oxygen is transported from the lungs to the tissues, where the oxygen is released. Compare methaemoglobin.

oxymesterone n. a synthetic male sex hormone with body-building action. It has the same action and uses as *methandienone.

oxyntic cells (parietal cells) cells of the *gastric glands that secrete hydrochloric acid in the fundic region of the stomach.

oxypertine n. a major *tranquillizer used to treat anxiety and tension in mental illnesses such as schizophrenia. It is administered by mouth and commonly causes drowsiness, dizziness, and restlessness, especially in high doses. Trade name: **Integrin**.

oxyphenbutazone n. an *analgesic that also reduces inflammation and fever. It is used mainly to relieve pain in rheumatoid arthritis, gout, and similar conditions. It is administered by mouth or in suppositories; common side-effects include nausea, rashes, dizziness, and mouth ulcers. Trade name: **Tanderil**.

oxyphencyclimine n. a drug with actions similar to *atropine. Since it slows down the digestive processes, it is used to treat stomach and duodenal ulcers and other digestive disorders. It is administered by mouth; side-effects include dry mouth, thirst, and disturbances of vision. Trade name: **Daricon**.

oxytetracycline n. an *antibiotic used to treat infections caused by a wide variety of bacteria. It is administered by mouth or injection or applied to the skin in a cream; side-effects are those of the other *tetracyclines. Trade names: **Abbocin, Berkmycen, Clinimycin, Galenomycin, Imperacin, Oxydon, Oxymycin, Stecsolin, Terramycin, Unimycin**.

oxytocia n. labour and childbirth of exceptionally short duration.

oxytocic n. a drug that induces or accelerates labour by stimulating the muscles of the womb to contract. See also oxytocin.

oxytocin n. a hormone, released by the pituitary gland, that causes increased contraction of the womb during labour and stimulates the ejection of milk from the breasts. Oxytocin may be given by mouth or injection to assist labour.

oxyuriasis n. see enterobiasis.

Oxyuris n. see pinworm.

ozaena n. a disorder of the nose in which the bones forming the sides of the nasal cavity become atrophied, with the production of an offensive discharge and crusts.

ozone n. a poisonous gas containing three oxygen atoms per molecule. Ozone is a very powerful oxidizing agent and is formed when oxygen or air is subjected to electric discharge. Ozone is found in the atmosphere at very high altitudes and is responsible for destroying a large proportion of the sun's ultraviolet radiation. Without this absorption by ozone the earth would be subjected to a lethal amount of ultra-violet radiation.

P

Pacchionian body *see* arachnoid villus.

pacemaker *n.* **1.** a device used to produce and maintain a normal heart rate in patients who have *heart block. The unit consists of a battery that stimulates the heart through an insulated electrode wire attached to the surface of the ventricle (*epicardial pacemaker*) or lying in contact with the lining of the heart (*endocardial pacemaker*). A pacemaker may be used as a temporary measure with an external battery or it may be permanent, when the whole apparatus is surgically implanted under the skin. Some pacemakers stimulate the heart at a fixed rate; others sense when the natural heart rate falls below a predetermined value and then stimulate the heart (*demand pacemaker*). **2.** the part of the heart that regulates the rate at which it beats: the *sinoatrial node.

pachy- *prefix denoting* **1.** thickening of a part or parts. **2.** the dura mater.

pachydactyly *n.* abnormal enlargement of the fingers and toes, occurring either as a congenital abnormality or as part of an acquired disease (such as *acromegaly).

pachydermia *n.* any abnormal thickening of the skin.

pachyglossia *n.* abnormal thickness of the tongue.

pachymeningitis *n.* inflammation of the dura mater, one of the membranes (meninges) covering the brain and spinal cord (*see* meningitis).

pachymeninx *n.* the *dura mater, outermost of the three meninges.

pachyonychia *n.* thickening of the nails. Rarely, this may occur as an inherited disease.

pachysomia *n.* thickening of parts of the body, which occurs in certain diseases.

pachytene *n.* the third stage of the first prophase of *meiosis, in which *crossing over begins.

Pacinian corpuscles sensory receptors for touch in the skin, consisting of sensory nerve endings surrounded by capsules of membrane in 'onion-skin' layers. They are especially sensitive to changes in pressure and so detect vibration particularly well.

pack *n.* a pad of folded moistened material, such as cotton-wool, applied to the body or inserted into a cavity.

packed cell volume (haematocrit) the volume of the red cells (erythrocytes) in blood, expressed as a fraction of the total volume of the blood. The packed cell volume is determined by centrifuging blood in a tube and measuring the height of the red-cell column as a fraction of the total.

pad *n.* cotton-wool, foam rubber, or other material used to protect a part of the body from friction, bruising, or other unwanted contact.

paed- (paedo-) *prefix denoting* children.

paederasty *n.* *sodomy with a boy or a young man.

paediatrics *n.* the general medicine of childhood. Handling the sick child requires a special approach at every age from birth (or premature birth) to adolescence and also a proper understanding of parents. It also requires detailed knowledge of genetics, obstetrics, psychological development, management of handicaps at home and in school, and effects of social conditions on child health. The preventive measures associated with all these aspects of paediatrics are the concern of *community physicians (child health) of area health authorities or community paediatricians (hospital-based *consultants). *See also* child health clinic. —**paediatrician** *n*.

paedodontics *n*. the branch of dentistry concerned with the care and treatment of children's teeth.

paedophilia *n*. sexual attraction to children (of either sex). Sexual activity with any children under the age of 16 is illegal in the UK. The condition is usually caused by psychological and social factors, which affect the development of sexuality. Paedophiles may seek treatment because of society's disapproval: *behaviour therapy can be used, or the sexual drive can be reduced by drug treatment. —**paedophile** *n*. —**paedophilic** *adj*.

Paget's disease 1. a chronic disease of bones, occurring in the elderly and most frequently affecting the skull, backbone, pelvis, and long bones. Affected bones become thickened and their structure disorganized: X-rays reveal patchy *sclerosis. Severe continuous pain may result, which is relieved by a prolonged course of *thyrocalcitonin injections. Medical name: **osteitis deformans. 2.** an inflammatory condition of the nipple, resembling eczema in appearance, associated with underlying cancer of the milk ducts of the breast. *See also* breast cancer.

paint *n*. (in pharmacy) a liquid preparation that is applied to the skin or mucous membranes. Paints usually contain antiseptics, astringents, caustics, or analgesics.

palaeo- *prefix denoting* **1.** ancient. **2.** primitive.

palaeocerebellum *n*. the anterior lobe of the cerebellum. In evolutionary

terms it is one of the earliest parts of the hindbrain to develop in mammals.

palaeopathology *n*. the study of the diseases of man and other animals in prehistoric times, from examination of their bones or other remains. By examining the bones of specimens of Neanderthal man it has been discovered that spinal arthritis was a disease that existed at least 50,000 years ago.

palaeostriatum *n*. *see* pallidum.

palaeothalamus *n*. the anterior and central part of the *thalamus, older in evolutionary terms than the lateral part, the neothalamus, which is well developed in apes and man.

palate *n*. the roof of the mouth, which separates the mouth from the nasal cavity and consists of two portions. The *hard palate*, at the front of the mouth, is formed by processes of the maxillae and palatine bones and is covered by mucous membrane. The *soft palate*, further back, is a movable fold of mucous membrane that tapers to the back of the mouth to form a fleshy hanging flap of tissue – the *uvula*.

palatine bone either of a pair of approximately L-shaped bones of the face that contribute to the hard *palate, the nasal cavity, and the orbits. *See* skull.

palato- *prefix denoting* **1.** the palate. **2.** the palatine bone.

palatoplasty *n*. plastic surgery of the roof of the mouth, usually to correct cleft palate or other defects present at birth.

palatorrhaphy *n*. *see* staphylorrhaphy.

pali- (palin-) *prefix denoting* repetition or recurrence.

palilalia *n*. a disorder of speech in which a word spoken by the individual is rapidly and involuntarily repeated. It is seen, with other tics, in the *Gilles de la Tourette syndrome. It is also encountered when encephalitis or other processes damage the *extrapyramidal system of the brain.

palindromic *adj.* relapsing: describing diseases or symptoms that recur or get worse.

palingraphia *n.* writing in which the words and letters are reversed so that they appear as mirror images. Adoption of this as a consistent style is usually a matter of voluntary choice or is *hysterical; very occasionally it follows brain damage. Mirror-image reversals of single letters are common in children learning to write and in older children whose language abilities are impaired.

paliphrasia *n.* repetition of phrases while speaking: a form of *stammering or a kind of *tic.

palliative *n.* a medicine that gives temporary relief from the symptoms of a disease but does not actually cure the disease. Palliatives are often used in the treatment of such diseases as cancer.

pallidectomy *n.* a neurosurgical operation to destroy or modify the effects of the globus pallidus (*see* basal ganglia). This operation was used for the relief of *parkinsonism and other conditions in which involuntary movements are prominent.

pallidum (palaeostriatum) *n.* one of the dense collections of grey matter, deep in each cerebral hemisphere, that go to make up the *basal ganglia.

pallium *n.* the outer wall of the cerebral hemisphere as it appears in the early stages of evolution of the mammalian brain. In the modern brain it corresponds to the *cerebral cortex.

pallor *n.* abnormal paleness of the skin, due to reduced blood flow or lack of normal pigments. Pallor may be associated with an indoor mode of life; it may also indicate shock, anaemia, cancer, or other diseases.

palmitic acid *see* fatty acid.

palpation *n.* the process of examining part of the body by careful feeling with the hands and fingertips. Using palpation it is possible, in many cases, to distinguish between swellings that are solid and those that are cystic (*see* fluctuation). Palpation is also used to discover the presence of a fetus in the womb (*see* ballottement).

palpebral *adj.* relating to the eyelid (palpebra).

palpitation *n.* an awareness of the heart beat. This is normal with fear, emotion, or exertion. It may also be a symptom of neurosis, arrhythmias, heart disease, and overactivity of the circulation (as in thyrotoxicosis).

palsy *n.* paralysis. This archaic word is retained in compound terms, such as *Bell's palsy, *cerebral palsy, and *Todd's palsy.

paludism *n. see* malaria.

pan- (pant(o)-) *prefix denoting* all; every: hence (in medicine) affecting all parts of an organ or the body; generalized.

panacea *n.* a medicine said to be a cure for all diseases and disorders, no matter what their nature. Unfortunately panaceas do not exist, despite the claims of many patent medicine manufacturers.

Panadol *n. see* paracetamol.

pancarditis *n. see* endomyocarditis.

pancreas *n.* a compound gland, about 15 cm long, that lies behind the stomach. One end lies in the curve of the duodenum; the other end touches the spleen. It is composed of clusters (*acini*) of cells that secrete *pancreatic juice. This contains a number of enzymes concerned in digestion. The juice drains into small ducts that open into the *pancreatic duct*. This unites with the common *bile duct and the secretions pass into the duodenum. Interspersed among the acini are the *islets of Langerhans – isolated groups of cells that secrete the hormones *insulin and *glucagon into the bloodstream.

pancreas divisum a congenital abnormality in which the pancreas develops in two parts draining separately into the duodenum, the small ventral pancreas through the main ampulla and the larger dorsal pancreas through an accessory papilla. In rare instances this is associated with recurrent abdominal pain, probably due to inadequate drainage of the dorsal pancreas. Diagnosis is made by *ERCP.

pancreatectomy *n.* surgical removal of the pancreas. *Total pancreatectomy* (*Whipple's operation*) involves the entire gland and part of the duodenum. In *subtotal pancreatectomy* most of the gland is removed, usually leaving a small part close to the duodenum. In *partial pancreatectomy* only a portion of the gland is removed. The operations are performed for tumours in the gland or because of chronic or relapsing *pancreatitis. After total or subtotal pancreatectomy it is necessary to administer pancreatic enzymes with food to aid its digestion and insulin injections to replace that normally secreted by the gland.

pancreatic juice the digestive juice secreted by the *pancreas. Its production is stimulated by hormones secreted by the duodenum, which in turn is stimulated by contact with food from the stomach. If the duodenum produces the hormone *secretin the pancreatic juice contains a large amount of sodium bicarbonate, which neutralizes the acidity of the stomach contents. Another hormone (*see* cholecystokinin-pancreozymin) causes the production of a juice rich in digestive enzymes, including trypsinogen and chymotrypsinogen (which are converted to *trypsin and *chymotrypsin in the duo-

denum), *amylase, *lipase, and *maltase.

pancreatin *n.* an extract obtained from the *pancreas, containing the pancreatic enzymes. Pancreatin is administered for conditions in which pancreatic secretion is deficient; for example, in pancreatitis.

pancreatitis *n.* inflammation of the pancreas. *Acute pancreatitis* is a sudden illness in which the patient experiences severe pain in upper abdomen and back, with shock; its cause is uncertain. It may be mistaken for a perforated peptic ulcer but differs from this condition in that the level of the enzyme *amylase in the blood is raised. The main complication is formation of a *pseudocyst. Treatment consists of intravenous feeding (no food or drink should be given by mouth), and *anticholinergic drugs. *Relapsing pancreatitis*, in which the above symptoms are recurrent and less severe, may be associated with gallstones or alcoholism; prevention is by removal of gallstones and avoidance of alcohol and fat. *Chronic pancreatitis* may produce symptoms similar to relapsing pancreatitis or may be painless; it leads to pancreatic failure causing *malabsorption and *diabetes mellitus. The pancreas often becomes calcified, producing visible shadowing on X-rays. The malabsorption is treated by a low-fat diet with pancreatic enzyme supplements, and the diabetes with insulin.

pancreatogram *n.* a radiographic image of the pancreatic ducts obtained by injecting a contrast medium into them by direct puncture under *ultrasound guidance, at the time of laparotomy or by *ERCP.

pancreatotomy *n.* surgical opening of the duct of the pancreas in order to inspect the duct, to join the duct to the intestine, or to inject contrast material in order to obtain X-ray pictures of the duct system.

pancreozymin *n. see* cholecystokinin-pancreozymin.

pancytopenia *n.* a simultaneous decrease in the numbers of red cells (*anaemia), white cells (*neutropenia), and platelets (*thrombocytopenia) in the blood. It occurs in a variety of disorders, including aplastic *anaemias, *hypersplenism, and tumours of the bone marrow.

pandemic *n.* an *epidemic so widely spread that vast numbers of people in different countries are affected. The Black Death, the epidemic plague that ravaged Europe in the fourteenth century and killed over one third of the population, was a classical pandemic. —**pandemic** *adj.*

panhysterectomy *n.* the surgical removal of the entire womb, including its neck (cervix). *See* hysterectomy.

panhysterocolpectomy *n.* surgical removal of the entire womb and the vagina.

panhystero-oophorectomy *n.* surgical removal of the entire womb and of one or both ovaries.

panhysterosalpingo-oophorectomy *n.* surgical removal of the entire womb, the ovaries, and the *Fallopian tubes.

panmixis *n.* random mating within a population, i.e. when there is no selection of partners on religious, racial, social, or other grounds.

panniculitis *n.* inflammation of the layer of fat beneath the skin (*panniculus adiposus*), leading to multiple tender nodules in the thighs, trunk, and breasts. When there are other features, including fever and enlargement of the liver and spleen, the condition is known as the *Weber-Christian disease*.

panniculus *n.* a membranous sheet of tissue. For example, the *panniculus adiposus* is the fatty layer of tissue underlying the skin.

pannus *n.* invasion of the outer layers of the cornea of the eye by tissue containing many blood vessels, which grows in from the conjunctiva. It is seen as a response to inflammation of the cornea or conjunctiva, particularly in *trachoma.

panophthalmitis *n.* inflammation involving the whole of the interior of the eye.

Panstrongylus *n.* a genus of large bloodsucking bugs (*see* reduviid). *P. megistus* is important in transmitting *Chagas' disease to man in Brazil.

pant- (panto-) *prefix. see* pan-.

pantothenic acid a B vitamin that is a constituent of *coenzyme A. It plays an important role in the transfer of acetyl groups in the body. Pantothenic acid is widely distributed in food and a deficiency is therefore unlikely to occur.

pantropic *adj.* describing a virus that can invade and affect many different tissues of the body, for example the nerves, skin, or liver, without showing a special affinity for any one of them.

papain *n.* a preparation that contains one or more protein-digesting enzymes. It is obtained from the pawpaw fruit and is used as a digestant.

Papanicolaou test (Pap test) a test to detect cancer of the neck (cervix) or lining (endometrium) of the womb. A specimen of tissue taken from the womb is stained and examined under the microscope for the presence of abnormal cells.

papaverine *n.* an alkaloid, derived from opium, that relaxes smooth muscle. It is administered by mouth or injection to treat muscle spasm in such conditions as colic and in sprays for the relief of asthma. It may cause abnormal heart rate.

papilla *n.* (*pl.* **papillae**) any small nipple-shaped protuberance. Several different kinds of papillae occur on the *tongue, in association with the taste buds. The *optic papilla* is an alternative name for the *optic disc.

papillitis *n.* inflammation of the first part of the optic nerve (the optic disc or optic papilla), i.e. where the nerve leaves the eyeball.

papilloedema *n.* swelling of the first part of the optic nerve (the optic disc or optic papilla).

papilloma *n.* a benign growth on the surface of skin or mucous membrane (for example, in the womb). Papillomas, which develop from the *epidermis, are usually in the form of a conical, flattish, or stalked protuberance, 2–5 mm in diameter. *Warts are a type of papilloma.

papillomatosis *n.* a condition in which many *papillomas grow on an area of skin or mucous membrane.

papillotomy *n.* the operation of cutting the *ampulla of Vater to widen its outlet in order to improve bile drainage and allow the passage of stones from the common bile duct. It is usually performed using a diathermy wire through a *duodenoscope following *ERCP.

papovavirus *n.* one of a group of small DNA-containing viruses producing tumours (usually malignant) in animals (subgroup *polyoma viruses*) and non-malignant tumours in animals and man (subgroup *papilloma viruses*).

Pappataci fever *see* sandfly fever.

papule *n.* a small superficial raised abnormality or spot on the skin. It usually forms part of a rash, such as appears with chickenpox.

papulo- *prefix denoting* a papule or pimple.

papulosquamous *adj.* **1.** describing a rash that is both papular and scaly. **2.** denoting a group of skin diseases that

have this characteristic, including *pityriasis rosea, seborrhoeic *dermatitis, *lichen planus, and *psoriasis.

para- *prefix denoting* **1.** beside or near. Example: *paranasal* (near the nasal cavity). **2.** resembling. Example: *paradysentery* (a mild form of dysentery). **3.** abnormal. Example: *paralalia* (abnormal speech).

para-aminobenzoic acid a naturally occurring drug used in lotions and creams to prevent sunburn. It was formerly administered by mouth to treat certain infections now treated with antibiotics. High doses may cause nausea, vomiting, itching, and rashes.

para-aminosalicylic acid (PAS) a drug, chemically related to aspirin, used – in conjunction with isoniazid or streptomycin – to treat various types of tuberculosis. It is administered by mouth and commonly causes nausea, vomiting, diarrhoea, and rashes.

paracentesis *n.* tapping: the process of drawing off excess fluid from a part of the body through a hollow needle or *cannula.

paracetamol *n.* an *analgesic drug that also reduces fever. It is used to treat mild or moderate pain, such as headache, toothache, and rheumatism. It is administered by mouth and may cause digestive upsets; overdosage causes liver damage. Trade names: **Panadol, Panasorb, Salzone.**

paracholia *n. Archaic.* disordered bile secretion.

Paracoccidioides *n.* a genus of yeast-like fungi causing infection of the skin and mucous membranes. The species *P. brasiliensis* causes a chronic skin disease, South American *blastomycosis.

paracusis *n.* any abnormality of hearing.

paradidymis *n.* the vestigial remains of part of the embryonic *mesonephros that are found near the testis of the adult. Some of the mesonephric collecting tubules persist as the functional *vasa efferentia but the rest degenerate almost completely. A similar vestigial structure (the *paroophoron*) is found in females.

paradoxical breathing breathing movements seen in patients with broken ribs: on inhalation the chest wall moves in instead of out, and vice versa on exhalation.

paraesthesiae *pl. n.* spontaneously occurring abnormal tingling sensations, sometimes described as *pins and needles.* They are symptoms of partial damage to a peripheral nerve, such as that caused by external pressure on the affected part. *Compare* dysaesthesiae.

paraffin *n.* one of a series of hydrocarbons derived from petroleum. *Paraffin wax (hard paraffin),* a whitish mixture of solid hydrocarbons melting at 45–60°C, is used in medicine mainly as a base for ointments; it is also used for *embedding specimens for microscopical study. *Liquid paraffin* is a mineral oil, which has been used as a laxative.

paraffinoma *n.* a type of tumour induced by the presence in the tissues of paraffin wax, formerly used in cosmetic surgery to increase the size of the female breasts.

paraformaldehyde *n.* a white crystalline polymer of formaldehyde, used as a disinfectant fumigant and in the treatment of certain skin disorders.

paraganglion *n.* one of the small oval masses of cells found in the walls of the ganglia of the sympathetic nervous system, near the spinal cord. They are *chromaffin cells, like those of the adrenal gland, and may secrete adrenaline.

parageusia (parageusis) *n.* abnormality of the sense of taste.

paragonimiasis (endemic haemoptysis) *n.* a tropical disease, occurring principally in the Far East, caused by the presence of the fluke *Paragonimus westermani* in the lungs. The infection is acquired by eating inadequately cooked shellfish, such as crayfish and crabs. Symptoms resemble those of chronic *bronchitis, including the coughing up of blood and difficulty in breathing (dyspnoea). Paragonimiasis is treated with the drugs bithionol and chloroquine.

Paragonimus *n.* a genus of large tropical parasitic *flukes that are particularly prevalent in the Far East. The adults of *P. westermani* live in the lungs of man, where they cause destruction and bleeding of the tissues (*see* paragonimiasis). However, they may also be found in other organs of the body. Eggs are passed out in the sputum and the larvae undergo their development in two other hosts, a snail and a crab.

paragranuloma *n.* an old term for one of the types of *Hodgkin's disease. It is now known as *lymphocyte-predominant Hodgkin's disease* and has the best prognosis of all the types.

paragraphia *n.* a disorder of writing, involving the omission or transposition of letters or of whole words. The appearance of this in adult life is usually due to damage to the brain. In childhood it usually reflects a developmental delay in learning to write correctly.

para-influenza viruses a group of large RNA-containing viruses that cause infections of the respiratory tract producing mild influenza-like symptoms. They are included in the paramyxovirus group (*see* myxovirus).

paraldehyde *n.* a *hypnotic and *anticonvulsant drug used to induce sleep in mental patients and to control convulsions in tetanus. It is administered by mouth, injection, or in suppositories;

side-effects may include digestive upsets and, in large doses, prolonged unconsciousness. *Tolerance and *dependence may result from prolonged use of the drug.

paralysis n. muscle weakness that varies in its extent, its severity, and the degree of *spasticity or flaccidity according to the nature of the underlying disease and its distribution in the brain, spinal cord, peripheral nerves, or muscles. See also diplegia, hemiplegia, paraplegia, poliomyelitis. —**paralytic** adj.

paramedian adj. situated close to or beside the *median plane.

paramedical adj. describing or relating to the professions closely linked to the medical profession and working in conjunction with them. Such professions require expert knowledge and experience in certain fields, but no medical degree. Paramedical personnel in a hospital include the nurses, radiographers, physiotherapists, and dietitians.

paramesonephric duct (Müllerian duct) either of the paired ducts that form adjacent to the *mesonephric ducts in the embryo. In the female these ducts develop into the Fallopian tubes, womb, and part of the vagina. However, in the male they degenerate almost completely.

parameter n. (in medicine) a measurement of some factor, such as blood pressure, pulse rate, or haemoglobin level, that may have a bearing on the condition being investigated.

paramethadione n. an *anticonvulsant drug used to prevent or reduce petit mal fits in epilepsy. It is administered by mouth; the commonest side-effects include drowsiness, digestive upsets, and blurred vision. Trade name: **Paradione**.

parametric test see significance.

parametritis (pelvic cellulitis) n. inflammation of the loose connective tissue and smooth muscle around the womb (the parametrium). The condition may be associated with *puerperal fever.

parametrium n. the layer of connective tissue surrounding the womb.

paramnesia n. a distorted memory, such as *confabulation or *déjà vu.

paramyoclonus multiplex a benign disorder of the nervous system that is characterized by brief irregular twitch-like contractions of the muscles of the limbs and trunk.

paramyotonia congenita a rare constitutional disorder in which prolonged contraction of muscle fibres (see myotonia) develops when the patient is exposed to cold. This may be due to a disorder of potassium metabolism.

paranasal sinuses the air-filled spaces, lined with mucous membrane, within some of the bones of the skull. They open into the nasal cavity, via the meatuses, and are named according to the bone in which they are situated. They comprise the frontal sinuses and the maxillary sinuses (one pair of each), the ethmoid sinuses (consisting of many spaces inside the ethmoid bone), and the two sphenoid sinuses. (See illustration.)

paranoia n. a mental disorder characterized by *delusions organized into a system, without hallucinations or other marked symptoms of mental illness. It is a rare chronic condition; most people with such delusions will in time develop signs of other mental illness.
The same term is sometimes used more loosely for a state of mind in which the individual has a strong belief that he is persecuted by others. His behaviour is therefore suspicious and isolated. This can be a result of *personality disorder as well as mental illnesses causing *paranoid states.

Paranasal sinuses projected to the surface

Labels: frontal, ethmoidal, sphenoidal, maxillary

paranoid *adj.* **1.** describing a mental state characterized by fixed and logically elaborated *delusions. There are many causes, including paranoid *schizophrenia, *manic-depressive psychosis, organic psychoses such as *alcoholism, *paraphrenia, and severe emotional stress. **2.** describing a personality distinguished by such traits as excessive sensitivity to rejection by others, suspiciousness, hostility, and self-importance.

paraparesis *n.* weakness of both legs, resulting from disease of the nervous system.

paraphasia *n.* a disorder of language in which unintended syllables, words, or phrases are interpolated in the patient's speech. A severe degree of paraphasia results in speech that is a meaningless jumble of words and sounds, called *jargon aphasia*.

paraphimosis *n.* retraction and constriction of the foreskin behind the glans penis. This occurs in some patients with *phimosis on erection of the penis: the tight foreskin cannot be drawn back over the glans and becomes painful and swollen. Manual replacement of the foreskin can usually be achieved under local or general anaes-

thesia, but *circumcision is required to prevent a recurrence.

paraphrenia *n.* a mental disorder characterized by systematic *delusions and prominent *hallucinations but without any other marked symptoms of mental illness. The only loss of contact with reality is in areas affected by the delusions and hallucinations. It is typically seen in the elderly and deaf. Some sufferers, if followed up over a period of years, eventually show other symptoms of *schizophrenia. It is therefore debatable whether paraphrenia constitutes a separate entity.

paraplegia *n.* *paralysis of both legs, usually due to disease or injury of the spinal cord. It is often accompanied by loss of sensation below the level of the injury and disturbed bladder function. —**paraplegic** *adj., n.*

paraprotein *n.* an abnormal protein of the *immunoglobulin series. Paraproteins appear in malignant disease of the spleen, bone marrow, liver, etc. Examples of paraproteins are *myeloma globulins, *macroglobulin, and *Bence-Jones protein.

parapsoriasis *n.* any one of a group of skin diseases (*erythrodermas) that develop slowly and are typified by chronic red scaly patches that resemble psoriasis.

parapsychology *n.* the study of *extrasensory perception, *psychokinesis, and other mental abilities that appear to defy natural law.

paraquat *n.* the chemical compound dimethyl dipyridilium, widely used as a weed-killer. When swallowed it exerts its most serious effects upon the lungs, the tissues of which it destroys after a few days. Paraquat poisoning is almost invariably fatal.

parasite *n.* any living thing that lives in (*see* endoparasite) or on (*see* ectoparasite) another living organism (*see* host). The parasite, which may spend all or only part of its existence with the host, obtains food and/or shelter from the host and contributes nothing to its welfare. Some parasites cause irritation and interfere with bodily functions; others destroy host tissues and release toxins into the body, thus injuring health and causing disease. Human parasites include fungi, bacteria, viruses, protozoa, and worms. *See also* commensal, symbiosis. —**parasitic** *adj.*

parasiticide *n.* an agent, such as *gamma benzene hexachloride, that destroys parasites (excluding bacteria and fungi). *See also* acaricide, anthelmintic, trypanocide.

parasitology *n.* the study and science of parasites.

parasternal *adj.* situated close to the sternum. The *parasternal line* is an imaginary vertical line parallel to and midway between the lateral margin of the sternum and the vertical line through the nipple.

parasuicide *n.* a self-injuring act (such as an overdose of sleeping tablets) that is not motivated by a genuine wish to die. It differs from attempted *suicide in being common in young people who are distressed but not seriously mentally ill. However, many people who have acted in this way go on to attempt, or even to achieve, suicide. Help in sorting out their difficulties should therefore be given. *See also* Samaritans.

parasympathetic nervous system one of the two divisions of the *autonomic nervous system, having fibres that leave the central nervous system from the brain and the lower portion of the spinal cord and are distributed to blood vessels, glands, and the majority of internal organs. The system works in balance with the *sympathetic nervous system, the actions of which it frequently opposes.

parasympatholytic *n.* a drug opposing the effects of the *parasympathetic nervous system. The actions of parasympatholytic drugs are *anticholinergic* (i.e. preventing acetylcholine from acting as a neurotransmitter); they include relaxation of smooth muscle, decreased secretion of saliva, sweat, and digestive juices, and dilation of the pupil of the eye. *Atropine and similar drugs have these effects; they are used in the treatment of peptic ulcers (e.g. *propantheline) and parkinsonism (e.g. *chlorphenoxamine), to relieve spasm of smooth muscle (*see* spasmolytic), and as *mydriatics. Characteristic side-effects include dry mouth, thirst, blurred vision, dry skin, increased heart rate, and difficulty in urination.

parasympathomimetic *n.* a drug that has the effect of stimulating the *parasympathetic nervous system. The actions of parasympathomimetic drugs are *cholinergic* (resembling those of *acetylcholine) and include stimulation of skeletal muscle, *vasodilatation, depression of heart rate, increasing the tension of smooth muscle, increasing secretions (such as saliva), and constricting the pupil of the eye. They are used in the treatment of *myasthenia gravis (*see* anticholinesterase), glaucoma (*see* miotic), and some heart and circulatory conditions (e.g. *carbachol) and to restore intestinal and bladder function after surgery (e.g. bethenecol).

paratenon *n.* the tissue of a tendon sheath that fills up spaces round the tendon.

parathion *n.* an organic phosphorus compound, used as a pesticide, that causes poisoning when inhaled, ingested, or absorbed through the skin. Like several other organic phosphorus compounds, it attacks the enzyme *cholinesterase and causes excessive stimulation of the parasympathetic nervous system. The symptoms are headache, sweating, salivation, lacrimation, vomiting, diarrhoea, and muscular spasms. Treatment is by administration of *atropine.

parathormone *n.* *see* parathyroid hormone.

parathyroidectomy *n.* surgical removal of the parathyroid glands, usually as part of the treatment of *hyperparathyroidism.

parathyroid glands two pairs of yellowish-brown *endocrine glands that are situated behind, or sometimes embedded within, the *thyroid gland. They are stimulated to produce *parathyroid hormone by a decrease in the amount of calcium in the blood.

parathyroid hormone (parathormone) a hormone, synthesized and released by the parathyroid glands, that controls the distribution of calcium and phosphate in the body. A high level of the hormone causes transfer of calcium from the bones to the blood; a deficiency lowers blood calcium levels, causing *tetany. This condition may be treated by injections of the hormone. *Compare* thyrocalcitonin.

paratyphoid fever an infectious disease caused by the bacterium *Salmonella paratyphi A, B,* or *C.* Bacteria are spread in the faeces of patients or carriers, and outbreaks occur as a result of poor sanitation or unhygienic food-handling. After an incubation period of 1–10 days, symptoms, including diarrhoea, mild fever, and a pink rash on the chest, appear and last for about a week. Treatment with chloramphenicol is effective. Vaccination with *TAB provides temporary immunity against paratyphoid A and B.

pareidolia *n.* misperception of random stimuli as real things or people, as when faces are vividly seen in the flames of a fire.

parenchyma *n.* the functional part of an organ, as opposed to the supporting tissue (*stroma*).

parenteral *adj.* administered by any way other than through the mouth: applied, for example, to the introduction of drugs or other agents into the body by injection.

paresis *n.* muscular weakness caused by disease of the nervous system. It implies a lesser degree of weakness than *paralysis*, although the two words are often used interchangeably.

paries *n.* (*pl.* **parietes**) 1. the enveloping or surrounding part of an organ or other structure. 2. the wall of a cavity.

parietal *adj.* 1. of or relating to the inner walls of a body cavity, as opposed to the contents: applied particularly to the membranes lining a cavity (*see* peritoneum, pleura). 2. of or relating to the parietal bone.

parietal bone either of a pair of bones forming the top and sides of the cranium. *See* skull.

parietal cells *see* oxyntic cells.

parietal lobe one of the major divisions of each cerebral hemisphere (*see* cerebrum), lying behind the frontal lobe, above the temporal lobe, and in front of the occipital lobe. It is thus beneath the crown of the skull. It contains the *sensory cortex and *association areas.

parity *n.* the condition of a woman with regard to the number of pregnancies she has had that have each resulted in the birth of an infant capable of survival.

parkinsonism *n.* a disorder of middle-aged and elderly people characterized by tremor, rigidity and a poverty of spontaneous movements. The first and most prominent symptom is tremor, which often affects one hand, spreading first to the leg on the same side and then to the other limbs. It is most pronounced in resting limbs, interfering with such actions as holding a cup. The patient has an expressionless face, an unmodulated voice, and an increasing tendency to stoop (a shuffling run is needed to maintain balance). Parkinsonism is a disease affecting the basal ganglia of the brain for which in many cases no cause can be found. Drug-induced parkinsonism may complicate the use of psychoactive substances, including the phenothiazines, butyrophenones, and metoclopramide. Uncommonly it can be attributed to the late effects of *encephalitis or coal-gas poisoning or to *Wilson's disease. Relief of the symptoms may be obtained with *anticholinergic drugs and *levodopa.

paromomycin *n.* an antibiotic, active against intestinal bacteria and amoebae used to treat dysentery and gastroenteritis. It is administered by mouth; side-effects include stomach pains, itching, and heartburn.

paronychia *n.* inflammation and swelling of the skin folds and tissues surrounding a fingernail or toenail. Chronic paronychia is usually caused by the fungus *Candida* or it can occur in psoriasis. Acute paronychia is the result of bacterial infection. *See also* whitlow.

paroophoron *n.* the vestigial remains of part of the *mesonephric duct in the female, situated next to each ovary. It is associated with a similar structure, the *epoophoron*. Both are without known function.

parosmia *n.* any disorder of the sense of smell.

parotid gland one of a pair of *salivary glands situated in front of each ear. The openings of the parotid ducts (*Stensen's ducts*) are on the inner sides of the cheeks, opposite the second upper molar teeth.

parotitis *n.* inflammation of the parotid salivary glands. *See* mumps (infectious parotitis).

parous *adj.* having given birth to one or more children.

paroxysm *n.* **1.** a sudden violent attack, especially a spasm or convulsion. **2.** the abrupt worsening of symptoms or recurrence of disease. —**paroxysmal** *adj.*

parrot disease an infectious disease of parrots and budgerigars due to a virus-like organism of the genus *Chlamydia*; it can be transmitted to man and causes headache, bleeding from the nose, shivering, fever, and complications involving the lungs. Untreated the disease can be fatal, but it responds to tetracyclines or penicillin. Medical name: **psittacosis**. *Compare* ornithosis.

pars *n.* a specific part of an organ or other structure, such as any of parts of the pituitary gland.

Part III accommodation *see* National Assistance Act.

parthenogenesis *n.* reproduction in which an organism develops from an unfertilized ovum. It is common in plants and occurs in some lower animals (e.g. aphids).

partially sighted register (in Britain) a list of persons who have poor sight but are not technically blind. In general their sight is adequate to permit the performance of tasks for which some vision is essential. *Compare* blind register.

parturition *n.* childbirth. *See* labour.

parvi- *prefix denoting* small size.

PAS *see* para-aminosalicylic acid.

pascal *n.* the *SI unit of pressure, equal to 1 newton per square metre. Symbol: Pa.

Paschen bodies particles that occur in the cells of skin rashes in patients with *cowpox or *smallpox; they are thought to be the virus particles.

passive movement movement not brought about by a patient's own efforts. Passive movements are induced by manipulation of the joints by a physiotherapist. They are useful in maintaining function when a patient has nerve or muscle disorders that prevent voluntary movement.

pass pointing (past pointing) failure to touch a chosen target with an outstretched hand when the eyes are closed. It is a sign of imbalance in the function of the labyrinth of the inner ear. The hand moves towards the side of the affected labyrinth.

paste *n.* (in pharmacy) a medicinal preparation of a soft sticky consistency, which is applied externally.

Pasteurella a genus of small rodlike Gram-negative bacteria that are parasites of animals and man. The species *P. pestis* causes *plague in man, and *P. tularensis* causes *tularemia.

pasteurization *n.* the treatment of milk by heating it to 65°C for 30 minutes, or to 72°C for 15 minutes, followed by rapid cooling, to kill such bacteria as those of tuberculosis and typhoid.

pastille *n.* a medicinal preparation containing gelatine and glycerine, usually coated with sugar, that is dissolved in the mouth so that the medication is applied to the mouth or throat.

patch test a test to discover which, if any, of a number of possible substances is responsible for a patient's allergy. Small quantities of different allergens are applied either to light scratches on the skin of the arm or back or beneath plaster. In common allergies the offending substance causes a patch of swelling and a typical red flare in the skin in 5 to 15 minutes. A delayed reaction may take 24 to 72 hours to develop.

patella *n.* the lens shaped bone that forms the kneecap. It is situated in front of the knee in the tendon of the quadriceps muscle of the thigh. *See also* sesamoid bone.

patellar reflex the knee jerk, in which stretching the muscle at the front of the thigh by tapping its tendon below the knee cap causes a *reflex contraction of the muscle, so that the leg kicks. This is a test of the connection between the sensory nerves attached to stretch receptors in the muscle, the spinal cord, and the motor neurones running from the cord to the thigh muscle, all of which are involved in the reflex. Disease or damage may result in absence of the reflex.

patent ductus arteriosus *see* ductus arteriosus.

path- (patho-) *prefix denoting* disease. Example: *pathophobia* (morbid fear of).

pathogen *n.* a microorganism, such as a bacterium, that parasitizes an animal (or plant) or man and produces a disease.

pathogenic *adj.* capable of causing disease. The term is applied to a parasitic microorganism (especially a bacterium) in relation to its host. —**pathogenicity** *n.*

pathognomonic *adj.* describing a symptom or sign that is characteristic of or unique to a particular disease. The presence of such a sign or symptom allows positive diagnosis of the disease.

pathological *adj.* relating to or arising from disease. For example, a pathological *fracture is one associated with disease of the bone.

pathology *n.* the study of disease processes with the aim of understanding their nature and causes. This is achieved by observing samples of blood, urine, faeces, and diseased tissue obtained from the living patient or at autopsy, by the use of X-rays, and by many other techniques. (*See* biopsy.) *Clinical pathology* is the application of the knowledge gained to the treatment of patients. —**pathologist** *n.*

-pathy *suffix denoting* **1.** disease. Example: *nephropathy* (of the kidney). **2.** therapy. Example: *osteopathy* (by manipulation).

pauciarthritis *n. see* arthritis.

pavementation (pavementing) *n.* the sticking of white blood cells to the linings of the finest blood vessels (capillaries) when inflammation occurs.

peau d'orange a dimpled appearance of the skin over a breast tumour, resembling the surface of an orange. The skin is thickened and the openings of hair follicles and sweat glands are enlarged.

pecten *n.* **1.** the middle section of the anal canal, below the anal valves (*see* anus). **2.** a sharp ridge on the upper branch of the pubis (part of the hip bone). —**pectineal** *adj.*

pectoral *adj.* relating to the chest.

pectoral girdle *see* shoulder girdle.

pectoral muscles the chest muscles (see illustration). The *pectoralis major* is a large fan-shaped muscle that works over the shoulder joint, drawing the arm forward across the chest and rotating it medially. Beneath it, the *pectoralis minor* depresses the shoulder and draws the scapula down towards the chest.

Pectoral muscles

pectoriloquy *n.* abnormal transmission of the patient's voice sounds through the chest wall so that they can be clearly heard through a stethoscope. Whispered sounds (*whispering pectoriloquy*) can be heard over the lung of a patient with pneumonia.

pectus *n.* the chest or breast.

pedicle *n.* **1.** the narrow neck of tissue connecting some tumours to the normal tissue from which they have developed. **2.** (in plastic surgery) a narrow folded tube of skin by means of which a piece of skin used for grafting remains attached to its original site. A pedicle graft is used when the recipient site is unsuited to take an independent skin graft (for example, because of poor blood supply). *See also* flap, skin graft. **3.** (in anatomy) any slender stemlike process.

pediculicide *n.* an agent that kills lice; for example *benzyl benzoate, and *gamma benzene hexachloride.

Pediculoides (Pyemotes) *n.* a genus of widely distributed tiny predaceous mites. *P. ventricosus* occasionally attacks man and causes an allergic dermatitis called *grain itch*. This complaint most usually affects those people coming into contact with stored cereal products, such as hay and grain.

pediculosis *n.* an infestation of the body and/or scalp with lice of the genus *Pediculus*, which causes intense itching; continued scratching by the patient may result in bacterial infection of the skin. Untreated pediculosis of the scalp can lead to a condition in which the hair becomes matted together by the exudate from weeping skin lesions. Body lice are destroyed by dusting the body and clothes with DDT powder; head lice are eliminated with gamma benzene hexachloride.

Pediculus *n.* a widely distributed genus of lice. There are two varieties of the species affecting man: *P. humanus capitis*, the head louse; and *P. humanus corporis*, the body louse. The presence of these parasites can irritate the skin (*see* pediculosis), and in some parts of the world body lice are involved in transmitting *relapsing fever and *typhus.

pedometer *n.* a small portable device that records the number of paces walked, and thus the approximate distance covered. A pedometer is usually attached to the leg or hung at the belt.

peduncle *n.* a narrow process or stalk-like structure, serving as a support or a connection. For example, the *middle*

cerebellar peduncle connects the pons and cerebellum.

pellagra *n.* a nutritional disease due to a deficiency of *nicotinic acid (a B vitamin). Pellagra results from the consumption of a diet that is poor in either nicotinic acid or the amino acid tryptophan, from which nicotinic acid can be synthesized in the body. It is common in maize-eating communities. The symptoms of pellagra are scaly dermatitis on exposed surfaces, diarrhoea, and depression.

pellicle *n.* a thin layer of skin, membrane, or any other substance.

pelvic girdle (hip girdle) the bony structure to which the bones of the lower limbs are attached. It consists of the right and left *hip bones.

pelvimetry *n.* the measurement of the four internal diameters of the pelvis (transverse, anteroposterior, left oblique, and right oblique). Pelvimetry helps in determining whether it will be possible for a fetus to be delivered in the normal way. Abnormality of the outlet of the pelvis may be an indication for Caesarean section.

pelvis *n.* (*pl.* **pelves**) **1.** the bony struc-

The male pelvis (ventral view)

ture formed by the *hip bones, *sacrum, and *coccyx: the bony pelvis (see illustration). The hip bones are fused at the back to the sacrum to form a rigid structure that protects the organs of the lower abdomen and provides attachment for the bones and muscles of the lower limbs. **2.** the lower part of the abdomen. **3.** the cavity within the bony pelvis. **4.** any structure shaped like a basin, e.g. the expanded part of the ureter in the kidney (*renal pelvis*). —**pelvic** *adj.*

pemphigoid *n.* any of a group of skin disorders that resemble pemphigus but are distinct from it. A common type affects the elderly, with large, sometimes bloody, blisters occurring on the trunk and limbs. Attacks may be short or recurrent.

pemphigus *n.* any of several distinctive skin diseases marked by successive outbreaks of blisters. There are several types; for example, *benign familial pemphigus*, which is a hereditary condition; and *pemphigus vulgaris*, a rare serious disease occurring in middle age and initially affecting the mucous membranes.

penetrance *n.* the frequency with which the characteristic controlled by a gene is seen in the individuals possessing it. Complete penetrance occurs when the characteristic is seen in all individuals known to possess the gene. If a percentage of individuals with the gene do not show its effects, penetrance is incomplete. In this way a characteristic in a family may appear to 'skip' a generation.

-penia *suffix denoting* lack or deficiency. Example: *neutropenia* (of neutrophils).

penicillamine *n.* a drug that binds metals and therefore aids their excretion (*see* chelating agent). It is used to treat *Wilson's disease, poisoning by metals such as lead, copper, and mer-

cury, and severe rheumatoid arthritis. It is administered by mouth and commonly causes digestive upsets and allergic reactions. Trade names: **Cuprimine, Distamine**.

penicillin (benzylpenicillin, penicillin G) *n.* an *antibiotic derived from the mould *Penicillium notatum* and used to treat infections caused by a wide variety of bacteria. It is usually administered by injection, but taken orally is widely used to treat dental abscesses and remains the antibiotic of choice for their treatment. There are few serious side-effects, but some patients are allergic to penicillin and develop such reactions as skin rashes, swelling of the throat, and fever. Trade names: **Crystapen, Falapen, Icipen, Stabillin**.
There are several similar drugs prepared from *P. notatum* (*see* benethamine penicillin, benzathine penicillin) and a number of antibiotics derived from the penicillins (including *ampicillin and *cloxacillin), known as *semisynthetic penicillins*.

penicillinase *n.* an enzyme-like substance, produced by some bacteria, that is capable of antagonizing the antibacterial action of *penicillin. Purified penicillinase, obtained from a strain of *Bacillus cereus*, may be used to treat reactions to penicillin. It is also used in diagnostic tests to isolate microorganisms from the blood of patients receiving penicillin.

Penicillium *n.* a genus of mouldlike fungi that commonly grow on decaying fruit, bread, or cheese. The species *P. chrysogenum* is the major natural source of the antibiotic *penicillin. Some species of *Penicillium* are pathogenic to man, causing diseases of the skin and respiratory tract.

penis *n.* the male organ that carries the *urethra, through which urine and semen are discharged (see illustration). Urination can occur in the normal hanging position. Most of the organ is composed of erectile tissue (*see* corpus cavernosum, corpus spongiosum), which becomes filled with blood under conditions of sexual excitement so that the penis is erected. In this position it can act as a sexual organ, capable of entering the vagina and ejaculating semen. *See also* glans, prepuce.

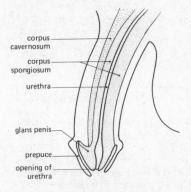

corpus cavernosum
corpus spongiosum
urethra
glans penis
prepuce
opening of urethra

The penis (median section)

pent- (penta-) *prefix denoting* five.

pentaerythritol *n.* a drug that dilates blood vessels and is used in the treatment of angina and other heart conditions. It is administered by mouth and may cause headache and indigestion. Trade names: **Cardiacap**, **Mycardol**, **Pentral**, **Peritrate**.

pentagastrin *n.* a synthetic hormone that has the same effects as *gastrin in stimulating the secretion of gastric juice from the stomach. It is injected to test for gastric secretion in the diagnosis of digestive disorders. Trade name: **Peptavlon**.

pentazocine *n.* a potent *analgesic drug used to relieve moderate or severe pain. It is administered by mouth, injection, or in suppositories; side-effects include dizziness and digestive upsets. Trade name: **Fortral**.

pentobarbitone *n.* a *barbiturate drug used to relieve insomnia and agitation and also as an *anticonvulsant. It is administered by mouth, injection, or in suppositories. Side-effects include rashes, digestive upsets, and lethargy, and prolonged use may lead to *dependence. Trade name: **Nembutal**.

pentose *n.* a simple sugar with five carbon atoms: for example, ribose and xylose.

pentosuria *n.* an inborn defect of sugar metabolism causing abnormal excretion of pentose in the urine. There are no serious ill-effects.

Pentothal *n. see* thiopentone.

pepsin *n.* an enzyme in the stomach that begins the digestion of proteins by splitting them into peptones (*see* peptidase). It is produced by the action of hydrochloric acid on *pepsinogen*, which is secreted by the gastric glands. Once made, pepsin itself can act on pepsinogen to produce more pepsin.

pepsinogen *n. see* pepsin.

peptic *adj.* **1.** relating to pepsin. **2.** relating to digestion.

peptic ulcer a breach in the lining (mucosa) of the digestive tract produced by digestion of the mucosa by pepsin and acid. This may occur when pepsin and acid are present in abnormally high concentrations or when some other mechanism reduces the normal protective mechanisms of the mucosa; bile salts may play a part, especially in stomach ulcers. A peptic ulcer may be found in the oesophagus (*oesophageal ulcer*, associated with reflux *oesophagitis); the stomach (*see* gastric ulcer); duodenum (*see* duodenal ulcer); jejunum (*jejunal ulcer*, usually in the *Zollinger-Ellison syndrome); in a Meckel's *diverticulum; and close to a *gastroenterostomy (*stomal ulcer, anastomatic ulcer, marginal ulcer*).

peptidase *n.* one of a group of digestive enzymes that split proteins in the stomach and intestine into their constituent amino acids. The group is divided into *endopeptidases and *exopeptidases.

peptide *n.* a molecule consisting of two or more *amino acids linked by bonds between the amino group (-NH) and the carboxyl group (-CO). This bond is known as a *peptide bond. See also* polypeptide.

peptone *n.* a large protein fragment produced by the action of enzymes on proteins in the first stages of protein digestion.

peptonuria *n.* the presence in the urine of *peptones, intermediate compounds formed during the digestion of proteins.

perception *n.* (in psychology) the process by which information about the world, received by the senses, is analysed and made meaningful. Abnormalities of perception include *hallucinations, *illusions, and *agnosia.

percussion *n.* the technique of examining part of the body by tapping it with the fingers or an instrument (*plessor*) and sensing the resultant vibrations. With experience it is possible to detect the presence of abnormal solidification or enlargement in different organs and the presence of fluid, for example in the lungs.

percutaneous *adj.* through the skin: often applied to the route of administration of drugs in ointments, etc., which are absorbed through the skin.

percutaneous nephrolithotomy a technique of removing stones from the kidney via an endoscope passed into the kidney through a track from the skin surface previously established by the presence of a catheter.

perforation *n.* the creation of a hole in an organ, tissue, or tube. This may occur in the course of a disease (e.g. a *duodenal ulcer, colonic *diverticulitis, or stomach cancer), allowing the contents of the intestine to enter the peritoneal cavity, which causes acute inflammation (*peritonitis) with sudden severe abdominal pain and shock. Treatment is usually by surgical repair of the perforation, but conservative treatment with antibiotics may result in spontaneous healing. Perforation may also be caused accidentally by instruments – for example a gastroscope may perforate the stomach, a curette may perforate the womb – or by injury; for example to the eardrum.

perfusion *n.* **1.** the passage of fluid through a tissue, especially the passage of blood through the lung tissue to pick up oxygen from the air in the alveoli, which is brought there by *ventilation, and release carbon dioxide. If ventilation is impaired deoxygenated venous blood is returned to the general circulation. If perfusion is impaired insufficient gas exchange takes place. **2.** the deliberate introduction of fluid into a tissue, usually by injection into the blood vessels supplying the tissue.

peri- *prefix denoting* near, around, or enclosing. Examples: *pericardial* (around the heart); *peritonsillar* (around a tonsil).

periadenitis *n.* inflammation of tissues surrounding a gland.

perianal haematoma (external haemorrhoid) a small painful swelling beside the anus, occurring after a bout of straining to pass faeces or coughing. Perianal haematomas are caused by the rupture of a small vein in the anus. They often heal spontaneously but occasionally rupture. Rarely this is followed by abscess formation. If severe pain continues, surgical removal can be undertaken. *See also* haemorrhoids.

periapical *adj.* around an apex, particularly the apex of a tooth. The term is applied to bone surrounding the apex and to X-ray views of this area.

periarteritis nodosa *see* polyarteritis nodosa.

periarthritis *n.* inflammation of tissues around a joint capsule, including tendons and *bursae. *Chronic periarthritis*, which may be spontaneous or follow injury, is a common cause of pain and stiffness of the shoulder; it usually responds to local steroid injections or physiotherapy.

pericard- (pericardio-) *prefix denoting* the pericardium.

pericardectomy *n.* surgical removal of the membranous sac surrounding the heart (pericardium). It is used in the treatment of chronic constrictive pericarditis and chronic pericardial effusion (*see* pericarditis).

pericardiocentesis *n.* removal of excess fluid from within the sac (pericardium) surrounding the heart by means of needle *aspiration. *See* pericarditis, hydropericardium.

pericardiolysis *n.* the surgical separation of *adhesions between the heart and surrounding structures within the ribcage (*adherent pericardium*). The operation has now fallen into disuse.

pericardiorrhaphy *n.* the repair of wounds in the membrane surrounding the heart (pericardium), such as those due to injury or surgery.

pericardiostomy *n.* an operation in which the membranous sac around the heart is opened and the fluid within drained via a tube. It is sometimes used in the treatment of septic pericarditis.

pericarditis *n.* acute or chronic inflammation of the membranous sac (pericardium) surrounding the heart. Pericarditis may be seen alone or as part of pancarditis (*see* endomyocarditis). It has numerous causes, including virus infections, uraemia, and cancer. *Acute* *pericarditis* is characterized by fever, chest pain, and a pericardial friction rub. Fluid may accumulate within the pericardial sac (*pericardial effusion*). Rarely, chronic thickening of the pericardium (*chronic constrictive pericarditis*) develops. This interferes with activity of the heart and has many features in common with *heart failure, including oedema, pleural effusions, ascites, and engorgement of the veins. Constrictive pericarditis most often results from tubercular infection.

The treatment of pericarditis is directed to the cause. Pericardial effusions may be aspirated by a needle inserted through the chest wall. Chronic constrictive pericarditis is treated by surgical removal of the pericardium (*pericardectomy*).

pericardium *n.* the membrane surrounding the heart, consisting of two portions. The outer *fibrous pericardium* completely encloses the heart and is attached to the large blood vessels emerging from the heart. The internal *serous pericardium* is a closed sac of *serous membrane: the inner visceral portion (*epicardium*) is closely attached to the muscular heart wall and the outer parietal portion lines the fibrous pericardium. Within the sac is a very small amount of fluid, which prevents friction as the two surfaces slide over one another as the heart beats. —**pericardial** *adj.*

pericardotomy *n.* surgical opening or puncture of the membranous sac (pericardium) around the heart. It is required to gain access to the heart in heart surgery and to remove excess fluid from within the pericardium.

perichondritis *n.* inflammation of cartilage and surrounding soft tissues, usually due to chronic infection. A common site is the external ear.

perichondrium *n.* the dense layer of fibrous connective tissue that covers the surface of *cartilage.

pericolpitis (paracolpitis) *n.* inflammation of the connective tissues around the vagina.

pericoronitis *n.* inflammation around the crown of a tooth, particularly a partially erupted third molar.

pericranium *n.* the *periosteum of the skull.

pericystitis *n.* inflammation in the tissues around the bladder, causing pain in the pelvis, fever, and symptoms of *cystitis. It usually results from infection in the Fallopian tubes or womb, but can occasionally arise from severe infection in a *diverticulum of the bladder itself. Treatment of pericystitis is directed to the underlying cause and usually involves antibiotic therapy. Pericystitis associated with a pelvic abscess clears when the abscess is surgically drained.

pericyte *n.* a type of cell surrounding the smallest blood vessels (terminal arterioles and venules and capillaries). It is not capable of contraction, and its function is uncertain.

periderm *n. see* epitrichium.

perifolliculitis *n.* inflammation around the hair follicles.

perihepatitis *n.* inflammation of the membrane covering the liver. It is usually associated with abnormalities of the liver (including liver abscess, cirrhosis, tuberculosis) or in chronic peritonitis.

perikaryon *n. see* cell body.

perilymph *n.* the fluid between the bony and membranous *labyrinths of the ear.

perimeter *n.* an instrument for mapping the absolute extent of the *visual field (see illustration). The patient looks steadily at a target in the centre of the inner surface of the hemisphere. Objects are presented on this surface and the patient says if he sees them. The edge of the visual field can be defined and any gaps in the field can be detected. There are several types of perimeter. In the *static perimeter* the movable object is replaced by a system of tiny lights, set in a black background, that can be flashed singly or in patterns. If the patient has a field defect he will fail to see the lights that flash in the area of the defect. —**perimetry** *n.*

arc that can be rotated about the pivot

movable object

33cm

central pivot

fixed central target

chin rest

table

A perimeter

perimetritis *n.* inflammation of the membrane on the outer surface of the womb. The condition may be associated with *parametritis.

perimetrium *n.* the *peritoneum of the womb (uterus).

perimysium *n.* the fibrous sheath that surrounds each bundle of *muscle fibres.

perinatal *adj.* relating to the period from about three months before to one month after birth.

perinatal mortality rate *see* infant mortality rate.

perineoplasty *n.* a tissue-grafting operation to repair the area between the vulva and anus (the perineum).

perineorrhaphy *n.* the stitching of a tear, possibly sustained during childbirth, in the region between the vulva and anus (the perineum). The operation may involve repair of the vaginal wall.

perinephritis *n.* inflammation of the tissues around the kidney. This is usually due to spread of infection from the kidney itself (*see* pyelonephritis, pyonephrosis). The patient has pain in the loins, fever, and fits of shivering. Prompt treatment of the underlying renal infection is required to prevent progression to an abscess.

perineum *n.* the region of the body between the anus and the urethral opening, including both skin and underlying muscle. In females it is perforated by the vaginal opening. —**perineal** *adj.*

perineurium *n.* the sheath of connective tissue that surrounds individual bundles (fascicles) of nerve fibres within a large *nerve.

periodic acid–Schiff (PAS) reaction a test for the presence of glycoproteins, polysaccharides, certain mucopolysaccharides, glycolipids, and certain fatty acids in tissue sections. The tissue is treated with periodic acid, followed by *Schiff's reagent. A positive reaction is the development of a red or magenta coloration.

periodic fever *see* malaria.

periodontal *adj.* denoting or relating to the tissues surrounding the teeth.

periodontal abscess an abscess that arises in the periodontal tissues and is invariably an acute manifestation of periodontal disease.

periodontal disease disease of the tissues that support and attach the teeth – the gums, periodontal membrane, and alveolar bone. It is caused by the metabolism of bacterial *plaque on the surfaces of the teeth adjacent to these tissues. Periodontal disease includes *gingivitis and the more advanced stage of *periodontitis*, which results in the formation of spaces between the gums and the teeth (*periodontal pockets*), the loss of some fibres that attach the tooth to the jaw, and the loss of bone. The disease is widespread and is the most common cause of tooth loss in older people. Poor oral hygiene is a major contributory factor, but the resistance of the patient has some influence.

periodontal membrane (periodontal ligament) the ligament around a *tooth, by which it is attached to the bone.

periodontal pocket a space between the gingival tissues and tooth occurring in periodontitis. See periodontal disease.

periodontium *n.* the tissues that support and attach the teeth: the gums (*see* gingiva), *periodontal membrane, alveolar bone, and *cementum.

periodontology *n.* the branch of dentistry concerned with the tissues that support and attach the teeth and the prevention and treatment of *periodontal disease.

periosteum *n.* a layer of dense connective tissue that covers the surface of a bone except at the articular surfaces. The outer layer of the periosteum is extremely dense and contains a large number of blood vessels. The inner layer is more cellular in appearance and contains osteoblasts and fewer blood vessels. The periosteum provides attachment for muscles, tendons, and ligaments.

periostitis *n.* inflammation of the membrane surrounding a bone (*see* periosteum). *Acute periostitis* results from direct injury to the bone and is associated with a *haematoma, which may later become infected. The uncomplicated condition subsides quickly with rest and anti-inflammatory anal-

peripheral nervous system

gesics. *Chronic periostitis* sometimes follows but is more often due to an inflammatory disease, such as tuberculosis or syphilis, or to a chronic ulcer overlying the bone involved. Chronic periostitis causes thickening of the underlying bone, which is evident on X-ray.

peripheral nervous system all parts of the nervous system lying outside the central nervous system (brain and spinal cord). It includes the *cranial nerves and *spinal nerves and their branches, which link the receptors and effector organs with the brain and spinal cord. *See also* autonomic nervous system.

periphlebitis *n*. inflammation of the tissues around a vein: seen as an extension of *phlebitis.

perisalpingitis *n*. inflammation of the membrane on the outer surface of a Fallopian tube.

perisplenitis *n*. inflammation of the external coverings of the spleen.

peristalsis *n*. a wavelike movement that progresses along some of the hollow tubes of the body. It occurs involuntarily and is characteristic of tubes that possess circular and longitudinal muscles, such as the *intestines. It is induced by distension of the walls of the tube. Immediately behind the distension the circular muscle contracts. In front of the distension the circular muscle relaxes and the longitudinal muscle contracts, which pushes the contents of the tube forward. —**peristaltic** *adj*.

peritendineum *n*. the fibrous covering of a tendon.

peritendinitis *n*. *see* tenosynovitis.

peritomy *n*. an eye operation in which an incision of the conjunctiva is made in a complete circle around the cornea. It is performed for the relief of *pannus.

peritoneoscope *n*. *see* laparoscope.

peritoneum *n*. the *serous membrane of the abdominal cavity (see illustration). The *parietal peritoneum* lines the walls of the abdomen, and the *visceral peritoneum* covers the abdominal organs. *See also* mesentery, omentum. —**peritoneal** *adj*.

liver
kidney
pancreas
stomach
duodenum
transverse colon
peritoneal cavity
mesentery
jejunum
ileum
bladder
pubic symphysis
rectum

Sagittal section of the abdomen to show arrangement of the peritoneum

peritonitis *n*. inflammation of the *peritoneum. *Primary peritonitis* is caused by bacteria spread via the bloodstream: examples are *pneumococcal peritonitis* and *tuberculous peritonitis*. Symptoms are diffuse abdominal pain and swelling, with fever and weight loss. Fluid may accumulate in the peritoneal cavity (*see* ascites) or the infection may complicate existing ascites. *Secondary peritonitis* is due to perforation or rupture of an abdominal organ (for example, a duodenal ulcer or the vermiform appendix), allowing access of bacteria and irritant digestive juices to the peritoneum. This produces sudden severe abdominal pain, first at the site of rupture but becoming generalized. Shock develops, and the abdominal wall becomes rigid; X-ray examination may reveal gas within the peritoneal cavity. Treatment is usually by surgical repair of the perforation, but in some cases conservative treatment using antibiotics and intravenous fluid may be used. *Subphrenic abscess is a possible complication.

peritonsillar abscess *see* quinsy.

peritrichous *adj.* describing bacteria in which the flagella cover the entire cell surface.

perityphlitis *n. Archaic.* inflammation of the tissues around the caecum. *See* typhlitis.

periureteritis *n.* inflammation of the tissues around a ureter. This is usually associated with inflammation of the ureter itself (*ureteritis) often behind an obstruction caused by a stone or stricture. Treatment is directed to relieving any obstruction of the ureter and controlling the infection with antibiotics.

perle *n.* a soft capsule containing medicine.

perleche *n.* dryness and cracking of the corners of the mouth, sometimes with infection. Perleche may be caused by persistent lip licking or by a vitamin-deficient diet.

pernicious *adj.* describing diseases that are highly dangerous or likely to result in death if untreated. *See also* pernicious anaemia.

pernicious anaemia a form of *anaemia resulting from deficiency of *vitamin B_{12}. This in turn results either from failure to produce the substance (*intrinsic factor) that facilitates absorption of B_{12} from the bowel or from dietary deficiency of the vitamin. Pernicious anaemia is characterized by defective production of red blood cells and the presence of *megaloblasts in the bone marrow. In severe forms the nervous system is affected (*see* subacute combined degeneration of the cord). The condition is treated by injections of vitamin B_{12}.

pernio *n. see* chilblain.

perniosis *n.* any one of a group of conditions caused by the effect of persistent cold on individuals whose skin blood vessels are especially sensitive. The small arteries constrict and the capillaries dilate slowing the blood flow. The blood loses all its oxygen and fluid passes from the stagnant capillary blood into the tissues. The affected area becomes blue, swollen, and cold. Perniosis includes such conditions as *chilblains, *acrocyanosis, *erythrocyanosis, and *Raynaud's disease.

pero- *prefix denoting* deformity; defect. Example: *peromelia* (of the limbs).

peroneal *adj.* relating to or supplying the outer (fibular) side of the leg.

peroneus *n.* one of the muscles of the leg that arises from the fibula. The *peroneus longus* and *peroneus brevis* are situated at the side of the leg and inserted into the metatarsal bones of the foot. They help to turn the foot outwards.

peroxidase *n.* an enzyme, found mainly in plants but also present in leucocytes and milk, that catalyses the dehydrogenation (oxidation) of various substances in the presence of hydrogen peroxide (which acts as a hydrogen acceptor, being converted to water in the process).

peroxisome *n.* a small structure within a cell that is similar to a *lysosome but contains different enzymes, some of which may take part in reactions involving hydrogen peroxide.

perphenazine *n.* a major *tranquillizer used to relieve anxiety, tension, and agitation and to prevent nausea and vomiting. It is administered by mouth or injection; side-effects are similar to those of *chlorpromazine. Trade name: **Fentazin**.

perseveration *n.* excessive persistence at a task that prevents the individual from turning his attention to new situations. It is a symptom of organic disease of the brain and sometimes of obsessional neurosis.

personality *n.* (in psychology) an enduring disposition to act and feel in particular ways that differentiate one individual from another. These patterns are sometimes conceptualized as different categories (*see* personality disorder) and sometimes as different dimensions (*see* extroversion, neuroticism).

personality disorder a deeply ingrained and maladjusted pattern of behaviour, persisting through many years. It is usually manifest by the time the individual is adolescent. The abnormality of behaviour must be sufficiently severe that it causes suffering, either to the patient or to other people (or to both). Some such personalities mature into happier people. Most forms of psychotherapy claim to be of therapeutic value, but the worth of any treatment remains debatable. *See* anankastic, asthenic, hysterical, paranoid, psychopath, schizoid.

perspiration *n.* *sweat or the process of sweating. *Insensible perspiration* is sweat that evaporates immediately from the skin and is therefore not visible; *sensible perspiration* is visible on the skin in the form of drops.

Perthes' disease *see* Legg-Calvé-Perthes disease.

pertussis *n. see* whooping cough.

perversion *n.* any abnormal sexual behaviour. (An equivalent term with less derogatory implications is *deviation*). The abnormality may be in the sexual object (as in *homosexuality and *fetishism) or in the activity engaged in (for example, *sadism and *exhibitionism). The activity is sexually pleasurable.
The definition of what is normal varies with different cultures. Treatment is necessary only when the perversion causes suffering. Some people may find that *counselling helps them to adjust to their deviation. Others may wish for treatment to change the deviation: *aversion therapy is used, also *conditioning normal sexual fantasies to pleasurable behaviour. The only helpful effect of drugs is to reduce sexual drive generally.

pes *n.* (in anatomy) the foot or a part resembling a foot.

pes cavus *see* claw-foot.

pes planus *see* flat-foot.

pessary *n.* **1.** a plastic or metal instrument, often ring-shaped, that fits into the vagina and keeps the womb in position: used to treat *prolapse. **2.** a plug or cylinder of cocoa butter or other soft material containing a drug that is fitted into the vagina for the treatment of gynaecological disorders, e.g. vaginitis. Also called: **vaginal suppository**.

pesticide *n.* a chemical agent used to kill insects or other organisms harmful to crops\ and other cultivated plants. Some pesticides, such as *parathion and *dieldrin, have caused poisoning in human beings and livestock after accidental exposure.

petechia *n.* (*pl.* **petechiae**) a small round flat dark-red spot caused by bleeding into the skin or beneath the mucous membrane. Petechiae occur, for example, in the *purpuras.

pethidine *n.* a potent *analgesic drug with mild sedative action, used to relieve moderate or severe pain. It is administered by mouth or injection; side-effects may include nausea, dizziness, and dry mouth, and *dependence may occur with prolonged use.

petit mal a form of idiopathic epilepsy in which there are brief spells of unconsciousness, lasting for a few seconds, during which posture and balance are maintained. The eyes stare blankly and there may be fluttering movements of the lids and momentary twitching of the fingers and mouth. The electroencephalogram characteristically shows bisynchronous wave and spike discharges (3 per second) during the attacks and at other times. Attacks are sometimes provoked by overbreathing or intermittent photic stimulation. As the stream of thought is completely interrupted, children with frequent petit mal may have learning difficulties. Petit mal seldom appears before the age of three or after adolescence.

Drug treatment (with *sodium valproate or *ethosuximide) is usually effective. Petit mal often subsides spontaneously in adult life. It may be accompanied or followed by grand mal.

Petri dish a flat shallow circular glass or plastic dish with a pillbox-like lid, used to hold solid agar or gelatin media for culturing bacteria.

petrissage n. kneading: a form of *massage in which the skin is lifted up, pressed down and squeezed, and pinched and rolled. Alternate squeezing and relaxation of the tissues stimulates the local circulation and may have a pain-relieving effect in muscular disorders.

petrositis n. inflammation of the petrous part of the *temporal bone (which encloses the inner ear), usually due to an extension of *mastoiditis.

petrous bone see temporal bone.

-pexy suffix denoting surgical fixation. Example: omentopexy (of the omentum).

Peyer's patches oval masses of *lymphoid tissue on the mucous membrane lining the small intestine.

Peyronie's disease a dense fibrous plaque in the penis, which can be felt in the erectile tissue as an irregular hard lump. The penis curves or angulates at this point on erection and pain often

results. The cause is unknown and treatment unsatisfactory. The pain usually subsides spontaneously, but impotence often results.

pH a measure of the concentration of hydrogen ions in a solution, and therefore of its acidity or alkalinity. A pH of 7 indicates a neutral solution, a pH below 7 indicates acidity, and a pH in excess of 7 indicates alkalinity.

phaco- prefix. see phako-.

phaeochromocytoma n. a small vascular tumour of the inner region (medulla) of the adrenal gland. By its uncontrolled and irregular secretion of the hormones *adrenaline and *noradrenaline, the tumour causes attacks of raised blood pressure, increased heart rate, palpitations, and headache.

phag- (phago-) prefix denoting 1. eating. 2. phagocytes.

phage n. see bacteriophage.

phagedaena n. rapidly spreading ulceration with sloughing of dead skin. See also bedsore.

-phagia suffix denoting a condition involving eating.

phagocyte n. a cell that is able to engulf and digest bacteria, protozoa, cells and cell debris, and other small particles. Phagocytes include many white blood cells (see leucocyte) and *macrophages, which play a major role in the body's defence mechanism. —**phagocytic** adj.

phagocytosis n. the engulfment and digestion of bacteria and other foreign particles by a cell (see phagocyte). Compare pinocytosis.

phako- (phaco-) prefix denoting the lens of the eye.

phakoemulsification n. the process of softening the lens of the eye before removing it in a method of surgery for cataract. A fine probe is inserted into the lens and the emulsification is commonly performed by ultrasonic vibration.

phalangeal cells rows of supporting cells between the sensory hair cells of the organ of Corti (*see* cochlea).

phalangectomy *n.* surgical removal of one or more of the small bones (phalanges) in the fingers or toes.

phalanges *n.* (*sing.* **phalanx**) the bones of the fingers and toes (digits). The first digit (thumb/big toe) has two phalanges. Each of the remaining digits has three phalanges. —**phalangeal** *adj.*

phalangitis *n.* inflammation of a finger or toe, causing swelling and pain. The condition may be caused by infection of the soft tissues, tendon sheaths, bone, or joints or by some rheumatic diseases, such as *psoriatic arthritis. *See also* dactylitis.

phalanx *n. see* phalanges.

phalloplasty *n.* surgical reconstruction or repair of the penis. It is required for congenital deformity of the penis, as in *hypospadias or *epispadias, and sometimes also following injury to the penis with loss of skin.

phallus *n.* the embryonic penis, before the urethral duct has reached its final state of development.

phanero- *prefix denoting* visible; apparent.

phaneromania *n.* an excessively strong impulse to touch or rub parts of one's own body.

phantasy *n. see* fantasy.

phantom limb the sensation that an arm or leg, or part of an arm or leg, is still attached to the body after it has been amputated. Pain may seem to come from the amputated part. This may arise because of stimulation of the amputation stump, which contains severed nerves that formerly carried messages from the removed portion.

phantom tumour a swelling, in the abdomen or elsewhere, caused by local muscular contraction or the accumulation of gases, that mimics a swelling caused by a tumour or other structural change. The condition is usually associated with emotional disorder, and the 'tumour' may disappear under anaesthesia.

pharmaceutical *adj.* relating to pharmacy.

pharmaceutical committee (local) *see* medical committee (local).

pharmacist *n.* a person who is qualified by examination and registered and authorized to dispense medicines or to keep open a shop for the sale and dispensing of medicines.

pharmaco- *prefix denoting* drugs. Example: *pharmacophobia* (morbid fear of).

pharmacognosy *n.* the knowledge or study of pharmacologically active principles derived from plants.

pharmacology *n.* the science of the properties of drugs and their effects on the body. —**pharmacological** *adj.*

pharmacomania *n.* an abnormal desire for taking medicines.

pharmacopoeia *n.* a book containing a list of the drugs used in medicine, with details of their formulae, methods of preparation, dosages, standards of purity, etc.

pharmacy *n.* **1.** the preparation and dispensing of drugs. **2.** premises registered to dispense medicines and sell poisons.

pharyng- (pharyngo-) *prefix denoting* the pharynx. Example: *pharyngopathy* (disease of).

pharyngeal arch (branchial or **visceral arch)** any of the paired segmented ridges of tissue in each side of the throat of the early embryo that correspond to the gill arches of fish. Each arch contains a cartilage, a cranial nerve, and a blood vessel. Between each arch there is a *pharyngeal pouch.

pharyngeal cleft (branchial or **visceral cleft)** any of the paired segmented clefts in each side of the throat of the early embryo that correspond to the gills of fish. Soon after they have formed they close to form the *pharyngeal pouches, except for the first cleft, which persists as the external auditory meatus.

pharyngeal pouch (branchial or **visceral pouch)** any of the paired segmented pouches in the side of the throat of the early embryo. They give rise to the tympanic cavity, the parathyroid glands, the thymus, and probably the thyroid gland.

pharyngectomy *n.* surgical removal of part of the pharynx.

pharyngismus *n.* spasmodic contraction of the muscles of the pharynx.

pharyngitis *n.* inflammation of the part of the throat behind the soft palate (pharynx). It produces *sore throat and is usually associated with *tonsillitis.

pharyngocele *n.* a pouch or cyst opening off the pharynx (*see* branchial cyst).

pharyngoplegia *n.* muscular paralysis of the pharynx.

pharyngoscope *n.* an *endoscope for the examination of the pharynx.

pharynx *n.* a muscular tube, lined with mucous membrane, that extends from the beginning of the oesophagus (gullet) up to the base of the skull. It is divided into the *nasopharynx, *oropharynx, and *laryngopharynx (see illustration) and it communicates with the posterior *nares, *Eustachian tube, the mouth, larynx, and oesophagus. The pharynx acts as a passageway for food from the mouth to the oesophagus, and as an air passage from the nasal cavity and mouth to the larynx. It also acts as a resonating chamber for the sounds produced in the larynx. —**pharyngeal** *adj.*

Longitudinal section of the pharynx

phenacemide *n.* an *anticonvulsant drug used in the treatment of epilepsy. It is administered by mouth; side-effects include digestive upsets, fever, and rash. Mental changes and damage to liver, kidneys, and bone marrow may also occur.

phenacetin *n.* an *analgesic drug that also reduces fever, used to relieve mild or moderate pain. It is administered by mouth; side-effects may include sweating and skin rashes. Because prolonged high doses may cause kidney damage, its use in Britain was restricted by law in 1974.

phenazocine *n.* an *analgesic drug used for rapid relief of moderate or severe pain. It is administered by mouth or injection; side-effects may include digestive upsets and dizziness, and prolonged use may lead to *dependence. Trade name: **Narphen**.

phenazopyridine *n.* an *analgesic drug used to relieve pain in inflammatory conditions of the bladder and urinary tract, such as cystitis and urethritis. It is administered by mouth and occasionally causes digestive upsets; in patients with kidney disease it may damage the red blood cells. Trade name: **Pyridium**.

phenelzine *n.* a drug used to relieve depression and anxiety (*see* MAO inhibitor). It is administered by mouth; side-effects include dizziness, drowsiness, tiredness, and digestive upsets. Trade name: **Nardil**.

pheneturide *n.* an *anticonvulsant drug used in the treatment of major types of epilepsy. It is administered by mouth; side-effects may include lack of muscular coordination, loss of appetite, and skin reactions. Trade name: **Benuride**.

phenformin *n.* a drug that reduces blood sugar levels and is used to treat *diabetes. It is administered by mouth; side-effects include a metallic taste in the mouth and digestive upsets. Trade names: **Dibotin**, **Dipar**, **Meltrol**.

phenindione *n.* an *anticoagulant drug used to treat thrombosis in the blood vessels of the heart and limbs. It is administered by mouth or injection; side-effects may include skin rashes, fever, and diarrhoea. Trade name: **Dindevan**.

pheniramine *n.* an *antihistamine used to treat allergic reactions such as hay fever and hives. It is administered by mouth or is applied to the skin in an ointment; side-effects may include drowsiness, digestive upsets, and skin reactions. Trade name: **Daneral**.

phenmetrazine *n.* a drug that reduces the appetite and was formerly used in the treatment of obesity. It is administered by mouth and its actions and side-effects are similar to those of *amphetamine. Prolonged use and large doses may cause mental depression and *dependence.

phenobarbitone *n.* a *barbiturate drug used to treat insomnia and anxiety and as an anticonvulsant in the treatment of epilepsy. It is administered by mouth or injection; side-effects may include drowsiness and skin sensitivity reactions, and dependence may result from continued use.

phenol (carbolic acid) *n.* a strong *disinfectant used for cleansing wounds, treating inflammations of the mouth, throat, and ear, and as a preservative in injections. It is administered as solution, ointments, and lotions and is highly toxic if taken by mouth.

phenolphthalein *n.* an irritant *laxative administered by mouth, usually given at night to act the following morning. Side-effects may include stomach cramps.

phenolsulphonphthalein *n.* a red dye administered by injection in a test for kidney function.

phenothiazines *n.* a group of chemically related compounds with various pharmacological actions. Some (e.g. *chlorpromazine and *trifluoperazine) are major *tranquillizers; others (e.g. *piperazine) are anthelmintics.

phenotype *n.* the observable characteristics of an individual, which result from interaction between the genes he possesses (*genotype) and the environment.

phenoxybenzamine *n.* a drug that dilates blood vessels (*see* vasodilator). It is used to reduce blood pressure and to treat conditions involving poor circulation, such as Raynaud's disease and chilblains. It is administered by mouth or injection and may cause dizziness and fast heart beat. Trade name: **Dibenyline**.

phenoxymethylpenicillin *n.* an *antibiotic, similar to *penicillin, used to treat infections caused by a wide variety of microorganisms. It is administered by mouth and may cause diarrhoea and allergic reactions.

phensuximide *n.* an *anticonvulsant drug used to prevent or reduce petit mal fits in epilepsy. It is administered by mouth; side-effects may include dizziness, drowsiness, nausea, and loss of appetite.

phentermine *n.* a *sympathomimetic drug that suppresses the appetite and is used in the treatment of obesity. It is administered by mouth; side-effects include dry mouth, nausea, and restlessness, and continued use produces *tolerance. Trade names: **Duromine**, **Ionamin**.

phentolamine *n.* a drug that dilates blood vessels (*see* vasodilator) and is used to reduce blood pressure in *phaeochromocytoma and to treat conditions of poor circulation such as Raynaud's disease and chilblains. It is administered by mouth or injection; side-effects include fast heart beat and digestive upsets. Trade name: **Rogitine**.

phenylalanine *n.* an *essential amino acid that is readily converted to tyrosine. Blockade of this metabolic pathway gives rise to *phenylketonuria, which is associated with the excretion of large amounts of phenylalanine and phenylpyruvic acid in the urine and retarded mental development.

phenylbutazone *n.* an *analgesic drug that reduces fever and inflammation and is used to relieve pain in rheumatic and related diseases. It is administered by mouth or injection; common side-effects include digestive upsets, rashes, and fluid retention. Trade names: **Butazolidin**, **Butazone**, **Flexazone**.

phenylephrine *n.* a drug that constricts blood vessels (*see* sympathomimetic). It is given by injection to increase blood pressure, in a nasal spray to relieve nasal congestion, and in eye-drops to dilate the pupils. Irritation may occur when applied. Trade name: **Neophryn**.

phenylketonuria *n.* an inborn defect of protein metabolism causing an excess of the amino acid phenylalanine in the blood, which damages the nervous system and leads to severe mental retardation. Screening of newborn infants by testing a blood sample for phenylalanine (the *Guthrie test*) enables the condition to be detected soon enough for dietary treatment to prevent any brain damage: the baby's diet contains proteins from which phenylalanine has been removed. The gene responsible for phenylketonuria is recessive, so that a child is affected only if both parents are carriers of the defective gene.

phenylpropanolamine *n.* a drug with actions similar to those of *ephedrine. It is used to relieve allergic conditions, such as asthma and hay fever, and nasal congestion, and is administered by mouth, injection, or by inhalation. Side-effects may include dizziness, headache, digestive disorders, sweating, and thirst.

phenylthiocarbamide (PTC) *n.* a substance that tastes bitter to some individuals but is tasteless to others. Response to PTC appears to be controlled by a single pair of genes (*alleles): ability to taste PTC is *dominant to the inability to taste it.

phenytoin *n.* an *anticonvulsant drug used to control major (grand mal) and focal fits. It is administered by mouth or injection; the side-effects include gum hypertrophy, hirsutism, and skin rashes. Overdosage causes unsteadiness. Trade name: **Epanutin**.

phial

phial *n.* a small glass bottle for storing medicines or poisons.

-philia *suffix denoting* morbid craving or attraction. Example: *nyctophilia* (for darkness).

phimosis *n.* narrowing of the opening of the foreskin, which cannot therefore be drawn back over the underlying glans penis. This predisposes to inflammation (*see* balanitis, balanoposthitis), which results in further narrowing. Treatment is by surgical removal of the foreskin (*circumcision).

phleb- (phlebo-) *prefix denoting* a vein or veins. Example: *phlebectopia* (abnormal position of).

phlebectomy *n.* the surgical removal of a vein (or part of a vein), sometimes performed for the treatment of varicose veins in the legs (*varicectomy*).

phlebitis *n.* inflammation of the wall of a vein, which is most commonly seen in the legs as a complication of *varicose veins. A segment of vein becomes painful and tender and the surrounding skin feels hot and appears red. Thrombosis (*thrombophlebitis*) commonly develops. Treatment consists of elastic support together with drugs, such as phenylbutazone, to relieve the inflammation and pain. Anticoagulants are not used (*compare* phlebothrombosis). Phlebitis may also complicate sepsis (*see* pylephlebitis) or cancer, especially of the stomach, bronchus, or pancreas. In pancreatic cancer the phlebitis may affect a variety of veins (*thrombophlebitis migrans*).

phlebography *n. see* venography.

phlebolith *n.* a stone-like structure, usually found incidentally on abdominal X-ray, that results from deposition of calcium in a venous blood clot. It appears as a small round white opacity in the pelvic region. It does not produce symptoms and requires no treatment.

phlebosclerosis (venosclerosis) *n.* a rare degenerative condition, of unknown cause, that affects the leg veins of young men. The vein walls become thickened and feel like cords under the skin. It is not related to arteriosclerosis and needs no treatment.

phlebothrombosis *n.* obstruction of a vein by a blood clot, without preceding inflammation of its wall. It is most common within the deep veins of the calf of the leg (in contrast to thrombophlebitis, which affects superficial leg veins (*see* phlebitis)). Prolonged bed rest, heart failure, pregnancy, injury, and surgery predispose to thrombosis by encouraging sluggish blood flow. Many of these conditions are associated with changes in the clotting factors in the blood that increase the tendency to thrombosis; these changes also occur in some women taking oral contraceptives.

The affected leg may become swollen and tender. The main danger is that the clot may become detached and give rise to *pulmonary embolism. Regular leg exercises help to prevent phlebothrombosis, and anticoagulant drugs (such as warfarin and heparin) are used in prevention and treatment. Large clots may be removed surgically in the operation of *thrombectomy* to relieve leg swelling.

Phlebotomus *n. see* sandfly.

phlebotomy (venesection) *n.* the surgical opening or puncture of a vein in order to remove blood (in the treatment of *polycythaemia) or to infuse fluids, blood, or drugs in the treatment of many conditions. It may also be required for cardiac *catheterization and *angiocardiography.

phlegm *n.* a nonmedical term for *sputum.

phlegmon *n. Archaic.* inflammation of connective tissue, leading to ulceration.

phlycten *n.* a small pinkish-yellow nodule surrounded by a zone of dilated blood vessels that occurs in the conjunctiva or in the cornea. It develops into a small ulcer that heals without trace in the conjunctiva but produces some residual scarring in the cornea. Phlyctens, which are prone to recur, are thought to be due to a type of allergy to the tubercle bacillus.

phobia *n.* a pathologically strong *fear of a particular event or thing. Avoiding the feared situation may severely restrict one's life and cause much suffering. The main kinds of phobia are *specific phobias*, (isolated fears of particular things, such as sharp knives); *agoraphobia; *social phobias* of encountering people; and *animal phobias*, as of spiders, rats, or dogs (*see also* preparedness). Treatment is with behaviour therapy, especially *desensitization and *flooding. *Psychotherapy and drug therapy are also useful.

-phobia *suffix denoting* morbid fear or dread.

phocomelia *n.* congenital absence of the upper arm and/or upper leg, the hands or feet or both being attached to the trunk by a short stump. The condition is extremely rare except as a side-effect of the drug *thalidomide taken during early pregnancy.

pholcodine *n.* a drug that suppresses coughs and reduces irritation in the respiratory system (*see* antitussive). It is administered by mouth in cough mixtures and sometimes causes nausea and drowsiness.

phon *n.* a unit of loudness of sound. The intensity of a sound to be measured is compared by the human ear to a reference tone of 2×10^{-5} pascal sound pressure and 1000 hertz frequency. The intensity of the reference tone is increased until it appears to be equal in loudness to the sound being measured; the loudness of this sound in phons is then equal to the number of decibels by which the reference tone has had to be increased.

phon- (phono-) *prefix denoting* sound or voice.

phonasthenia *n.* weakness of the voice, especially when due to fatigue.

phonation *n.* the production of vocal sounds, particularly speech.

phonocardiogram *n. see* electrocardiophonography. —**phonocardiography** *n.*

-phoria *suffix denoting* (in ophthalmology) an abnormal deviation of the eyes or turning of the visual axis. Example: *heterophoria* (tendency to squint).

Phormia *n.* a genus of non-bloodsucking flies, commonly known as blowflies. The maggot of *P. regina* normally breeds in decaying meat but it has occasionally been found in suppurating wounds, giving rise to a type of *myiasis.

phosgene *n.* a poisonous gas developed during World War I. It is a choking agent, acting on the lungs to produce *oedema, with consequent respiratory and cardiac failure.

phosphagen *n.* creatine phosphate (*see* creatine).

phosphataemia *n.* the presence of phosphates in the blood. Sodium, calcium, potassium, and magnesium phosphates are normal constituents.

phosphatase *n.* one of a group of enzymes capable of catalysing the hydrolysis of phosphoric acid esters. An example is glucose-6-phosphatase, which catalyses the hydrolysis of glucose-6-phosphate to glucose and phosphate. Phosphatases are important in the absorption and metabolism of carbohydrates, nucleotides, and phospholipids and are essential in the calcification of bone. *Acid phosphatase* is present in kidney, semen, serum, and the prostate gland. *Alkaline phosphatase* occurs in teeth, developing bone, plasma, kidney, and intestine.

phosphatidylcholine *n. see* lecithin.

phosphatidylserine *n.* a cephalin-like phospholipid containing the amino acid serine. It is found in brain tissue. *See also* cephalin.

phosphaturia (phosphuria) *n.* the presence of an abnormally high concentration of phosphates in the urine, making it cloudy. The condition may be associated with the formation of stones (calculi) in the kidneys or bladder.

phosphocreatine *n.* creatine phosphate (*see* creatine).

phosphofructokinase *n.* an enzyme that catalyses the conversion of fructose-6-phosphate to fructose-1,6-diphosphate. This is an important reaction occurring during the process of *glycolysis.

phospholipid *n.* a *lipid containing a phosphate group as part of the molecule. Phospholipids are constituents of all tissues and organs, especially the brain. They are synthesized in the liver and small intestine and are involved in many of the body's metabolic processes. Examples are *cephalins, *lecithins, plasmalogens, and phosphatidylserine.

phosphonecrosis *n.* the destruction of tissues caused by excessive amounts of phosphorus in the system. The tissues likely to suffer in phosphorus poisoning are the liver, kidneys, muscles, bones, and the cardiovascular system.

phosphorus *n.* a nonmetallic element. Phosphorus compounds are major constituents in the tissues of both plants and animals. In man, phosphorus is mostly concentrated in *bone. However, certain phosphorus-containing compounds – for example adenosine triphosphate (*ATP) and *creatine

phosphate – play an important part in energy conversions and storage in the body. In a pure state, phosphorus is toxic.

phosphorylase *n.* any enzyme that catalyses the combination of an organic molecule (usually glucose) with a phosphate group (phosphorylation). Phosphorylase is found in the liver and kidney, where it is involved in the breakdown of glycogen to glucose-1-phosphate.

phot- (photo-) *prefix denoting* light.

photalgia *n.* pain in the eye caused by very bright light.

photocoagulation *n.* the destruction of tissue by heat released from the absorption of light shone on it. In eye disorders the technique is used to destroy diseased retinal tissue, occurring, for example, as a complication of diabetes; and to produce scarring between the retina and choroid, thus binding them together, in cases of *detached retina. Several instruments are available for producing the intense light needed; the principle is similar when lasers are used.

photodermatitis *n.* a condition in which the skin becomes sensitized to a substance (certain antiseptics used in soaps may be a trigger) but only those parts of the skin subsequently exposed to light react by developing *dermatitis.

photomicrograph *n.* an enlarged photographic record of an object taken through an optical or electron microscope. *Compare* microphotograph.

photophobia *n.* an abnormal intolerance of light, in which exposure to light produces intense discomfort of the eyes with tight contraction of the eyelids and other reactions aimed at avoiding the light. In most cases the light simply aggravates already existing discomfort from eye disease. Photophobia may be associated with dilation of the pupils as a result of drug administration or with migraine, measles, German measles, or meningitis.

photophthalmia *n.* inflammation of the eye due to exposure to light. It is usually caused by the damaging effect of ultraviolet light on the cornea, for example in snow blindness.

photopic *adj.* relating to or describing conditions of bright illumination. For example, *photopic vision* is vision in bright light, in which the *cones of the retina are responsible for visual sensation. —**photopia** *n.*

photopsia *n.* the sensation of flashes of light caused by irritation of the retina of the eye, usually due to inflammation or slight movements of the retina.

photoretinitis *n.* damage to the retina of the eye caused by looking at the sun without adequate protection for the eyes. The retina may be burnt by the intense light focused on it; this affects the central part of the visual field, which may be permanently lost (*sun blindness*).

photosensitivity *n.* abnormal and severe reaction of the skin to sunlight. —**photosensitive** *adj.*

photosynthesis *n.* the process whereby green plants and some bacteria manufacture carbohydrates from carbon dioxide and water, using energy absorbed from sunlight by the green pigment chlorophyll. In green plants this complex process may be summarized thus:

$$6CO_2 + 6H_2O \rightarrow C_6H_{12}O_6 + 6O_2$$

phototaxis *n.* movement of a cell or organism in response to a stimulus of light.

photuria *n.* the excretion of phosphorescent urine, which glows in the dark, due to the presence of certain phosphorus-containing compounds derived from phosphates.

phren- (phreno-) *prefix denoting* **1.** the mind or brain. **2.** the diaphragm. **3.** the phrenic nerve.

phrenemphraxis (phreniclasia) *n.* surgical crushing of a portion of the *phrenic nerve. This paralyses the diaphragm on the side operated upon, which is then pushed up by the abdominal contents, so pressing on the lung and partially collapsing it. Deliberate collapsing of the lung was a technique formerly used in the treatment of pulmonary tuberculosis.

-phrenia *suffix denoting* a condition of the mind. Example: *hebephrenia* (schizophrenia affecting young adults).

phrenic avulsion the surgical removal of a section of the *phrenic nerve, which paralyses the diaphragm. The procedure was used as a means of resting a lung infected with tuberculosis.

phrenicectomy *n.* surgical division or removal of part of the phrenic nerve. Partial removal of the nerve produces the same results as *phrenemphraxis and division (phrenicotomy); it is done because the nerve sometimes regenerates after the other procedures.

phreniclasia *n. see* phrenemphraxis.

phrenic nerve the nerve that supplies the muscles of the diaphragm. On each side it arises in the neck from the third, fourth, and fifth cervical spinal roots and passes downwards between the lungs and the heart to reach the diaphragm. Impulses through the nerves from the brain bring about the regular contractions of the diaphragm during breathing.

phrenology *n.* the study of the bumps on the outside of the skull in order to determine a person's character. It is based on the mistaken theory that the skull becomes modified over the different functional areas of the cortex of the brain.

phthiriasis *n.* infestation of the crab louse, *Phthirus pubis*, which causes intense itching; continued scratching by the patient may result in bacterial infection of the skin. Phthiriasis can be treated with applications containing gamma benzene hexachloride.

Phthirus *n.* a widely distributed genus of lice. The crab (or pubic) louse, *P. pubis*, is a common parasite of man that lives permanently attached to the body hair, particularly that of the pubic or perianal regions but also on the eyelashes and the hairs in the armpits. Crab lice are not known to transmit disease but their bites can irritate the skin (*see* phthiriasis). An infestation may be acquired during sexual intercourse or from hairs left on clothing, towels, and lavatory seats.

phthisis *n.* a former name for: **1.** any disease resulting in wasting of tissues; **2.** pulmonary *tuberculosis.

phycomycosis *n.* a disease caused by parasitic fungi of the genera *Rhizopus*, *Absidia*, and *Mucor*. The disease affects the sinuses, the central nervous system, the lungs, and the skin tissues. The fungi are able to grow within the blood vessels of the lungs and nervous tissue, thus causing blood clots which cut off the blood supply (*see* infarction). Treatment with the antibiotic *amphotericin has proved effective.

phylogenesis *n.* the evolutionary history of a species or individual.

physi- (physio-) *prefix denoting* **1.** physiology. **2.** physical.

physical *adj.* (in medicine) relating to the body rather than to the mind. For example, a *physical sign* is one that a doctor can detect when examining a patient, such as abnormal dilation of the pupils or the absence of a knee-jerk reflex (*see also* functional disorder, organic disorder).

physical medicine a medical specialty established by the Royal Society of Medicine in 1931. Initially the members pioneered clinics devoted to the diagnosis and management of rheumatic diseases, but later extended their interests to the *rehabilitation of patients with physical disabilities ranging from asthma and hand injuries to back trouble and poliomyelitis. The term has caused confusion in recent years, with many doctors preferring the description *rheumatology and rehabilitation* for this specialist activity. Since 1972, however, when the Royal College of Physicians approved it, physical medicine has become the generally accepted term. *See also* rheumatology.

physician *n.* a registered medical practitioner who specializes in the diagnosis and treatment of disease by other than surgical means. In the USA the term is applied to any authorized medical practitioner. *See also* Doctor.

physiological solution one of a group of solutions used to maintain tissues in a viable state. These solutions contain specific concentrations of substances that are vital for normal tissue function (e.g. sodium, potassium, calcium, chloride, magnesium, bicarbonate, and phosphate ions, glucose, and oxygen). An example of such a solution is *Ringer's solution.

physiology *n.* the science of the functioning of living organisms and of their component parts. —**physiological** *adj.* —**physiologist** *n.*

physiotherapy *n.* the branch of treatment that employs physical methods to promote healing, including the use of light, infrared and ultraviolet rays, heat, electric current, massage, manipulation, and remedial exercise.

physo- *prefix denoting* air or gas.

physostigmine (eserine) *n.* a *parasympathomimetic drug used mainly to constrict the pupil of the eye and to reduce pressure inside the eye in glaucoma. It is administered by injection, in eye-drops, or in an ointment; side-effects include digestive upsets and salivation.

phyt- (phyto-) *prefix denoting* plants; of plant origin.

phytomenadione *n.* a form of *vitamin K occurring naturally in green plants but usually synthesized for use as an antidote to overdosage with anticoagulant drugs. It promotes the production of prothrombin, essential for the normal coagulation of blood.

phytophotodermatitis *n.* an eruption of large blisters occurring after exposure to light in people who have been in contact with certain plants, such as wild parsnip or cow parsley, to which they are sensitive.

phytotoxin *n.* any poisonous substance (toxin) produced by a plant, such as any of the toxins produced by fungi of the genus *Amanita.

pia (pia mater) *n.* the innermost of the three *meninges surrounding the brain and spinal cord. The membrane is closely attached to the surface of the brain and spinal cord, faithfully following each fissure and sulcus. It contains numerous finely branching blood vessels that supply the nerve tissue within. The subarachnoid space separates it from the arachnoid.

pian *n. see* yaws.

pica *n.* the indiscriminate eating of non-nutritious or harmful substances, such as grass, stones, or clothing. It is common in early childhood but may also be found in mentally handicapped and psychotic patients. Although thought to be completely nonadaptive, recent evidence suggests that some patients showing pica may have particular mineral deficiencies (such as iron deficiency).

Pick's disease a rare cause of dementia in middle-aged people. The damage is mainly in the frontal and temporal lobes of the brain, in contrast with the diffuse degeneration of *Alzheimer's disease.

pico- *prefix denoting* one million-millionth (10^{-12}).

picornavirus *n.* one of a group of small RNA-containing viruses (pico = small; hence pico-RNA-virus). The group includes *Coxsackie viruses, *echoviruses, *polioviruses, and *rhinoviruses.

picric acid (trinitrophenol) a yellow crystalline solid used as a dye and as a tissue *fixative.

piedra *n.* a fungal disease of the hair in which the hair shafts carry hard masses of black or white fungus. The black fungus, *Piedraia hortai*, is found mainly in the tropics and the white variety, *Trichosporon cutaneum*, in temperate regions.

pigeon chest forward protrusion of the breastbone resulting in deformity of the chest. The condition is painless and harmless.

pigeon toes an abnormal posture in which the toes are turned inwards. It is often associated with *knock-knee.

pigment *n.* a substance giving colour. Physiologically important pigments include the blood pigments (especially *haemoglobin), *bile pigments, and retinal pigment (*see* rhodopsin). The pigment *melanin occurs in the skin and in the iris of the eye. Important plant pigments include *chlorophyll and the *carotenoids.

pigmentation *n.* coloration produced in the body by the deposition of one pigment, especially in excessive amounts. Pigmentation may be produced by natural pigments, such as bile pigments (as in jaundice) or melanin, or by foreign material, such as lead or arsenic in chronic poisoning.

piles *n. see* haemorrhoids.

pili (fimbriae) *pl. n.* (*sing.* **pilus, fimbria**) hairlike processes present on the surface of certain bacteria. They are thought to be involved in adhesion of bacteria to other cells and in transfer of DNA during *conjugation.

pill *n.* **1.** a small round ball, sometimes coated with sugar, that contains one or more medicinal substances in solid form. It is taken by mouth. **2. the Pill** *see* oral contraceptive.

pillar *n.* (in anatomy) an elongated apparently supportive structure. For example, the *pillars of the fauces* are folds of mucous membrane on either side of the opening from the mouth to the pharynx.

pilo- *prefix denoting* hair. Example: *pilosis* (excessive development of).

pilocarpine *n.* a drug with actions and uses similar to those of *physostigmine. It is administered as eye-drops and may cause digestive upsets and salivation if absorbed into the system.

pilomotor nerves sympathetic nerves that supply muscle fibres in the skin, around the roots of hairs. Activity of the sympathetic nervous system causes the muscles to contract, raising the hairs and giving the 'gooseflesh' effect of fear or cold.

pilonidal sinus a short tract leading from an opening in the skin in or near the cleft at the top of the buttocks and containing hairs. The sinus may be recurrently infected, leading to pain and the discharge of pus. Treatment is by surgical opening and cleaning of the sinus.

pilosebaceous *adj.* relating to the hair follicles and their associated sebaceous glands.

pilus *n.* a hair. *See also* pili.

pimel- (pimelo-) *prefix denoting* fat; fatty.

pimozide *n.* a major *tranquillizer used to relieve hallucinations and delusions occurring in schizophrenia. It is administered by mouth; side-effects may include skin rashes, tremors, and abnormal movements. Trade name: **Orap**.

pimple *n.* a small inflamed swelling on the skin that contains pus. It may be the result of bacterial infection of a skin pore that has become obstructed with fatty secretions from the sebaceous glands. Pimples occurring in large numbers on the chest, back, and face are usually described as *acne, a common condition of adolescence.

pincement *n.* one of the techniques used in massage, in which pinches of the patient's flesh are taken between finger and thumb and twisted or rolled before release. This is said to improve the tone of the skin, improve circulation, and alleviate underlying pain.

pineal body (pineal gland) a pea-sized mass of tissue attached by a stalk to the posterior wall of the third ventricle of the brain, deep between the cerebral hemispheres at the back of the skull. It may play a part in initiating the development of the gonads, but this is uncertain; in other mammals it secretes the hormone-like substance *melatonin*. The gland becomes calcified as age progresses, providing a useful landmark in X-rays of the skull. Anatomical name: **epiphysis**.

pinguecula *n.* a degenerative change in the conjunctiva of the eye, seen most commonly in the elderly and in those who live in hot dry climates. Thickened yellow triangles develop on the conjunctiva at the inner and outer margins of the cornea.

pink disease a severe illness of children of the teething age, marked by pink cold clammy hands and feet, heavy sweating, raised blood pressure, rapid pulse, photophobia, loss of appetite, and insomnia. It has been suggested that the condition is an allergic reaction to mercury, since it used to occur when teething powders, lotions, and ointments containing mercury were used. Although there is no definite proof of this, the disease has virtually disappeared since all mercury-containing paediatric preparations have been banned. Medical names: **acrodynia**, **erythroedema**, **erythromelalgia**.

pink eye *see* conjunctivitis.

pinna (auricle) *n.* the flap of skin and cartilage that projects from the head at the exterior opening of the external auditory meatus of the *ear (see illustration). In man the pinna is largely vestigial but it may be partly concerned with detecting the direction of sound sources.

The pinna

pinocytosis *n.* the intake of small droplets of fluid by a cell by cytoplasmic engulfment. It occurs in many white blood cells and in certain kidney and liver cells. *Compare* phagocytosis.

pinta *n.* a skin disease, prevalent in tropical America, that seems to affect only the dark-skinned races. It is caused by the *spirochaete *Treponema carateum*, a microorganism similar to those causing *yaws and *syphilis. The disease is thought to be transmitted either by direct contact between individuals or by flies that carry the infective

spirochaetes on their bodies. Symptoms include thickening and eventual loss of pigment of the skin, particularly on the hands, wrists, feet, and ankles. Pinta is rarely disabling or fatal and is treated successfully with *penicillin.

pinworm (threadworm) *n.* a parasitic nematode worm of the genus *Enterobius* (*Oxyuris*), which lives in the upper part of the large intestine of man. The threadlike female worm, some 12 mm long, is larger than the male; it emerges from the anus in the evening to deposit its eggs, and later dies. If the eggs are swallowed by man and reach the intestine they develop directly into adult worms. Pinworms cause *enterobiasis, a disease common in children throughout the world.

piperazine *n.* a drug used to treat infestations by roundworms and threadworms. It is administered by mouth; side-effects do not usually occur, but continued treatment at high doses may cause nausea, vomiting, headache, tingling sensations, and rashes. Trade names: **Antepar**, **Pripsen**.

piperidolate *n.* a drug, similar to *atropine, used to treat colic and other conditions involving spasm of the stomach and intestine. It is administered by mouth. Trade name: **Dactil**.

piriform fossae two pear-shaped depressions that lie on either side of the opening to the larynx.

pisiform bone the smallest bone of the wrist (*carpus): a pea-shaped bone that articulates with the triquetral bone and, indirectly by cartilage, with the ulna.

pit *n.* (in anatomy) a hollow or depression, such as any of the depressions on the surface of an embryo marking the site of future organs.

pithiatism *n.* the treatment of certain disorders by persuading the patient that all is well. Disorders that disappear in these circumstances are regarded as manifestations of psychological disturbance and are classified as hysterical disorders.

pithing *n.* the laboratory procedure in which a part or the whole of the central nervous system of an experimental animal (such as a frog) is destroyed, usually by inserting a probe through the foramen magnum, in preparation for physiological or pharmacological experiments.

pitting *n.* the formation of depressed scars, as occurs on the skin following smallpox or acne. *Pitting oedema* is swelling of the tissues due to excess fluid in which fingertip pressure leaves temporary indentations in the skin.

pituicyte *n.* a type of cell found in the posterior lobe of the pituitary gland, similar in appearance to an *astrocyte, with numerous fine branches that end in contact with the lining membrane of the blood channels in the gland.

pituitary gland (hypophysis) the master endocrine gland: a pea-sized body attached beneath the *hypothalamus in a bony cavity at the base of the skull. It has an anterior lobe (*adenohypophysis*), which secretes *thyroid-stimulating hormone, *ACTH (adrenocorticotrophic hormone), *gonadotrophins, *growth hormone, *prolactin, *lipotrophin, and *melanocyte-stimulating hormone. The secretion of all these hormones is regulated by specific *hormone releasing factors*, which are produced in the hypothalamus. The posterior lobe (*neurohypophysis*) secretes *vasopressin and *oxytocin, which are synthesized in the hypothalamus and transported to the pituitary, where they are stored before release.

pityriasis *n.* (originally) any of a group of skin diseases typified by the development of fine branlike scales. The term is now used only with a modifying adjective. For instance, *pityriasis rosea* is a common skin complaint, of unknown

cause, in which flat pink oval spots (macules) develop on the trunk and upper parts of the limbs. It occurs mainly in young people in spring and autumn and typically starts with a localized patch of spots that precedes the general eruption by about seven days. *Pityriasis alba* is a very common condition in children and adolescents in which uneven round pale macules appear on the face. This disease may persist until adulthood. *See also* dandruff (pityriasis capitis), liver spot.

pivot joint *see* trochoid joint.

placebo *n.* a medicine that is ineffective but may help to relieve a condition because the patient has faith in its powers. New drugs are tested against placebos in clinical trials: the drug's effect is compared with the *placebo response*, which occurs even in the absence of any pharmacologically active substance in the placebo.

placenta *n.* an organ within the uterus (womb) by means of which the embryo is attached to the wall of the uterus. Its primary function is to provide the embryo with nourishment, eliminate its wastes, and exchange respiratory gases. This is accomplished by the close proximity of the maternal and fetal blood systems within the placenta. It also functions as a gland, secreting *chorionic gonadotrophin, *progesterone, and oestrogens, which regulate the maintenance of pregnancy. *See also* afterbirth. —**placental** *adj.*

placenta praevia the attachment of the placenta to the lower part of the womb (instead of to the upper part, as is normal). As it grows, the placenta may partially or completely cover the outlet from the womb to the vagina. Slight bleeding may occur from about the seventh month of pregnancy, and anaemia may develop. Childbirth may be made difficult because the placenta hinders the movement of the infant through the vagina and delivery by Caesarean section may be necessary.

placentography *n.* *radiography of the pregnant womb in order to determine the position of the *placenta. *See also* placenta praevia.

placode *n.* any of the thickened areas of ectoderm in the embryo that will develop into nerve ganglia or the special sensory structures of the eye, ear, or nose.

plagiocephaly *n.* any distortion or lack of symmetry in the shape of the head, usually due to irregularity in the closure of the sutures between the bones of the skull.

plague *n.* **1.** any epidemic disease with a high death rate. **2.** an acute epidemic disease of rats and other wild rodents caused by the bacterium *Pasteurella pestis*, which is transmitted to man by rat fleas. *Bubonic plague*, the most common form of the disease, has an incubation period of 2–6 days. Headache, fever, weakness, aching limbs, and delirium develop and are followed by acute painful swellings of the lymph nodes (*see* bubo). In favourable cases the buboes burst after about a week, releasing pus, and then heal. In other cases bleeding under the skin, producing black patches, can lead to ulcers, which may prove fatal (hence the former name *Black Death*). In the most serious cases bacteria enter the bloodstream (*septicaemic plague*) or lungs (*pneumonic plague*); if untreated, these are nearly always fatal. Treatment with tetracycline, streptomycin, and chloramphenicol is effective; vaccination against the disease provides only partial protection.

plane *n.* a level or smooth surface, especially any of the hypothetical flat surfaces – orientated in various directions – used to divide the body; for example, the *coronal and *sagittal planes.

planoconcave *adj.* describing a structure, such as a lens, that is flat on one side and concave on the other.

planoconvex *adj.* describing a structure, such as a lens, that is flat on one side and convex on the other.

plantar *adj.* relating to the sole of the foot (*planta*). *See also* flexion.

plantar arch the arch in the sole of the foot formed by anastomosing branches of the plantar arteries.

plantar reflex a reflex obtained by drawing a bluntly pointed object along the outer border of the sole of the foot from the heel to the little toe. The normal *flexor response* is a bunching and downward movement of the toes. An upward movement of the great toe is called an *extensor response* (or *Babinski reflex*). In all persons over the age of 18 months this is a sensitive indication of disease in the brain or spinal cord.

plantar wart a wart occurring in the skin on the sole of the foot, usually at the base of the toes. *See* wart.

plantigrade *adj.* walking on the entire sole of the foot: a habit of man and some animals.

plaque *n.* **1.** a layer that forms on the surface of a tooth, principally at its neck, composed of bacteria in an organic matrix. Under certain conditions the plaque may cause *gingivitis, *periodontal disease, or *dental caries. The purpose of oral hygiene is to remove plaque. **2.** a raised circular patch of skin or mucous membrane resulting from local damage, usually due to infection.

-plasia *suffix denoting* formation; development. Example: *hyperplasia* (excessive tissue formation).

plasm- (plasmo-) *prefix denoting* **1.** blood plasma. **2.** protoplasm or cytoplasm.

plasma (blood plasma) *n.* the straw-coloured fluid in which the blood cells are suspended. It consists of a solution of various inorganic salts of sodium, potassium, calcium, etc., with a high concentration of protein (approximately 70 g/1) and a variety of trace substances.

plasmacytoma *n.* a malignant tumour of plasma cells, very closely allied to *myeloma. It usually occurs as a solitary tumour of bone, but may be multiple. Less frequently it affects soft tissues, usually the upper air passages. All of these tumours may produce the abnormal gamma globulins that are characteristic of myeloma, and they may progress to widespread myeloma. The soft-tissue tumours often respond to radiotherapy and to such drugs as melphalan and cyclophosphamide; the bone tumours are less responsive. Tumours originating in soft tissue may spread to bone, producing an appearance on X-ray identical to myeloma deposits; these secondary growths often resolve completely after radiological treatment.

plasmalogen *n.* a phospholipid, found in brain and muscle, similar in structure to *lecithin and *cephalin.

plasmapheresis *n.* a method of removing a quantity of plasma from the blood. Blood is withdrawn from the patient and allowed to settle in a container. The plasma is drawn off the top of the blood, and the blood cells are then transfused back into the patient.

plasmidotrophoblast (syncytiotrophoblast) *n.* that part of the *trophoblast that loses its cellular structure and becomes a *syncytium. This is the invasive part of the trophoblast, which erodes the maternal tissues and forms the villi of the placenta.

plasmin (fibrinolysin) *n.* an enzyme that digests the protein fibrin. Its function is the dissolution of blood clots (*see* fibrinolysis). Plasmin is not normally present in the blood but exists as an inactive precursor, *plasminogen*.

plasminogen *n.* a substance normally present in the blood plasma that may be activated to form *plasmin. *See* fibrinolysis.

Plasmodium *n.* a genus of protozoans (*see* Sporozoa) that live as parasites within the red blood cells and liver cells of man. The parasite undergoes its asexual development (*see* schizogony) in man and completes the sexual phase of its development (*see* sporogony) in the stomach and digestive glands of a bloodsucking *Anopheles* mosquito. Four species cause *malaria in man: *P. vivax*, *P. ovale*, *P. falciparum*, and *P. malariae*.

plasmolysis *n.* a process occurring in bacteria and plants in which the protoplasm shrinks away from the rigid cell wall when the cell is placed in a *hypertonic solution. This is due to withdrawal of water from the cell by *osmosis.

plaster *n.* adhesive tape used in shaped pieces or as a bandage to keep a dressing in place.

plaster model (in dentistry) an accurate cast of the teeth and jaws made from modified plaster of Paris. A pair of models are used to study the dentition, particularly before treatment. Models are also used to construct dentures, orthodontic appliances, or such restorations as crowns.

plaster of Paris a preparation of gypsum (calcium sulphate) that sets hard when water is added. It is used in various modified forms in dentistry to make *plaster models. It is also used in orthopaedics for preparing plaster *casts.

plastic lymph a transparent yellowish liquid produced in a wound or other site of inflammation, in which connective tissue cells and blood vessels develop during healing.

plastic surgery a branch of surgery dealing with the reconstruction of deformed or damaged parts of the body. It also includes the replacement of parts of the body that have been lost. If performed simply to improve appearances plastic surgery is called *cosmetic surgery*, but most plastic surgery involves the treatment and repair of burns or accidents and the correction of congenital defects, such as harelip and cleft palate.

plastron *n.* the breastbone (*sternum) together with the costal cartilages attached to it.

-plasty *suffix denoting* plastic surgery. Example: *labioplasty* (of the lips).

platelet (thrombocyte) *n.* a disc-shaped structure, 1–2 μm in diameter, present in the blood. With *Romanowsky stains platelets appear as fragments of pale-blue cytoplasm with a few red granules. They have several functions, all relating to the arrest of bleeding (*see* blood coagulation). There are normally 150–400 × 10^9 platelets per litre of blood. *See also* thrombopoiesis.

platy- *prefix denoting* broad or flat.

platyhelminth *n. see* flatworm.

platysma *n.* a broad thin sheet of muscle that extends from below the collar bone to the angle of the jaw. It depresses the corner of the mouth.

pledget *n.* a small wad of dressing material, such as lint, used either to cover a wound or sore or as a plug.

-plegia *suffix denoting* paralysis. Example: *hemiplegia* (of one side of the body).

pleio- (pleo-) *prefix denoting* 1. multiple. 2. excessive.

pleiotropy *n.* a situation in which a single gene is responsible for more than

one effect in the *phenotype. The mutation of such a gene will therefore have multiple effects. —**pleiotropic** *adj.*

pleocytosis *n.* the presence of an abnormally large number of lymphocytes in the cerebrospinal fluid, which bathes the brain and spinal cord.

pleomastia (polymastia) *n.* multiple breasts or nipples. These are usually symmetrically arranged along a line between the mid point of the collar bone and the pelvis (the nipple line).

pleomorphism *n.* the condition in which an individual assumes a number of different forms during its life cycle. The malarial parasite (*Plasmodium*) displays pleomorphism.

pleoptics *n.* special techniques practised by orthoptists (*see* orthoptics) for developing normal function of the macula (the most sensitive part of the retina), in people whose macular function has previously been disturbed because of strabismus (squint).

plerocercoid *n.* a larval stage of certain tapeworms, such as *Diphyllobothrium latum*. It differs from the *cysticercus (another larval form) in being solid and in lacking a cyst or bladder.

plessimeter (pleximeter) *n.* a small plate of bone, ivory, or other material pressed against the surface of the body and struck with a *plessor in the technique of *percussion.

plessor (plexor) *n.* a small hammer used to investigate nervous reflexes and in the technique of *percussion.

plethora *n.* any excess of any bodily fluid, especially blood (*see* hyperaemia). —**plethoric** *adj.*

plethysmography *n.* the process of recording the changes in the volume of a limb caused by alterations in blood pressure. The limb is inserted into a fluid-filled watertight casing (*oncom-*

eter) and the pressure variations in the fluid are recorded.

pleur- (pleuro-) *prefix denoting* **1.** the pleura. **2.** the side of the body.

pleura *n.* the covering of the lungs (*visceral pleura*) and of the inner surface of the chest wall (*parietal pleura*). (See illustration.) The covering consists of a closed sac of *serous membrane, which has a smooth shiny moist surface due to the secretion of small amounts of fluid. This fluid lubricates the opposing visceral and parietal surfaces so that they can slide painlessly over each other during breathing. —**pleural** *adj.*

parietal pleura
pleural cavity
chest wall
visceral pleura
diaphragm

The pleura

pleuracentesis *n. see* pleurocentesis.

pleural cavity the space between the visceral and parietal *pleura, which is normally very small as the pleural membranes are in close contact. The introduction of fluid (*pleural effusion*) or gas separates the pleural surfaces and increases the volume of the pleural space.

pleurectomy *n.* surgical removal of part of the *pleura, which is sometimes done to overcome recurrent *pneumothorax or to remove diseased areas of pleura.

pleurisy *n.* inflammation of the *pleura, usually due to pneumonia in the underlying lung. The normally shiny and slippery pleural surfaces lose their sheen and become slightly sticky, so that there is pain on deep breathing and a characteristic 'rub' can be heard

through a stethoscope. Pleurisy is always associated with some other disease in the lung, chest wall, diaphragm, or abdomen.

pleurocele *n.* herniation of the pleura. *See* hernia.

pleurocentesis (pleuracentesis, thoracentesis, thoracocentesis) *n.* insertion of a hollow needle into the *pleural cavity through the chest wall in order to withdraw fluid, blood, pus, or air.

pleurodesis *n.* the artificial production of pleurisy by chemical or mechanical means to obliterate the *pleural cavity, in order to prevent recurrent, usually malignant, pleural effusions.

pleurodynia *n.* severe paroxysmal pain arising from the muscles between the ribs. It is often thought to be of rheumatic origin.

pleurolysis (pneumolysis) *n.* surgical stripping of the parietal *pleura from the chest wall to allow the lung to collapse. The procedure was used in the days before effective antituberculous drugs to help tuberculosis to heal.

pleuropneumonia *n.* inflammation involving both the lung and pleura. *See* pleurisy, pneumonia.

pleuropneumonia-like organisms (PPLO) *n. see* mycoplasma.

pleurotomy *n.* surgical incision of the pleura. *See* pleurectomy.

pleurotyphoid *n.* *typhoid fever involving the lungs.

pleximeter *n. see* plessimeter.

plexor *n. see* plessor.

plexus *n.* a network of nerves or blood vessels. *See* brachial plexus.

plica *n.* a fold of tissue; for example, the *plica sublingualis*, the mucous fold in the floor of the mouth. —**plicate** *adj.*

plication *n.* a surgical technique in which the size of a hollow organ is reduced by taking tucks or folds in the walls.

plombage *n.* **1.** a technique used in surgery for the correction of a *detached retina. A small piece of silicone plastic is sewn on the outside of the eyeball to produce an indentation over the region where a retinal hole has been found. **2.** the insertion of plastic balls into the pleural cavity to cause collapse of the lung. This was done in the days before effective antituberculous drugs to help tuberculosis to heal.

plumbism *n.* lead poisoning. *See* lead¹.

pluri- *prefix denoting* more than one; several.

pneo- *prefix denoting* breathing; respiration.

pneum- (pneumo-) *prefix denoting* **1.** the presence of air or gas. Example: *pneumocolon* (within the colon). **2.** the lung(s). Example: *pneumogastric* (relating to the lungs and stomach). **3.** respiration.

pneumat- (pneumato-) *prefix denoting* **1.** the presence of air or gas. **2.** respiration.

pneumatization *n.* the presence of air-filled cavities in bone, such as the sinuses of the skull.

pneumatocele *n.* herniation of lung tissue. *See* hernia.

pneumaturia *n.* the presence in the urine of bubbles of air or other gas, due to the formation of gas by bacteria infecting the urinary tract or to an abnormal connection (fistula) between the urinary tract and bowel.

pneumo- *prefix. see* pneum-.

pneumocephalus (pneumocele) *n.* the presence of air within the skull, usually resulting from a fracture passing through one of the air sinuses.

There may be a leak of cerebrospinal fluid at the site of the fracture, manifested as a watery discharge from the nose. Pneumocephalus can best be detected by plain X-rays of the skull, which show air and a fluid level inside a cavity.

pneumococcus *n.* (*pl.* **pneumococci**) the bacterium associated with pneumonia: *Streptococcus pneumoniae.*—**pneumococcal** *adj.*

pneumoconiosis *n.* a lung disease caused by inhaling dust. The dust particles must be less than 0.5 μm in diameter to reach the depths of the lung and there is usually a long period after initial exposure before shadows appear on the chest X-ray and breathlessness develops. In practice industrial exposure to coal dust (*anthracosis*), silica (*see* silicosis), and asbestos (*see* asbestosis) produces most of the cases of pneumoconiosis. In Britain such cases are examined by the Pneumoconiosis Medical Panels, on whose advice statutory compensation for industrial injury is awarded.

Pneumocystis *n.* a genus of protozoans. The species *P. carinii* causes pneumonia in immunosuppressed patients, usually following intensive chemotherapy (*see also* AIDS). The infection is fatal if untreated, but it can be overcome with high doses of *co-trimoxazole.

pneumocyte *n.* a type of cell that lines the walls separating the air sacs (*see* alveolus) in the lungs. Type I pneumocytes are flat and inconspicuous. Type II pneumocytes are cuboidal and secrete *surfactant.

pneumoencephalography *n.* a technique used in the X-ray diagnosis of disease within the skull. Air is introduced into the cavities (ventricles) of the brain to displace the cerebrospinal fluid, thus acting as a *contrast medium. X-ray photographs show the size and disposition of the ventricles and the subarachnoid spaces.

pneumograph *n.* an instrument used to record the movements made during respiration.

pneumohaemothorax *n. see* haemopneumothorax.

pneumohydrothorax *n. see* hydropneumothorax.

pneumolysis *n. see* pleurolysis.

pneumon- (pneumono-) *prefix denoting* the lung(s). Example: *pneumonopexy* (surgical fixation to the chest wall).

pneumonectomy *n.* surgical removal of a lung, usually for cancer.

pneumonia *n.* inflammation of the lung caused by bacteria, in which the air sacs (*alveoli) fill up with pus so that air is excluded and the lung becomes solid (*see* consolidation). The symptoms depend on the amount of lung involved and the virulence of the bacteria, but they generally include cough and chest pain, with shadows on the chest X-ray. The most common type is *bronchopneumonia*, which starts around the bronchi and bronchioles. *Lobar pneumonia* affects whole lobes of either or both lungs and is caused by certain strains of *Streptococcus pneumoniae*; *hypostatic pneumonia* develops in dependant parts of the lung in people who are otherwise ill, chilled, or immobilized. The bacteria that cause pneumonia are usually sensitive to *antibiotics, and recovery is usually quick. *Compare* pneumonitis.

pneumonitis *n.* inflammation of the lung that is confined to the walls of the air sacs (alveoli) and often caused by viruses or unknown agents. It may be acute and transient or chronic, leading to increasing respiratory disability. It does not respond to antibiotics but corticosteroids may be helpful. *Compare* pneumonia.

pneumopericardium *n.* the presence of air within the membranous sac surrounding the heart. *See* hydropneumopericardium.

pneumoperitoneum *n.* air or gas in the peritoneal or abdominal cavity, usually due to a perforation of the stomach or bowel. A former treatment of tuberculosis was the deliberate injection of air into the peritoneal cavity to allow the tuberculous lung to be rested (*artificial pneumoperitoneum*).

pneumoradiography *n.* X-ray examination of part of the body using a gas, such as air or carbon dioxide, as a *contrast medium. For example, introduction of air into the ventricles of the brain enables them to be distinguished by X-rays; in their normal (fluid-filled) state they are not sufficiently contrasted with the brain tissue itself.

pneumothorax *n.* air in the *pleural cavity. Any breach of the lung surface or chest wall allows air to enter the pleural cavity, causing the lung to collapse. The leak can occur without apparent cause, in otherwise healthy people (*spontaneous pneumothorax*), or result from injuries to the chest (*traumatic pneumothorax*). In *tension pneumothorax* a breach in the lung surface acts as a valve, admitting air into the pleural cavity when the patient breathes in but preventing its escape when he breathes out. This air must be let out by surgical incision.
A former treatment for pulmonary tuberculosis – *artificial pneumothorax* – was the deliberate injection of air into the pleural cavity to collapse the lung and allow the tuberculous areas to heal.

-pnoea *suffix denoting* a condition of breathing. Example: *dyspnoea* (breathlessness).

pock *n.* a small pus-filled eruption on the skin characteristic of *chickenpox and *smallpox rashes. *See also* pustule.

pocket *n.* (in dentistry) *see* periodontal pocket.

pod- *prefix denoting* the foot.

podagra *n.* gout of the foot, especially the big toe.

podalic version altering the position of a fetus in the womb so that its feet will emerge first at birth. *See also* version.

-poiesis *suffix denoting* formation; production. Example: *haemopoiesis* (of blood cells).

poikilo- *prefix denoting* variation; irregularity.

poikilocyte *n.* an abnormally shaped red blood cell (*erythrocyte). Poikilocytes may be classified into a variety of types on the basis of their shape; for example elliptocytes (ellipsoid) and schistocytes (semilunar). *See also* poikilocytosis.

poikilocytosis *n.* the presence of abnormally shaped red cells (*poikilocytes) in the blood. Poikilocytosis is particularly marked in *myelofibrosis but can occur to some extent in almost any blood disease.

poikiloderma *n.* a condition in which the skin atrophies and becomes pigmented, giving it a mottled appearance.

poikilothermic *adj.* cold-blooded: being unable to regulate the body temperature, which fluctuates according to that of the surroundings. Reptiles and amphibians are cold-blooded. *Compare* homoiothermic. —**poikilothermy** *n.*

pointillage *n.* a procedure in massage in which the operator's fingers are pressed, fingertip first, deep into the patient's skin. This is done to manipulate underlying structures and break up adhesions that may have formed following injury.

poison *n.* any substance that irritates, damages, or impairs the activity of the body's tissues. In large enough doses almost any substance acts as a poison, but the term is usually reserved for substances, such as arsenic, cyanide, and strychnine, that are harmful in relatively small amounts.

Poisson distribution *see* frequency distribution.

polar body one of the small cells produced during the formation of an ovum from an *oocyte that does not develop into a functional egg cell.

poldine *n.* a drug, similar to *atropine, that inhibits gastric secretion and is used to treat such disorders as gastric and duodenal ulcers. It is administered by mouth; side-effects may include dry mouth, blurred vision, difficulty in urination, and fast heart beat. Trade name: **Nacton**.

pole *n.* (in anatomy) the extremity of the axis of the body, an organ, or a cell.

poli- (polio-) *prefix denoting* the grey matter of the nervous system.

polioencephalitis (viral encephalitis) *n.* a virus infection of the brain, causing particular damage to the *grey matter of the cerebral hemispheres and the brainstem. The infection is usually transmitted to man by the bite of a mosquito or tick. Some forms of this illness are endemic in a particular locality (e.g. Japanese (B) encephalitis); others have occurred as epidemics, e.g. encephalitis lethargica (sleepy sickness). *See also* encephalitis.

polioencephalomyelitis *n.* any virus infection of the central nervous system affecting the grey matter of the brain and spinal cord. *Rabies is the outstanding example.

poliomyelitis (infantile paralysis, polio) *n.* an infectious virus disease affecting the central nervous system. The virus is excreted in the faeces of an infected person and the disease is therefore most common where sanitation is poor. However, epidemics may occur in more hygienic conditions, where individuals have not acquired immunity to the disease during infancy. Symptoms commence 7–12 days after infection. In most cases paralysis does not occur: in *abortive poliomyelitis* only the throat and intestines are infected and the symptoms are those of a stomach upset or influenza; in *nonparalytic poliomyelitis* these symptoms are accompanied by muscle stiffness, particularly in the neck and back. *Paralytic poliomyelitis* is much less common. The symptoms of the milder forms of the disease are followed by weakness and eventual paralysis of the muscles: in *bulbar poliomyelitis* the muscles of the respiratory system are involved and breathing is affected.

There is no specific treatment, apart from measures to relieve the symptoms: cases of bulbar polio may require the use of a *respirator. Immunization, using the *Sabin vaccine (taken orally) or the *Salk vaccine (injected), is highly effective.

poliosis *n.* premature greying of the hair.

poliovirus *n.* one of a small group of RNA-containing viruses causing *poliomyelitis. They are included within the *picornavirus group.

pollex *n.* (*pl.* **pollices**) the thumb.

pollinosis *n.* a more precise term than *hayfever for an allergy due to the pollen of grasses, trees, or shrubs.

poly- *prefix denoting* **1.** many; multiple. **2.** excessive. **3.** generalized; affecting many parts.

polyarteritis nodosa (periarteritis nodosa) a disease of unknown cause in which there is patchy inflammation of the walls of the arteries. It is one of the *collagen diseases. Common manifestations are arthritis, neuritis, asthma, skin rashes, hypertension, kidney failure, and fever. The inflammation is suppressed by corticosteroid drugs (such as prednisolone).

polyarthritis *n.* rheumatic disease involving several to many joints, either together or in sequence, causing pain, stiffness, swelling, tenderness, and loss of function. *Rheumatoid arthritis is the most common cause.

polychromasia (polychromatophilia) *n.* the presence of certain blue red blood cells (*erythrocytes) seen in blood films stained with *Romanowsky stains, as well as the normal pink cells. The cells that appear blue are juvenile erythrocytes (*see* reticulocyte).

polycoria *n.* a rare congenital abnormality of the eye in which there are one or more holes in the iris in addition to the pupil.

polycystic disease of the kidneys an inherited disorder, transmitted as an autosomal *dominant, in which the substance of both kidneys is largely replaced by numerous cysts. Symptoms – including *haematuria, urinary tract infection, and hypertension-appear between the ages of 20 and 40 and are associated with chronic kidney failure.

polycythaemia *n.* an increase in the haemoglobin concentration of the blood. This may be due either to a decrease in the total volume of the plasma (*relative polycythaemia*) or to an increase in the total volume of the red cells (*absolute polycythaemia*). The latter may occur as a primary disease (*see* polycythaemia vera) or as a secondary condition in association with various respiratory or circulatory disorders that cause deficiency of oxygen in the tissues and with certain tumours, such as carcinoma of the kidney.

polycythaemia vera (erythraemia, Vaquez-Osler disease) a disease in which the number of red cells in the blood is greatly increased (*see also* polycythaemia). There is often also an increase in the numbers of white blood cells and platelets. Symptoms include headache, thromboses, *cyanosis, and *plethora. Polycythaemia vera may be treated by blood-letting, but more severe cases are best treated by radiotherapy. The cause of the disease is not known.

polydactylism *n. see* hyperdactylism.

polydipsia *n.* abnormally intense thirst, leading to the drinking of large quantities of fluid. This is a symptom typical of diabetes mellitus and diabetes insipidus.

polygene *n.* one of a number of genes that together control a single characteristic in an individual. Each polygene has only a slight effect and the expression of a set of polygenes is the result of their combined interaction. Characteristics controlled by polygenes are usually of a quantitative nature, e.g. height. *See also* multifactorial. —**polygenic** *adj.*

polymastia *n. see* pleomastia.

polymer *n.* a substance formed by the linkage of a large number of smaller molecules known as *monomers*. An example of a monomer is glucose, whose molecules link together to form glycogen, a polymer. Polymers may have molecular weights from a few thousands to many millions. Polymers made up of a single type of monomer are known as *homopolymers*; those of two or more monomers as *heteropolymers*.

polymorph (**polymorphonuclear leucocyte**) *n. see* neutrophil.

polymorphism *n.* (in genetics) a condition in which a chromosome or a genetic character occurs in more than one form, resulting in the coexistence of more than one morphological type in the same population.

polymyalgia rheumatica a rheumatic disease causing aching and progressive stiffness of the muscles of the shoulders and hips. The condition is most com-mon in the elderly, rarely occurring before the age of 50. The symptoms respond rapidly and effectively to corticosteroid treatment, which must usually be continued for several years. It is often associated with temporal *arteritis.

polymyositis *n.* a generalized disease of the muscles that may be acute or chronic. It particularly affects the muscles of the shoulder and hip girdles, which are weak and tender to the touch. Microscopic examination of the affected muscles shows diffuse inflammatory changes, and relief of the symptoms is obtained with *corticosteroid drugs. The skin may be reddened and atrophic. *See also* dermatomyositis.

polymyxin B an *antibiotic used to treat infections caused by Gram-negative bacteria, especially *Pseudomonas*. It is usually administered by injection but is also taken by mouth or applied as a solution or ointment for ear and eye infections. The drug may cause mild dizziness. Trade name: **Aerosporin**.

polyneuritis *n.* any disorder involving all the peripheral nerves. The term is often used interchangeably with *polyneuropathy although its specific use implies inflammation of the nerves.

polyneuropathy *n.* any disease involving all of the peripheral nerves. The symptoms first affect the tips of the fingers and toes (i.e. the extremities of the nerve fibres) and subsequently spread towards the trunk. The symptoms are usually roughly symmetrical. *See* neuropathy.

polynucleotide *n.* a long chain of linked *nucleotides, of which molecules of DNA and RNA are made.

polyopia *n.* the sensation of multiple images of one object. It is sometimes experienced by people with early cataract. *See also* diplopia.

polyorchidism *n.* a congenital abnormality resulting in more than two testes.

polyp (polypus) *n.* a growth, usually benign, protruding from a mucous membrane. Polyps are commonly found in the nose and sinuses, giving rise to obstruction, chronic infection, and discharge. They are often present in patients with allergic rhinitis, in whom they may develop in response to long-term antigenic stimulation. Other sites of occurrence include the ear, the stomach, and the bowel. Polyps are usually removed surgically (*see* polypectomy).

polypectomy *n.* the surgical removal of a *polyp. The technique used depends upon the site and size of the polyp, but it is often done by cutting across the base using a wire loop (snare) through which is passed a coagulating *diathermy current.

polypeptide *n.* a molecule consisting of three or more amino acids linked together by *peptide bonds. *Protein molecules are polypeptides.

polyphagia *n.* gluttonous excessive eating.

polypharmacy *n.* treatment of a patient with more than one type of medicine.

polyphyletic *adj.* describing a number of individuals, species, etc., that have evolved from more than one ancestral group. *Compare* monophyletic.

polyploid *adj.* describing cells, tissues, or individuals in which there are three or more complete sets of chromosomes. *Compare* diploid, haploid. —**polyploidy** *n.*

polypoid *adj.* having the appearance of a *polyp.

polyposis *n.* a condition in which numerous polyps form in an organ or tissue. *Familial polyposis coli* is a hereditary disease in which multiple polyps develop in the colon at puberty. As these polyps often become malignant, patients are usually advised to undergo total removal of the colon. *Compare* pseudopolyposis.

polypus *n. see* polyp.

polyradiculitis (polyradiculopathy) *n.* any disorder of the peripheral nerves (*see* neuropathy) in which the brunt of the disease falls on the nerve roots where they emerge from the spinal cord. An abnormal allergic response in the nerve fibres is thought to be the cause of this condition. The *Guillain-Barré syndrome is an example.

polyribosome *n. see* polysome.

polysaccharide *n.* a *carbohydrate formed from many monosaccharides joined together in long linear or branched chains. Polysaccharides have two important functions: (1) as storage forms of energy; for example *glycogen in animals and man and *starch in plants, and (2) as structural elements; for example *mucopolysaccharides in animals and man and *cellulose in plants.

polyserositis *n.* inflammation of the membranes that line the chest, abdomen, and joints, with accumulation of fluid in the cavities. Commonly the condition is inherited and intermittent and is termed *familial Mediterranean fever*. If complicated by infiltration of major organs by a glycoprotein (*see* amyloidosis) the disease usually proves fatal.

polysome (polyribosome) *n.* a structure that occurs in the cytoplasm of cells and consists of a group of *ribosomes linked together by *messenger RNA molecules: formed during protein synthesis.

polyspermia *n.* **1.** excessive formation of semen. **2.** *see* polyspermy.

polyspermy (polyspermia) *n.* fertilization of a single ovum by more than one spermatozoon: the development is abnormal and the embryo dies.

polythelia *n.* a congenital excess of nipples (*see* pleomastia).

polyuria *n.* the production of large volumes of urine, which is dilute and of a pale colour. The phenomenon may be due simply to excessive liquid intake or to disease, particularly diabetes mellitus, diabetes insipidus, and kidney disorders.

pompholyx *n.* *eczema of the hands and feet. Because the horny layer of the skin in these parts is so thick the vesicles typical of eczema cannot rupture; they therefore persist in the skin, looking like rice grains. There is intense itching until the skin eventually peels. There may be secondary infection due to scratching. Pompholyx is commonest in early adulthood and attacks occur suddenly, lasting up to six weeks. The disease may be recurrent or persist as a chronic condition.

pons *n.* **1.** *see* pons Varolii. **2.** any portion of tissue that joins two parts of an organ.

pons Varolii (pons) the part of the *brainstem that links the medulla oblongata and the thalamus, bulging forwards in front of the cerebellum, from which it is separated by the fourth ventricle. It contains numerous nerve tracts between the cerebral cortex and the spinal cord and several nuclei of grey matter. From its front surface the *trigeminal nerves emerge.

popliteus *n.* a flat triangular muscle at the back of the knee joint, between the femur and tibia, that helps to flex the knee. —**popliteal** *adj.*

porcelain *n.* (in dentistry) a ceramic material used to construct tooth-coloured crowns.

pore *n.* a small opening; for example, *sweat pores* are the openings of the sweat glands on the surface of the skin.

porencephaly *n.* an abnormal communication between the lateral *ventricle and the surface of the brain. This is usually a consequence of brain injury or cerebrovascular disease; uncommonly it may be a developmental defect, when it would most likely affect both lateral ventricles.

porocephaliasis *n.* a rare infestation of the nasal cavities, windpipe, lungs, liver, or spleen by the nymphs of the parasitic arthropod *Porocephalus. Man becomes infected on consumption of water or uncooked vegetables contaminated with the parasite's eggs. There may be some abdominal pain while the parasite is in the gut but generally there are no symptoms. Porocephaliasis has been occasionally reported in negroes of central Africa.

Porocephalus *n.* a genus of wormlike arthropods occurring mainly in tropical Africa and India. The legless adults are parasites in the lungs of snakes. The eggs, which are ejected with the snake's bronchial secretions, may be accidentally swallowed by man. The larva bores through the gut wall and usually migrates to the liver, where it develops into a nymph (*see* porocephaliasis).

porphin *n.* a complex nitrogen-containing ring structure and parent compound of the *porphyrins.

porphobilinogen *n.* a pigment that appears in the urine of individuals with acute *porphyria, causing it to darken if left standing.

porphyria *n.* one of a group of rare inherited disorders due to disturbance of the metabolism of the breakdown products (*porphyrins) of the red blood pigment haemoglobin. The defect may be primarily in the liver (*hepatic porphyria*) or in the bone marrow (*erythropoietic porphyria*) or both. The prominent features include the excretion of porphyrins and their derivatives in the urine, which may change colour on standing (*see* porphobilinogen); sensitivity of the skin to sunlight causing chronic inflammation or blistering; inflammation of the nerves (neuritis); mental disturbances; and attacks of abdominal pain.

porphyrin *n.* one of a number of pigments derived from *porphin, which are widely distributed in living things. All porphyrins form chelates with iron, magnesium, zinc, nickel, copper, and cobalt. These chelates are constituents of *haemoglobin, *myoglobin, the *cytochromes, and chlorophyll, and are thus important in many oxidation/reduction reactions in all living organisms. *See also* protoporphyrin IX.

porphyrinuria *n.* the presence in the urine of breakdown products of the red blood pigment haemoglobin (porphyrins), sometimes causing discoloration. *See* porphyria, porphobilinogen.

porta *n.* the aperture in an organ through which its associated vessels pass. Such an opening occurs in the liver (*porta hepatis*).

portacaval anastomosis (portacaval shunt) **1.** a surgical technique in which the hepatic portal vein is joined to the inferior vena cava. Blood draining from the abdominal viscera is thus diverted past the liver. It is used in the treatment of *portal hypertension, since – by lowering the pressure within the veins of the stomach and oesophagus – it prevents serious bleeding into the gastrointestinal tract. **2.** any of the natural communications between the branches of the hepatic portal vein in the liver and the inferior vena cava.

portal *adj.* **1.** relating to the portal vein or system. **2.** relating to a porta.

portal hypertension a state in which the pressure within the hepatic *portal vein is increased, causing enlargement

of the spleen, enlargement of veins in the oesophagus (gullet) (which may rupture to cause severe bleeding), and accumulation of fluid in the peritoneal cavity (ascites). The commonest cause is *cirrhosis, but other diseases of the liver or thrombosis of the portal vein will also produce it. Treatment is by *diuretic drugs, but under some circumstances surgery to join the portal vein to the inferior vena cava (bypassing the liver) may be necessary (*see* portacaval anastomosis).

portal system a vein or group of veins that terminates at both ends in a capillary bed. The best known is the *hepatic portal system*, which consists of the *portal vein and its tributaries (see illustration). Blood is drained from the spleen, stomach, pancreas, and small and large intestines into veins that merge to form the portal vein leading to the liver. Here the portal vein branches, ending in many small capillaries called *sinusoids. These permit the passage into the liver cells of nutrients absorbed by blood from the intestines.

portal vein a short vein, about 8 cm long, forming part of the hepatic *portal system. It receives many tributaries, including the splenic vein from the spleen and pancreas, the gastric vein from the stomach, the mesenteric vein from the small and large intestines, and the rectal vein from the rectum and anus.

positron emission tomography (PET) a technique used to evaluate activity of brain tissues by measuring the emission of radioactive particles from molecules of radiation-labelled 2-deoxyglucose. This substance is accepted by brain cells in much the same way as glucose, but it is metabolized very slowly after uptake by functioning neurones. Metabolic activity is reduced in damaged brain tissues and radioactive emissions from these areas is absent or reduced considerably if

The hepatic portal system

scanned by tomography equipment designed to detect radiation. The 2-deoxy-glucose, usually tagged with radioactive oxygen, is injected into the patient to be examined. PET examinations are employed in the diagnosis and treatment of patients suffering from cerebral palsy and similar types of brain damage. *See also* tomography. *Compare* computerized axial tomography (CAT).

posology *n.* the science of the dosage of medicines.

Possum *n.* a device that enables severely paralysed patients to use typewriters, adding machines, telephones, and a wide variety of other machines. Modern Possums are operated by micro-switches that require only the slightest movement in any limb. The original device worked by blowing and sucking a mouthpiece. The name derives from *Patient-Operated Selector Mechanism* (*POSM*).

post- *prefix denoting* **1.** following; after. Example: *postepileptic* (after an epilep-

tic attack). **2.** (in anatomy) behind. Example: *postoral* (behind the mouth).

postcentral *adj.* **1.** situated behind any centre. **2.** situated behind the central fissure of the brain.

postcibal *adj.* occurring after eating.

posterior *adj.* situated at or near the back of the body or an organ.

postero- *prefix denoting* posterior. Example: *posterolateral* (behind and at the side of).

posteroanterior *adj.* from the back to the front. In radiology it denotes a view in the *coronal plane.

postganglionic *adj.* describing a neurone in a nerve pathway that starts at a ganglion and ends at the muscle or gland that it supplies. In the sympathetic nervous system, postganglionic fibres are *adrenergic, unlike those in the parasympathetic system, which are *cholinergic. *Compare* preganglionic.

posthetomy *n.* an obsolete term for *circumcision.

posthitis *n.* inflammation of the foreskin. This usually occurs in association with inflammation of the glans penis (*balanitis*; *see* balanoposthitis). Pain, redness, and swelling of the foreskin occurs due to bacterial infection. Treatment is by antibiotic administration, and subsequent *circumcision prevents further attacks.

posthumous birth 1. delivery of a child by *Caesarean section after the mother's death. **2.** birth of a child after the father's death.

post mortem Latin: after death. *See* autopsy.

postoperative *adj.* following operation: referring to the condition of a patient or to the treatment given at this time.

postpartum *adj.* relating to the period of a few days immediately after birth.

postprandial *adj.* occurring after eating.

postural muscles (antigravity muscles) muscles (principally extensors) that serve to maintain the upright posture of the body against the force of gravity.

potassium chloride a salt of potassium used to prevent and treat potassium deficiency, especially during treatment with certain diuretics. It is administered by mouth or injection; some irritation in the digestive system may occur after oral administration. Trade names: **Kalium, Kay-Cee-L, K-Contin, Slow-K**.

potassium hydroxyquinoline a salt of potassium that has antifungal, antibacterial, and deodorant activities. It is applied to the skin in creams or lotions to treat skin infections and occasionally causes skin irritation.

potassium perchlorate a salt of potassium that is used to treat overactivity of the thyroid gland (thyrotoxicosis). It is administered by mouth; side-effects may include digestive upsets and rashes. Trade name: **Peroidin**.

potassium permanganate a salt of potassium used for disinfecting and cleansing wounds and as a general skin *antiseptic. It irritates mucous membranes and is poisonous if taken into the body.

Pott's disease *tuberculosis of the backbone, usually transmitted by infected cows' milk. Untreated, it can lead to a hunchback deformity.

pouch *n.* (in anatomy) a small sac-like structure, especially occurring as an outgrowth of a larger structure.

poultice (fomentation) *n.* a preparation of hot moist material applied to any part of the body to increase local circulation, alleviate pain, or soften the skin to allow matter to be expressed from a boil. Poultices containing kaolin

retain heat for a considerable period during use.

Poupart's ligament *see* inguinal ligament.

powder *n.* (in pharmacy) a medicinal preparation consisting of a mixture of two or more drugs in the form of fine particles.

pox *n.* **1.** an infectious disease causing a skin rash. **2.** a rash of pimples that become pus-filled, as in *chickenpox and *smallpox.

poxvirus *n.* one of a group of large DNA-containing viruses including those that cause *smallpox (variola) and *cowpox (vaccinia) in man, and pox and tumours in animals.

PPLO *see* mycoplasma.

practolol *n.* a drug administered by mouth or injection to control abnormal heart rhythm (*see* beta blocker). It has the side-effects of *propranolol and, in addition, more serious side-effects, particularly affecting the eyes and skin, which led to its withdrawal in 1975. Trade name: **Eraldin**.

pre- *prefix denoting* **1.** before; preceding. Example: *premenstrual* (before menstruation); *prenatal* (before birth). **2.** (in anatomy) in front of; anterior to. Example: *precardiac* (in front of the heart); *prepatellar* (in front of the patella).

pre-agonal *adj.* relating to the phenomena that precede the moment of death. *See also* agonal.

precancerous *adj.* describing a growth that is not yet malignant but that is known to become so if left untreated. *Leukoplakia of the vulva is known to be a precancerous condition. *See also* metaplasia.

precipitin *n.* any antibody that combines with its antigen to form a complex that comes out of solution and is seen as a precipitate. The antibody-antigen reaction is specific; the precipitin reaction is therefore a useful means of confirming the identity of an unknown antigen or establishing that a serum contains antibodies to a known disease. This test may be performed in watery solution or in a semisolid medium such as agar gel. *See also* agglutination.

precipitinogen *n.* any antigen that is precipitated from solution by a *precipitin.

precision attachment (in dentistry) a special machined joint that holds certain types of partial *dentures in place. The attachment is in two parts, one fixed to the denture and the other fixed to a crown on one of the teeth abutting the denture.

precocity *n.* an acceleration of normal development. The intellectually precocious child has a high IQ and may become isolated from his contemporaries or frustrated at school. Mental illness is less common than in those who develop normally. —**precocious** *adj.*

precordium *n.* the region of the thorax immediately over the heart. —**precordial** *adj.*

precuneus *n.* an area of the inner surface of the cerebral hemisphere on each side, above and in front of the *corpus callosum. *See* cerebrum.

predisposition *n.* a tendency to be affected by a particular disease or kind of disease. Such a tendency may be hereditary or may arise because of such factors as lack of vitamins, food, or sleep. *See also* diathesis.

prednisolone *n.* a synthetic *corticosteroid used to treat rheumatic diseases and inflammatory and allergic conditions. It is administered by mouth, injected into joints, or applied in creams, lotions, and ointments (for skin conditions). Side-effects are those of *cortisone. Trade names: **Codelcortone,**

Delta-Cortef, Deltacortril, Deltastab, Precortisyl, Prednesol.

prednisone *n.* a synthetic *corticosteroid used to treat rheumatic diseases, severe allergic conditions, inflammatory conditions, and leukaemia. It is administered by mouth and side-effects are those of *cortisone. Trade names: **Deltacortone, Di-Adreson.**

pre-eclampsia *n.* a condition that affects women at an advanced stage of pregnancy and is marked by high blood pressure, swelling of the ankles, and the presence of protein in the urine. Pre-eclampsia sometimes develops into a much more serious condition involving convulsions (*see* eclampsia). *See also* toxaemia of pregnancy.

prefrontal lobe the region of the brain at the very front of each cerebral hemisphere (*see* frontal lobe). The functions of the lobe are concerned with emotions, memory, learning, and social behaviour. Nerve tracts in the lobe are cut during the operation of prefrontal *leucotomy.

preganglionic *adj.* describing fibres in a nerve pathway that end in a ganglion, where they form synapses with *postganglionic fibres that continue the pathway to the effector organ, muscle or gland.

pregnancy *n.* the period during which a woman carries a developing fetus. Pregnancy lasts for approximately 266 days, from *conception until the baby is born, and the fetus normally develops in the womb (*compare* ectopic pregnancy). During pregnancy menstruation is absent, there may be a great increase in appetite, and the breasts increase in size; the woman may also experience *morning sickness. These and other changes are brought about by a hormone (*progesterone) produced at first by the ovary and later by the *placenta. Definite evidence of pregnancy is provided by various *pregnancy tests and by the detection of the heart beat of the fetus. Medical name: **cyesis**. *See also* pseudocyesis (phantom pregnancy). —**pregnant** *adj.*

pregnancy test any of several methods used to demonstrate whether or not a woman is pregnant. A commonly used laboratory test of early pregnancy is based on detection of a hormone, *chorionic gonadotrophin, in the urine. Mixture of a few drops of urine with a test solution containing an antibody that reacts with the hormone gives an almost immediate result. The test becomes positive within a month of conception and false-positive results are very rare. Alternative tests that require a woman to take hormonal drugs should be avoided if the pregnancy is intended, since there is a risk of damage to the developing embryo.

pregnanediol *n.* a steroid that is formed during the metabolism of the female sex hormone *progesterone. It occurs in the urine during pregnancy and certain phases of the menstrual cycle.

pregnenolone *n.* a steroid synthesized in the adrenal glands, ovaries, and testes. Pregnenolone is an important intermediate product in steroid hormone synthesis and can – depending on the pathways followed – be converted to corticosteroids (glucocorticoids or mineralocorticoids), androgens, or oestrogens.

premature beat *see* ectopic beat.

premature birth birth of a baby before full term. Since the date of conception is often not precisely known, a premature baby is defined as one weighing less than 2500 g (5½ lb) at birth. If such babies are unable to maintain a normal body temperature they require special care in an incubator.

premature ejaculation emission of semen (and consequent loss of erection)

during the initial stages of preparation for sexual intercourse, before insertion into the vagina or immediately afterwards.

premedication *n.* drugs administered to a patient before an operation (usually one in which an anaesthetic is used). Premedication usually comprises injection of a *sedative, to calm the patient down, together with a drug, such as *atropine, to dry up the secretions of the lungs (which might otherwise be inhaled during anaesthesia).

premenstrual tension a condition of nervousness, irritability, emotional disturbance, headache, and/or depression affecting some women for up to about ten days before menstruation. The condition is associated with the accumulation of salt and water in the tissues. It usually disappears soon after menstruation begins.

premenstruum *n.* the stage of the *menstrual cycle immediately preceding menstruation.

premolar *n.* either of the two teeth on each side of each jaw behind the canines and in front of the molars in the adult *dentition.

premyelocyte *n. see* promyelocyte.

prenatal diagnosis (antenatal diagnosis) diagnostic procedures carried out on pregnant women in order to discover genetic or other abnormalities in the developing fetus. The investigations involve the use of X-rays, *ultrasound scanning, *thermography, and analysis of amniotic fluid (obtained by *amniocentesis) or of fetal blood (obtained by *fetoscopy). Some of the techniques, including amniocentesis, involve possible risks to the mother and/or fetus and should not be undertaken without good cause. If the results indicate that the child is likely or certain to be born with severe malformation or abnormality, the possibility of abortion is discussed by the doctors involved and the parents.

prenylamine *n.* a drug that dilates blood vessels (*see* vasodilator). It is administered by mouth to treat angina; side-effects at high doses may include digestive upsets, skin reactions, and drowsiness. Trade name: **Synadrin**.

preoperative *adj.* before operation: referring to the condition of a patient or to treatment, such as sedation, given at this time.

preparedness *n.* (in psychology) a quality of some stimuli that makes them much more likely to give rise to a pathological fear. For example, animals or high places are much more likely to become the subject of a *phobia than are plants or clothes. One theory is that individuals are genetically predisposed to *conditioning of fear to objects that have been a biological threat during the evolution of mankind.

prepubertal *adj.* relating to or occurring in the period before puberty.

prepuce (foreskin) *n.* the fold of skin that grows over the end (glans) of the penis. On its inner surface modified sebaceous glands (*preputial glands*) secrete a lubricating fluid over the glans. The accumulation of this secretion is known as *smegma. The foreskin is often surgically removed in infancy (*see* circumcision). The fold of skin that surrounds the clitoris is also called the prepuce. —**preputial** *adj.*

preputial glands modified sebaceous glands on the inner surface of the *prepuce.

prepyramidal *adj.* **1.** situated in the middle lobe of the cerebellum, in front of the *pyramid. **2.** describing nerve fibres in tracts that descend from the cerebral cortex to the spinal cord, before the crossing over that occurs at the pyramid of the medulla oblongata.

presby- (presbyo-) *prefix denoting* old age.

presbyacusis *n.* the progressive perceptive *deafness that occurs with age.

presbyopia *n.* difficulty in reading at the usual distance (about one foot from the eyes) and in performing other close work, due to the decline with age in the ability of the eye to alter its focus to see close objects clearly. This is caused by gradual loss of elasticity of the lens of the eye which thus becomes progressively less able to increase its curvature in order to focus on near objects.

prescribed disease one of a number of illnesses (currently 48) arising as a result of employment requiring close contact with a hazardous substance or circumstance. Examples include poisoning by such chemicals as mercury or benzene, decompression sickness in divers, and infections such as *anthrax in those handling wool. Some diseases that occur widely in the population may be prescribed in relation to a specific occupation (e.g. deafness in those working with pneumatic drills or tuberculosis in mortuary attendants).

prescription *n.* a written direction from a registered medical practitioner to a pharmacist for preparing and dispensing a drug.

presenility *n.* premature ageing of the mind and body, so that a person shows the reduction in mental and physical abilities normally found only in old age. *See also* dementia, progeria. —**presenile** *adj.*

presentation *n.* the part of the infant's body that appears first at the opening from the neck of the womb during childbirth, as perceived on inserting the finger into the vagina. Normally the head appears first (*cephalic presentation*). However, the infant's buttocks (*see* breech presentation), its side (*transverse presentation*), its feet, or the placenta (*see* placenta praevia) may be the first parts to appear. These and other abnormal presentations may cause complications during childbirth, and an attempt may be made to correct them (*see* cephalic version).

pressor *n.* an agent that raises blood pressure. *See* vasoconstrictor.

pressure point a point at which an artery lies over a bone on which it may be compressed by finger pressure, to arrest haemorrhage beyond. For example, the femoral artery may be compressed against the pelvic bone in the groin.

pressure sore *see* bedsore.

presymptomatic *adj.* describing or relating to a symptom that occurs before the typical symptoms of a disease. *See also* prodromal.

presystole *n.* the period in the cardiac cycle just preceding systole.

prevalence rate a measure of morbidity based on current sickness in a population, estimated either at a particular time (*point prevalence*) or over a stated period (*period prevalence*). It can be expressed either in terms of sick people (persons) or episodes of sickness per 1000 individuals at risk. *Compare* incidence rate.

preventive dentistry the branch of dentistry concerned with the prevention of dental disease. It includes dietary counselling, advice on oral hygiene, and the application of *fluoride and *fissure sealants to the teeth.

preventive medicine the branch of medicine whose main aim is the prevention of disease. This is a wide field, in which workers tackle problems ranging from the immunization of persons against infectious diseases, such as diphtheria or whooping-cough, to finding methods of eliminating *vectors, such as malaria-carrying mosquitoes.

priapism *n.* persistent erection of the penis. It is commonly due to a blood clot in the erectile tissue of the penis and is most often encountered in patients with kidney failure undergoing intermittent *dialysis. Treatment is by early surgical removal of the blood clot and the construction of a venous shunt to permit blood flow from the penis.

prickle cells cells with cytoplasmic processes that form intercellular bridges. The germinative layer of the *epidermis is sometimes called the prickle cell layer.

prickly heat (heat rash) an itchy rash of small raised red spots. It occurs usually on the face, neck, back, chest, and thighs. Infants and obese people are susceptible to prickly heat, which is most common in hot moist weather. Medical name: **miliaria**.

prilocaine *n.* a local *anaesthetic used particularly in ear, nose, and throat surgery and in dentistry. It is applied in a solution to mucous membranes or injected. High doses may cause methaemoglobinaemia and cyanosis. Trade name: **Citanest**.

primaquine *n.* a drug used to treat malaria. It is administered by mouth, usually in combination with other antimalarial drugs, such as *chloroquine. High doses may cause blood disorders (such as methaemoglobinaemia or haemolytic anaemia) and digestive upsets. Trade name: **Mysoline**.

primary medical care *see* general practitioner.

prime *vb.* (in chemotherapy) to administer small doses of *cyclophosphamide prior to high-dose chemotherapy and/or radiotherapy. This causes proliferation of the primitive bone marrow cells and aids subsequent regeneration of the bone marrow.

prime mover *see* agonist.

primidone *n.* an *anticonvulsant drug used to treat major (grand mal) epilepsy. It is administered by mouth; common side-effects, which are usually transient, include drowsiness, muscle incoordination, digestive upsets, vertigo, and sight disturbances. Trade name: **Mysoline**.

primigravida (unigravida) *n.* a woman experiencing her first pregnancy.

primipara (unipara) *n.* a woman who has given birth to one infant capable of survival.

primitive streak the region of the embryo that proliferates rapidly, producing mesoderm cells that spread outwards between the layers of ectoderm and endoderm.

primordial *adj.* (in embryology) describing cells or tissues that are formed in the early stages of embryonic development.

pro- *prefix denoting* **1.** before; preceding. **2.** a precursor. **3.** in front of.

probability *n. see* significance.

proband *n. see* propositus.

probang *n.* a long flexible rod with a small sponge, ball, or tuft at the end, used to remove obstructions from the larynx or oesophagus (gullet). A probang is also used to apply medication to these structures.

probe *n.* a thin rod of pliable metal, such as silver, with a blunt swollen end. The instrument is used for exploring cavities, wounds, *fistulas, or sinus channels.

probenecid *n.* a drug that reduces the level of uric acid in the blood (*see* uricosuric drug) and is used chiefly in the treatment of gout. It is administered by mouth; mild side-effects, such as digestive upsets, dizziness, and skin rashes, may occur. Trade name: **Benemid**.

procainamide *n.* a drug that slows down the activity of the heart and is used to control abnormal heart rhythm. It is administered by mouth or injection; side-effects may include digestive upsets, dizziness, and allergic reactions. Trade name: **Pronestyl**.

procaine *n.* a local *anaesthetic administered by injection for *spinal anaesthesia. It was formerly used in dentistry. Side-effects are uncommon, but allergic reactions may occur. Trade name: **Novutex**.

procaine penicillin an *antibiotic, consisting of penicillin and procaine, used to treat infections caused by organisms sensitive to penicillin. It is injected into muscle so that the penicillin is released slowly and remains effective for some time. Trade names: **Bicillin, Depocillin**.

procarbazine *n.* a drug that inhibits growth of cancer cells by preventing cell division and is used to treat such cancers as Hodgkin's disease. It is administered by mouth; common side-effects include loss of appetite, nausea, vomiting, diarrhoea, and mouth sores. Trade name: **Natulan**.

process *n.* (in anatomy) a thin prominence or protuberance; for example, any of the processes of a vertebra.

prochlorperazine *n.* a major *tranquillizer used to treat schizophrenia and other mental disorders, migraine, vertigo, nausea, and vomiting. It is administered by mouth, injection, or in suppositories; side-effects include drowsiness and dry mouth, and high doses may cause tremors and abnormal muscle movements. Trade name: **Stemetil**.

procidentia *n.* the complete downward displacement (*prolapse) of an organ, especially the womb (*uterine procidentia*), which protrudes from the vaginal opening. Uterine procidentia may result from injury to the floor of the pelvic cavity.

proct- (procto-) *prefix denoting* the anus and/or rectum.

proctalgia (proctodynia) *n.* pain in the rectum or anus. In *proctalgia fugax* severe pain suddenly affects the rectum and may last for minutes or hours; attacks may be days or months apart. There is no structural disease and the pain is probably due to muscle spasm. Relief is sometimes obtained from a bowel action, inserting a finger into the rectum, or from a hot bath.

proctatresia *n. see* imperforate anus.

proctectasia *n.* enlargement or widening of the rectum, usually due to long-standing constipation (*see* dyschezia).

proctectomy *n.* surgical removal of the rectum. It is usually performed for cancer of the rectum and requires the construction of a permanent opening in the colon (*see* colostomy).

proctitis *n.* inflammation of the rectum. Symptoms are ineffectual straining to empty the bowels (*tenesmus), diarrhoea, and often bleeding. Proctitis is invariably present in ulcerative *colitis and sometimes in *Crohn's disease, but may occur independently (*idiopathic proctitis*). Rarer causes include damage by irradiation (for example in radiation therapy for cervical cancer) or by *lymphogranuloma venereum.

proctocele (rectocele) *n.* bulging or pouching of the rectum, usually a forward protrusion of the rectum into the vagina in association with prolapse of the womb.

proctoclysis *n.* an infusion of fluid into the rectum: formerly used to replace fluid but rarely employed now.

proctocolectomy *n.* a surgical operation in which the rectum and colon are removed. In *panproctocolectomy* the whole rectum and colon are removed,

necessitating a permanent opening of the ileum (*see* ileostomy). This is usually performed for ulcerative *colitis.

proctocolitis *n.* inflammation of the rectum and colon, usually due to ulcerative *colitis. *See also* proctitis.

proctodeum *n.* the site of the embryonic anus, marked by a depression lined with ectoderm. The membrane separating it from the hindgut breaks down in the third month of gestation. *Compare* stomodeum.

proctodynia *n. see* proctalgia.

proctology *n.* the study of disorders of the rectum and anus.

proctorrhaphy *n.* a surgical operation to stitch tears of the rectum or anus.

proctoscope *n.* an illuminated instrument through which the lower part of the rectum and the anus may be inspected and minor procedures (such as injection therapy for haemorrhoids) carried out. —**proctoscopy** *n.*

proctosigmoiditis *n.* inflammation of the rectum and the sigmoid (lower) colon. *See also* proctocolitis.

proctotomy *n.* incision into the rectum or anus to relieve *stricture (narrowing) of these canals or to open an imperforate (closed) anus.

procyclidine *n.* a drug, similar in its effects to *atropine, used to reduce muscle tremor and rigidity in parkinsonism. It is administered by mouth or injection; common side-effects include dry mouth, blurred vision, and giddiness. Trade name: **Kemadrin**.

prodromal *adj.* relating to the period of time between the appearance of the first symptoms of an infectious disease and the development of a rash or fever. A *prodromal rash* is one preceding the full rash of an infectious disease.

prodrome *n.* a symptom indicating the onset of a disease.

proenzyme (zymogen) *n.* the inactive form in which certain enzymes (e.g. digestive enzymes) are originally produced and secreted. The existence of this inactive form prevents the enzyme from breaking down the cells in which it was made. Once the proenzyme has been secreted it is converted to the active form.

proerythroblast *n.* the earliest recognizable precursor of the red blood cell (erythrocyte). It is found in the bone marrow and has a large nucleus and a cytoplasm that stains deep blue with *Romanowsky stains. *See also* erythroblast, erythropoiesis.

profunda *adj.* describing blood vessels that are deeply embedded in the tissues they supply.

progeria *n.* a very rare condition in which all the signs of old age appear and progress in a child, so that 'senility' is reached before puberty.

progesterone *n.* a steroid hormone secreted by the *corpus luteum of the ovary, the placenta, and also (in small amounts) by the adrenal cortex and testes. It is responsible for preparing the inner lining (endometrium) of the womb for pregnancy. If fertilization occurs it maintains the womb throughout pregnancy and prevents the further release of eggs from the ovary. *See also* menstrual cycle.

progestogen *n.* one· of a group of naturally occurring or synthetic steroid hormones, including *progesterone, that maintain the normal course of pregnancy. Progestogens are used to treat threatened or habitual abortion, premenstrual tension, *amenorrhoea, and abnormal bleeding from the womb. Because they prevent ovulation, progestogens are a major constituent of *oral contraceptives. Synthetic progestogens may be taken by mouth but the naturally occurring hormone must be given by intramuscular injection.

proglottis *n.* (*pl.* **proglottids** or **proglottides**) one of the segments of a *tapeworm. Mature segments, situated at the posterior end of the worm, each consist mainly of a branched uterus packed with eggs.

prognathism *n.* the state of one jaw being markedly larger than the other and therefore in front of it. —**prognathic** *adj.*

prognosis *n.* an assessment of the future course and outcome of a patient's disease, based on knowledge of the course of the disease in other patients together with the general health, age, and sex of the patient.

proguanil *n.* a drug that kills malaria parasites and is used in the prevention and treatment of malaria. It is administered by mouth and rarely causes side-effects. Trade name: **Paludrine**.

proinsulin *n.* a substance produced in the pancreas from which the hormone *insulin is derived.

projection *n.* (in psychology) the attribution of one's own qualities to other people. In psychoanalytic psychology this is one of the *defence mechanisms; people who cannot tolerate their own feelings (e.g. anger) may cope by imagining that other people have those feelings (e.g. are persecuting).

projective test a way of measuring aspects of personality, in which the subject is asked to talk freely about ambiguous objects. His responses are then analysed. Examples are the *Rorschach test and the Thematic Apperception Test (in which the subject invents stories about a set of pictures).

prolactin (lactogenic hormone, luteotrophic hormone, luteotrophin) *n.* a hormone, synthesized and stored in the anterior pituitary gland, that stimulates milk production after childbirth and also stimulates production of *progesterone by the *corpus luteum in the ovary. In both sexes excessive secretion of prolactin gives rise to abnormal production of milk (galactorrhoea).

prolapse n. downward displacement of an organ or a part from its normal position. This may happen if the supporting tissues are weak. The womb (see metroptosis) and rectum are most commonly affected by this condition.

prolapsed intervertebral disc (PID) a 'slipped disc': protrusion of the pulpy inner material of an *intervertebral disc through the fibrous outer coat, causing pressure on adjoining nerve roots, ligaments, etc. The condition often results from sudden twisting or bending of the backbone. Pressure on a nerve root causes *sciatica, and if severe may damage the nerve's function, leading to abnormalities or loss of sensation, muscle weakness, or loss of tendon reflexes. Treatment is by complete bed rest on a firm surface, manipulation, *traction, and analgesics; if these fail, the protruding portion of the disc is surgically removed (see laminectomy).

proline n. an *amino acid found in many proteins.

promazine n. a major *tranquillizer used to relieve agitation, confusion, severe pain, anxiety, nausea, and vomiting and in the treatment of alcoholism and drug withdrawal symptoms. It is administered by mouth or injection; common side-effects are drowsiness and dizziness. Trade name: **Sparine**.

promegakaryocyte n. an immature cell, found in the bone marrow, that develops into a *megakaryocyte.

promethazine n. a powerful *antihistamine drug used to treat allergic conditions and – because of its sedative action – insomnia. It is also used as an *antitussive in cough mixtures. Promethazine is administered by mouth or injection; side-effects include drowsiness, dizziness, and confusion. Trade name: **Phenergan**.

prominence n. (in anatomy) a projection, such as a projection on a bone.

promontory n. (in anatomy) a projecting part of an organ or other structure.

prompting n. a technique used in *behaviour modification to elicit a response not previously present. The subject is made to engage passively in the required behaviour by instructions or by being physically put through the movements. The behaviour can then be rewarded (see reinforcement). This is followed by *fading*, in which the prompting is gradually withdrawn and the reinforcement maintained.

promyelocyte (premyelocyte) n. one of the series of cells that gives rise to the *granulocytes (a type of white blood cell). It has abundant cytoplasm that, with *Romanowsky stains, appears blue with reddish granules (compare myeloblast, myelocyte). Promyelocytes are normally found in the blood-forming tissue of the bone marrow but may appear in the blood in a variety of diseases. See also granulopoiesis.

pronation n. the act of turning the hand so that the palm faces downwards. In this position the bones of the forearm (radius and ulna) are crossed. Compare supination.

pronator n. any muscle that causes pronation of the forearm and hand; for example, the pronator teres, a two-headed muscle arising from the humerus and ulna, close to the elbow, and inserted into the radius.

prone adj. **1.** lying with the face downwards. **2.** (of the forearm) in the position in which the palm of the hand faces downwards (see pronation). Compare supine.

pronephros n. the first kidney tissue that develops in the embryo. It is not functional and soon disappears. Compare mesonephros, metanephros.

pronucleus *n.* (*pl.* **pronuclei**) the nucleus of either the ovum or spermatozoon after fertilization but before the fusion of nuclear material. The pronuclei are larger than the normal nucleus and have a diffuse appearance.

propanidid *n.* an *anaesthetic that is injected to give rapid complete anaesthesia for a short period of time, for use in minor surgical operations. Side-effects may include digestive upsets, abnormal muscle movements, and a fall in blood pressure. Trade name: **Epontol**.

propantheline *n.* a drug that decreases activity of smooth muscle (*see* parasympatholytic) and is used to treat disorders of the digestive system, including stomach and duodenal ulcers, and enuresis (bed wetting). It is administered by mouth or injection; side-effects include dry mouth and blurred vision. Trade name: **Pro-Banthine**.

properdin *n.* a group of substances in blood plasma that, in combination with *complement and magnesium ions, is capable of destroying certain bacteria and viruses. The properdin complex occurs naturally, rather than as the result of previous exposure to microorganisms, and its activity is not directed against any particular species. *Compare* antibody.

Proper Officer *see* community physician.

prophase *n.* the first stage of *mitosis and of each division of *meiosis, in which the chromosomes become visible under the microscope. The first prophase of meiosis takes place in five stages (*see* leptotene, zygotene, pachytene, diplotene, diakinesis).

prophylactic *n.* an agent that prevents the development of a condition or disease. An example is *glyceryl trinitrate, which is used to prevent attacks of angina.

prophylaxis *n.* any means taken to prevent disease, such as immunization against diphtheria or whooping cough, or *fluoridation to prevent dental decay in children. —**prophylactic** *adj.*

propositus (proband) *n.* the first individual studied in an investigation of several related patients with an inherited or familial disorder.

propranolol *n.* a drug (*see* beta blocker) used to treat abnormal heart rhythm, angina, and high blood pressure and also taken to relieve anxiety. It is administered by mouth or injection; common side-effects include digestive upsets, insomnia, and lassitude. Trade name: **Inderal**.

proprietary name (in pharmacy) the trade name of a drug: the name assigned to it by the firm that manufactured it. For example, Mogadon is the proprietary name for nitrazepam.

proprioceptor *n.* a specialized sensory nerve ending (*see* receptor) that monitors internal changes in the body brought about by movement and muscular activity. Proprioceptors located in muscles and tendons transmit information that is used to coordinate muscular activity (*see* stretch receptor, tendon organ). *See also* mechanoreceptor.

proptometer *n. see* exophthalmometer.

proptosis *n.* forward displacement of an organ, especially the eye (*see* exophthalmos).

propylthiouracil *n.* a drug that reduces thyroid activity and is used to treat *thyrotoxicosis and to prepare patients for surgical removal of the thyroid gland. It is administered by mouth; side-effects may include rashes and digestive upsets.

prorennin *n. see* rennin.

prosencephalon *n.* the forebrain.

prosop- (prosopo-) *prefix denoting* the face. Example: *prosopodynia* (pain in).

prospective study 1. a forward-looking review of a group of individuals in relation to morbidity. **2.** *see* cohort study.

prostaglandin *n.* one of a group of hormone-like substances present in a wide variety of tissues and body fluids (including the womb, brain, lungs, kidney, and semen). Prostaglandins have many actions, one of which is to cause contraction of the womb: for this reason they have been used therapeutically to aid labour and induce abortion.

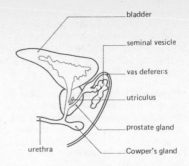

The prostate gland and associated structures (median view)

prostatectomy *n.* surgical removal of the prostate gland. The operation is necessary to relieve retention of urine due to enlargement of the prostate or to cure the symptoms of frequency and poor urinary flow due to the same cause. The operation can be performed through the bladder (*transvesical prostatectomy*) or through the surrounding capsule of the prostate (*retropubic prostatectomy*). In the operation of *transurethral prostatectomy* (*transurethral resection*) the obstructing prostate can be removed through the urethra using a *resectoscope.

prostate gland a male accessory sex gland that opens into the urethra just below the bladder and vas deferens (see illustration). During ejaculation it secretes an alkaline fluid that forms part of the *semen. The prostate may become enlarged in elderly men. This obstructs the neck of the bladder, impairing urination. The bladder dilates and the increased pressure is transmitted through the ureters to the kidney nephrons, leading to damage and impaired function of the kidneys. Treatment is by *prostatectomy.

prostatitis *n.* inflammation of the prostate gland. This may be due to bacterial infection and can be either acute or chronic. In acute prostatitis the patient has all the symptoms of a urinary infection, including pain in the perineal area, temperature, and shivering. Treatment is by antibiotic administration. In chronic prostatitis the urinary symptoms are variable; if urinary obstruction develops, transurethral *prostatectomy is indicated.

prostatorrhoea *n.* an abnormal discharge of fluid from the prostate gland. This occurs in some patients with acute *prostatitis, who complain of a profuse discharge from the urethra. The discharge is usually thin and watery and is often sterile on culture. The discharge usually subsides when the underlying prostatitis is controlled.

prosthesis (*pl.* **prostheses**) *n.* any artificial device that is attached to the body as an aid. Prostheses include dentures, artificial limbs, hearing aids, implanted pacemakers, and many other substitutes for parts of the body that are missing or nonfunctional. —**prosthetic** *adj.*

prosthetic dentistry the branch of dentistry concerned with the provision of dentures.

protamine *n.* one of a group of simple proteins that can be conjugated with nucleic acids to form nucleoproteins. Protamine can also be combined with *insulin to form *protamine zinc insulin,* which – when injected – is absorbed much more slowly than ordinary insulin and thus reduces the frequency of injections.

protanopia *n.* a defect in colour vision in which affected persons are insensitive to red light and confuse reds, yellows, and greens. *Compare* deuteranopia, tritanopia.

protease *n. see* proteolytic enzyme.

protein *n.* one of a group of organic compounds of carbon, hydrogen, oxygen, and nitrogen (sulphur and phosphorus may also be present). The protein molecule is a complex structure made up of one or more chains of *amino acids, which are linked by peptide bonds. Proteins are essential constituents of the body; they form the structural material of muscles, tissues, organs, etc., and are equally important as regulators of function, as enzymes and hormones. Proteins are synthesized in the body from their constituent amino acids, which are obtained from the digestion of protein in the diet. Excess protein, not required by the body, can be converted into glucose and used as an energy source.

proteinuria *n.* the presence of protein in the urine. This may indicate the presence of damage to, or disease of, the kidneys. *See also* albuminuria.

proteolysis *n.* the process whereby complex protein molecules, obtained from the diet, are broken down by digestive enzymes in the stomach and small intestine into their constituent amino acids, which are then absorbed into the bloodstream. *See* endopeptidase, exopeptidase. —**proteolytic** *adj.*

proteolytic enzyme (protease) a digestive enzyme that causes the breakdown of protein. *See* endopeptidase, exopeptidase.

proteose *n.* a product of the hydrolytic decomposition of protein.

Proteus *n.* a genus of rodlike Gram-negative flagellate highly motile bacteria common in the intestines and in decaying organic material. All species can decompose urea. Some species may cause disease in man: *P. morganii* is associated with acute enteritis in children, and *P. vulgaris* can cause urinary tract infections.

prothionamide *n.* a drug used in the treatment of tuberculosis. It is administered by mouth, usually together with other antituberculosis drugs; side-effects may include loss of appetite and digestive upsets. Trade name: **Trevintix**.

prothipendyl *n.* a *tranquillizer and *sedative drug used to relieve anxiety, agitation, restlessness, and excitement, to induce sleep, and to prevent nausea and vomiting. It is administered by mouth or injection; common side-effects are dry mouth and abdominal pains. Trade name: **Tolnate**.

prothrombin *n.* a substance, present in blood plasma, that is the inactive precursor from which the enzyme *thrombin is derived during the process of *blood coagulation. *See also* coagulation factors.

proto- *prefix denoting* 1. first. 2. primitive; early. 3. a precursor.

protodiastole *n.* the short period in the cardiac cycle between the end of systole and the closure of the *aortic valve marking the start of diastole.

protopathic *adj.* describing the ability to perceive only strong stimuli of pain, heat, etc. *Compare* epicritic.

protoplasm *n.* the material of which living cells are made, which includes the cytoplasm and nucleus. —**protoplasmic** *adj.*

protoplast

protoplast *n.* a bacterial or plant cell without its cell wall.

protoporphyrin IX the most common type of *porphyrin found in nature. It is a constituent of haemoglobin, myoglobin, most of the cytochromes, and the commoner chlorophylls.

Protozoa *n.* a group of microscopic single-celled animals. Most Protozoa are free-living but some are important disease-causing parasites of man; for example, *Plasmodium, *Leishmania, and *Trypanosoma cause *malaria, *kala-azar, and *sleeping sickness respectively. *See also* amoeba.

protozoan *n.* a single-celled animal. *See* Protozoa.

protozoology *n.* the study of single-celled animals (*Protozoa).

protriptyline *n.* a tricyclic *antidepressant drug used to treat moderate or severe depression, especially in apathetic and withdrawn patients. It is administered by mouth; side-effects include dry mouth, blurred vision, fast heart beat, digestive disturbances, and skin rashes. Trade name: **Concordin**.

protrusion *n.* (in dentistry) **1.** forward movement of the lower jaw. **2.** a *malocclusion in which some of the teeth are further forward than usual. *Compare* retrusion.

protuberance *n.* (in anatomy) a rounded projecting part, e.g. the projecting part of the chin (*mental protuberance*).

provitamin *n.* a substance that is not itself a vitamin but can be converted to a vitamin in the body. An example is β-carotene, which can be converted into vitamin A.

proximal *adj.* (in anatomy) situated close to the origin or point of attachment or close to the median line of the body. *Compare* distal.

prurigo *n.* a chronic itchy skin disease of unknown cause. It usually starts in childhood with small pale pimples arising deep in the skin. Prurigo may occur in association with hay fever or asthma or start in warm weather. Treatment is unsatisfactory and relapses are frequent.

pruritus *n.* itching, caused by local irritation of the skin or sometimes nervous disorders. Severe itching is a symptom of some forms of jaundice. Pruritus of the vulva in women may be due to vaginal infection, in some cases caused by yeast organisms that flourish in diabetes, when the urine contains sugar. Pruritus of the anal region may be due to poor hygiene, haemorrhoids, or the presence of intestinal worms.

prussic acid *see* hydrocyanic acid.

psammoma *n.* a tumour containing gritty sandlike particles (*psammoma bodies*). Such tumours may be found in the meninges (the membranes surrounding the brain), the ovary, etc.

psellism *n.* a deficiency of articulation of speech, such as *stammering.

pseud- (pseudo-) *prefix denoting* superficial resemblance to; false.

pseudarthrosis (nearthrosis) *n.* a 'false' joint, formed around a displaced bone end after dislocation. Congenital hip dislocation may result in a pseudarthrosis.

pseudoagglutination *n.* the misleading appearance of clumping during an antiserum-antigen test as a result of incorrect temperature or acidity of the solutions used.

pseudocholinesterase *n.* an enzyme found in the blood and other tissues that – like *cholinesterase – breaks down acetylcholine, but much more slowly. Not being localized at nerve endings, it plays little part in the normal breakdown of acetylcholine in synapses and at neuromuscular junctions.

pseudocoxalgia *n. see* Legg-Calvé-Perthes disease.

pseudocrisis *n.* a false crisis: a sudden but temporary fall of temperature in a patient with fever. The pseudocrisis is followed by a return to the fever.

pseudocroup *n.* spasmodic contraction of the larynx that is not caused by inflammation of the glottis or associated with coughing. It occurs particularly in children with rickets.

pseudocryptorchidism *n.* apparent absence of the testes. This is quite common in young boys, who retract their testes into the groin due to involuntary or reflex contraction of the cremasteric muscle of the suspensory cord. The condition is only important in that it needs to be distinguished from true failure of descent of the testes into the scrotum, which requires early surgical treatment (*see* cryptorchidism).

pseudocyesis (phantom pregnancy) *n.* a condition in which a nonpregnant woman exhibits symptoms of pregnancy, e.g. enlarged abdomen, increased weight, morning sickness, and absence of menstruation. The condition usually has an emotional basis and is determined by hormones secreted by the pituitary gland.

pseudocyst *n.* a fluid-filled space without a proper wall or lining, within an organ. A *pancreatic pseudocyst* may develop in cases of chronic pancreatitis or as a complication of acute pancreatitis. As the pseudocyst, which is filled with enzyme-rich pancreatic juice, slowly expands it may cause episodes of abdominal pain accompanied by a rise in the level of enzymes in the blood. It may be felt by abdominal examination, or may be seen by radiology as it displaces other organs. Treatment is by surgical drainage, usually by the technique of joining the pseudocyst to the stomach (*marsupialization).

pseudogout *n.* joint pain and swelling, resembling gout, caused by crystals of calcium pyrophosphate in the synovial membrane and fluid. *See also* chondrocalcinosis.

pseudohermaphroditism *n.* a congenital abnormality in which the external genitalia of a male or a female resemble those of the opposite sex; for example, a woman would have enlarged labia and clitoris, resembling a scrotum and penis respectively.

pseudohypertrophy *n.* increase in the size of an organ or structure caused by excessive growth of cells that have a packing or supporting role but do not contribute directly to its functioning. The result is usually a decline in the efficiency of the organ although it becomes larger. —**pseudohypertrophic** *adj.*

pseudohypoparathyroidism *n.* a syndrome of mental retardation, restricted growth, and bony abnormalities due to a genetic defect that causes lack of response to the hormone secreted by the *parathyroid glands. Treatment with calcium and vitamin D can reverse most of the features.

pseudologia fantastica the telling of elaborate and fictitious stories as if they were true. Often some facts are woven into the tissue of lies. While not necessarily a symptom of illness, it is sometimes a feature of chronic mental illness and of personality disorders, particularly psychopathy.

pseudomembrane *n.* a false membrane, consisting of a layer of exudate on the surface of the skin or a mucous membrane. In diphtheria a pseudomembrane forms in the throat.

Pseudomonas *n.* a genus of rodlike motile pigmented Gram-negative bacteria. Most live in soil and decomposing organic matter; they are involved in recycling nitrogen, converting nitrates to ammonia or free nitrogen. The species *P. aeruginosa* is pathogenic to man, occurring in pus from wounds; it is associated with urinary tract infections. *P. pseudomallei* is the causative agent of *melioidosis.

pseudomutuality *n.* a disorder of communication within a family in which a superficial pretence of closeness and reciprocal understanding belies a lack of real feeling. It has been alleged, but not proved, to be a factor in the backgrounds of schizophrenics.

pseudomyxoma *n.* a mucoid tumour of the peritoneum, often seen in association with *myxomas of the ovary. In *pseudomyxoma peritonei* material from a myxoma, usually in the ovary, is spilled into the peritoneal cavity and continues to be produced within the abdomen, often to massive proportions.

pseudoneuritis *n.* a condition that resembles *retrobulbar neuritis but is not due to inflammation. The most usual cause is blockage of blood vessels in the optic nerve (*ischaemic optic neuropathy*).

pseudophakos *n.* the state of the eye after the natural lens has been replaced by a plastic lens implanted inside the eye, approximately in the position previously occupied by the natural lens. This is a modern form of surgery for cataract.

pseudoplegia *n.* paralysis of the limbs not associated with organic abnormalities. *See also* hysterical.

pseudopodium *n.* (*pl.* **pseudopodia**) a temporary and constantly changing extension of the body of an amoeba or an amoeboid cell (*see* phagocyte). Pseudopodia engulf bacteria and other particles as food and are responsible for the movements of the cell.

pseudopolyposis *n.* a condition in which the bowel lining (mucosa) is covered by elevated or protuberant plaques (*pseudopolyps*) that are not true *polyps but abnormal growth of inflamed mucosa. It is usually found in chronic ulcerative *colitis. The pseudopolyps may be seen with the *sigmoidoscope or *colonoscope (through which they may be sampled for microscopic examination) or by barium enema examination.

pseudopseudohypoparathyroidism *n.* a condition in which all the symptoms of *pseudohypoparathyroidism are present but the patient's response to parathyroid hormone is normal. It is often found in families affected with pseudohypoparathyroidism.

pseudotumour cerebri *see* benign intracranial hypertension.

psilosis *n.* *see* sprue.

psittacosis *n.* *see* parrot disease.

psoas (psoas major) *n.* a muscle in the groin that acts jointly with the iliacus muscle to flex the hip joint (see illustration). A smaller muscle, *psoas minor*, has the same action but is often absent.

Psoas and iliacus muscles

psoriasis *n.* a chronic skin disease in which itchy scaly red patches form on the elbows, forearms, knees, legs, scalp, and other parts of the body. Psoriasis is one of the commonest skin diseases in Britain, affecting about 1% of the population, but its cause is not known. The disorder often runs in families and may be brought on by anxiety; it is rare in infants and the elderly, the commonest time of onset being in childhood or adolescence. It sometimes occurs in association with arthritis (*see* psoriatic arthritis). Occasionally the disease may be very severe, affecting much of the skin and causing considerable disability in the patient. There is no known cure and treatment is palliative with lotions or ointments.

psoriatic arthritis arthritis associated with *psoriasis. It occurs in only a small minority of patients with psoriasis but may be painful and disabling. It often affects small joints, such as the terminal joints of the fingers and toes, or the spine (*spondylitis) and sacroiliac joints (*sacroiliitis).

psych- (psycho-) *prefix denoting* 1. the mind; psyche. 2. psychology.

psychasthenia *n.* an obsolete term for a group of neuroses including phobias, anxiety states, and obsessions. The psychiatrist P. Janet divided the neuroses into *hysterias and psychasthenias.

psyche *n.* the mind or the soul; the mental (as opposed to the physical) functioning of the individual.

psychedelic *adj.* describing drugs that induce changes in the level of consciousness of the mind. Psychedelic drugs, which include *lysergic acid diethylamide (LSD) and *cannabis, are *hallucinogens and are used legally only for experimental purposes.

psychiatrist *n.* a medically qualified physician who specializes in the study and treatment of mental disorders.

psychiatry *n.* the study of mental disorders and their diagnosis, management, and prevention. —**psychiatric** *adj.*

psychic *adj.* 1. of or relating to the *psyche. 2. relating to parapsychological phenomena. 3. describing a person who is endowed with extrasensory or psychokinetic powers.

psychoanalysis *n.* a school of psychology and a method of treating mental disorders based upon the teachings of Sigmund Freud (1856–1939). Psychoanalysis employs the technique of *free association in the course of intensive *psychotherapy in order to bring repressed fears and conflicts to the conscious mind, where they can be dealt with (*see* repression). It stresses the dynamic interplay of unconscious forces and the importance of sexual development in childhood for personality development. —**psychoanalyst** *n.* —**psychoanalytic** *adj.*

psychodrama *n.* a form of group psychotherapy in which individuals acquire insight into themselves by acting out situations from their past with other group members. *See* group therapy.

psychogenic *adj.* having an origin in the mind rather than in the body. The term is applied particularly to symptoms and illnesses.

psychogeriatrics *n.* the branch of psychiatry that deals with the mental disorders of old people. —**psychogeriatric** *adj.*

psychokinesis *n.* a supposed ability of some individuals to alter the state of an object by the power of the mind alone, without any physical intervention. *See also* parapsychology.

psychologist *n.* a person who is engaged in the scientific study of the mind. He may work in a university, in industry, in schools, or in a hospital. A *clinical psychologist* has been trained in aspects of the assessment and treatment of the ill and handicapped. He usually works in a hospital, often as one of a multidisciplinary team. An *educational psychologist* has been trained in aspects of the cognitive and emotional development of children. He usually works in close association with schools and advises on the management of children.

psychology *n.* the science concerned with the behaviour of man and animals. Different schools of psychology have used different methods and theories. *Experimental psychology* uses laboratory experiments to study processes such as motivation and learning. *Ethology* investigates animal behaviour by observation in the natural environment. *Introspectionist psychology* used the method of trained subjects describing their own mental states. Other schools include *behaviourism, *gestaltism, and *psychoanalysis. —**psychological** *adj.*

psychometrics *n.* the measurement of individual differences in psychological functions (such as intelligence and personality) by means of standardized tests. —**psychometric** *adj.*

psychomotor *adj.* relating to muscular and mental activity. The term is applied to disorders in which muscular activities are affected by cerebral disturbance.

psychomotor epilepsy *see* epilepsy.

psychoneurosis *n.* a *neurosis that is manifest in psychological rather than organic symptoms.

psychopath *n.* a person who behaves in an antisocial way and shows little or no guilt for antisocial acts and little capacity for forming emotional relationships with others. There is some evidence that EEG patterns of psychopaths are abnormal. Psychopaths tend to respond poorly to treatment but many mature as they age. *See also* personality disorder. —**psychopathic** *adj.* —**psychopathy** *n.*

psychopathology *n.* **1.** the study of mental disorders, with the aim of explaining and describing aberrant behaviour. *Compare* psychiatry. **2.** the symptoms, collectively, of a mental disorder. —**psychopathological** *adj.*

psychopharmacology *n.* the study of the effects of drugs on mental processes and behaviour, particularly *psychotropic drugs.

psychophysiology *n.* the branch of psychology that records physiological measurements, such as the electrical resistance of the skin, the heart rate, the size of the pupil, and the electroencephalogram, and relates them to psychological events. —**psychophysiological** *adj.*

psychosexual development the process by which an individual becomes more mature in his sexual feelings and behaviour. Gender identity, sex-role behaviour, and choice of sexual partner are the three major areas of development. The phrase is sometimes used specifically for a sequence of stages, supposed by psychoanalytic psychologists to be universal, in which oral, anal, phallic, latency, and genital stages successively occur. These stages reflect the parts of the body on which sexual interest is concentrated during childhood development.

psychosis *n.* a severe mental illness in which the sufferer loses contact with reality. *Delusions and *hallucinations occur and thought processes may be altered. The major varieties are *organic* and *functional*; in the latter no physical cause has been demonstrated. The most important functional psychoses are *schizophrenia and *manic-depressive psychosis. Psychoses not typical of either of these also occur: *oneiroid psychosis* is characterized by an acute dreamlike confused state; *cycloid psychosis* by a tendency to recur; and *schizoaffective psychosis* by the presence of both schizophrenic and manic-depressive qualities. —**psychotic** *adj.*

psychosomatic *adj.* relating to or involving both the mind and body: usually applied to illnesses that are caused by the interaction of mental and physical factors. Certain physical illnesses, including asthma, eczema, and peptic ulcer, are thought to be in part a response to psychological and social stresses. Psychological treatments sometimes have a marked effect, but are usually much less effective than physical treatments for such illnesses.

psychosurgery *n.* surgery of the brain to relieve psychological symptoms. The operation most commonly performed is *leucotomy, but *cingulectomy and amygdalectomy are sometimes also used. These are all irreversible treatments and are therefore reserved for the most severe and intractable of symptoms, particularly severe chronic anxiety, depression, and untreatable pain. Side-effects can be severe but are less common with modern selective operations. —**psychosurgical** *adj.*

psychotherapy *n.* psychological (as opposed to physical) methods for the treatment of mental disorders and psychological problems. There are many different approaches to psychotherapy, including *psychoanalysis, *client-centred therapy, and *group therapy. These approaches share the views that the relationship between therapist and client is of prime importance, that the goal is to help personal development and self-understanding generally rather than to remove symptoms, and that the therapist does not direct the client's decisions. They have all been very widely applied to differing clinical conditions but are of unknown value as treatments of mental illness. *See also* behaviour therapy, counselling. —**psychotherapeutic** *adj.* —**psychotherapist** *n.*

psychoticism *n.* a dimension of personality derived from psychometric tests, which appears to indicate a degree of emotional coldness and some cognitive impairment.

psychotropic *adj.* describing drugs that affect mood. *Antidepressants, *sedatives, *stimulants, and *tranquillizers are psychotropic.

psychro- *prefix denoting* cold.

psychrophilic *adj.* describing organisms, especially bacteria, that grow best at temperatures of 0–25°C. *Compare* mesophilic, thermophilic.

PTC *see* phenylthiocarbamide.

pterion *n.* the point on the side of the skull at which the sutures between the *parietal, *temporal, and *sphenoid bones meet.

pteroylglutamic acid *see* folic acid.

pterygium *n.* a triangular overgrowth of the cornea, usually the inner side, by thickened and degenerative conjunctiva. It is most commonly seen in people from dry hot dusty climates, and only rarely interferes with vision.

pterygo- *prefix denoting* the pterygoid process of the sphenoid bone. Example: *pterygomaxillary* (of the pterygoid process and the maxilla).

pterygoid process either of two large processes of the *sphenoid bone.

ptomaine *n.* any of various substances produced in decaying foodstuffs and responsible for the unpleasant taste and smell of such foods. These compounds – which include putrescine, cadaverine, and neurine – were formerly thought to be responsible for food poisoning, but although they are often associated with toxic bacteria they themselves are harmless.

ptosis *n.* drooping of the upper eyelid, for which there are several causes. It may be due to a disorder of the third cranial nerve (*oculomotor nerve), in which case it is likely to be accompanied by paralysis of eye movements causing double vision and an enlarged pupil. When part of *Horner's syndrome, ptosis is accompanied by a small pupil and an absence of sweating on that side of the face. It may be due to *myasthenia gravis, in which the ptosis increases with fatigue and is part of a more widespread fatiguable weakness. Ptosis may also occur as an isolated congenital feature or as part of a disease of the eye muscles, when it is associated with weak or absent eye movements.

-ptosis *suffix denoting* a lowered position of an organ or part; prolapse. Example: *colpoptosis* (of the vagina).

ptyal- (ptyalo-) *prefix denoting* saliva. Example: *ptyalorrhoea* (excessive flow of).

ptyalin *n.* an enzyme (an *amylase) found in saliva.

ptyalism (sialorrhoea) *n.* the excessive production of saliva: a symptom of certain nervous disorders, poisoning (by mercury, mushrooms, or organophosphates), or infection (rabies). *Compare* xerostomia.

ptyalith *n.* a stone (*calculus) in a salivary gland or duct.

ptyalography *n. see* sialography.

puberty *n.* the time at which the onset of sexual maturity occurs and the reproductive organs become functional. This is manifested in both sexes by the appearance of *secondary sexual characteristics (e.g. deepening of the voice in boys; growth of breasts in girls) and in girls by the start of *menstruation. These changes are brought about by an increase in sex hormone activity due to stimulation of the ovaries and testes by pituitary hormones. *See also* androgen, oestrogen. —**pubertal** *adj.*

pubes *n.* **1.** the body surface that overlies the pubis, at the front of the pelvis. It is covered with *pubic hair*. **2.** *see* pubis. —**pubic** *adj.*

pubiotomy *n.* an operation to divide the pubic bone near the symphysis, the front midline where the left and right pubic bones meet. Pubiotomy is performed during childbirth if it is necessary to increase the size of an abnormally small pelvis to allow passage of the child.

pubis *n.* (*pl.* **pubes**) a bone forming the lower and anterior part of each side of the *hip bone (*see also* pelvis). The two pubes meet at the front of the pelvis at the *pubic symphysis. See also* pubes.

Public Health Inspector the former title of the Environmental Health Officer.

Public Health Laboratory (in Britain) a regional service, with headquarters at Colindale, to assist with the investigation and control of infections. Such laboratories are a separate organization from hospital laboratories, which are under the control of District Health Authorities, but they can be located within a hospital and can contribute to the day-to-day diagnosis of hospital in-patients and out-patients.

pudendum *n.* (*pl.* **pudenda**) the external genital organs, especially those of the female (*see* vulva). —**pudendal** *adj.*

puerpera *n.* a woman who has recently given birth and whose womb has not yet returned to its normal nonpregnant dimensions.

puerperal (puerperous) *adj.* relating to childbirth or the period that immediately follows it.

puerperal fever (childbed fever) blood poisoning (*septicaemia) in a mother shortly after childbirth resulting from infection of the lining of the womb or the vagina, which have been torn or bruised during labour. Increased standards of hygiene in midwifery and the use of such antibiotics as penicillin have reduced the numbers of deaths caused by puerperal fever from the formerly high level almost to nil.

puerperalism *n.* illness of a mother or her baby associated with childbirth.

puerperium (childbed) *n.* the period of up to about six weeks after childbirth, during which the size of the womb decreases to normal.

Pulex *n.* a genus of widely distributed *fleas. *P. irritans*, the human flea, is a common parasite of man and its bite may give rise to intense irritation and bacterial infection. It is an intermediate host for larvae of the tapeworms *Hymenolepis* and *Dipylidium*, which it can transmit to man, and it may also be involved in the transmission of plague.

pulicide *n.* any chemical agent, for example *DDT or malathion, used for killing fleas.

pulmo- (pulmon(o)-) *prefix denoting* the lung(s).

pulmonary *adj.* relating to, associated with, or affecting the lungs.

pulmonary artery the artery that conveys blood from the heart to the lungs for oxygenation: the only artery in the body containing deoxygenated blood. It leaves the right ventricle and passes upwards for 5 cm before dividing into two, one branch going to each lung. Within the lungs each pulmonary artery divides into many fine branches, which end in capillaries in the alveolar walls. *See also* pulmonary circulation.

pulmonary circulation a system of blood vessels effecting transport of blood between the heart and lungs. Deoxygenated blood leaves the right ventricle by the pulmonary artery and is carried to the alveolar capillaries of the lungs. Gaseous exchange occurs, with carbon dioxide leaving the circulation and oxygen entering. The oxygen-

ated blood then passes into small veins leading to the pulmonary veins, which leave the lungs and return blood to the left atrium of the heart. The oxygenated blood can then be pumped around the body via the *systemic circulation.

pulmonary embolism obstruction of the *pulmonary artery or one of its branches by an *embolus, usually a blood clot derived from *phlebothrombosis of the leg veins. Large pulmonary emboli result in acute heart failure or sudden death. Smaller emboli cause death of sections of lung tissue, pleurisy, and haemoptysis (coughing of blood). Minor pulmonary emboli respond to the *anticoagulant drugs heparin and warfarin. Major pulmonary embolism is treated by *embolectomy or by dissolution of the blood clot with an infusion of *streptokinase. Recurrent pulmonary embolism may result in *pulmonary hypertension.

pulmonary hypertension a condition in which there is raised blood pressure within the blood vessels supplying the lungs (the pulmonary artery blood pressure is normally much lower than the pressure within the aorta and its branches). Pulmonary hypertension may complicate pulmonary embolism, *septal defects, heart failure, diseases of the mitral valve, and chronic lung diseases. It may also develop without any known cause (*primary pulmonary hypertension*). The right ventricle enlarges and heart failure, fainting, and chest pain occur. The treatment is that of the cause; drugs used to control *hypertension are ineffective.

pulmonary stenosis congenital narrowing of the outlet of the right ventricle of the heart to the pulmonary artery. The defect may be in the pulmonary valve (*valvular stenosis*) or in the outflow tract of the right ventricle below the valve (*infundibular stenosis*). It may be isolated or combined with other heart defects (e.g. *tetralogy of

Fallot). Severe pulmonary stenosis may produce angina pectoris, faintness, and heart failure. The defect is corrected by surgery.

pulmonary tuberculosis *see* tuberculosis.

pulmonary vein a vein carrying oxygenated blood from the lung to the left atrium. *See* pulmonary circulation.

pulp *n.* **1.** a soft mass of tissue (for example, of the spleen). **2.** the mass of connective tissue in the *pulp cavity*, at the centre of a *tooth. It is surrounded by dentine except where it communicates with the rest of the body at the apex.

pulpitis *n.* inflammation of the pulp of a tooth: a frequent cause of toothache.

pulse *n.* a series of pressure waves within an artery caused by contractions of the left ventricle and corresponding with the heart rate (the number of times the heart beats per minute). It is easily detected on such superficial arteries as the radial artery near the wrist and the carotid artery in the neck. The average adult pulse rate at rest is 60–80 per minute, but exercise, injury, illness, and emotion may produce much faster rates.

pulsus paradoxus a large fall in systolic blood pressure and pulse volume when the patient breathes in. It is seen in constrictive *pericarditis, pericardial effusion, and asthma.

pulvinar *n.* the expanded posterior end of the *thalamus.

punch-drunk syndrome a group of symptoms consisting of progressive *dementia, tremor of the hands, and epilepsy. It is a consequence of repeated blows to the head that have been severe enough to cause *concussion.

punctum *n.* (*pl.* **puncta**) (in anatomy) a point or small area, especially the *puncta lacrimalia* – the two openings of

the tear ducts in the inner corners of the upper and lower eyelids (*see* lacrimal apparatus).

puncture 1. *n.* a wound made accidentally or deliberately by a sharp object or instrument. Puncture wounds need careful treatment as a small entry hole in the skin can disguise serious injury in an underlying organ or tissue. Punctures are also performed for diagnostic purposes, in order to withdraw tissue or fluid for examination. *See also* lumbar puncture. **2.** *vb.* to pierce a tissue with a sharp instrument.

pupil *n.* the circular opening in the centre of the *iris, through which light passes into the lens of the eye. —**pupillary** *adj.*

pupillary reflex (light reflex) the reflex change in the size of the pupil according to the amount of light entering the eye. Bright light reaching the retina stimulates nerves of the *parasympathetic nervous system, which cause the pupil to contract. In dim light the pupil opens, due to stimulation of the *sympathetic nervous system. *See also* iris.

purgation *n.* the use of drugs to stimulate intestinal activity and clear the bowels. *See* laxative.

purgative *n. see* laxative.

purine *n.* a nitrogen-containing compound with a two-ring molecular structure. Examples of purines are adenine and guanine, which form the *nucleotides of nucleic acids, and uric acid, which is the end-product of purine metabolism.

Purkinje cells nerve cells found in great numbers in the cortex of the cerebellum. The cell body is flask-shaped, with numerous dendrites branching from the neck and extending fanwise among other cells towards the surface and a long axon that runs from the base deep into the cerebellum (see illustration).

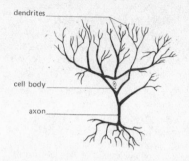

dendrites

cell body

axon

A Purkinje cell

Purkinje fibres *see* atrioventricular bundle.

purpura *n.* a skin rash resulting from bleeding into the skin from small blood vessels (capillaries); the individual purple spots of the rash are called *petechiae*. Purpura may be due either to defects in the capillaries (*nonthrombocytopenic purpura*) or to a deficiency of blood platelets (*thrombocytopenic purpura*). *Acute idiopathic thrombocytopenic purpura* is a disease of children in which antibodies are produced that destroy the patient's platelets. The child usually recovers without treatment. *See also* thrombocytopenia, Schönlein-Henoch purpura.

purulent *adj.* forming, consisting of, or containing pus.

pus *n.* a thick yellowish or greenish liquid formed at the site of an established infection. Pus contains dead white blood cells, both living and dead bacteria, and fragments of dead tissue. *See also* mucopus, seropus.

pustule *n.* a small pus-containing blister on the skin.

putamen *n.* a part of the lenticular nucleus (*see* basal ganglia).

putrefaction *n.* the process whereby proteins are decomposed by bacteria. This is accompanied by the formation of amines (such as *putrescine* and *cadaverine*) having a strong and very unpleasant smell.

putrescine *n.* an amine formed during *putrefaction.

py- (pyo-) *prefix denoting* pus; a purulent condition. Example: *pyoureter* (pus in a ureter).

pyaemia *n.* blood poisoning by pus-forming bacteria released from an abscess. Widespread formation of abscesses may develop, with fatal results. *Compare* sapraemia, septicaemia, toxaemia.

pyarthrosis *n.* an infected joint filled with pus. Drainage, combined with antibiotic treatment, is necessary, though the joint may already be severely damaged if diagnosis is late.

pyel- (pyelo-) *prefix denoting* the pelvis of the kidney. Example: *pyelectasis* (dilation of).

pyelitis *n.* inflammation of the pelvis of the kidney (the part of the kidney from which urine drains into the ureter). This is usually caused by a bacterial infection, which may develop in any condition causing obstruction to the flow of urine. The patient experiences pain in the loins, shivering, and a high temperature. Treatment is by the administration of a suitable antibiotic, together with analgesics and a high fluid intake. Any underlying abnormality of the urinary system must be relieved to prevent further attacks.

pyelocystitis *n.* inflammation of the renal pelvis and urinary bladder (*see* pyelitis, cystitis).

pyelogram *n. see* intravenous pyelogram, pyelography.

pyelography (urography) *n.* X-ray examination of the kidneys using *ra-

pyelolithotomy

dio-opaque contrast material. In *intravenous pyelography* (*excretion urography*) the contrast medium is injected into a vein and is concentrated and excreted by the kidneys (*see* intravenous pyelogram). In *retrograde pyelography*, fine catheters are passed up the ureter to the kidneys at *cystoscopy and contrast material is injected directly into the renal pelvis to allow X-ray examination. The X-ray pictures obtained from these procedures are called *pyelograms*.

pyelolithotomy *n.* surgical removal of a stone from the kidney through an incision made in the pelvis of the kidney. The incision is usually made into the posterior surface of the pelvis (*posterior pyelotomy*) to gain access to the stone, which can then be lifted clear.

pyelonephritis *n.* bacterial infection of the kidney substance. In *acute pyelonephritis*, the patient has pain in the loins, a high temperature, and shivering fits. Treatment is by the administration of an appropriate antibiotic, and a full urological investigation is conducted to determine any underlying abnormality and prevent recurrence. In *chronic pyelonephritis*, the kidneys become small and scarred and kidney failure ensues. *Vesicoureteric reflux in childhood is one of the causes.

pyeloplasty *n.* an operation to relieve obstruction at the junction of the pelvis kidney and the ureter. *See* hydronephrosis, Dietl's crisis.

pyelotomy *n.* surgical incision into the pelvis of the kidney. This operation is usually undertaken to remove a stone (*see* pyelolithotomy) but is also necessary when surgical drainage of the kidney is required by a catheter or tube.

Pyemotes *n. see* Pediculoides.

pyg- (pygo-) *prefix denoting* the buttocks.

pykno- *prefix denoting* thickness or density.

pyknolepsy *n. Obsolete.* a very high frequency of *petit mal attacks.

pyknosis *n.* the process in which the cell nucleus is thickened into a dense mass, which occurs when cells die. —**pyknotic** *adj.*

pyl- (pyle-) *prefix denoting* the portal vein.

pylephlebitis (portal pyaemia) *n.* septic inflammation and thrombosis of the hepatic portal vein. This is a rare result of the spread of infection within the abdomen (as from appendicitis). The condition causes severe illness, with fever, liver abscesses, and *ascites. Treatment is by antibiotic drugs and surgical drainage of abscesses.

pylethrombosis *n.* obstruction of the portal vein by a blood clot (*see* thrombosis). It can result from infection of the umbilicus in infants, pylephlebitis, cirrhosis of the liver, and liver tumours. *Portal hypertension is a frequent result.

pylor- (pyloro-) *prefix denoting* the pylorus. Example: *pyloroduodenal* (of the pylorus and duodenum).

pylorectomy *n.* a surgical operation in which the muscular outlet of the stomach (*pylorus) is removed. *See* antrectomy, pyloroplasty.

pyloric stenosis narrowing of the muscular outlet of the stomach (*pylorus). This causes delay in passage of the stomach contents to the duodenum, which leads to repeated vomiting (sometimes of food eaten more than 24 hours earlier), and sometimes visible distension and movement of the stomach. If the condition persists the patient loses weight, becomes dehydrated, and develops *alkalosis. *Congenital hypertrophic pyloric stenosis* occurs in babies about 10 to 14 days old (particularly boys) in which the thickened pyloric muscle can be felt as a nodule. Treatment is by the surgical operation of *pyloromyotomy (Ramstedt's operation). Recovery is usually complete and the condition does not recur. Pyloric stenosis in adults is caused either by a *peptic ulcer close to the pylorus or by a cancerous growth invading and obstructing the pylorus. Treatment is by surgical removal or bypass (see gastroenterostomy).

pyloromyotomy (Ramstedt's operation) n. a surgical operation in which the muscle around the outlet of the stomach (pylorus) is divided down to the lining (mucosa) in order to relieve congenital *pyloric stenosis.

pyloroplasty n. a surgical operation in which the outlet of the stomach (pylorus) is widened by a form of reconstruction. It is done to allow the contents of the stomach to pass more easily into the duodenum, particularly after *vagotomy to treat peptic ulcers (which would otherwise cause delay in gastric emptying).

pylorospasm n. closure of the outlet of the stomach (pylorus) due to muscle spasm, leading to delay in the passage of stomach contents to the duodenum and vomiting. It is usually associated with duodenal or pyloric ulcers.

pylorus n. the lower end of the *stomach, which leads to the duodenum. It terminates at a ring of muscle – the pyloric sphincter – which contracts to close the opening by which the stomach communicates with the duodenum. —**pyloric** adj.

pyo- prefix. see py-.

pyocele n. a swelling caused by an accumulation of pus in a part of the body.

pyocolpos n. the presence of pus in the vagina.

pyocyanin n. an antibiotic substance produced by the bacterium *Pseudomonas aeruginosa and active principally against Gram-positive bacteria.

pyoderma n. any infected skin disease in which pus is produced.

pyogenic adj. causing the formation of pus. Pyogenic bacteria include Staphylococcus aureus, Streptococcus hemolyticus, and Neisseria gonorrhoeae.

pyometra n. the presence of pus in the womb.

pyometritis n. inflammation of the womb, with the formation of pus.

pyomyositis n. bacterial or fungal infection of a muscle resulting in painful inflammation.

pyonephrosis n. obstruction and infection of the kidney resulting in pus formation. A kidney stone is the usual cause of the obstruction, and the kidney becomes distended by pus and destroyed by the inflammation, which extends into the kidney substance itself and sometimes into the surrounding tissues (see perinephritis). Treatment is urgent *nephrectomy under antibiotic cover.

pyopneumothorax n. pus and gas or air in the *pleural cavity. The condition can arise if gas is produced by gas-forming bacteria as part of an *empyema or if air is introduced during attempts to drain the pus from an empyema. Alternatively a *hydropneumothorax may become infected.

pyorrhoea n. a former name for *periodontal disease.

pyosalpingitis n. inflammation of a Fallopian tube, with the formation of pus.

pyosalpingo-oophoritis n. inflammation of an ovary and Fallopian tube, with the formation of pus.

pyosalpinx n. the accumulation of pus in a Fallopian tube.

pyosis *n.* the formation and discharge of pus.

pyothorax *n. see* empyema.

pyr- (pyro-) *prefix denoting* **1.** fire. **2.** a burning sensation. **3.** fever.

pyramid *n.* **1.** one of the conical masses that make up the medulla of the *kidney, extending inwards from a base inside the cortex towards the pelvis of the kidney. **2.** one of the elongated bulging areas on the anterior surface of the *medulla oblongata in the brain, extending downwards to the spinal cord. **3.** one of the divisions of the vermis of the *cerebellum in the middle lobe. **4.** a protrusion of the medial wall of the vestibule of the middle ear.

pyramidal cell a type of neurone found in the *cerebral cortex, with a pyramid-shaped cell body, a branched dendrite extending from the apex towards the brain surface, several dendrites extending horizontally from the base, and an axon running in the white matter of the hemisphere (see illustration).

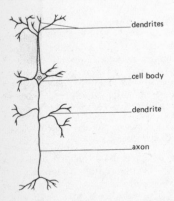

A pyramidal cell

pyramidal system a collection of nerve tracts within the *pyramid of the medulla oblongata, en route from the cerebral cortex to the spinal cord. Within the pyramid fibres cross from one side of the brain to the opposite of the spinal cord; this is called the *decussation of the pyramids*.

pyrazinamide *n.* a drug administered by mouth, usually in combination with other drugs, to treat tuberculosis. Side-effects may include digestive upsets, joint pains, gout, fever, and rashes, and high doses may cause liver damage. Trade name: **Zinamide**.

pyret- (pyreto-) *prefix denoting* fever.

pyrexia *n. see* fever.

pyridoxal phosphate a derivative of vitamin B_6 that is an important *coenzyme in certain reactions of amino-acid metabolism. *See* transamination.

pyridoxine *n. see* vitamin B_6.

pyrimidine *n.* a nitrogen-containing compound with a ring molecular structure. The commonest pyrimidines are cytosine, thymine, and uracil, which form the *nucleotides of nucleic acids.

pyrogen *n.* any substance or agent producing fever. —**pyrogenic** *adj.*

pyromania *n.* an excessively strong impulse to set things on fire. —**pyromaniac** *adj., n.*

pyrosis *n.* another term (chiefly US) for *heartburn.

pyruvic acid (pyruvate) a compound, derived from carbohydrates, that may be oxidized via a complex series of reactions in the *Krebs cycle to yield carbon dioxide and energy in the form of ATP.

pyuria *n.* the presence of pus in the urine, making it cloudy. This is a sign of bacterial infection in the urinary tract.

Q

Q fever an acute infectious disease of cattle, sheep, and goats that is caused by a *rickettsia, *Coxiella burnetti*, and can be transmitted to man primarily through contaminated unpasteurized milk. The disease lasts about two weeks and causes fever, severe headache, and respiratory problems. Treatment with tetracyclines or chloramphenicol is effective. *See also* typhus.

quadrantanopia *n.* absence or loss of one quarter of the *visual field (i.e. upper nasal (inner), upper temporal (outer), lower nasal (inner), or lower temporal (outer)). In *homonymous quadrantanopia* the same quarter is lost in the field of vision of each eye.

quadrate lobe one of the lobes of the *liver.

quadratus *n.* any of various four-sided muscles. The *quadratus femoris* is a flat muscle at the head of the femur, responsible for lateral rotation of the thigh.

quadri- *prefix denoting* four. Example: *quadrilateral* (having four sides).

quadriceps *n.* one of the great extensor muscles of the legs. It is situated in the thigh and is subdivided into four distinct portions: the *rectus femoris* (which also flexes the thigh), *vastus lateralis*, *vastus medialis*, and *vastus intermedius* (see illustration).

quadripara *n.* a woman who has been pregnant at least four times and who has given birth to an infant capable of survival after each of four pregnancies.

quadriplegia (tetraplegia) *n.* paralysis affecting all four limbs. —**quadriplegic** *adj., n.*

pelvic bone

rectus femoris

vastus lateralis

vastus medialis

common tibial tendon

head of femur

vastus intermedius

cut end of rectus femoris

Components of the quadriceps femoris

quarantine *n.* the period for which a person (or animal) is kept in isolation to prevent the spread of a contagious disease. The original quarantine was a period of 40 days, but different diseases now have different quarantine periods.

quartan fever *see* malaria.

Queckenstedt test a part of the routine *lumbar puncture procedure. It

quellung reaction

is used to determine whether or not the flow of cerebrospinal fluid is blocked in the spinal canal.

quellung reaction a reaction in which antibodies against the bacterium *Streptococcus pneumoniae* combine with the bacterial capsule, which becomes swollen and visible to light microscopy.

quickening *n.* the first movement of a baby in the womb that is felt by the mother. Quickening is usually experienced after about four months of pregnancy, although it may occur up to about two months earlier. In some normal pregnancies fetal movements may never be felt.

quiescent *adj.* describing a disease that is in an inactive or undetectable phase.

quinestradol *n.* a synthetic female sex hormone (*see* oestrogen) administered by mouth to treat inflammation of the vagina, particularly after the menopause. Side-effects do not usually occur. Trade name: **Pentovis**.

quinestrol *n.* a synthetic female sex hormone (*see* oestrogen) used to inhibit lactation in mothers not breast feeding. It is administered by mouth; side-effects are uncommon, though nausea and vomiting sometimes occur. Trade name: **Estrovis**.

quinidine *n.* a drug that slows down the activity of the heart and is administered by mouth to control abnormal and increased heart rhythm. Digestive upsets and symptoms of *cinchonism may occur as side-effects. Trade names: **Kinidin, Natisedine, Quinicardine**.

quinine *n.* a drug formerly used to prevent and treat *malaria, now largely replaced by more effective less toxic drugs. It is administered by mouth or injection; large doses can cause severe poisoning, symptoms of which include headache, fever, vomiting, confusion and damage to the eyes and ears (*see* cinchonism).

quinism *n.* the symptoms of overdosage or too prolonged treatment with quinine. *See* cinchonism.

quinsy *n.* a pus-filled swelling in the soft palate around the tonsil: a complication of *tonsillitis. The patient has great difficulty in swallowing and surgical incision of the abscess may be necessary to release the collection of pus. Medical name: **peritonsillar abscess**.

quotidian fever *see* malaria.

R

rabbit fever *see* tularaemia.

rabies (hydrophobia) *n.* an acute virus disease of the central nervous system that affects all warm-blooded animals and is usually transmitted to man by a bite from an infected dog. Symptoms appear after an incubation period ranging from 10 days to over a year and include malaise, fever, difficulty in breathing, salivation, periods of intense excitement, and painful muscle spasms of the throat induced by swallowing. In the later stages of the disease the mere sight of water induces convulsions and paralysis; death occurs within 4–5 days.
Daily injections of rabies vaccine, together with an injection of rabies antiserum, may prevent the disease from developing in a person bitten by an infected animal. —**rabid** *adj.*

racemose *adj.* resembling a bunch of grapes. The term is applied particularly to a compound gland the secretory part of which consists of a number of small sacs.

rachi- (rachio-) *prefix denoting* the spine.

rachianaesthesia *n.* *spinal anaesthesia.

rachiotomy *n. see* laminectomy.

rachis *n. see* backbone.

rachischisis *n. see* spina bifida.

rachitic *adj.* afflicted with rickets.

rad *n.* a former unit of absorbed dose of ionizing radiation. It has been replaced by the *gray.

radial *adj.* relating to or associated with the radius (a bone in the forearm).

radial artery a branch of the brachial artery, beginning at the elbow and passing superficially down the forearm to the styloid process of the radius at the wrist. It then winds around the wrist and enters the palm of the hand, sending out branches to the fingers.

radial nerve an important mixed sensory and motor nerve of the arm, forming the largest branch of the *brachial plexus. It extends downwards behind the humerus, supplying muscles of the upper arm, to the elbow, which it supplies with branches, and then runs parallel with the radius. It supplies sensory branches to the base of the thumb and a small area of the back of the hand.

radial reflex flexion of the forearm (and sometimes also of the fingers) that occurs when the lower end of the radius is tapped. It is due to contraction of the brachioradialis muscle, which is stimulated by tapping its point of insertion in the radius.

radiation *n.* energy in the form of waves or particles, especially *electromagnetic radiation*, which includes (in order of increasing wavelength), *gamma rays, *X-rays, *ultraviolet rays, visible light, and infrared rays (radiant heat), and the particles.

radiation sickness any acute illness caused by exposure to rays emitted by radioactive substances, e.g. X-rays or gamma rays. Very high doses cause death within hours from destructive lesions of the central nervous system. Lower doses, which may still prove fatal, cause immediate symptoms of nausea, vomiting, and diarrhoea followed after a week or more by bleeding and other symptoms of damage to the bone marrow, loss of hair, and bloody diarrhoea.

radical treatment vigorous treatment that aims at the complete cure of a disease rather than the mere relief of symptoms. *Compare* conservative treatment.

radicle *n.* (in anatomy) **1.** a small *root. **2.** the initial fibre of a nerve or the origin of a vein. —**radicular** *adj.*

radiculitis *n.* inflammation of the root of a nerve. *See* polyradiculitis.

radio- *prefix denoting* **1.** radiation. **2.** radioactive substances.

radioactivity *n.* disintegration of the nuclei of certain elements, with the emission of energy in the form of alpha, beta, or gamma rays. As particles are emitted the elements 'decay' into other elements. Naturally radioactive elements include radium and uranium. There are many artificially produced isotopes, including iodine-131 and cobalt-60, which are used in radiotherapy. *See* radioisotope. —**radioactive** *adj.*

radioautography *n. see* autoradiography.

radiodermatitis *n.* inflammation of the skin after its exposure to ionizing radiation. This may occur after a short dose of heavy radiation (radiotherapy or atomic explosions) or to prolonged exposure to small doses, as may happen accidentally to X-ray workers. The skin becomes dry, hairless, and atrophied, losing its colouring. Infection is common.

radiograph *n.* an image produced on a film by X-rays: an X-ray picture. *See* radiography.

radiographer *n.* a person trained in the technique of taking X-ray pictures of parts of the body. *See* radiography.

radiography *n.* the technique of examining the body by directing *X-rays through it to produce images (*radiographs*) on photographic plates or fluorescent screens. Radiography is used in the diagnosis of such disorders as broken bones, gastric ulcers, and stones in the gall bladder or kidney, when inspection from outside the body is insufficient for diagnosis. It is also widely used in dentistry for detecting dental caries, periodontal disease, periapical disease, the presence and position of unerupted teeth, and disease of the jaws.

radioimmunoassay *n.* the technique of using radioactive *tracers to determine the levels of particular antibodies in the blood. For example, radioactive iodine may be used to 'label' the hormone insulin. In some diabetic patients insulin provokes the formation of anti-insulin antibodies, which combine with the insulin. After the injection of the tracer insulin, samples of the patient's blood are analysed by *electrophoresis or *chromatography, and the antibody components of the blood are tested for the presence of radioactivity.

radioisotope *n.* an *isotope of an element that emits alpha, beta, or gamma radiation during its decay into another element. Artificial radioisotopes, produced by bombarding elements with beams of neutrons, are widely used in medicine as *tracers and as sources of radiation for the different techniques of *radiotherapy.

radiologist *n.* a doctor specialized in the interpretation of X-ray photographs for the diagnosis of disorders.

radiology *n.* the branch of medicine concerned with the use of radiation, including X-rays, and radioactive substances in the diagnosis and treatment of disease. *See also* radiotherapy. *Compare* radiography.

radionecrosis *n.* necrosis (death) of tissue, most commonly bone, whose ability to heal has been markedly reduced by radiotherapy for a tumour. It is easily induced by injury or surgery (such as tooth extraction) after irradiation.

radio-opaque *adj.* having the property of absorbing, and therefore being opaque to, X-rays. Radio-opaque materials, many of them containing iodine, are used as *contrast media in radiography (*see* diodone, iopanoic acid). Barium salts are also radio-opaque and used in barium 'meals' and enemas for the investigation of the digestive tract by X-rays.

radio pill a capsule containing a miniature radio transmitter that can be swallowed by a patient. During its passage through the digestive tract it transmits information about internal conditions (acidity, etc.) that can be monitored by means of a radio receiver near the patient.

radioscopy *n.* examination of an X-ray image on a fluorescent screen (*see* fluoroscope).

radiosensitive *adj.* describing certain forms of cancer cell that are particularly susceptible to radiation and are likely to be dealt with successfully by radiotherapy.

radiosensitizer *n.* a substance that increases the sensitivity of cells to radiation. The presence of oxygen and other compounds with a high affinity for electrons will increase radiosensitivity.

radiotherapy *n.* the treatment of disease with penetrating radiation, such as X-rays, beta rays, or gamma rays, which may be produced by machines or given off by radioactive isotopes. Beams of radiation may be directed at a diseased part from a distance (*see* tele-curietherapy), or radioactive material, in the form of needles, wires, or pellets, may be implanted in the body. Many forms of cancer are destroyed by radiation, the chief problem being the risk of damage to normal tissues.

radium *n.* a radioactive metallic element that emits alpha and gamma rays during its decay into other elements. The gamma radiation is employed in *radiotherapy for the treatment of cancer. Because *radon, a radioactive gas, is released from radium, the metal must be enclosed in gas-tight containers during use. Radium is stored in lead-lined containers, which give protection from the radiation. Symbol: Ra. *See also* thorium-X.

radius *n.* the outer and shorter bone of the forearm (*compare* ulna). It partially revolves about the ulna, permitting *pronation and *supination of the hand. The head of the radius articulates with the *humerus. The lower end articulates both with the scaphoid and lunate bones of the *carpus (wrist) and with the ulna (via the *ulnar notch* on the side of the bone). —**radial** *adj.*

radix *n. see* root.

radon *n.* a radioactive gaseous element that is produced during the decay of *radium. Sealed in small capsules called *radon seeds*, it is used in *radiotherapy for the treatment of cancer. It emits alpha and gamma radiation. Symbol: Rn.

rale *n. see* crepitation.

Ramsay Hunt syndrome a form of *herpes zoster affecting the facial nerve, associated with facial paralysis and loss of taste. It also produces pain in the ear and other parts supplied by the nerve.

Ramstedt's operation *see* pyloromyotomy.

ramus *n.* (*pl.* **rami**) **1.** a branch, especially of a nerve fibre or blood vessel. **2.** a thin process projecting from a bone, e.g. the rami of the *mandible.

randomized controlled trial *see* intervention study.

random sample a subgroup of a large population (the so-called *universe*) selected by a random process ensuring that each member of the universe has an equal chance of being included in the sample. It is sometimes *stratified* so that separate samples are drawn from each of several layers of the universe, usually on the basis of age, sex, and *social class.

ranula *n.* a cyst found under the tongue, formed when the duct leading from a salivary or mucous gland is obstructed and distended.

raphe *n.* a line, ridge, seam, or crease in a tissue or organ, especially the line marking the junction of two embryologically distinct parts that have fused to form a single structure in the adult. For example, the *raphe of the tongue* is the furrow that passes down the centre of the dorsal surface of the tongue.

rarefaction *n.* thinning of bony tissue sufficient to cause decreased density of bone to X-rays, as in osteoarthritis.

rash *n.* a temporary eruption on the skin, usually typified by reddening – either discrete red spots or generalized reddening – and itching. A rash may be a local skin reaction or the outward sign of a disorder affecting the body. Rashes commonly occur with infectious diseases, such as chickenpox and measles.

raspatory *n.* a filelike surgical instrument used for scraping the surface of bone (see illustration).

A rib raspatory

rat-bite fever (sodokosis) a disease, contracted from the bite of a rat, due to infection by either the bacterium *Spirillum minus*, which causes ulceration of the skin and recurrent fever, or by the fungus *Streptobacillus moniliformis*, which causes inflammation of the skin, muscular pains, and vomiting. Both infections respond well to penicillin.

rationalization *n.* (in psychiatry) the explanation of events or behaviour in terms that avoid giving the true reasons. For example, a patient may explain not going to a party in terms of being too tired whereas he did not go because he was afraid of meeting new people.

rauwolfia *n.* the dried root of the shrub *Rauwolfia serpentina*, which contains several alkaloids, including *reserpine. Rauwolfia and its alkaloids lower blood pressure and depress activity of the central nervous system. They were formerly used as tranquillizers in the treatment of mental illness but have been replaced by more effective and reliable drugs. Rauwolfia is still sometimes used to lower blood pressure.

Raynaud's disease a condition of unknown cause in which the arteries of the fingers are unduly reactive and enter spasm (*angiospasm* or *vasospasm*) when the hands are cold. This produces attacks of pallor, numbness, and discomfort in the fingers. A similar condition (*Raynaud's phenomenon*) may result from atherosclerosis, collagen diseases, ingestion of ergot derivatives, or the frequent use of vibrating tools. Gangrene or ulceration of the finger tips may result from lack of blood to the affected part. Warm gloves and antispasmodic drugs (such as phenoxybenzamine) may relieve the condition. In unresponsive cases *sympathectomy is of value.

reaction formation (in psychoanalysis) a *defence mechanism by which unacceptable unconscious ideas are replaced by the opposite conscious attitude. For instance, a man might make an ostentatious show of affection to a person for whom he has an unconscious hatred.

reactive *adj.* describing mental illnesses that are precipitated by events in the psychological environment. For example, *reactive depression* is distinguished in this way from *endogenous depression.

reagin *n.* a type of *antibody, formed against an allergen, that has special affinity for cell membranes and remains fixed in various tissues. Subsequent contact with the allergen causes damage to the tissue when the antigen-antibody reaction occurs. The damaged cells, particularly *mast cells, release histamine and serotonin, which are responsible for the local inflammation of an allergy or the very severe effects of anaphylactic shock (*see* anaphylaxis). Reagins belong to the IgE class of *immunoglobulins.

reamer *n.* an instrument used in *endodontics to prepare the walls of a root canal.

receptaculum *n.* the dilated portion of a tubular anatomical part. The *receptaculum* (or *cisterna*) *chyli* is the dilated end of the *thoracic duct, into which lymph vessels from the lower limbs and intestines drain.

receptor *n.* a cell or group of cells specialized to detect changes in the environment and trigger impulses in the sensory nervous system. All sensory nerve endings act as receptors, whether they simply detect touch, as in the skin, or chemical substances, as in the nose and tongue, or sound or light, as in the ear and eye. *See* exteroceptor, interoceptor, mechanoreceptor, proprioceptor.

recess *n.* (in anatomy) a hollow chamber or a depression in an organ or other part.

recessive *adj.* describing a gene (or its corresponding characteristic) whose effect is shown in the individual only when its *allele is the same. *Compare* dominant. —**recessive** *n.*

recipient *n.* a person who receives something from a *donor, such as a blood transfusion or a kidney transplant.

record linkage the means by which information about health events from several different sources (e.g. hospital attendance, vaccination, and consultation with general practitioners) are all related to a specific individual in a common file or more usually a computerized record. This contrasts with data in which events only are recorded (*see* Hospital In-Patient Enquiry) and two separate individuals treated for the same disease cannot be distinguished from one individual treated on two separate occasions.

recrudescence *n.* a fresh outbreak of a disorder in a patient after a period during which its signs and symptoms had died down and recovery seemed to be taking place.

recruitment *n.* **1.** (in physiology) the phenomenon whereby an increase in the strength of a stimulus or repetition of the stimulus will stimulate increasing numbers of nerve cells to respond. **2.** the *loudness recruitment test*: a test of hearing used to distinguish deafness due to disease of the *cochlea (in the inner ear) from other causes of deafness. In cochlear deafness, while quiet sounds are heard with difficulty in the deaf ear compared with the normal one, louder sounds are heard equally well in both ears.

rect- (recto-) *prefix denoting* the rectum. Examples: *rectouterine* (relating to the rectum and womb); *rectovesical* (relating to the rectum and bladder).

rectocele *n. see* proctocele.

rectosigmoid *n.* the region of the large intestine around the junction of the sigmoid colon and the rectum.

rectum *n.* the terminal part of the large *intestine, about 12 cm long, which runs from the sigmoid colon to the anal canal. Faeces are stored in the rectum before defecation. —**rectal** *adj.*

rectus *n.* any of several straight muscles. The *rectus muscles of the orbit* are some of the extrinsic *eye muscles. *Rectus abdominis* is a long flat muscle that extends bilaterally along the entire length of the front of the abdomen. The rectus muscles acting together serve to bend the trunk forwards; acting separately they bend the body sideways. The *rectus femoris* forms part of the *quadriceps.

recurrent *adj.* (in anatomy) describing a structure, such as a nerve or blood vessel, that turns back on its course, forming a loop.

red blood cell *see* erythrocyte.

redia *n.* (*pl.* **rediae**) the third-stage larva of a parasitic *fluke. Rediae develop within the body of a freshwater snail and undergo a process of asexual reproduction, giving rise to many fourth-stage larvae called *cercariae. *See also* miracidium, sporocyst.

reduction *n.* (in surgery) the restoration of a displaced part of the body to its normal position by manipulation or operation. The fragments of a broken bone are reduced before a splint is applied; a dislocated joint is reduced to its normal seating; or a hernia is reduced when the displaced organ or tissue is returned to its usual anatomical site.

reduction division the first division of *meiosis, in which the chromosome number is halved. The term is sometimes used as a synonym for the whole of meiosis.

reduplication

reduplication *n.* doubling of the heart sounds, which may be heard in healthy individuals and shows variation with respiration due to the slightly asynchronous closure of the heart valves.

reduviid *n.* any one of a group of winged insects (Reduviidae) whose mouthparts – adapted for piercing and sucking – take the form of a long proboscis that is tucked beneath the head when not in use. Some South American genera, notably *Panstrongylus*, *Rhodnius*, and *Triatoma* – the kissing bugs, are nocturnal bloodsucking insects that transmit the parasite causing *Chagas' disease in man.

Reduvius *n.* a genus of predatory bloodsucking reduviid bugs. *R. personatus*, widely distributed in Europe, normally preys upon insects but occasionally attacks man. Its bite causes various allergic symptoms, including rash (*see also* urticaria), nausea, and palpitations.

referred pain (synalgia) pain felt in a part of the body other than where it might be expected. An abscess beneath the diaphragm, for example, may cause a referred pain in the shoulder area, while heart disorders may cause pain in the left arm and fingers. The confusion arises because sensory nerves from different parts of the body share common pathways when they reach the spinal cord.

reflex *n.* an automatic or involuntary activity brought about by relatively simple nervous circuits, without consciousness being necessarily involved. Thus a painful stimulus such as a pinprick will bring about the reflex of withdrawing the finger before the brain has had time to send a message to the muscles involved. *See* conditioned reflex, patellar reflex, plantar reflex.

reflex arc the nervous circuit involved in a *reflex, being at its simplest a sensory nerve with a receptor, linked at

a synapse in the brain or spinal cord with a motor nerve, which supplies a muscle or gland (see illustration). In a simple reflex (such as the *patellar reflex) only two neurones may be involved, but in other reflexes there may be several *interneurones in the arc.

A reflex arc

reflux *n.* a backflow of liquid, against its normal direction of movement. *See also* (reflux) oesophagitis, vesicoureteric reflux.

refraction *n.* **1.** the change in direction of light rays when they pass obliquely from one transparent medium to another, of a different density. Refraction occurs as light enters the eye, when it passes from air to the media of the eye, i.e. cornea, aqueous humour, lens, and vitreous humour, to come to a focus on the retina. Errors of refraction, in which light rays do not come to a focus on the retina due to defects in the refracting media or shape of the eyeball, include astigmatism and long- and short-sightedness. **2.** determination of the power of refraction of the eye. This gives the degree to which the eye differs from normal, which determines whether or not the patient needs glasses and, if so, how strong they should be.

refractometer *n. see* optometer.

refractory *adj.* unresponsive: applied to a condition that fails to respond satisfactorily to a given treatment.

refractory period (in neurology) the time of recovery needed for a nerve cell that has just transmitted a nerve impulse or for a muscle fibre that has just contracted. During the refractory period a normal stimulus will not bring about excitation of the cell, which is undergoing *repolarization.

refrigeration *n.* lowering the temperature of a part of the body to reduce the metabolic activity of its tissues or to provide a local anaesthetic effect.

regimen *n.* (in therapeutics) a prescribed systematic form of treatment, such as a diet, course of drugs, or special exercises, for curing disease or improving health.

Regional Health Authority *see* National Health Service.

regional ileitis *see* Crohn's disease.

Regional Manpower Committee *see* manpower committee.

Regional Medical Committee *see* medical committee.

Regional Medical Officer *see* community physician.

registrar *n.* (in a hospital) an experienced physician or surgeon responsible for the care of a number of patients with the assistance of junior doctors, whom he instructs. A registrar may work with one or more senior surgeons, physicians, or *consultants.

regression *n.* 1. (in psychiatry) reversion to a more immature level of functioning. The term may be applied to the state of a patient in hospital who becomes incontinent and demanding. It may also be applied to a single psychological function; for example, psychoanalysts speak of the *libido regressing

to an early stage of development. 2. the stage of a disease during which the signs and symptoms disappear and the patient recovers.

regurgitation *n.* 1. the bringing up of undigested material from the stomach to the mouth (*see* vomiting). 2. the flowing back of a liquid in a direction opposite to the normal one, as when blood surges back through a defective valve in the heart after the heart has contracted.

rehabilitation 1. (in *physical medicine) the treatment of an ill, injured, or disabled patient by massage, electrotherapy, and graduated exercises to restore normal health and functions or to prevent the disability from getting worse. 2. any means for restoring the independence of a patient after diseases or injury, including employment retraining.

reimplant (replant) *vb.* to reinsert a tooth into its socket after its accidental or deliberate removal.

reinforcement *n.* (in psychology) the strengthening of a conditioned reflex (*see* conditioning). In classical conditioning this takes place when a conditioned stimulus is presented simultaneously with – or just before – the unconditioned stimulus. In operant conditioning it takes place when a pleasurable event (or *reinforcer*), such as a reward, follows immediately after some behaviour. The *reinforcement schedule* governs how often and when such behaviour is rewarded. Different schedules produce different effects on behaviour.

Reissner's membrane the membrane that separates the scala vestibuli and the scala media of the *cochlea of the ear.

Reiter's syndrome a disease of men involving diarrhoea, inflammation of the urethra (*see* urethritis) and conjunctiva (*see* conjunctivitis), and arthritis.

Horny areas may develop on the skin. The symptoms resemble those of *gonorrhoea. No causative agent has been positively identified, although a virus may be implicated.

relapse *n.* a return of disease symptoms after recovery had apparently been achieved or the worsening of an apparently recovering patient's condition during the course of an illness.

relapsing fever an infectious disease caused by bacteria of the genus *Borrelia*, which is transmitted by ticks or lice and results in recurrent fever. The first episode of fever occurs about a week after infection: it is accompanied by severe headache and aching muscles and joints and lasts 2–8 days. Subsequent attacks are milder and occur at intervals of 3–10 days; untreated, the attacks may continue for up to 12 weeks. Treatment with antibiotics, such as tetracycline or chloramphenicol, is effective.

relative analgesia a sedation technique, used particularly in dentistry, in which a mixture of *nitrous oxide and oxygen is given. The patient remains conscious throughout; the technique is used to supplement local anaesthesia in nervous patients.

relaxant *n.* an agent that reduces tension and strain, particularly in muscles (*see* muscle relaxant).

relaxation *n.* (in physiology) the diminution of tension in a muscle, which occurs when it ceases to contract: the state of a resting muscle.

relaxation therapy treatment by teaching a patient to decrease his anxiety by reducing the tone in his muscles. This can be used by itself to help people cope with stressful situations or as a part of *desensitization to specific fears.

relaxin *n.* a hormone, secreted by the placenta in the terminal stages of pregnancy, that causes the neck (cervix) of the womb to dilate and prepares the womb for the action of *oxytocin during labour.

reline *n.* the procedure by which the fitting surface of a denture is rebased to make it fit a jaw that has undergone resorption since the denture was originally made. The procedure is often necessary for dentures that were fitted immediately after extraction of the teeth.

rem *n.* roentgen equivalent man: a former unit dose of ionizing radiation equal to the dose that gives the same biological effect as that due to one roentgen of X-rays. The rem has been replaced by the *sievert.

REM rapid eye movement: describing a stage of *sleep during which the muscles of the eyeballs are in constant motion behind the eyelids. People woken up during this stage of sleep generally report that they were dreaming at the time.

remedial profession any profession (including occupational therapy, physiotherapy and speech therapy) in which the therapists use their skills to assist those with *handicap to achieve living and working standards as near normal as possible.

remission *n.* a lessening in the severity of symptoms or their temporary disappearance during the course of an illness.

remittent fever *see* fever.

Remploy *n.* (in Britain) a nationally financed system of sheltered employment for those with severe *handicap in specially designed workshops managed and financed by the Department of Employment. Limited numbers of able-bodied craftsmen are included on the payroll to assist with administration and supervision and also to carry out tasks that would be potentially dangerous for those with handicap. Goods produced (especially furniture and luggage) are sold on the open market.

renal *adj.* relating to or affecting the kidneys.

renal artery either of two large arteries arising from the abdominal aorta and supplying the kidneys. Each renal artery divides into an anterior and a posterior branch before entering the kidney.

renal cell carcinoma *see* hypernephroma.

renal tubule (uriniferous tubule) the fine tubular part of a *nephron, through which water and certain dissolved substances are reabsorbed back into the blood.

reni- (reno-) *prefix denoting* the kidney.

renin *n.* a substance released into the blood by the kidney in response to stress. It reacts with a substrate from the liver to produce *angiotensin, which causes constriction of blood vessels and thus an increase in blood pressure. Excessive production of renin results in the syndrome of renal *hypertension.

rennin *n.* an enzyme produced in the stomach that coagulates milk. It is secreted by the gastric glands in an inactive form, *prorennin*, which is activated by hydrochloric acid. Rennin converts caseinogen (milk protein) into insoluble casein in the presence of calcium ions. This ensures that the milk remains in the stomach, exposed to protein-digesting enzymes, for as long as possible. Rennin is present in the largest amounts in the stomachs of young mammals.

renography *n.* the radiological study of the kidneys by a *gamma camera following the intravenous injection of a radioactive substance, which is concentrated and excreted by the kidneys. The radioactive isotope (usually *technetium-131) emits gamma rays, which are recorded by the camera positioned over the kidneys. The resultant graph of each kidney gives information regarding function and rate of drainage.

reovirus *n.* one of a group of small RNA-containing viruses that infect both respiratory and intestinal tracts without producing specific or serious diseases (and were therefore termed *respiratory enteric orphan viruses). Compare* echovirus.

replacement bone a bone that is formed by replacing cartilage with bony material.

replant *vb. see* reimplant.

replication *n.* the process by which *DNA makes copies of itself when the cell divides. The two strands of the DNA molecule unwind and each strand directs the synthesis of a new strand complementary to itself (see illustration).

A adenine
C cytosine
G guanine
T thymine

Replication of a DNA molecule

repolarization *n.* the process in which the membrane of a nerve cell returns to its normal electrically charged state

531

repositor

after a nerve impulse has passed. During the passage of a nerve impulse a temporary change in the molecular structure of the membrane allows a surge of ions across the membrane (*see* action potential). During repolarization ions diffuse back to restore the charge and the nerve becomes ready to transmit further impulses. *See* refractory period.

repositor *n.* an instrument used to return a displaced part of the body – for instance, a prolapsed womb – to its normal position.

repression *n.* (in *psychoanalysis) the process of excluding an unacceptable wish or an idea from conscious mental life. The repressed material continues to control behaviour and may give rise to symptoms. One goal of psychoanalysis is to return repressed material to conscious awareness so that it may be dealt with rationally.

reproduction rate *see* fertility rate.

reproductive system the combination of organs and tissues associated with the process of reproduction. In males it includes the testes, vasa deferentia, prostate gland, seminal vesicles, urethra, and penis; in females it includes the ovaries, Fallopian tubes, womb (uterus), vagina, and vulva. (See illustration.)

resection *n.* surgical removal of a portion of any part of the body. For example, a section of diseased intestine may be removed and the healthy ends sewn together. A *submucous resection* is removal of part of the cartilage septum (central division) of the nose that has become deviated, usually by injury. *Transurethral resection* (*TUR, resection of the prostate*) – an operation performed when the prostate gland becomes enlarged – involves removal of the gland through the urethra using an instrument called a *resectoscope*.

resectoscope *n.* a type of surgical instrument (an *endoscope) used in resection of the prostate or in the removal of bladder tumours.

reserpine *n.* a drug extracted from *rauwolfia and used to lower high blood pressure and, occasionally, to relieve anxiety. It is administered by mouth or injection; side-effects often include mental depression, nasal congestion, and digestive upsets. Trade name: **Serpasil**.

reserve volume the extra volume of air that an individual could inhale or

Male reproductive system

Female reproductive system

exhale if he is not breathing to the limit of his capacity.

residual volume the volume of air that remains in the lungs after the individual has breathed out as much as he can. This volume is increased in *emphysema.

resistance n. **1.** the degree of *immunity that the body possesses: a measure of its ability to withstand disease. **2.** the degree to which a disease or disease-causing organism remains unaffected by antibiotics or other drugs.

resolution n. **1.** the stage during which inflammation gradually disappears. **2.** the degree to which individual details can be distinguished by the eye, as through a *microscope.

resorcinol n. a drug that causes the skin to peel. It is applied to the skin in ointments to treat such conditions as acne, and used in hair lotions for dandruff. If the drug is absorbed into the body, it causes underactivity of the thyroid gland (myxoedema) and convulsions.

resorption n. loss of substance through physiological or pathological means.

respiration n. the process of gaseous exchange between an organism and its environment. This includes both *external respiration*, which involves *breathing, in which oxygen is taken up by the capillaries of the lung *alveoli and carbon dioxide is released from the blood, and *internal respiration*, during which oxygen is released to the tissues and carbon dioxide absorbed by the blood. Blood provides the transport medium for the gases between the lungs and tissue cells. In addition, it contains a pigment, *haemoglobin, with special affinity for oxygen. Once inside the cell oxygen is utilized in metabolic processes resulting in the production of energy (*see* ATP), water, and waste materials (including carbon dioxide). *See also* lung. —**respiratory** *adj.*

respirator n. **1.** a device used to maintain the breathing movements of paralysed patients. In the *positive-pressure respirator* air is blown into the patient's lungs via a tube passed either through the mouth into the trachea or through a *tracheostomy. Air is released from the lungs when the pressure from the respirator is relaxed. The *iron lung* is a type of respirator in which the patient is enclosed, except for the head, in an airtight container in which the air pressure is decreased and increased mechanically. This draws air into and out of the lungs, through the normal air passages. The *cuirass respirator* works on a similar principle, but leaves the limbs free. **2.** a face mask for administering oxygen or other gas or for filtering harmful fumes, dust, etc. *See also* artificial respiration.

respiratory distress syndrome (hyaline membrane disease) the condition of a newborn infant in which the lungs are imperfectly expanded. Initial inflation and normal expansion of the lungs requires the presence of a substance (*surfactant) that reduces the surface tension of the air sacs (alveoli). The condition is most common and serious among premature infants (especially between the 32nd and 37th weeks of gestation), in whom *surfactant is liable to be deficient. Breathing is rapid, laboured, and shallow, and microscopic examinations of lung tissue in fatal cases has revealed the presence of *hyaline material in the collapsed air sacs. The condition is treated by careful nursing, intravenous fluids, and oxygen, with or without positive pressure by a *respirator.

respiratory quotient (RQ) the ratio of the volume of carbon dioxide transferred from the blood into the alveoli to the volume of oxygen absorbed into the alveoli. The RQ is usually about 0.8 because more oxygen is taken up than carbon dioxide excreted.

respiratory syncytial virus (RSV) a paramyxovirus (*see* myxovirus) that causes infections of the nose and throat. It is a major cause of bronchiolitis and pneumonia in young children. In tissue cultures infected with the virus, cells merge together to form a conglomerate (*syncytium*).

respiratory system the combination of organs and tissues associated with *breathing. It includes the nasal cavity, pharynx, larynx, trachea, bronchi, bronchioles, and lungs and also the diaphragm and other muscles associated with breathing movements.

response *n.* the way in which the body or part of the body reacts to a *stimulus. For example, a nerve impulse may produce the response of a contraction in a muscle that the nerve supplies.

restiform body a thick bundle of nerve fibres that conveys impulses from tracts in the spinal cord to the cortex of the anterior and posterior lobes of the cerebellum.

resting cell a cell that is not undergoing division. *See* interphase.

restoration *n.* (in dentistry) any type of dental *filling or *crown, which is aimed at restoring a tooth to its normal form, function, and appearance.

retainer *n.* (in dentistry) **1.** a component of a partial *denture that keeps it in place. **2.** an *orthodontic appliance that holds the teeth in position. **3.** a component of a *bridge that is fixed to a natural tooth.

retardation *n.* the slowing up of a process. The term *mental retardation* is used as a synonym for mental *subnormality; it implies that the subnormality is regarded as a delay in development rather than a qualitative defect. *Psychomotor retardation* is a marked slowing down of activity and speech, which can reach a degree where a patient can no longer care for himself. It is a symptom of severe *depression.

retching *n.* repeated unavailing attempts to vomit.

rete *n.* a network of blood vessels, nerve fibres, or other strands of interlacing tissue in the structure of an organ. The *rete testis* is a network of tubules conducting sperm from the seminiferous tubules of the *testis to the vasa efferentia.

retention *n.* inability to pass urine, which is retained in the bladder. The condition may be acute and painful or chronic and painless. The commonest cause is enlargement of the prostate gland in men, although many other conditions may result in obstruction of bladder outflow. Retention is relieved by catheter drainage of the bladder before dealing with the underlying problem.

retention appliance *see* dental appliance.

retention defect (in psychology) a memory defect in which items that have been registered in the memory are lost from storage. It is a feature of *dementia.

reticular activating system the system of nerve pathways in the brain concerned with the level of consciousness – from the states of sleep, drowsiness, and relaxation to full alertness and attention. The system integrates information from all of the senses and from the cerebrum and cerebellum and determines the overall activity of the brain and the autonomic nervous system and patterns of behaviour during waking and sleeping.

reticular fibres microscopic, almost nonelastic, branching fibres of *connective tissue that join together to form a delicate supportive meshwork around blood vessels, muscle fibres, glands, nerves, etc. They are composed of a collagen-like protein (*reticulin*) and are particularly common in lymph nodes, the spleen, liver, kidneys, and muscles.

reticular formation a network of nerve pathways and nuclei throughout the *brainstem, connecting motor and sensory nerves to and from the spinal cord, the cerebellum and the cerebrum, and the cranial nerves. It is estimated that a single neurone in this network may have synapses with as many as 25,000 other neurones.

reticulin *n.* a protein that is the major constituent of *reticular fibres.

reticulocyte *n.* an immature red blood cell (erythrocyte). Reticulocytes may be detected and counted by staining living red cells with certain basic dyes that result in the formation of a blue precipitate (*reticulum*) within the reticulocytes. They normally comprise about 1% of the total red cells and are increased (*reticulocytosis*) whenever the rate of red cell production increases.

reticulocytosis *n.* an increase in the proportion of immature red blood cells (reticulocytes) in the bloodstream. It is a sign of increased output of new red cells from the bone marrow.

reticuloendothelial system (RES) a community of cells – *phagocytes – spread throughout the body. It includes *macrophages and *monocytes. The RES is concerned with defence against microbial infection and with the removal of worn-out blood cells from the bloodstream. *See also* spleen.

reticuloendotheliosis (histiocytosis X) *n.* overgrowth of cells of the *reticuloendothelial system, causing either isolated swelling of the bone marrow (*eosinophilic granuloma*) or destruction of the bones of the skull (*Hand-Schüller-Christian disease*). The most acute form, starting in infancy and usually rapidly fatal, is associated with tumours containing histiocytes in the internal organs (*Letterer-Siwe disease*).

reticulosis *n.* abnormal overgrowth, usually malignant, of any of the cells of the lymphatic glands or the immune system. *See* lymphoma, Hodgkin's disease, Burkitt's tumour.

reticulum *n.* a network of tubules or blood vessels. *See* endoplasmic reticulum, sarcoplasmic reticulum.

retin- (retino-) *prefix denoting* the retina. Example: *retinopexy* (fixation of a detached retina).

retina *n.* the light-sensitive layer that lines the interior of the eye. The outer

The structure of the retina

part of the retina, next to the *choroid, is pigmented to prevent the passage of light. The inner part, next to the cavity of the eyeball, contains *rods and *cones (light-sensitive cells) and their associated nerve fibres (see illustration). A large number of cones is concentrated in a depression in the retina at the back of the eyeball called the *fovea. —**retinal** *adj.*

retinaculum *n.* (*pl.* **retinacula**) a thickened band of tissue that serves to hold various tissues in place. For example, *flexor retinacula* are found over the flexor tendons in the wrist and ankle.

retinal (retinene) *n.* the aldehyde of retinol (*vitamin A). *See also* rhodopsin.

retinene *n. see* retinal.

retinitis *n.* inflammation of the retina. In practice, the term is often used for conditions not strictly inflammatory; for example *retinitis pigmentosa*, a noninflammatory hereditary condition involving progressive degeneration of the retina. For such conditions the term *retinopathy is becoming more widely used.

retinoblastoma *n.* a rare malignant tumour of the retina, occurring in infants.

retinol *n. see* vitamin A.

retinopathy *n.* any disorder of the retina resulting in impairment or loss of vision. It is usually due to damage to the blood vessels of the retina, occurring (for example) as a complication of diabetes (*diabetic retinopathy*) or high blood pressure.

retinoscope *n.* an instrument used to determine the power of *refraction of the eye. It is held in the hand and casts a beam of light into the subject's eye. The examiner looks along the beam and sees the shadows it produces in the subject's pupil. By interpreting the way

the shadows move when he moves the instrument, and by altering them by lenses held in his other hand near the subject's eye, he is able to detect long- or short-sightedness or astigmatism and to determine its degree. —**retinoscopy** *n.*

retraction *n.* **1.** (in obstetrics) the permanent shortening of the muscle fibres of the womb wall that occurs each time they contract during labour. **2.** (in dentistry) the drawing back of one or more teeth into a better position by an *orthodontic appliance.

retraction ring 1. a depression on the surface of the womb that may be detected during labour by applying the hand to the lower part of the abdomen. It occurs in the region of the neck (cervix) of the womb when the circular muscle fibres fail to relax and it indicates the presence of a constriction around the womb, which tends to prevent the infant from emerging into the cervical canal. Also called: **Bandl's ring**. **2.** the dividing line between the upper contracting part of the womb in labour and the lower dilating part.

retractor *n.* a surgical instrument used to expose the operation site by drawing aside the cut edges of skin, muscle, or other tissues. There are several types of retractors for different operations (see illustration).

wound retractor

abdominal retractor

Retractors

retro- *prefix denoting* at the back or behind. Examples: *retrobulbar* (at the back of the eyeball); *retroperitoneal* (behind the peritoneum).

retrobulbar neuritis (optic neuritis) inflammation of the optic nerve behind the eye, causing increasingly blurred vision. When the inflammation involves the first part of the nerve and can be seen at the optic disc, it is called *optic papillitis*. Retrobulbar neuritis is one of the symptoms of multiple sclerosis but it can also occur as an isolated lesion, in the absence of any other involvement of the nervous system, with the patient recovering vision completely.

retroflexion *n.* the bending backward of an organ or part of an organ, especially of the upper part of the womb (*uterine retroflexion*) in relation to the lower part (cervix).

retrograde *adj.* going backwards, or moving in the opposite direction to the normal. (*See* (retrograde) pyelography.) *Retrograde amnesia* is a failure to remember events immediately preceding an illness or injury.

retropulsion *n.* a compulsive tendency to walk backwards. It is a symptom of *parkinsonism.

retrospective study a backward-looking review of the characteristics of a group of individuals in relation to morbidity, embracing some aspects of *cross-sectional and/or *case control studies. The term is sometimes loosely used as a synonym for such studies.

retroversion *n.* the backward inclination of an organ, especially of the womb (*uterine retroversion*), when it is tipped back so that the neck (cervix) points towards the pubic symphysis (the bone under the pubic hair).

retrovirus *n.* an RNA-containing virus that can transfer its genetic material into the DNA of its host's cells. Retroviruses have been implicated in the development of some cancers.

retrusion *n.* (in dentistry) **1.** backward movement of the lower jaw. **2.** a malocclusion in which some of the teeth are further back than usual. *Compare* protrusion.

rhabdomyoma *n.* a rare benign tumour of skeletal muscle or heart muscle.

rhabdomyosarcoma *n.* a malignant tumour originating in, or showing the characteristics of, striated muscle. *Pleomorphic rhabdomyosarcoma* occurs in late middle age, in the muscles of the limbs. *Embryonal rhabdomyosarcomas*, affecting infants, children, and young adults, are classified as *botryoid* (in the vagina, bladder, ear, etc.), *embryonal* (most common in the head and neck, particularly the orbit); and *alveolar* (at the base of the thumb). The pleomorphic and alveolar types respond poorly to treatment; botryoid tumours are treated with a combination of radiotherapy, surgery, and drugs. The embryonal type, if treated at an early stage, can often be cured with a combination of radiotherapy and drugs (including vincristine, actinomycin-D, and cyclophosphamide).

rhagades *pl. n.* cracks or long thin scars in the skin, particularly around the mouth or other areas of the body subjected to constant movement. The fissures around the mouth and nose of babies with congenital syphilis eventually heal to form rhagades.

rheo- *prefix denoting* **1.** a flow of liquid. **2.** an electric current.

rhesus factor (Rh factor) a group of *antigens that may or may not be present on the surface of the red blood cells; it forms the basis of the rhesus blood group system. Most people have the rhesus factor, i.e. they are *Rh-positive*. People who lack the factor are termed *Rh-negative*. Incompatibility between Rh-positive and Rh-negative blood is an important cause of blood transfusion reactions and *haemolytic disease of the newborn. *See also* blood group.

rheumatic fever (acute rheumatism) a disease affecting mainly children and young adults that arises as a delayed complication of infection of the upper respiratory tract with haemolytic streptococci (*see* Streptococcus). The main features are fever, arthritis progressing from joint to joint, reddish circular patches on the skin, small painless nodules formed on bony prominences such as the elbow, abnormal involuntary movements of the limbs and head (*chorea), and inflammation of the membrane surrounding the heart. The condition may progress to *chronic rheumatic heart disease*, with scarring and chronic inflammation of the heart and its valves leading to heart failure, murmurs, and damage to the valves. The initial infection is treated with antibiotics (e.g. penicillin) and bed rest, with aspirin for the joint pain.

rheumatism *n.* any disorder in which aches and pains affect the muscles and joints. *See* rheumatoid arthritis, rheumatic fever, osteoarthritis, gout.

rheumatoid arthritis a form of *arthritis that is the second most common rheumatic disease (after *osteoarthritis). It typically involves the joints of the fingers, wrists, feet, and ankles and often the hips and shoulders: the joints are affected symmetrically and there is a considerable range of severity. The condition is diagnosed by a blood test, which shows the presence of the *rheumatoid factor*, and by X-rays revealing typical changes (*rheumatoid erosions*) around the affected joints.
A wide variety of treatments, usually based on anti-inflammatory analgesics, provide relief of symptoms. The condition may resolve spontaneously and often undergoes periods of remission of symptoms.

rheumatology *n.* the medical specialty concerned with the diagnosis and management of disease involving joints, tendons, muscles, ligaments, and associated structures. *See also* physical medicine. —**rheumatologist** *n.*

rhexis *n.* the breaking apart of a blood vessel, organ, or tissue.

Rh factor *see* rhesus factor.

rhin- (rhino-) *prefix denoting* the nose.

rhinencephalon *n.* the parts of the brain, collectively, that in early stages of evolution were concerned mainly with the sense of smell. The rhinencephalon includes the olfactory nerve, olfactory tract, and the regions now usually classified as belonging to the *limbic system.

rhinitis *n.* inflammation of the mucous membrane of the nose. It may be caused by virus infection (*acute rhinitis*; *see* (common) cold) or an allergic reaction (*allergic rhinitis*; *see* hay fever). In *atrophic rhinitis* the mucous membrane becomes thinned and fragile; in *chronic catarrhal rhinitis* there is overgrowth of, and increased secretion by, the membrane.

rhinolith *n.* a stone (calculus) in the nose.

rhinology *n.* the branch of medicine concerned with disorders of the nose and nasal passages.

rhinomycosis *n.* fungal infection of the lining of the nose.

rhinophyma *n.* permanent redness and swelling of the nose. It commonly occurs with *rosacea, in which the characteristic nodular swelling may produce grotesque deformity. Surgery may be necessary for cosmetic purposes.

rhinoplasty *n.* reparative or cosmetic surgery of the nose, sometimes by the repair of a defect with tissue (skin or bone) taken from elsewhere in the body.

rhinorrhoea *n.* a persistent watery mucous discharge from the nose, as in the common cold.

rhinoscleroma *n.* the formation of nodules in the interior of the nose and *nasopharynx, which become thickened. It is caused by bacterial infection (with *Klebsiella rhinoscleroma*).

rhinoscopy *n.* examination of the interior of the nose.

rhinosporidiosis *n.* an infection of the mucous membranes of the nose, larynx, eyes, and genitals that is caused by the fungus *Rhinosporidium seeberi* and is characterized by the formation of tiny growths called *polyps. It occurs most commonly in Asia.

rhinovirus *n.* any one of a group of RNA-containing viruses that cause respiratory infections in man resembling the common cold. They are included in the *picornavirus group.

Rhipicephalus *n.* a genus of hard *ticks widely distributed in the tropics. The dog tick (*R. sanguineus*) can suck the blood of man and is commonly involved in the transmission of diseases caused by rickettsiae (*see* typhus).

rhiz- (rhizo-) *prefix denoting* a root. Example: *rhizonychia* (the root of a nail).

rhizotomy *n.* a surgical procedure in which selected nerve roots are cut at the point where they emerge from the spinal cord. In *posterior rhizotomy* the posterior (sensory) nerve roots are cut for the relief of intractable pain in the organs served by these nerves. An *anterior rhizotomy* – the cutting of the anterior (motor) nerve roots – is sometimes done for the relief of severe muscle spasm.

Rhodnius *n.* a genus of large bloodsucking bugs (*see* reduviid). *R. prolixus*

is important in the transmission of *Chagas' disease in Central America and the northern part of South America.

rhodopsin (visual purple) *n.* a pigment in the retina of the eye, within the *rods, consisting of *retinal* – an aldehyde of retinol (*vitamin A) – and a protein. The presence of rhodopsin is essential for vision in dim light. It is bleached in the presence of light and this stimulates nervous activity in the rods.

rhombencephalon *n. see* hindbrain.

rhomboid *n.* either of two muscles (*rhomboid major* and *rhomboid minor*) situated in the upper part of the back, between the backbone and shoulder blade. They help to move the shoulder blade backwards and upwards.

rhonchus *n.* (*pl.* **rhonchi**) an abnormal musical noise produced by air passing through narrowed bronchi. It is heard through a stethoscope, usually when the patient breathes out.

rhythm method a contraceptive method in which sexual intercourse is restricted to the *safe period* at the beginning and end of the *menstrual cycle. The safe period is calculated either on the basis of the length of the menstrual cycle or by reliance on the change of body temperature that occurs at ovulation. A third possible indicator is the change that occurs with ovulation in the stickiness of the mucus at the neck (cervix) of the womb. The method depends for its reliability on the woman having uniform regular periods and its failure rate is higher than with mechanical methods, approaching 25 pregnancies per 100 woman-years.

rib *n.* a curved, slightly twisted, strip of bone forming part of the skeleton of the thorax, which protects the heart and lungs. There are 12 pairs of ribs. The head of each rib articulates with one of the 12 thoracic vertebrae of the back-

riboflavin

bone; the other end is attached to a section of cartilage (*see* costal cartilage). The first seven pairs – the *true ribs* – are connected directly to the sternum by their costal cartilages. The next three pairs – the *false ribs* – are attached indirectly: each is connected by its cartilage to the rib above it. The last two pairs of ribs – the *floating ribs* – end freely in the muscles of the body wall. Anatomical name: **costa**.

riboflavin *n. see* vitamin B₂.

riboflavin *n. see* vitamin B_2.

ribonuclease *n.* an enzyme, located in the *lysosomes of cells, that splits RNA at specific places in the molecule.

ribonucleic acid *see* RNA.

ribose *n.* a pentose sugar (i.e. one with free carbon atoms) that is a component of *RNA and several coenzymes. Ribose is also involved in intracellular metabolism.

ribosome *n.* a particle, consisting of RNA and protein, that occurs in cells and is the site of protein synthesis in the cell (*see* translation). Ribosomes are either attached to the *endoplasmic reticulum or free in the cytoplasm as *polysomes. —**ribosomal** *adj.*

ricin *n.* a highly toxic albumin obtained from castor-oil seeds (*Ricinus communis*) that inhibits protein synthesis and becomes attached to the surface of cells, resulting in gastroenteritis, hepatic congestion and jaundice, and cardiovascular collapse. It is lethal to most species, even in minute amounts (1 μg/kg body weight); it is most toxic if injected intravenously or inhaled as fine particles.

rickets *n.* a disease of children in which the bones do not harden and are malformed due to a deficiency of *vitamin D. Without vitamin D not enough calcium salts are deposited in the bones to make them rigid. They are therefore softer than normal and bend out of shape. *See also* osteomalacia.

Renal rickets is due to impaired kidney function: the bones are malformed as bone-forming minerals are excreted in the urine.

rickettsiae *pl. n.* (*sing.* **rickettsia**) a group of very small nonmotile spherical or rodlike parasitic organisms. They resemble bacteria in their cellular structure and method of asexual reproduction, but – like viruses – they cannot reproduce outside the bodies of their hosts. Rickettsiae infect arthropods (ticks, mites, etc.), through whom they can be transmitted to mammals (including man), in which they can cause severe illness. The species *Rickettsia akari* causes *rickettsial pox; *R. conori*, *R. mooseri*, *R. prowazeki*, *R. quintana*, and *R. tsutsugamushi* cause different forms of *typhus, and *R. rickettsii* causes *Rocky Mountain spotted fever. *See also* Coxiella. —**rickettsial** *adj.*

rickettsial pox a disease of mice caused by the microorganism *Rickettsia akari* and transmitted to man by mites: it produces chills, fever, muscular pain, and a rash similar to that of *chickenpox. The disease is mild and runs its course in 2–3 weeks. *See also* typhus.

ridge *n.* **1.** (in anatomy) a crest or a long narrow protuberance, e.g. on a bone. **2.** (in dental anatomy) *see* alveolus.

rifampicin *n.* an *antibiotic used to treat various infections, particularly tuberculosis. It is administered by mouth; digestive upsets and sensitivity reactions sometimes occur. Trade names: **Rifadin, Rimactane**.

rifamycin *n.* an *antibiotic used to treat certain infections, particularly tuberculosis. It is administered by injection, inhalation, or in a solution applied to the infected area. Side-effects are uncommon.

Rift Valley fever a virus disease of East Africa transmitted from animals to man by mosquitoes and causing symptoms resembling those of *influenza.

rigidity *n.* (in neurology) resistance to the passive movement of a limb that persists throughout its range. It is a symptom of *parkinsonism. A smooth resistance is called *plastic* or *lead-pipe rigidity* while intermittent resistance is called *cogwheel rigidity*. *Compare* spasticity.

rigor *n.* **1.** an abrupt attack of shivering and a sensation of coldness, accompanied by a rapid rise in body temperature. This often marks the onset of a fever and may be followed by a feeling of heat, with copious sweating. **2.** *see* rigor mortis.

rigor mortis the stiffening of a body that occurs within some eight hours of death, due to chemical changes in muscle tissue. It starts to disappear after about 24 hours.

rima *n.* (in anatomy) a cleft. The *rima glottidis* (or glottis) is the space between the vocal cords.

rimiterol *n.* a drug, similar to *isoprenaline, used as a *bronchodilator to relieve asthma and chronic bronchitis. It is administered by inhalation; side-effects, following large doses, may include dizziness, fainting, tremor, anxiety, and fast heart rate. Trade name: **Pulmadil**.

ring *n.* (in anatomy) *see* annulus.

Ringer's solution (Ringer's mixture) a clear colourless *physiological solution of sodium chloride (common salt), potassium chloride, and calcium chloride prepared with recently boiled pure water. The osmotic pressure of the solution is the same as that of blood serum. Ringer's solution is used for maintaining organs or tissues alive outside the animal or human body for limited periods. Sterile Ringer's solution is injected intravenously to treat dehydration.

ringworm (tinea) *n.* a fungus infection of the surface of the skin, particularly the scalp and feet, and occasionally of the nails. Ringworm is caused by various species of the fungi *Microsporum*, *Trichophyton*, and *Epidermophyton* and it also affects animals: a source of infection for man. Ringworm is highly contagious and can be spread by direct contact or via infected materials. As its name suggests, the infection is ringlike and it causes intense itching. The commonest form of ringworm is *athlete's foot* (*tinea pedis*), which affects the skin between the toes. Another common type is ringworm of the scalp (*tinea capitis*), of which there is a severe form – *favus. Ringworm also affects the skin under a beard (*tinea barbae*). The disease is treated with antifungal agents taken by mouth (such as griseofulvin) or applied locally.

Rinne's test a test to determine whether *deafness is conductive or perceptive. A vibrating tuning fork is held first in the air, close to the ear, and then with its base placed on the bone (mastoid process) behind the ear. If the sound conducted by air is heard for a longer time than the sound conducted by bone the test is positive and the deafness perceptive; a negative result, when the sound conducted by the bone lasts longer, indicates conductive deafness.

risk factor an attribute (such as a habit (e.g. cigarette smoking) or exposure to some environmental hazard) that leads the individual concerned to have a greater likelihood of developing an illness. The relationship is one of probability and as such can be distinguished from a *causal agent.

risk register a list of infants who have experienced some event in their obstetric and/or perinatal history known to be correlated with a higher than average likelihood of serious abnormality. Such children are subjected to extra surveillance. Problems associated with risk registers include limiting the designation of predisposing conditions so as to contain the number on the register within reasonable proportions and ensuring that children not on the register receive adequate surveillance.

risus sardonicus an abnormal grinning expression resulting from involuntary prolonged contraction of facial muscles, as seen in *tetanus.

river blindness *see* onchocerciasis.

RNA (ribonucleic acid) a *nucleic acid, occurring in the nucleus and cytoplasm of cells, that is concerned with synthesis of proteins (*see* messenger RNA, ribosome, transfer RNA, translation). In some viruses RNA is the genetic material. The RNA molecule is a single strand made up of units called *nucleotides.

Rocky Mountain spotted fever (spotted fever, tick fever) a disease of rodents and other small mammals in the USA caused by the microorganism *Rickettsia rickettsii* and transmitted to man by ticks. Symptoms include fever, muscle pains, and a profuse reddish rash like that of measles. If untreated the disease may be fatal, but treatment with tetracycline or chloramphenicol is effective. *See also* typhus.

rod *n.* one of the two types of light-sensitive cells in the *retina of the eye (*compare* cone). The human eye contains about 125 million rods, which are necessary for seeing in dim light. They contain a pigment, *visual purple* (*rhodopsin*), which is broken down (bleached) in the light and regenerated in the dark. Breakdown of visual purple gives rise to nerve impulses; when all the pigment is bleached (i.e. in bright light) the rods no longer function. *See also* dark adaptation, light adaptation.

rodent ulcer a slow-growing malignant tumour of the face, usually at the edge of the eyelids, lips, or nostrils.

Rodent ulcers occur in middle age or later; if untreated, they destroy skin muscle and bone but they do not spread to other parts of the body. Europeans persistently exposed to hot sun may develop the disease and it is a complication of chronic *radiodermatitis. It can be treated by surgery or radiotherapy. Medical name: **basal cell carcinoma**.

roentgen *n.* a unit of exposure dose of X- or gamma-radiation equal to the dose that will produce 2.58×10^{-4} coulomb on all the ions of one sign, when all the electrons released in a volume of air of mass 1 kilogram are completely stopped.

roentgenology *n.* the study of the applications of X-rays (roentgen rays) in medicine.

role playing acting out another person's expected behaviour, usually in a contrived situation, in order to understand them better. It is used in family psychotherapy, in teaching social skills to patients, and also in the training of psychiatric (and other) staff.

Romaña's sign an early clinical sign of *Chagas' disease, appearing some three weeks after infection. There is considerable swelling of the eyelids of one or both eyes. This may be due to the presence of the parasites causing the disease but it may also be an allergic reaction to the repeated bites of their insect carriers.

Romanowsky stains a group of stains used for microscopical examination of blood cells, consisting of variable mixtures of thiazine dyes, such as azure B, with eosin. Romanowsky stains give characteristic staining patterns, on the basis of which blood cells are classified. The group includes the stains of Leishmann, Wright, May-Grunwald, Giemsa, etc.

Romberg's sign evidence of a sensory disorder affecting those nerves that transmit information to the brain about the position of the limbs and joints and the tension in the muscles. The patient is asked to stand upright. Romberg's sign is positive if he maintains his posture when his eyes are open but sways and falls when his eyes are closed.

rongeur *n.* powerful biting forceps for cutting tissue, particularly bone.

root *n.* **1.** (in neurology) a bundle of nerve fibres at its emergence from the spinal cord. The 31 pairs of *spinal nerves have two roots on each side, an anterior root containing motor nerve fibres and a posterior root containing sensory fibres. The roots merge outside the cord to form mixed nerves. **2.** (in dentistry) the part of a *tooth that is not covered by enamel and is normally attached to the alveolar bone by periodontal fibres. **3.** the origin of any structure, i.e. the point at which it diverges from another structure. Anatomical name: **radix**.

root filling 1. the final stage of *root treatment, in which the prepared canal inside a tooth root is filled with a suitable material. **2.** the material used to fill the canal in the root, usually a core of *gutta-percha with a thin coating of sealing cement.

root induction (in *endodontics) a procedure to allow continued root formation in an immature tooth with a damaged pulp.

root treatment (in *endodontics) the procedure of removing the remnants of the pulp of a tooth, cleaning and shaping the canal inside the tooth, and filling the root canal (*see* root filling). The entire treatment usually extends over several visits. It is used to treat toothache and apical abscesses.

Rorschach test a test to measure aspects of personality, consisting of ten inkblots, half of which are in various colours and the other half in black and white. The responses to the different inkblots are used to derive hypotheses about the subject. The use of the test for the diagnosis of brain damage is no longer generally supported. *See also* projective test.

rosacea *n.* a skin disease of the face in which the blood vessels enlarge, giving the cheeks and nose a flushed appearance. The cause is uncertain but irritant foods or drinks or too much alcohol may play a part, and extremes of climate may aggravate the condition. The nose may enlarge (*see* rhinophyma). Rosacea usually occurs after the age of 30 and affects women more often than men, with the menopause sometimes acting as a trigger.

roseola *n.* any rose-coloured rash, such as occurs in measles, the secondary stage of syphilis, or typhoid fever.

rostellum *n.* (*pl.* **rostella**) a mobile and retractable knob bearing hooks, present on the head (scolex) of certain *tapeworms, e.g. *Taenia* and *Echinococcus*.

rostrum *n.* (*pl.* **rostra**) (in anatomy) a beaklike projection, such as that on the sphenoid bone. —**rostral** *adj.*

rotator *n.* a muscle that brings about rotation of a part. The *rotatores* are small muscles situated deep in the back between adjacent vertebrae. They help to extend and rotate the vertebrae.

Rothera's test a method of testing urine for the presence of acetone or acetoacetic acid: a sign of *diabetes mellitus. Strong ammonia is added to a sample of urine saturated with ammonium sulphate crystals and containing a small quantity of sodium nitroprusside. A purple colour confirms the presence of acetone or acetoacetic acid.

Roth spot a pale area surrounded by haemorrhage sometimes seen in the retina, with the aid of an *ophthalmoscope, in those who have bacterial endocarditis, septicaemia, or leukaemia.

roughage *n.* *see* dietary fibre.

rouleau *n.* (*pl.* **rouleaux**) a cylindrical structure in the blood formed from several red blood cells piled one upon the other and adhering by their rims.

round window *see* fenestra (rotunda).

roundworm *n. see* nematode.

-rrhagia (-rrhage) *suffix denoting* excessive or abnormal flow or discharge from an organ or part. Examples: *haemorrhage* (excessive bleeding); *menorrhagia* (excessive menstrual flow).

-rrhaphy *suffix denoting* surgical sewing; suturing. Example: *herniorrhaphy* (of a hernia).

-rrhexis *suffix denoting* splitting or rupture of a part.

-rrhoea *suffix denoting* a flow or discharge from an organ or part. Example: *rhinorrhoea* (from the nose).

RSV *see* respiratory syncytial virus.

rubber dam (in dentistry) a sheet of rubber used to isolate one or more teeth during treatment.

rubefacient *n.* an agent that causes reddening and warming of the skin. Rubefacients are often used as *counterirritants for the relief of muscular pain.

rubella *n. see* German measles.

rubeola *n. see* measles.

rubidium-81 *n.* an artificial radiactive isotope that has a half-life of about four hours and decays into the radioactive gas *krypton-81m, emitting radiations as it does so.

rubor *n.* redness: one of the classical signs of inflammation in a tissue, the other three being *calor (heat), *dolor (pain) and *tumor (swelling). The redness of inflamed tissue is due to the increase in size of the small blood vessels in the area, which therefore contain more blood.

rubrospinal tract a tract of *motor neurones that extends from the midbrain down to different levels in the spinal cord, carrying impulses that have travelled from the cerebral and cerebellar cortex via the nucleus ruber (red nucleus). The tract plays an important part in the control of skilled and dextrous movements.

ruga *n.* (*pl.* **rugae**) a fold or crease, especially one of the folds of mucous membrane that line the stomach.

rumination *n.* (in psychiatry) an obsessional type of thinking in which the same thoughts or themes are experienced repetitively, to the exclusion of other forms of mental activity. The patient commonly feels depressed and guilty after rumination. Rumination may be distinguished from morbid preoccupation in that the thoughts are irrational and resisted by the patient; they often involve abhorrent or aggressive feelings about events in the remote past and are accompanied by a lack of confidence in memory.

rupture 1. *n. see* hernia. **2.** *n.* the bursting apart or open of an organ or tissue; for example, the splitting of the membranes enclosing an infant during childbirth. **3.** *vb.* (of tissues, etc.) to burst apart or open.

Russian spring-summer encephalitis an influenza-like viral disease that affects the brain and nervous system and occurs in Russia and central Europe. It is transmitted to man either through the bite of forest-dwelling ticks of the species *Ixodes persulcatus* or by drinking the milk of infected goats. Infection of the meninges results in paralysis of the limbs and of the muscles of the neck and back. The disease, which is often fatal, can be prevented by vaccination.

Ryle's tube a thin flexible tube of rubber or plastic, inserted through the mouth or nose of a patient and used for withdrawing fluid from the stomach or giving a test meal.

S

Sabin vaccine an oral vaccine against poliomyelitis, prepared by culture of the virus under special conditions so that it loses its virulence (i.e. it becomes attenuated) but retains its ability to stimulate antibody production.

sac *n.* a pouch or baglike structure. Sacs can enclose natural cavities in the body, e.g. in the lungs (*see* alveolus) or in the *lacrimal apparatus of the eye, or they can be pathological, as in a hernia.

sacchar- (saccharo-) *prefix denoting* sugar.

saccharide *n.* a carbohydrate. *See also* disaccharide, monosaccharide, polysaccharide.

saccharine *n.* a sweetening agent. Saccharine is 400 times as sweet as sugar and has no energy content. It is very useful as a sweetener in diabetic and low-calorie foods. Saccharine is destroyed by heat and is not therefore used in cooking.

Saccharomyces *n. see* yeast.

saccule (sacculus) *n.* the smaller of the two membranous sacs within the vestibule of the ear: it forms part of the membranous *labyrinth. It is filled with fluid (endolymph) and contains a *macula. This responds to gravity and relays information to the brain about the position of the head.

saccus *n.* a sac or pouch. The *saccus endolymphaticus* is the small sac connected to the saccule and utricle of the inner ear by the *endolymphatic duct.

sacralization *n.* abnormal fusion of the fifth lumbar vertebra with the sacrum.

sacral nerves the five pairs of *spinal nerves that emerge from the spinal column in the sacrum. The nerves carry sensory and motor fibres from the upper and lower leg and from the anal and genital regions.

sacral vertebrae the five vertebrae that are fused together to form the *sacrum.

sacro- *prefix denoting* the sacrum. Examples: *sacrococcygeal* (relating to the sacrum and coccyx); *sacrodynia* (pain in); *sacroiliac* (relating to the sacrum and ilium).

sacroiliitis *n.* inflammation of the sacroiliac joint. Involvement of both joints is a common feature of ankylosing *spondylitis and associated rheumatic diseases, including *Reiter's syndrome and *psoriatic arthritis. The resultant low back pain and stiffness may be alleviated by rest and analgesics.

sacrum *n.* (*pl.* **sacra**) a curved triangular element of the *backbone consisting of five fused vertebrae (*sacral vertebrae*). It articulates with the last lumbar vertebra above, the coccyx below, and the hip bones laterally. *See also* vertebra. —**sacral** *adj.*

saddle joint a form of *diarthrosis (freely movable joint) in which the articulating surfaces of the bones are reciprocally saddle-shaped. It occurs at the carpometacarpal joint of the thumb.

sadism *n.* sexual excitement in response to inflicting or thinking about inflicting pain upon other people. *See also* masochism, perversion. —**sadist** *n.* —**sadistic** *adj.*

safe period the days in each *menstrual cycle when conception is least likely. Ovulation generally occurs at the midpoint of each cycle, and in women with regular periods it is possible to calculate the days at the beginning and end of the cycle when coitus is unlikely to result in pregnancy. *See* rhythm method.

safranin (safranine) *n.* a group of water- and alcohol-soluble basic dyes used to stain cell nuclei and as counterstains for Gram-negative bacteria.

sagittal *adj.* describing the dorsoventral plane that extends down the long axis of the body, dividing it into right and left halves (see illustration).

Sagittal plane of section through the body

sagittal suture *see* suture (def. 1).

salbutamol *n.* a drug, similar to *isoprenaline, used as a *bronchodilator to relieve asthma, chronic bronchitis, and emphysema. It is administered by mouth, injection, or inhalation; side-effects may include dizziness, tremor, and fast heart rate, particularly after large doses. Trade name: **Ventolin**.

salicylamide *n.* an analgesic drug with effects and uses similar to those of *aspirin. It is administered by mouth and may cause dizziness, sweating, and digestive upsets at high doses. Trade name: **Salimed**.

salicylic acid a drug that causes the skin to peel and destroys bacteria and fungi. It is applied to the skin to treat ulcers, dandruff, eczema, psoriasis, warts, and corns. Skin sensitivity reactions may occur after continued use.

salicylism *n.* poisoning due to an overdose of aspirin or other salicylate-containing compounds. The main symptoms are headache, dizziness, ringing in the ears (tinnitus), disturbances of vision, vomiting, and – in severe cases – delirium and collapse. There is often severe *acidosis.

saline (normal saline) *n.* a solution containing 0.9% sodium chloride. Saline may be used clinically as a diluent for drugs administered by injection and as a plasma substitute.

saliva *n.* the alkaline liquid secreted by the *salivary glands and the mucous membrane of the mouth. Its principal constituents are water, mucus, buffers, and enzymes (e.g. amylase). The functions of saliva are to keep the mouth moist, to aid swallowing of food, to minimize changes of acidity in the mouth, and to digest starch. —**salivary** *adj.*

salivary gland a gland that produces *saliva. There are three pairs of salivary glands: the *parotid glands, *sublingual glands, and *submandibular glands (see illustration). They are stimulated by reflex action, which can be initiated by the taste, smell, sight, or thought of food.

parotid gland

parotid duct
(Stensen's duct)

tongue

sublingual
gland

submandibular
gland

Salivary glands

salivation *n.* the secretion of saliva by the salivary glands of the mouth, increased in response to the chewing action of the jaws or to the thought, taste, smell, or sight of food. A small but regular flow of saliva is maintained to promote cleanliness in the mouth even when food is not being eaten. *See also* ptyalism.

Salk vaccine a vaccine against poliomyelitis, formed by treating the virus with formalin, which prevents it from causing disease but does not impair its ability to stimulate antibody production. It is administered by injection.

Salmonella *n.* a genus of Gram-negative motile rodlike bacteria that inhabit the intestines of animals and man and cause disease. They ferment glucose, usually with the formation of gas. The species *S. paratyphi* causes *paratyphoid fever, and *S. typhi* causes *typhoid fever. Other species of *Salmonella* cause *food poisoning, gastroenteritis, and septicaemia.

salmonellosis *n.* an infestation of the digestive system by bacteria of the genus *Salmonella. *See also* food poisoning.

salping- (salpingo-) *prefix denoting* **1.** the Fallopian tube. **2.** the auditory tube (meatus).

salpingectomy *n.* the surgical removal or cutting of a Fallopian tube. The operation involving both tubes is a permanent and completely effective method of contraception (*see* sterilization) since it prevents the egg cells passing from the ovaries to the womb.

salpingitis *n.* inflammation of a tube, most commonly applied to inflammation of one or both of the Fallopian tubes caused by bacterial infection spreading from the vagina or womb or carried in the blood. In *acute salpingitis* there is a sharp pain in the lower abdomen, which may be mistaken for that of appendicitis, and the infection may spread to the membrane lining the abdominal cavity (*see* peritonitis). In severe cases the tubes may become blocked with scar tissue and the patient will be unable to conceive. The condition is treated with antibiotics or by surgical removal of the diseased tube(s).

salpingography *n.* *radiography of one or both Fallopian tubes after a *radio-opaque substance has been introduced into them via an injection into the womb.

salpingo-oophoritis (salpingo-oothecitis) *n.* inflammation of a Fallopian tube and an ovary.

salpingo-oophorocele (salpingo-oothecocele) *n.* hernia involving a Fallopian tube and an ovary.

salt depletion excessive loss of sodium chloride (common salt) from the body. This may result from sweating, persistent vomiting or diarrhoea, or loss of fluid in wounds. The main symptoms are muscular weakness and cramps. Miners and workers in hot climates are particularly at risk, and salt tablets are often taken as a preventive measure.

Samaritans *n.* a British voluntary organization providing a telephone service for the suicidal and despairing. Started in 1953 by the Rev. Chad

Varah in the cellars of a London church (St. Stephens, Walbrook) with one telephone, it now has over 170 branches throughout the country manned by some 20,000 volunteers. It offers a nonprofessional, confidential, and (if required) anonymous service at all hours. Samaritans will listen for as long as they are needed and the service is free. They offer little advice, believing that their clients will be helped to make their own decisions by talking to someone who cares. They also offer a befriending service to support exceptionally distressed clients through a serious crisis.

sanatorium *n.* **1.** a hospital or institution for the rehabilitation and convalescence of patients of any kind. **2.** an institution for patients who have suffered from pulmonary tuberculosis.

sandfly *n.* a small hairy fly of the widely distributed genus *Phlebotomus*. Adult sandflies rarely exceed 3 mm in length and have long slender legs. The blood-sucking females of certain species transmit various diseases, including *leishmaniasis, *sandfly fever, and *bartonellosis.

sandfly fever (Pappataci fever) a viral disease transmitted to man by the bite of the sandfly *Phlebotomus papatasii*. Sandfly fever occurs principally in countries surrounding the Persian Gulf and the tropical Mediterranean; it occurs during the warmer months, does not last long, and is never fatal. Symptoms resemble those of influenza. There is no specific treatment apart from aspirin and codeine to relieve the symptoms.

sangui- (sanguino-) *prefix denoting* blood.

sanguineous *adj.* **1.** containing, stained, or covered with blood. **2.** (of tissues) containing more than the normal quantity of blood.

sanies *n.* a foul-smelling watery discharge from a wound or ulcer, containing serum, blood, and pus.

saphena *n. see* saphenous vein.

saphenous nerve a large branch of the *femoral nerve that arises in the upper thigh, travels down on the inside of the leg, and supplies the skin from the knee to below the ankle with sensory nerves.

saphenous vein (saphena) either of two superficial veins of the leg, draining blood from the foot. The *long saphenous vein* – the longest vein in the body – runs from the foot, up the medial side of the leg, to the groin, where it joins the femoral vein. The *short saphenous vein* runs up the back of the calf to join the popliteal vein at the back of the knee.

sapr- (sapro-) *prefix denoting* **1.** putrefaction. **2.** decaying matter.

sapraemia *n.* blood poisoning by toxins of saprophytic bacteria (bacteria living on dead or decaying matter). *Compare* pyaemia, septicaemia, toxaemia.

saprophyte *n.* any free-living organism that lives and feeds on the dead and putrefying tissues of animals or plants. *Compare* parasite. —**saprophytic** *adj.*

sarc- (sarco-) *prefix denoting* **1.** flesh or fleshy tissue. **2.** muscle.

sarcocele *n.* an obsolete term for a fleshy tumour (sarcoma) of the testis.

Sarcocystis *n.* a genus of parasitic protozoans (*see* Sporozoa) that infect birds, reptiles, and herbivorous mammals. *S. lindemanni*, which occasionally infects man, forms cylindrical cysts (*sarcocysts*) in the muscle fibres. In heavy infections these cysts can cause tissue degeneration and so provoke muscular pain and weakness. Sarcocysts have, in the few positively diagnosed cases, been located in the heart muscles, arm muscles, and larynx.

sarcoid 1. *adj.* fleshy. **2.** *n.* a fleshy tumour.

sarcoidosis *n.* a chronic disorder of unknown cause in which the lymph nodes in many parts of the body are enlarged and small fleshy nodules (*see* granuloma) develop in the lungs, liver, and spleen. The skin, nervous system, and the eyes and salivary glands are also commonly affected (*see* uveoparotitis), and the condition has features similar to *tuberculosis. Recovery is complete with minimal after-effects in two-thirds of all cases.

sarcolemma *n.* the cell membrane that encloses a muscle cell (muscle fibre).

sarcoma *n.* any *cancer of connective tissue. These tumours may occur in any part of the body, as they arise in the tissues that make up an organ rather than being restricted to a particular organ. They can arise in fibrous tissue, muscle, fat, bone, cartilage, synovium, blood and lymphatic vessels, and various other tissues. *See also* chondrosarcoma, fibrosarcoma, leiomyosarcoma, liposarcoma, lymphangiosarcoma, osteosarcoma, rhabdomyosarcoma. —**sarcomatous** *adj.*

sarcoma botryoides *see* carcinosarcoma.

sarcomatosis *n.* *sarcoma that has spread widely throughout the body, most commonly through the bloodstream. It is treated with drugs, typically one or a combination of the following: cyclophosphamide, vincristine, actinomycin-D, methotrexate, or doxorubicin.

sarcomere *n.* one of the basic contractile units of which *striated muscle fibres are composed.

Sarcophaga *n.* a genus of widely distributed non-bloodsucking flies, the flesh flies. Maggots are normally found in carrion or excrement but occasionally females will deposit their eggs in wounds or ulcers giving off a foul-smelling discharge; the presence of the maggots causes a serious *myiasis. Rarely, maggots may be ingested with food and give rise to an intestinal myiasis.

sarcoplasm (myoplasm) *n.* the cytoplasm of muscle cells.

sarcoplasmic reticulum an arrangement of membranous vesicles and tubules found in the cytoplasm of striated muscle fibres. The sarcoplasmic reticulum plays an important role in the transmission of nervous excitation to the contractile parts of the fibres.

Sarcoptes *n.* a genus of small oval mites. The female of *S. scabiei*, the human itch mite, tunnels into the skin, where it lays its eggs. The presence of the mites causes severe irritation, which eventually leads to *scabies.

sarcostyle *n.* a bundle of muscle fibrils.

sartorius *n.* a narrow ribbon-like muscle at the front of the thigh, arising from the anterior superior spine of the ilium and extending to the tibia, just below the knee. The longest muscle in the body, the sartorius flexes the leg on the thigh and the thigh on the abdomen.

satyriasis *n.* an extreme degree of promiscuous heterosexual activity in men. *Compare* nymphomania.

saucerization *n.* **1.** an operation in which tissue is cut away from a wound to form a saucer-like depression. It is carried out to facilitate healing and is commonly used to treat injuries or disorders in which bone is infected. **2.** the concave appearance of the upper surface of a vertebra that has been fractured by compression.

Sayre's jacket a plaster of Paris cast shaped to fit around and support the backbone. It is used in cases where the vertebrae have been severely damaged by disease, such as tuberculosis.

scab *n.* a hard crust of dried blood, serum, or pus that develops during the body's wound-healing process over a sore, cut, or scratch.

scabicide *n.* a drug that kills the mites causing *scabies.

scabies *n.* a skin infection caused by the itch mite, *Sarcoptes scabiei*. Scabies is typified by severe itching (particularly at night), red papules, and often secondary infection. The female mite tunnels in the skin to lay her eggs and the newly hatched mites pass easily from person to person by contact. The intense itching is caused by the mite's secretion. Commonly infected areas are the groin, penis, nipples, and the skin between the fingers. Local treatment is with hexachlorophane or benzyl benzoate creams, which kill the mites. All members of a family may need treatment, and clothing and bedding should be disinfested.

scala *n.* one of the spiral canals of the *cochlea. The *scala media* (*cochlear duct*) is the central membranous canal, containing the sensory apparatus of the cochlea; the *scala vestibuli* and *scala tympani* are the two bony canals of the cochlea.

scald *n.* a *burn produced by a hot liquid or vapour, such as boiling water or steam.

scale 1. *n.* any of the flakes of dead epidermal cells shed from the skin. **2.** *vb.* to scrape deposits of calculus (tartar) from the teeth (*see* scaler).

scalenus *n.* one of four paired muscles of the neck (*scalenus anterior*, *medius*, *minimus*, and *posterior*), extending from the cervical (neck) vertebrae to the first and second ribs. They are responsible for raising the first and second ribs in inspiration and for bending the neck forward and to either side.

scalenus syndrome (thoracic outlet syndrome) the group of symptoms caused by the scalenus anterior muscle compressing the subclavian artery and the lower roots of the brachial plexus against the fibrous and bony structures of the outlet of the upper thoracic vertebrae. Loss of sensation, wasting, and vascular symptoms may be found in the affected arm.

scaler *n.* an instrument for removing calculus from the teeth. It may be a hand instrument or one energized by rapid ultrasonic vibrations.

scalpel *n.* a small pointed surgical knife used by surgeons for cutting tissues. It has a straight handle with detachable disposable blades of different shapes.

scanning speech a disorder of articulation in which the syllables are inappropriately separated and equally stressed. It is caused by disease of the cerebellum or its connecting fibres in the brainstem.

scaphocephaly *n.* an abnormally long and narrow skull due to premature closure of the suture between the two parietal bones, along the top of the skull. It is usually associated with mental retardation. —**scaphocephalic** *adj.*

scaphoid bone a boat-shaped bone of the wrist (*see* carpus). It articulates with the trapezium and trapezoid bones in front and with the radius behind.

scapul- (scapulo-) *prefix denoting* the scapula.

scapula *n.* (*pl.* **scapulas** *or* **scapulae**) the shoulder blade: a triangular bone, a pair of which form the back part of the shoulder girdle (see illustration). The *spine* on its dorsal (back) surface ends at the *acromion process* at the top of the shoulder. This process turns forward and articulates with the collar bone (*clavicle) at the *acromioclavicular joint*; it overhangs the *glenoid fossa*, into which the humerus fits to form the socket of the shoulder joint. The *cora-*

coid process curves upwards and forwards from the neck of the scapula and provides attachment for ligaments and muscles. —**scapular** *adj.*

Right scapula (dorsal surface)

acromion
coracoid process
spine of scapula
superior angle
glenoid fossa
medial border
lateral border
inferior angle

scar *n. see* cicatrix.

scarification *n.* the process of making a series of shallow cuts or scratches in the skin to allow a substance to penetrate the body. This is commonly performed during vaccination against smallpox; the vaccine is administered as a droplet left in contact with the scarified area.

scarlatina *n. see* scarlet fever.

scarlet fever a highly contagious disease, mainly of childhood, caused by bacteria of the genus *Streptococcus. It is transmitted either from a patient or carrier (by coughing) or through contaminated milk. Symptoms commence 2–4 days after exposure and include fever, sickness, sore throat, and a widespread scarlet rash that spreads from the armpits and groin to the neck, chest, back, and limbs and also affects the tongue. Treatment with antibiotics shortens the disease and prevents such complications as ear and kidney infections and swollen neck glands. An infection usually confers life-long immunity. Medical name: **scarlatina**. *Compare* German measles.

Scarpa's triangle *see* femoral triangle.

scat- (scato-) *prefix denoting* faeces.

scatter diagram (in statistics) *see* correlation.

Schick test a test to determine whether a person is susceptible to diphtheria. A small quantity of diphtheria toxin is injected under the skin; a patch of reddening and swelling shows that the person has no immunity and – if at particular risk – should be immunized.

Schiff's reagent aqueous *fuchsin solution decolourized with sulphur dioxide. A blue coloration develops in the presence of aldehydes.

Schilling test a test used to assess a patient's capacity to absorb vitamin B_{12} from the bowel. Radioactive vitamin B_{12} is given by mouth and urine collected for 24 hours. A normal individual will excrete at least 10% of the original dose over this period; a patient with *pernicious anaemia will excrete less than 5%.

schindylesis *n.* a form of *synarthrosis (immovable joint) in which a crest of one bone fits into a groove of another.

-schisis *suffix denoting* a cleft or split.

schism *n.* a disorder of relationships within a family, in which parents quarrel and children are made to take sides. It was proposed as a cause of later schizophrenia in the children, but is more likely to be a nonspecific cause of psychological vulnerability.

schisto- *prefix denoting* a fissure; split.

schistoglossia *n.* fissuring of the tongue. Congenital fissures are transverse, whereas those due to disease (such as syphilis) are usually longitudinal.

Schistosoma (Bilharzia) *n.* a genus of blood *flukes, three species of which are important parasites of man causing one of the most serious of tropical diseases (*see* schistosomiasis). *S. japonicum* is common in the Far East; *S. mansoni* is widespread in Africa, the West Indies, and South and Central America; and *S. haematobium* occurs in Africa and the Middle East.

schistosomiasis (bilharziasis) *n.* a tropical disease caused by blood flukes of the genus *Schistosoma*. Eggs present in the stools or urine of infected people undergo part of their larval development within freshwater snails living in water contaminated with human sewage. The disease is contracted when *cercaria larvae, released from the snails, penetrate the skin of anyone bathing in infected water. Adult flukes eventually settle in the blood vessels of the intestine (*S. mansoni* and *S. japonicum*) or bladder (*S. haematobium*); the release of their spiked eggs causes anaemia, inflammation, and the formation of scar tissue. Additional intestinal symptoms are diarrhoea, dysentery, enlargement of the spleen and liver, and cirrhosis of the liver. If the bladder is affected, blood is passed in the urine and cystitis and cancer of the bladder may develop. The disease is treated with various drugs, including *stibophen and other antimony-containing preparations and *niridazole.

schiz- (schizo-) *prefix denoting* a split or division.

schizogony *n.* a phase of asexual reproduction in the life cycle of a sporozoan (protozoan parasite) that occurs in the liver or red blood cells. The parasite grows and divides many times to form a *schizont*, which contains many *merozoites. The eventual release of merozoites of *Plasmodium*, the malaria parasite, from the blood cells produces fever in the patient.

schizoid personality a personality characterized by solitariness, emotional coldness to others, excessive introspection, and eccentricity of behaviour. Some schizophrenics have this personality before their illness, but most schizoid personalities do not become schizophrenic. *See* personality disorder.

schizont *n.* one of the stages that occurs during the asexual phase of the life cycle of a sporozoan. *See* schizogony.

schizonticide *n.* any agent used for killing *schizonts.

schizophrenia *n.* a severe mental disorder (or group of disorders) characterized by a disintegration of the process of thinking, of contact with reality, and of emotional responsiveness. *Delusions and *hallucinations (especially of voices) are usual features, and the patient usually feels that his thoughts, sensations, and actions are controlled by, or shared with, others. He becomes socially withdrawn and loses energy and initiative. The main types of schizophrenia are *simple*, in which increasing social withdrawal and personal ineffectiveness are the major changes; *hebephrenic*, which starts in adolescence or young adulthood (*see* hebephrenia); *paranoid*, characterized by prominent delusions; and *catatonic*, with marked motor disturbances (*see* catatonia). Schizophrenia commonly – but not inevitably – runs a progressive course. The prognosis has been improved in recent years with drugs such as *phenothiazines and vigorous psychological and social management and rehabilitation. There are strong genetic factors in the causation, and environmental stress can precipitate illness. —**schizophrenic** *adj.*

Schlemm's canal a channel in the eye, at the junction of the cornea and the sclera, through which the aqueous humour drains.

Schönlein-Henoch purpura a blood disease that affects young children; its cause is not known. It is characterized by a purple skin rash due to bleeding into the skin from defective capillaries; abdominal pain; and kidney disturbance. Spontaneous recovery is the usual outcome. *See also* purpura.

school health service (in Britain) a service concerned with the early detection of physical, mental, and emotional abnormalities in schoolchildren and their subsequent treatment and surveillance. The service was formerly based on an ideal of three examinations at 5, 11, and 15 years by doctors and nurses specially employed by the Local Education Authority (LEA). It has now been changed to a system of selective examinations based on recommendations by teachers, *school nurses, or parental requests. The service is now the responsibility of the District Health Authority, but ascertainment and responsibility for allocation to *special schools remain the responsibility of the LEA.

school nurse a member of the *school health service who conducts routine examinations and/or treats minor ailments. *Health visitors may sometimes work in this capacity but State Registered and State Enrolled Nurses may also perform these tasks.

Schwann cells the cells that lay down the *myelin sheath around the axon of a medullated nerve fibre. Each cell is responsible for one length of axon, around which it twists as it grows, so that concentric layers of membrane envelop the axon. The gap between adjacent Schwann cells forms a *node of Ranvier.

Schwannoma *n. see* neurofibroma.

sciatica *n.* pain felt down the back and outer side of the thigh, leg, and foot. It is usually caused by degeneration of an intervertebral disc, which protrudes laterally to compress a lower lumbar or an upper sacral spinal nerve root. The onset may be sudden, brought on by an awkward lifting or twisting movement. The back is stiff and painful. There may be numbness and weakness in the leg. Bed rest will often relieve the pain but any persistence of numbness or weakness is an indication for surgical treatment.

sciatic nerve the major nerve of the leg and the nerve with the largest diameter. It runs down behind the thigh from the lower end of the spine; above the knee joint it divides into two main branches, the *tibial* and *common peroneal nerves*, which are distributed to the muscles and skin of the lower leg.

scintigram *n.* a diagram showing the distribution of radioactive *tracer in a part of the body, produced by recording the flashes of light given off by a *scintillator as it is struck by radiation of different intensities. By scanning the body, section by section, a 'map' of the radioactivity in various regions is built up, aiding the diagnosis of cancer or other disorders. Such a record is known as a *scintiscan*.

scintillascope *n.* the instrument used to produce a *scintigram. It incorporates a *scintillator, a device to magnify the fluorescence produced in it by radiations, and a means of recording the results, often aided by a computer. *See also* gamma camera.

scintillation counter (scintimeter) a device to measure and record the fluorescent flashes in a *scintillator exposed to high-energy radiation, as in a *scintillascope.

scintillator *n.* a substance that produces a fluorescent flash when struck by high-energy radiation, such as beta or gamma rays. In medicine the most commonly used scintillator is a crystal of thallium-activated sodium iodide. The fluorescence, magnified by a phototube multiplier, may be recorded photographically or electronically during the production of a *scintigram or scintiscan.

scintiscan *n. see* scintigram.

scirrhous *adj.* describing carcinomas that are stony hard to the touch. Such a carcinoma (for example of the breast) is known as a *scirrhus*.

scissor leg a disability in which one leg becomes permanently crossed over the other as a result of spasticity of its *adductor muscles. The condition occurs in children with brain damage and in adults after strokes. A *tenotomy sometimes reduces the degree of disability.

scissura (scissure) *n.* a cleft or splitting, such as the splitting of the tip of a hair or the splitting open of tissues when a hernia forms.

scler- (sclero-) *prefix denoting* **1.** hardening or thickening. **2.** the sclera. **3.** sclerosis.

sclera (sclerotic coat) *n.* the white fibrous outer layer of the eyeball. At the front of the eye it becomes the cornea. *See* eye. —**scleral** *adj.*

sclerectomy *n.* an operation in which a portion of the sclera (the outer white layer of the eyeball) is removed.

scleritis *n.* inflammation of the sclera (the white of the eye).

scleroderma *n.* persistent hardening and contraction of the body's connective tissue. It can affect any part, including the skin, heart, kidney, lung, or oesophagus (gullet). Scleroderma may be localized (*see* morphoea) or it can spread slowly throughout the body, eventually causing death (there is no effective treatment). The skin is thickened and tough, often with pigmented patches.

scleroma *n.* a hardened patch of skin or mucous membrane, consisting of *granulation tissue.

scleromalacia *n.* thinning of the sclera (white of the eye) as a result of inflammation. The involved area becomes bluish in colour. Sometimes the sclera fades away completely in an area, and the underlying tissue (usually the ciliary body) bulges beneath the conjunctiva. This state is known as *scleromalacia perforans*.

scleronychia *n.* hardening and thickening of the nails.

sclerosis *n.* hardening of tissue, usually due to scarring (fibrosis) after inflammation. It can affect the lateral columns of the spinal cord and the medulla of the brain (*amyotrophic lateral sclerosis*), causing progressive muscular paralysis (*see* motor neurone disease). It can also occur in scattered patches throughout the brain and spinal cord (*see* multiple sclerosis) or in the walls of the arteries (*see* arteriosclerosis, atherosclerosis). *See also* tuberous sclerosis.

sclerotherapy *n.* treatment of varicose veins by the injection of an irritant solution. This causes thrombophlebitis, which encourages obliteration of the varicose vein by thrombosis and subsequent scarring.

sclerotic 1. (*or* **sclerotic coat**) *n. see* sclera. **2.** *adj.* affected with *sclerosis.

sclerotome *n.* **1.** a surgical knife used in the operation of *sclerotomy. **2.** (in embryology) the part of the segmented mesoderm (*see* somite) in the early embryo that gives rise to all the skeletal tissue of the body. The vertebrae and ribs retain the segmented structure, which is lost in the skull and limbs.

sclerotomy *n.* an operation in which an incision is made in the sclera (white of the eye).

scrub typhus

scolex *n.* (*pl.* **scolices**) the head of a *tapeworm. The presence of suckers and/or hooks on the scolex enables the worm to attach itself to the wall of its host's gut.

scoliosis *n.* lateral (sideways) deviation of the backbone, caused by congenital or acquired abnormalities of the vertebrae, muscles, and nerves. Treatment is with spinal braces and, in cases of severe deformity, surgical correction by fusion or *osteotomy. *See also* kyphosis, kyphoscoliosis.

-scope *suffix denoting* an instrument for observing or examining. Example: *gastroscope* (instrument for examining the stomach).

scopolamine *n. see* hyoscine.

scorbutic *adj.* affected with scurvy.

scoto- *prefix denoting* darkness.

scotoma *n.* (*pl.* **scotomata**) a small area of abnormally decreased or absent vision in the visual field, surrounded by normal sight. All people have a *blind spot in the visual field of each eye due to the small area of retina occupied by the optic disc, which is not sensitive to light. Similar islands of total visual loss in other parts of the field are referred to as *absolute scotomata*. A *relative scotoma* is a spot where the vision is decreased but still present.

scotometer *n.* an instrument used for mapping defects in the visual field. *See also* campimetry, perimeter.

scotopic *adj.* relating to or describing conditions of poor illumination. For example, *scotopic vision* is vision in dim light in which the *rods of the retina are involved (*see* dark adaptation).

screening test a simple test carried out on a large number of apparently healthy people to separate those who probably have a specified disease from those who do not. Examples are mass X-rays and cervical smears. Limitations depend on the severity and *frequency distribution of the disease and the efficiency and availability of treatment. Other factors to be taken into account are the safety, convenience, cost, and *sensitivity of the test.

scrofula *n.* *tuberculosis of lymph nodes, usually those in the neck, causing the formation of abscesses. Untreated, these burst through the skin and form running sores, which leave scars when they heal. Treatment with antituberculous drugs is effective. The disease, which is now rare, most commonly affects young children. —**scrofulous** *adj.*

scrofuloderma *n.* tuberculosis of the skin in which the skin breaks down over suppurating tuberculous glands, with the formation of irregular-shaped ulcers with blue-tinged edges. Treatment is with antituberculous drugs, to which scrofuloderma responds better than *lupus vulgaris, another type of skin tuberculosis.

scrotum *n.* the paired sac that holds the testes and epididymides outside the abdominal cavity. Its function is to allow the production and storage of spermatozoa to occur at a lower temperature than that of the abdomen. Further temperature control is achieved by contraction or relaxation of muscles in the scrotum. —**scrotal** *adj.*

scrub typhus (tsutsugamushi disease) a disease, widely distributed in SE Asia, caused by the parasitic microorganism *Rickettsia tsutsugamushi* and transmitted to man through the bite of mites. Only larval mites of the genus *Trombicula* are involved as vectors. Symptoms include headache, chills, high temperature (104°F), a red rash over most of the body, a cough, and delirium. A small ulcer forms at the site of the bite. Scrub typhus is treated with tetracycline antibiotics. *See also* rickettsiae, typhus.

scruple *n.* a unit of weight used in pharmacy. 1 scruple = 1.295 g (20 grains). 3 scruples = 1 drachm.

sculpting *n.* a technique of family psychotherapy, in which all the family members are seen together and one member is asked to arrange the others' physical positions to express their relationships and feelings. *See also* group therapy.

scurf *n. see* dandruff.

scurvy *n.* a disease that is caused by a deficiency of *vitamin C (ascorbic acid). It results from the consumption of a diet devoid of fresh fruit and vegetables. The first sign of scurvy is swollen bleeding gums. This may be followed by subcutaneous bleeding and the opening of previously healed wounds; prolonged deficiency of the vitamin may eventually lead to death. Treatment with vitamin C soon reverses the effects.

scybalum *n.* a lump or mass of hard faeces.

seasickness *n. see* travel sickness.

sebaceous cyst (steatoma, wen) a cyst arising in an oil-secreting (sebaceous) gland of the skin. It may grow to a considerable size and be filled with yellowish cheesy sebum, which sometimes becomes infected. Sebaceous cysts are found most commonly on the scalp, scrotum, and vulva and rarely occur before puberty. Treatment is by surgical excision.

sebaceous gland any of the simple or branched glands in the *skin that secrete an oily substance, *sebum. They open into hair follicles and their secretion is produced by the disintegration of their cells. Some parts of the skin have many sebaceous glands, others few. Activity varies with age: the glands are most active at puberty.

seborrhoea *n.* excessive secretion of sebum by the *sebaceous glands. The glands are enlarged, especially beside the nose and other parts of the face. The condition predisposes to acne and is common at puberty, usually lasting for a few years. Seborrhoea is sometimes associated by a kind of *eczema (seborrhoeic dermatitis). —**seborrhoeic** *adj.*

sebum *n.* the oily substance secreted by the *sebaceous glands and reaching the skin surface through small ducts that lead into the hair follicles. Sebum provides a thin film of fat over the skin, which slows the evaporation of water; it also has an antibacterial effect.

second *n.* the *SI unit of time, equal to the duration of 9,192,631,770 periods of the radiation corresponding to the transition between two hyperfine levels of the ground state of the caesium-133 atom. This unit is now the basis of all time measurements. Symbol: s.

secondary medical care *see* general practitioner.

secondary prevention the avoidance or alleviation of the serious consequences of disease by early detection. Best known methods include routine examinations, as in *child health clinics and the *school health service, or *screening tests applied to populations regarded as having a high risk of contracting specific diseases.

secondary sexual characteristics the physical characteristics that develop after puberty as a result of sexual maturation. In boys they include the growth of facial and pubic hair and the breaking of the voice. In girls they include the growth of pubic hair and the development of the breasts.

secretagogue *n.* a substance that stimulates secretion. An example is *pentagastrin, which stimulates the secretion of gastric juice.

secretin *n.* a hormone secreted from the small intestine (duodenum) when acidified food leaves the stomach. It stimulates the secretion of relatively enzyme-free alkaline juice by the pancreas (*see* pancreatic juice) and of bile by the liver.

secretion *n.* **1.** the process by which a gland isolates constituents of the blood or tissue fluid and chemically alters them to produce a substance that it discharges for use by the body or excretes. The principal methods of secretion – *apocrine, *holocrine, and *merocrine – are illustrated in the diagram. **2.** the substance that is produced by a gland.

merocrine

apocrine

holocrine

Methods of secretion

secretor *n.* a person in whose saliva and other body fluids are found traces of the water-soluble A, B, or O agglutinogens that determine *blood group.

section 1. *n.* (in surgery) the act of cutting (the cut or division made is also called a section). For example, an *abdominal section* is performed for surgical exploration of the abdomen (*see* laparotomy). A *transverse section* is a cut made at right angles to a structure's long axis. *See also* Caesarean section. **2.** *n.* (in microscopy) a thin slice of the specimen to be examined under a microscope. **3.** *vb.* to issue an order for *compulsory admission to a psychiatric hospital under the appropriate section of the *Mental Health Act.

secundigravida *n.* a woman who has been pregnant twice.

secundipara *n.* a woman who has been pregnant at least twice and who has given birth to an infant capable of survival after each of two pregnancies.

sedation *n.* the production of a restful state of mind, particularly by the use of drugs (*see* sedative).

sedative *n.* a drug that has a calming effect, relieving anxiety and tension. Sedatives are *hypnotic drugs, such as *barbiturates, administered at lower doses than those needed for sleep (drowsiness is a common side-effect). They have largely been replaced by *tranquillizers, which are less likely to cause drowsiness or dependence.

sedimentation rate the rate at which solid particles sink in a liquid under the influence of gravity. *See also* ESR (erythrocyte sedimentation rate).

segment *n.* (in anatomy) a portion of a tissue or organ, usually distinguishable from other portions by lines of demarcation. *See also* somite.

sella turcica a depression in the body of the sphenoid bone that encloses the pituitary gland.

semeiology *n. see* symptomatology.

semen (seminal fluid) *n.* the fluid ejaculated from the penis at sexual climax. Each ejaculate may contain 300–500 million sperms suspended in a fluid secreted by the *prostate gland and *seminal vesicles with a small contribution from *Cowper's glands. It contains fructose, which provides the sperms with energy, and *prostaglandins, which affect the muscles of the womb and may therefore assist transport of the sperms. —**seminal** *adj.*

semi- *prefix denoting* half.

semicircular canals three tubes that form part of the membranous *labyrinth of the ear. They are concerned

557

with balance and each canal registers movement in a different plane. At the base of each canal is a small swelling (an *ampulla*), which contains a *crista. When the head moves the fluid (endolymph) in the canals presses on the cristae, which register the movement and send nerve impulses to the brain.

semilunar cartilage one of a pair of crescent-shaped cartilages in the knee joint situated between the femur and tibia.

semilunar valve either of the two valves in the heart situated at the origin of the aorta (*aortic valve*) and the pulmonary artery (*pulmonary valve*). Each consists of three flaps (cusps), which maintain the flow of blood in one direction.

seminal vesicle either of a pair of male accessory sex glands that open into the vas deferens before it joins the urethra. The seminal vesicles secrete most of the liquid component of *semen.

seminiferous tubule any of the long convoluted tubules that make up the bulk of the *testis.

seminoma *n.* a malignant tumour of the testis, appearing as a swelling, often painless, in the scrotum. It tends to occur in an older age group than the *teratomas. The best treatment for localized disease is surgery involving removal of the testis (*see* orchidectomy). Secondary tumours in the lungs can be treated with intravenous cyclophosphamide followed by low-dose irradiation to the lungs. A similar tumour occurs in the ovary (*see* dysgerminoma).

semipermeable membrane a membrane that allows the passage of some molecules but not others. *Cell membranes are semipermeable. Semipermeable membranes are used clinically in *haemodialysis for patients with kidney failure.

semiprone *adj.* describing the position of a patient lying face downwards, but with one or both knees flexed to one side so that the body is not lying completely flat. *Compare* prone, supine.

senescence *n.* the condition of ageing, which is often marked by a decrease in physical and mental abilities. —**senescent** *adj.*

senile dementia loss of the intellectual faculties, beginning for the first time in old age. *See also* dementia.

senior house officer *see* consultant.

senna *n.* the dried fruits of certain shrubs of the genus *Cassia*, used as an irritant *laxative to relieve constipation and to empty the bowels before X-ray examination. It is administered by mouth; side-effects do not usually occur, but severe diarrhoea may follow large doses.

sensation *n.* a feeling: the result of messages from the body's sensory receptors registering in the brain as information about the environment. Messages from *exteroceptors are interpreted as specific sensations – smell, taste, temperature, pain, etc. – in the conscious mind. Messages from *interoceptors, however, rarely reach the consciousness to produce sensation.

sense *n.* one of the faculties by which the qualities of the external environment are appreciated – sight, hearing, smell, taste, or touch.

sense organ a collection of specialized cells (*receptors), connected to the nervous system, that is capable of responding to a particular stimulus from either outside or inside the body. Sense organs can detect light (the eyes), heat, pain, and touch (the skin), smell (the nose), and taste (the taste buds).

sensibility *n.* the ability to be affected by, and respond to, changes in the surroundings (*see* stimulus). Sensibility is a characteristic of cells of the nervous system.

sensitive *adj.* possessing the ability to respond to a *stimulus. The cells of the retina, for example, are sensitive to the stimulus of light and respond by sending nerve impulses to the brain. Other *receptors are sensitive to different specific stimuli, such as pressure or the presence of chemical substances.

sensitivity *n.* (in preventive medicine) a measure of the reliability of a *screening test based on the proportion of people with a specific disease who react positively to the test (the higher the sensitivity the fewer false negatives). This contrasts with *specificity*, which is the proportion of people free from disease who react negatively to the test (i.e. the higher the specificity the fewer the false positives). Though these are theoretically independent variables, most screening tests are so designed that if the sensitivity is increased the specificity is reduced and the number of false positives may rise to wasteful proportions.

sensitization *n.* **1.** alteration of the responsiveness of the body to the presence of foreign substances. In the development of an *allergy, an individual becomes sensitized to a particular allergen and reaches a state of *hypersensitivity. The phenomena of sensitization are due to the production of antibodies. **2.** (in behaviour therapy) a form of *aversion therapy in which anxiety-producing stimuli are associated with the unwanted behaviour. In *covert sensitization* the behaviour and an unpleasant feeling (such as disgust) are evoked simultaneously by verbal cues.

sensory *adj.* relating to the input division of the nervous system, which carries information from *receptors throughout the body towards the brain and spinal cord.

sensory cortex the region of the *cerebral cortex responsible for receiving incoming information relayed by sensory nerve pathways from all parts of the body. Different areas of cortex correspond to different parts of the body and to the various senses. *Compare* motor cortex.

sensory nerve a nerve that carries information inwards, from an outlying part of the body towards the central nervous system. Different sensory nerves convey information about temperature, pain, touch, taste, etc., to the brain. *Compare* motor nerve.

separation anxiety a state of distress and fear at the prospect of leaving secure surroundings, such as is experienced by some children when they must leave parents to go to school. It is often caused by insecure *attachment.

sepsis *n.* the putrefactive destruction of tissues by disease-causing bacteria or their toxins.

sept- (septi-) *prefix denoting* **1.** seven. **2.** (*or* septo-) a septum, especially the nasal septum. **3.** sepsis.

septal defect a hole in the partition (septum) between the left and right halves of the heart. This abnormal communication is congenital due to an abnormality of heart development in the fetus. It may be found between the two atria (*atrial septal defect*) or between the ventricles (*ventricular septal defect*). A septal defect permits abnormal circulation of blood from the left side of the heart, where pressures are higher, to the right. This abnormal circulation is called a *shunt* and results in excessive blood flow through the lungs. *Pulmonary hypertension develops and *heart failure may occur with large shunts. A heart *murmur is normally present. Large defects are closed surgically but small defects do not require treatment.

septic *adj.* relating to or affected with *sepsis.

septicaemia *n.* widespread destruction of tissues due to absorption of disease-causing bacteria or their toxins from the bloodstream. The term is also used loosely for any form of *blood poisoning. *Compare* pyaemia, sapraemia, toxaemia.

Septrin *n. see* co-trimoxazole.

septum *n.* (*pl.* **septa**) a partition or dividing wall within an anatomical structure. For example, the *atrioventricular septum* divides the atria of the heart from the ventricles. —**septal** *adj.* —**septate** *adj.*

sequela *n.* (*pl.* **sequelae**) any disorder or pathological condition that results from a preceding disease or accident.

sequestration *n.* the formation of a fragment of dead bone (*see* sequestrum) and its separation from the surrounding tissue.

sequestrectomy *n.* surgical removal of a *sequestrum.

sequestrum *n.* (*pl.* **sequestra**) a portion of dead bone formed in an infected bone in chronic *osteomyelitis. It is surrounded by an envelope (*involucrum*) of sclerotic bone and fibrous tissue and can be seen as a dense area within the bone on X-ray. It can cause irritation and the formation of pus, which may discharge through a *sinus, and is usually surgically removed (*sequestrectomy*).

ser- (sero-) *prefix denoting* **1.** serum. **2.** serous membrane.

serine *n. see* amino acid.

serofibrinous *adj.* describing an exudate of serum that contains a high proportion of the protein fibrin.

serology *n.* the study of blood serum and its constituents, particularly their contribution to the protection of the body against disease. *See* agglutination, complement fixation, precipitin. —**serological** *adj.*

seropus *n.* a mixture of serum and pus, which forms, for example, in infected blisters.

serosa *n. see* serous membrane.

serositis *n.* inflammation of a *serous membrane, such as the lining of the thoracic cavity (pleura). *See* polyserositis.

serotherapy *n.* the use of serum containing known antibodies (*see* antiserum) to treat a patient with an infection or to confer temporary passive *immunity upon a person at special risk. The use of antisera prepared in animals carries its own risks (for example, a patient may become hypersensitive to horse protein); the risk is reduced if the serum is taken from an immune human being.

serotonin (5-hydroxytryptamine) *n.* a compound widely distributed in the tissues, particularly in the blood platelets, intestinal wall, and central nervous system. It is thought to play a role in inflammation similar to that of *histamine and it also possibly acts as a *neurotransmitter, especially concerned with the process of sleep.

serotype *n.* a category into which material is placed based on its serological activity, particularly in terms of the antigens it contains or the antibodies that may be produced against it. Thus bacteria of the same species may be subdivided into serotypes that produce slightly different antigens. The serotype of an infective organism is important when treatment or prophylaxis with a vaccine is being considered.

serous *adj.* **1.** relating to or containing serum. **2.** resembling serum or producing a fluid resembling serum.

serous membrane (serosa) a smooth transparent membrane, consisting of *mesothelium and underlying elastic fibrous connective tissue, lining certain large cavities of the body. The *peritoneum of the abdomen, *pleura of the chest, and *pericardium of the heart are all serous membranes. Each consists of two portions: the *parietal* portion lines the walls of the cavity, and the *visceral* portion covers the organs concerned. The two are continuous, forming a closed sac with the organs essentially outside the sac. The inner surface of the sac is moistened by a thin fluid derived from blood serum, which allows frictionless movement of organs within their cavities. *Compare* mucous membrane.

serpiginous *adj.* having an indented or wavy margin: applied to certain skin lesions.

serratus *n.* any of several muscles arising from or inserted by a series of processes that resemble the teeth of a saw. An example is the *serratus anterior*, a muscle situated between the ribs and shoulder blade in the upper and lateral parts of the thorax. It is the chief muscle responsible for pushing and punching movements.

Sertoli cells cells found in the walls of the seminiferous tubules of the *testis. Compared with the germ cells they appear large and pale. They anchor and probably nourish the developing germ cells, especially the *spermatids, which become partly embedded within them.

serum (blood serum) *n.* the fluid that separates from clotted blood or blood plasma that is allowed to stand. Serum is essentially similar in composition to *plasma but lacks fibrinogen and other substances that are used in the coagulation process.

serum hepatitis *see* hepatitis.

serum sickness a reaction that sometimes occurs 7–12 days after injection of a quantity of foreign serum, such as horse serum used in the preparation of antitetanus injections. The usual symptoms are rashes, fever, joint pains, and enlargement of the lymph nodes. The reaction is due to the presence of antigenic material still in the circulation by the time that the body has started producing antibodies against it; it is therefore a form of delayed *hypersensitivity reaction. The condition is rarely serious.

sesamoid bone an oval nodule of bone that lies within a tendon and slides over another bony surface. The patella (kneecap) and certain bones in the hand and foot are sesamoid bones.

sessile *adj.* (of a tumour) having no stalk.

seton *n.* an outmoded form of treatment in which a thread was passed through a pinch of skin and tied in a loop. This acted as a counterirritant to pain elsewhere and produced a running sore thought to be useful for the drainage of harmful materials from the body.

sex chromatin *chromatin found only in female cells and believed to represent a single X chromosome in a nondividing cell. It can be used to discover the sex of a baby before birth by examination of cells obtained by *amniocentesis. There are two main kinds: (1) the *Barr body*, a small object that stains with basic dyes, found on the edge of the nucleus just inside the nuclear membrane; (2) a drumstick-like appendage to the nucleus in neutrophils (a type of white blood cell).

sex chromosome a chromosome that is involved in the determination of the sex of the individual. Women have two *X chromosomes; men have one X chromosome and one *Y chromosome. *Compare* autosome.

sex hormone any steroid hormone, produced mainly by the ovaries or testes, that is responsible for controlling sexual development and reproductive function. *Oestrogens and *progesterone are the female sex hormones; *androgens are the male sex hormones.

sex-limited *adj.* describing characteristics that are expressed differently in the two sexes but are controlled by genes not on the sex chromosomes, e.g. baldness in men.

sex-linked *adj.* describing genes (or the characteristics controlled by them) that are carried on the sex chromosomes, usually the *X chromosome. The genes for certain disorders, e.g. *haemophilia, are carried on the X chromosome. Since these sex-linked genes are *recessive, men are more likely to have the diseases since they have only one X chromosome; women can carry the genes but their harmful effects are usually masked by the dominant (normal) alleles on their second X chromosome.

sexology *n.* the study of sexual matters, including anatomy, physiology, behaviour, and techniques.

sex ratio the proportion of males to females in a population, usually expressed as the number of males per 100 females. The *primary sex ratio*, at the time of fertilization, is in theory 50% male. The *secondary sex ratio*, found at birth, usually indicates slightly fewer girls than boys.

sextigravida *n.* a woman who has been pregnant six times.

sextipara *n.* a woman who has been pregnant at least six times and who has given birth to an infant capable of survival after each of six pregnancies.

sexual abuse sexual activity by an adult involving a child. *See also* paedophilia.

SGOT serum glutamic oxaloacetic transaminase. *See* glutamic oxaloacetic transaminase.

SGPT *n.* serum glutamic pyruvic transaminase. *See* glutamic pyruvic transaminase.

shaking palsy an archaic name for *parkinsonism.

shaping *n.* a technique of *behaviour modification used in the teaching of complex skills or in encouraging rare forms of behaviour. At first the therapist rewards actions that are similar to the desired behaviour; thereafter the therapist rewards successively closer approximations, until eventually only the desired behaviour is rewarded and thereby learned.

sheath *n.* (in anatomy) the layer of connective tissue that envelops structures such as nerves, arteries, tendons, and muscles.

sheltered housing specially converted (or adapted) accommodation, often in the form of a flatlet, designed to meet the special needs of the elderly who are capable of self-care. A warden is generally in attendance. The extent to which meals and other services are provided on a continuous basis varies; so too in Britain does the *per capita* payment from the appropriate social service department.

Shigella *n.* a genus of nonmotile rod-like Gram-negative bacteria normally present in the intestinal tract of warm-blooded animals and man. They ferment carbohydrates without the formation of gas. Some species are pathogenic. *S. dysenteriae* is associated with bacillary *dysentery.

shigellosis *n.* an infestation of the digestive system by bacteria of the genus *Shigella*, causing bacillary *dysentery.

shingles *n.* herpes zoster (*see* herpes).

shock *n.* the condition associated with circulatory collapse, when the arterial blood pressure is too low to maintain an adequate supply of blood to the tissues.

The patient has a cold sweaty pallid skin, a weak rapid pulse, irregular breathing, dry mouth, dilated pupils, and a reduced flow of urine.

Shock may be due to a decrease in the volume of blood, as occurs after internal or external *haemorrhage, dehydration, burns, or severe vomiting or diarrhoea. It may be caused by reduced activity of the heart, as in coronary thrombosis, myocardial infarction, or pulmonary embolism. It may also be due to widespread dilation of the veins so that there is insufficient blood to fill them. This may be caused by the presence of bacteria in the bloodstream (*bacteraemic shock*), a severe allergic reaction (*anaphylactic shock*: see anaphylaxis), overdosage with such drugs as narcotics or barbiturates, or the emotional shock due to a personal tragedy or disaster (*neurogenic shock*). Sometimes shock may result from a combination of any of these causes, as in *peritonitis. The treatment of shock is determined by the cause.

short-sightedness *n. see* myopia.

shoulder girdle (pectoral girdle) the bony structure to which the bones of the upper limbs are attached. It consists of the right and left *scapulas (*shoulder blades*) and clavicles (collar bones).

shunt *n.* (in medicine) a passage connecting two anatomical channels and diverting blood from one to the other. It may occur as a congenital abnormality or be surgically created. *See also* anastomosis.

sial- (sialo-) *prefix denoting* 1. saliva. 2. a salivary gland.

sialadenitis *n.* inflammation of a salivary gland.

sialic acid an amino sugar. Sialic acid is a component of some *glycoproteins, *gangliosides, and bacterial cell walls.

sialogogue *n.* a drug that promotes the secretion of saliva. *Parasympathomimetic drugs have this action.

sialography (ptyalography) *n.* X-ray examination of the salivary glands, after introducing a quantity of radioopaque material into the ducts of the salivary glands in the mouth. It enables the presence of any obstruction to be detected.

sialolith *n.* a stone (calculus) in a salivary gland or duct, most often the duct of the submaxillary gland. The flow of saliva is obstructed, causing swelling and intense pain.

sialorrhoea *n. see* ptyalism.

Siamese twins identical twins that are physically joined together at birth. The condition ranges from twins joined only by the umbilical blood vessels (i.e. *allantoido-angiopagous twins*) to those in whom conjoined heads or trunk are inseparable.

sib *n. see* sibling.

sibilant *adj.* whistling or hissing. The term is applied to certain abnormal sounds heard through a stethoscope.

sibling (sib) *n.* one of a number of children of the same parents, i.e. a brother or sister.

sickle-cell disease (drepanocytosis) *n.* a hereditary blood disease that affects negroes. It is characterized by the production of an abnormal type of *haemoglobin – *sickle-cell haemoglobin* (*Hbs*) – in the red blood cells. Hbs becomes insoluble when the blood is deprived of oxygen and precipitates, forming elongated crystals that distort the blood cell into the characteristic sickle shape: this process is known as *sickling*. Sickle cells are rapidly removed from the circulation, leading to anaemia. There is no satisfactory treatment, but patients with this disease are resistant to infection with *Plasmodium* *falciparum*, which causes a serious form of malaria.

sickling *n. see* sickle-cell disease.

sickness benefit (in Britain) weekly payments made to those who are unable to work through illness, provided they have made the necessary number of consecutive contributions under the terms of the National Insurance Act. The rate is higher for married men and there is also increased payment for each dependent child. Those who claim may do so initially on the basis of a personal affidavit. However, in the long term they are required to provide supporting evidence of incapacity, normally a *medical certificate provided by their general practitioner. Those who do not qualify may be eligible for similar payments as supplementary benefits under the terms of the *National Assistance Act. When incapacity arises from an injury at work or through contact with toxic substances (e.g. lead) at work, payment is made at a higher rate and there is also no qualifying period (*injury benefit*). The same conditions apply to those incapacitated by certain industrial diseases where the nature of the work is a recognized hazard (e.g. tuberculosis in mortuary attendants).

side-effect *n.* an unwanted effect produced by a drug in addition to its desired therapeutic effects. Side-effects are often undesirable and may be harmful.

sidero- *prefix denoting* iron.

sideroblast *n.* a red blood cell precursor (*erythroblast) in which iron-containing granules can be demonstrated by suitable staining techniques. Sideroblasts may be seen in normal individuals and are absent in iron deficiency. A certain type of anaemia (*sideroblastic anaemia*) is characterized by the presence of abnormal *ringed sideroblasts*. —**sideroblastic** *adj.*

siderocyte *n.* a red blood cell in which granules of iron-containing protein (*Pappenheimer bodies*) can be demonstrated by suitable staining techniques. These granules are normally removed by the spleen and siderocytes are characteristically seen when the spleen is absent.

sideropenia *n.* iron deficiency. This may result from dietary inadequacy; increased requirement of iron by the body, as in pregnancy or childhood; or increased loss of iron from the body, usually due to chronic bleeding. The most important manifestation of iron deficiency is *anaemia, which is readily corrected by iron therapy.

siderosis *n.* the deposition of iron oxide dust in the lungs, occurring in silver finishers, arc welders, and haematite miners. Iron oxide itself is inert, but pulmonary *fibrosis may develop if fibrogenic dusts such as silica are also inhaled.

siemens *n.* the *SI unit of electrical conductance, equal to the conductance between two points on a conductor when a potential difference of 1 volt between these points causes a current of 1 ampere to flow between them. Symbol: S.

sievert *n.* the *SI unit of dose equivalent, being the dose equivalent when the absorbed dose of ionizing radiation multiplied by the stipulated dimensionless factors is 1 J kg^{-1}. As different types of radiation cause different effects in biological tissue a weighted absorbed dose, called the dose equivalent, is used in which the absorbed dose is modified by multiplying it by dimensionless factors stipulated by the International Commission on Radiological Protection. The sievert has replaced the *rem. Symbol: Sv.

sigmoid- *prefix denoting* the sigmoid colon. Example: *sigmoidotomy* (incision into).

sigmoid colon (sigmoid flexure) the S-shaped terminal part of the descending *colon, which leads to the rectum.

sigmoidectomy *n.* removal of the sigmoid colon by surgery. It is performed for tumours, severe *diverticular disease, or for an abnormally long sigmoid colon that has become twisted (*see* volvulus).

sigmoidoscope *n.* an instrument inserted through the anus in order to inspect the interior of the rectum and sigmoid colon. In its commonest form it consists of a steel or chrome tube, 25 cm long and 3 cm in diameter, with some form of illumination and a bellows to inflate the bowel.

sigmoidoscopy *n.* examination of the rectum and sigmoid colon with a *sigmoidoscope. It is used in the investigation of diarrhoea or rectal bleeding, particularly to detect colitis or cancer of the rectum. A general anaesthetic is sometimes given, especially if the procedure is expected to be painful or uncomfortable.

sign *n.* an indication of a particular disorder that is observed by a physician but is not apparent to the patient. *Compare* symptom.

significance *n.* (in statistics) a relationship between two groups of observations indicating that the difference between them (e.g. between the percentages of smokers and nonsmokers respectively who die from lung cancer) is unlikely to have occurred by chance alone. An assumption is made that there is no difference between the two populations from which the two groups come (*null hypothesis*). This is tested, and a calculation indicating that there is a *probability* of less than 5% ($P < 0.05$) that the observed difference or a larger one could have arisen by chance is regarded as being *statistically significant* and the null hypothesis is rejected. Some tests are *parametric*,

based on the assumption that the range of observations are distributed by chance in a *normal* or *Gaussian distribution*, with 95% within two *standard deviations of the *mean (*Student's t test* to compare means). Nonparametric tests (*Mann-Whitney U tests*) make no assumptions about distribution patterns. *See also* frequency distribution, standard error.

silicosis *n.* a lung disease – a form of *pneumoconiosis – produced by inhaling silica dust particles. It affects workers in mineral mining, quarrying, stone dressing, sand blasting, and boiler scaling. Silica stimulates *fibrosis of lung tissue, which produces progressive breathlessness and considerably increased susceptibility to tuberculosis (but not to lung cancer).

silver nitrate a salt of silver with *caustic, *astringent, and *disinfectant properties. It is applied in solutions or creams to destroy warts and to treat skin injuries, including burns. Continued application discolours the skin black, and ingestion of silver nitrate may cause severe poisoning.

Simmond's disease loss of sexual function, loss of weight, and other features of failure of the pituitary gland (*hypopituitarism) occurring in women after childbirth complicated by bleeding (postpartum haemorrhage).

Simulium *n. see* black fly.

sinew *n.* a tendon.

singultus *n. see* hiccup.

sinistr- (sinistro-) *prefix denoting* left or the left side.

sino- (sinu-) *prefix denoting* **1.** a sinus. **2.** the sinus venosus.

sinoatrial node (SA node) the pacemaker of the heart: a microscopic area of specialized cardiac muscle located in the upper wall of the right atrium near the entry of the vena cava. Fibres of the

SA node are self-excitatory, contracting rhythmically at around 70 times per minute. Following each contraction, the impulse spreads throughout the atrial muscle and into fibres connecting the SA node with the *atrioventricular node. The SA node is supplied by fibres of the autonomic nervous system; impulses arriving at the node accelerate or decrease the heart rate.

sinus *n.* **1.** an air cavity within a bone, especially any of the cavities within the bones of the face or skull (*see* paranasal sinus). **2.** any wide channel containing blood, usually venous blood. *Venous sinuses* occur, for example, in the dura mater and drain blood from the brain. **3.** a pocket or bulge in a tubular organ, especially a blood vessel; for example, the *carotid sinus. **4.** an infected tract leading from a focus of infection to the surface of the skin or a hollow organ. *See* pilonidal sinus.

sinus arrhythmia a normal variation in the heart rate, which accelerates slightly on inspiration and slows on expiration. It is common in healthy individuals.

sinusitis *n.* inflammation of one or more of the mucous-lined air spaces in the facial bones that communicate with the nose (the paranasal sinuses). It is often caused by infection spreading from the nose. Symptoms include headache and tenderness over the affected sinus, which may become filled with a purulent material that is discharged through the nose. In persistent cases treatment may require the affected sinus to be washed out or drained by a surgical operation.

sinusoid *n.* a small blood vessel found in certain organs, such as the adrenal gland and liver. Large numbers of sinusoids occur in the liver. They receive oxygen-rich blood from the hepatic artery and nutrients from the intestines via the portal vein. Oxygen and nutrients diffuse through the capillary

walls into the liver cells. The sinusoids are drained by the hepatic veins. *See also* portal system.

sinus venosus a chamber of the embryonic heart that receives blood from several veins. In the adult heart it becomes part of the right atrium.

siphonage *n.* the transfer of liquid from one container to another by means of a bent tube. The procedure is used in gastric *lavage, when the stomach is filled with water through a funnel and rubber tube, and the tube is then bent downwards to act as a siphon and empty the stomach of its contents.

Siphunculina *n.* a genus of flies. *S. funicola*, the eye fly of India, feeds on the secretions of the tear glands and in landing on or near the eyes contributes to the spread of *conjunctivitis.

sirenomelia *n. see* sympodia.

sito- *prefix denoting* food.

sitz bath a fairly shallow hip bath in which the person is seated. Sitz baths of cold and hot water, rapidly alternated, were formerly used for the treatment of a variety of sexual disorders.

SI units (Système International d'Unités) the internationally agreed system of units now in use for all scientific purposes. Based on the metre-kilogram-second system, SI units have seven base units and two supplementary units. Measurements of all other physical quantities are expressed in derived units, consisting of two or more base units. Tables 1 and 2 (Appendix) list the base units and the derived units having special names; all these units are defined in the dictionary.

Decimal multiples of SI units are expressed using specified prefixes; where possible a prefix representing 10 raised to a power that is a multiple of three should be used. Prefixes are listed in Table 3 (Appendix).

skull

mandible

cervical vertebrae

clavicle

scapula

ribs

sternum

humerus

thoracic vertebrae

lumbar vertebrae

ilium

ulna

sacrum

radius

metacarpals

carpals

phalanges

coccyx

patella

femur

tibia

fibula

tarsals

phalanges

metatarsals

The skeleton

Sjögren's syndrome a condition in which the patient complains of a dry mouth, caused by wasting of the salivary glands. It is associated with rheumatoid arthritis and dryness of the eyes.

skatole (methyl indole) *n.* a derivative of the amino acid tryptophan, excreted in the urine and faeces.

skeletal muscle *see* striated muscle.

skeleton *n.* the rigid framework of connected *bones that gives form to the body, protects and supports its soft organs and tissues, and provides attachments for muscles and a system of levers essential for locomotion. The 206 named bones of the body are organized into the *axial skeleton* (of the head and trunk) and the *appendicular skeleton* (of the limbs). (See illustration.) —**skeletal** *adj.*

skew *n.* a disorder of relationships within a family, in which one parent is overpowering and the other is submissive and there is a general avoidance of anxiety-provoking situations. It was proposed as a specific cause of schizophrenia in the children, but this has not been confirmed.

skew deviation a rare condition of the eyes in which one eye turns down and inwards while the other turns up and outwards. It is sometimes seen in disorders of the *cerebellum.

skia- *prefix denoting* shadow.

skiagram *n.* a 'shadow-photograph', such as an X-ray photograph produced in radiography. —**skiagraphy** *n.*

skin *n.* the outer covering of the body, consisting of an outer layer, the *epidermis, and an inner layer, the *dermis (see illustration). Beneath the dermis is a layer of fatty tissue. The skin has several functions. The epidermis protects the body from injury and from invasion by parasites. It also helps to prevent the body from becoming dehydrated. The combination of erectile hairs, *sweat glands, and blood capillaries in the skin form part of the temperature-regulating mechanism of the body. When the body is too hot, loss of heat is increased by sweating and by the dilation of the capillaries. When the body is too cold the sweat glands are inactive, the capillaries contract, and a layer of air is trapped over the epidermis by the erected hairs. The skin also acts as an organ of excretion (by the secretion of *sweat) and as a sense organ (it contains receptors that are sensitive to heat, cold, touch, and pain). The layer of fat underneath the dermis can act as a reservoir of food and water. Anatomical name: **cutis**.

skin graft a portion of healthy skin cut from one area of the body and used to cover a part that has lost its skin, usually as a result of injury, burns, or operation. A skin graft is normally taken from another part of the body of the same patient (an *autograft), but occasionally skin may be grafted from one person to another as a temporary healing measure (a *homograft). The full thickness of skin may be taken for a graft (*see* flap) or the surgeon may use three-quarters thickness, thin sheets of skin (*see* Thiersch's graft), or a pinch skin graft. The type used depends on the condition and size of the damaged area to be treated.

skull *n.* the skeleton of the head and face, which is made up of 22 bones. It can be divided into the cranium, which encloses the brain, and the face (including the lower jaw (mandible)). (See illustration.) The *cranium* consists of eight bones. The frontal, parietals (two), occipital, and temporals (two) form the vault of the skull (*calvaria*) and are made up of two thin layers of compact bone separated by a layer of spongy bone (*diploë*). The remaining bones of the cranium – the sphenoid and ethmoid – form part of its base. The 14 bones that make up the face are the nasals, lacrimals, inferior nasal con-

Section through the skin

Side view of the skull

chae, maxillae, zygomatics, and palatines (two of each), the vomer, and the mandible. All the bones of the skull except the mandible are connected to each other by immovable joints (*see* suture). The skull contains cavities for the eyes (*see* orbit) and nose (*see* nasal cavity) and a large opening at its base (*foramen magnum*) through which the spinal cord passes.

sleep *n.* a state of natural unconsciousness, during which the brain's activity is not apparent (apart from the continued maintenance of basic bodily functions, such as breathing) but can be detected by means of an electroencephalogram (EEG). Different stages of sleep are recognized by different EEG wave patterns. Drowsiness is marked by short irregular waves; as sleep deepens the waves become slower, larger, and more irregular. This slow-wave sleep is periodically interrupted by episodes of paradoxical, or *REM (rapid-eye-movement), sleep, when the EEG pattern is similar to that of an awake and alert person. Dreaming occurs during REM sleep. The two states of sleep alternate in cycles of from 30 to 90 minutes, REM sleep constituting about a quarter of the total sleeping time.

sleeping sickness (African trypanosomiasis) a disease of tropical Africa caused by the presence in the blood of the parasitic protozoans *Trypanosoma gambiense* or *T. rhodesiense*. The parasites are transmitted to man through the bite of *tsetse flies. Initial symptoms include fever, headache, and chills, followed later by enlargement of the lymph nodes, anaemia, and pains in the limbs and joints. After a period of several months or even years, the parasites invade the minute blood vessels supplying the central nervous system. This causes drowsiness and lethargy, and ultimately – if untreated – the patient dies. Rhodesian sleeping sickness is the more virulent form of the disease. The drugs *suramin and pentamidine are used to treat the early curable stages of sleeping sickness; drugs containing arsenic (*see* tryparsamide) are administered after the brain is affected. Eradication of tsetse flies helps prevent spread of the infection.

sleep-walking *n. see* somnambulism.

sling *n.* a bandage arranged to support and rest an injured limb so that healing is not hindered by activity. The most common sling is a *triangular bandage tied behind the neck to support the weight of a broken arm. The arm is bent at the elbow and held across the body.

slipped disc a colloquial term for a *prolapsed intervertebral disc.

slit lamp a device for providing a narrow beam of light, used in conjunction with a special microscope. It can be used to examine minutely the structures within the eye, one layer at a time.

slough *n.* dead tissue, such as skin, that separates from healthy tissue after inflammation or infection.

smallpox *n.* an acute infectious virus disease causing high fever and a rash that scars the skin. It is transmitted chiefly by direct contact with a patient. Symptoms commence 8–18 days after exposure and include headache, backache, high fever, and vomiting. On the third day, as the fever subsides, red spots appear on the face and spread to the trunk and extremities. Over the next 8–9 days all the spots (macules) change to pimples (papules), then to pea-sized blisters that are at first watery (vesicles) but soon become pus-filled (pustules). The fever returns, often causing delirium. On the eleventh or twelfth day the rash and fever abate. Scabs formed by drying out of pustules fall off 7–20 days later, leaving permanent scars. The patient remains infectious until all scabs have been shed. Most patients recover but serious complications such as nephritis or pneumonia may develop. Treatment with *thiosemicarbazone is effective. An attack usually confers immunity; immunization against smallpox has now totally eradicated the disease. Medical name: **variola**. *See also* alastrim, cowpox.

smear *n.* a specimen of tissue or other material taken from part of the body and smeared on a microscope slide for examination. *See* cervical smear.

smegma *n.* the secretion of the glands of the foreskin (*prepuce), which accumulates under the foreskin and has a white cheesy appearance. It becomes readily infested by a harmless bacterium that resembles the tubercle bacillus.

smooth muscle (involuntary muscle) muscle that produces slow long-term contractions of which the individual is unaware. Smooth muscle occurs in hollow organs, such as the stomach, intestine, blood vessels, and bladder. It consists of spindle-shaped cells within a network of connective tissue (see illustration) and is under the control of the autonomic nervous system. *Compare* striated muscle.

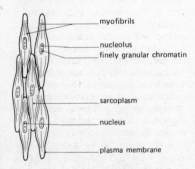

Arrangement of smooth muscle cells

snare *n.* an instrument consisting of a wire loop designed to remove polyps, tumours, and other projections of tissue, particularly those occurring in body cavities (see illustration). The loop is used to encircle the base of the tumour and is then pulled tight. *See also* diathermy.

A nasal snare

sneeze 1. *n.* an involuntary violent reflex expulsion of air through the nose and mouth provoked by irritation of the mucous membrane lining the nasal cavity. **2.** *vb.* to produce a sneeze.

Snellen chart the commonest chart used for testing sharpness of distant vision (*see* visual acuity). It consists of rows of capital letters, called *test types*, the letters of each row becoming smaller down the chart. The large letter at the top is of such a size that it can be read by a person with normal sight from a distance of 60 metres. A normally sighted person can read successive lines of letters from 36, 24, 18, 12, 9, 6, and 5 metres respectively, There is sometimes a line for 4 metres. The subject sits 6 metres from the chart and one eye is tested at a time. If he can only read down as far as the 12-metre line the visual acuity is expressed as 6/12. Normally sighted people can read the 6-metre line, i.e. normal acuity is 6/6, and many people read the 5-metre line with ease. A smaller chart on the same principle is available for testing near vision.

snore 1. *vb.* to breathe in such a way as to cause vibration of the soft palate of the roof of the mouth, resulting in a hoarse noise. Snoring usually occurs during sleep. **2.** *n.* the sound made by breathing in this way.

snow blindness a painful disorder of the cornea of the eye due to excessive exposure to ultraviolet light reflected

571

from the snow. Recovery usually follows within 24 hours of covering the eyes.

snuffles *n.* **1.** partial obstruction of breathing in infants, caused by the common cold. **2.** (formerly) discharge through the nostrils associated with necrosis of the nasal bones: seen in infants with congenital syphilis.

social class any one of the subdivisions of the population made by the Office of Population Censuses and Surveys based on occupation, as indicated in the ten-yearly census. Such groupings are intended to stratify the population according to standard of living and income (married women and children up to school-leaving age are classified in accordance with the occupation of husband/father). Five classes are recognized: I professional/self employed; II administrative; III (non-manual) clerical and (manual) skilled manual workers; IV semi-skilled; V unskilled. An alternative subdivision into *socio-economic groups* is believed by many sociologists to reflect employment grades more accurately, but it is more complicated and tends to be less generally applied.

social medicine *see* community medicine.

social services advice and practical help with problems due to social circumstances. Every local authority is responsible for establishing and starting a social service department, though block exchequer grants meet some of the costs. An increasing proportion of the *social workers* in these departments are professionally trained. The present policy is to train generic social workers, but there are special social workers with medical and psychiatric training who are seconded for work in hospitals (*see* medical social worker). Social workers assess eligibility of clients for such social services as home helps and meals on wheels or refer them to the appropriate statutory or voluntary services. *Case work* involves identifying the cause of the client's problem and, where appropriate, advising how best to correct it and/or adapt to the circumstances.

social worker *see* social services.

socio-economic group *see* social class.

socket *n.* (in anatomy) a hollow or depression into which another part fits, such as the cavity in the alveolar bone of the jaws into which the root of a tooth fits. *See also* dry socket.

sodium *n.* a mineral element and an important constituent of the human body (average sodium content of the adult body is 4000 mmol). Sodium controls the volume of extracellular fluid in the body and maintains the acid-base balance. It also helps maintain electrical potentials in the nervous system and is thus necessary for the functioning of nerves and muscles. Sodium is contained in most foods and is well absorbed, the average daily intake in the UK being 200 mmol. The amount of sodium in the body is controlled by the kidneys. An excess of sodium leads to the condition of *hypernatraemia*, which often results in *oedema. This may develop in infants fed on bottled milk, which has a much higher sodium content than human milk. Since babies are less able to remove sodium from the body than adults the feeding of a high-sodium diet to babies is dangerous and may lead to dehydration. Sodium is also implicated in hypertension: a high-sodium diet is thought to increase the risk of hypertension in later life.

sodium aminosalicylate a drug with effects and uses similar to those of *para-aminosalicylic acid. Trade name: **Paramisan**.

sodium bicarbonate a salt of sodium that neutralizes acid and is used to treat stomach and digestive disorders, *acidosis, and sodium deficiency. It is administered by mouth or injection; high doses may cause digestive upsets. *See also* antacid.

sodium fluoride a salt of sodium used to prevent tooth decay. It is administered by mouth or applied to the teeth as paste or solution. Taken by mouth, it may cause digestive upsets and large doses may cause fluorine poisoning. *See also* fluoridation.

sodium fusidate an *antibiotic used mainly to treat infections caused by *Staphylococcus*. It is administered by mouth or injection or applied in an ointment for skin infections; common side-effects are mild digestive upsets. Trade name: **Fucidin**.

sodium hydroxide (caustic soda) a powerful alkali in widespread use as a cleaning agent. It attacks the skin, causing severe chemical burns that are best treated by washing the area with large quantities of water. When swallowed it causes burning of the mouth and throat, which should be treated by giving water, milk, or other fluid to dilute the stomach contents and by gastric lavage.

sodium nitrite a sodium salt used, with sodium thiosulphate, to treat cyanide poisoning. It is administered by injection and may cause digestive upsets, dizziness, headache, fainting, and cyanosis. It also has effects similar to *glyceryl trinitrate and has been used to treat angina.

sodium salicylate a drug with actions and side-effects similar to those of *aspirin. It is used mainly to treat rheumatic fever. Trade name: **Entrosalyl**.

sodium thiosulphate a salt of sodium used, with *sodium nitrite, to treat cyanide poisoning. It is administered by intravenous injection.

sodium valproate an *anticonvulsant drug used to treat all types of epilepsy. It is administered by mouth; side-effects may include digestive upsets, drowsiness, and muscle incoordination. Trade name: **Epilim**.

sodokosis *n. see* rat-bite fever.

sodomy *n.* sexual intercourse using the anus. This may be homosexual, heterosexual, or between man and beast. *See also* perversion.

soft sore (chancroid) a venereal disease caused by the bacterium *Haemophilus ducreyi*, resulting in enlargement and ulceration of lymph nodes in the groin. Treatment with sulphonamides is effective.

solarium *n.* a room in which patients are exposed to either sunlight or artificial sunlight (a blend of visible light and infrared and ultraviolet radiation directed from special lamps).

solar plexus (coeliac plexus) a network of sympathetic nerves and ganglia high in the back of the abdomen.

soleus *n.* a broad flat muscle in the calf of the leg, beneath the *gastrocnemius muscle. The soleus flexes the foot, so that the toes point downwards.

soma *n.* **1.** the entire body excluding the germ cells. **2.** the body as distinct from the mind.

somat- *prefix denoting* **1.** the body. **2.** somatic.

somatic *adj.* **1.** relating to the nonreproductive parts of the body. A somatic mutation cannot be inherited. **2.** relating to the body wall (i.e. excluding the viscera), e.g. somatic *mesoderm. *Compare* splanchnic. **3.** relating to the body rather than the mind.

somatopleure *n.* the body wall of the early embryo, which consists of a simple layer of ectoderm lined with mesoderm. The amnion is a continuation of this structure outside the embryo. *Compare* splanchnopleure.

somatotrophin *n. see* growth hormone.

somatotype *n. see* body type.

somite *n.* any of the paired segmented divisions of *mesoderm that develop along the length of the early embryo. The somites differentiate into voluntary muscle, bones, connective tissue, and the deeper layers of the skin (*see* dermatome, myotome, sclerotome).

somnambulism (noctambulation) *n.* sleep-walking: walking about and performing other actions in a semiautomatic way during sleep without later memory of doing so. It is common during childhood and may persist into adult life. It can also arise spontaneously, as the result of stress or hypnosis. —**somnambulistic** *adj.*

somniloquence *n.* talking in one's sleep. *See also* somnambulism.

somnolism *n.* a hypnotic trance. *See* hypnosis.

sonoplacentography *n.* the technique of using *ultrasound waves to determine the position of the placenta during pregnancy. This has the advantage over using X-rays that the fetus is not subjected to possibly harmful radiation.

sonotopography *n.* the use of *ultrasound waves to determine the position of structures within the body, such as the position of a fetus within the womb or the midline of the brain within the skull.

soporific *n. see* hypnotic.

sorbitol *n.* a carbohydrate with a sweet taste, used by diabetics as a substitute for cane sugar. It is also used in disorders of carbohydrate metabolism and in drip feeding. It is administered by mouth or injection; large doses taken by mouth may cause digestive upsets.

sordes *pl. n.* the brownish encrustations that form around the mouth and teeth of patients suffering from fevers.

sore *n.* a lay term for any ulcer or other open wound of the skin or mucous membranes, which may be caused by injury or infection. *See also* bedsore, soft sore.

sore throat pain at the back of the mouth, commonly due to bacterial or viral infection of the tonsils (*tonsillitis) or the pharynx (*pharyngitis). If infection persists the lymph nodes in the neck may become tender and enlarged (cervical adenitis).

sotalol *n.* a drug (*see* beta blocker) used to treat abnormal heart rhythm, angina, and high blood pressure and to relieve symptoms in *thyrotoxicosis. It is administered by mouth or injection; side-effects may include digestive upsets, tiredness, and dizziness. Trade names: **Beta-Cardone, Sotacor**.

souffle *n.* a soft blowing sound heard through the stethoscope, usually produced by blood flowing in vessels.

sound (in surgery) **1.** *n.* a long rodlike instrument, often with a curved end, used to explore body cavities (such as the bladder) or to dilate *strictures in the urethra or other canals. **2.** *vb.* to explore a cavity using a sound.

Southey's tubes fine-calibre tubes for insertion into subcutaneous tissue to drain excess fluid. They are rarely used in practice today.

space maintainer an orthodontic appliance that maintains an existing space in the dentition.

Spanish fly the blister beetle, *Lytta vesicatoria*: source of the irritant and toxic chemical compound *cantharidin.

sparganosis *n.* a disease caused by the migration of certain tapeworm larvae (*see* Sparganum) in the tissues beneath the skin, between the muscles, and occasionally in the viscera and brain. The larvae, which normally develop in frogs and reptiles, are accidentally transferred to man by eating the uncooked flesh of these animals or by drinking water contaminated with minute crustaceans infected with the tapeworm larvae. The larvae cause inflammation, swelling, and fibrosis of the tissues. Treatment of the condition, common in the Far East, involves intravenous injections of neosalvarsan and surgical removal of the larvae.

Sparganum *n.* the larvae of certain tapeworms, including species of *Diphyllobothrium* and *Spirometra*, which may accidentally infect man (*see* sparganosis). They are actually *plerocercoids, but the generic name *Sparganum* is given to them since they fail to develop into adults and definite classification of the species is not possible from the larvae alone.

spasm *n.* a sustained involuntary muscular contraction, which may occur either as part of a generalized disorder, such as a *spastic paralysis, or as a local response to an otherwise unconnected painful condition. *Carpopedal spasm* affects the muscles of the hands and feet and is caused by a deficiency of available calcium in the body.

spasmo- *prefix denoting* spasm.

spasmodic *adj.* occurring in spasms or resembling a spasm.

spasmolytic *n.* a drug that relieves spasm of smooth muscle, e.g. *aminophylline, *papaverine, or *piperidolate. Spasmolytics may be used as *bronchodilators to relieve spasm in bronchial muscle, to stimulate the heart in the treatment of angina, or to relieve colic due to spasm of the digestive system.

spasmus nutans a combination of symptoms including a slow nodding movement of the head, *nystagmus (involuntary movements of the eyes), and spasm of the neck muscles. It

affects infants and it normally disappears within a year or two.

spastic colon *see* irritable bowel syndrome.

spasticity *n.* resistance to the passive movement of a limb that is maximal at the beginning of the movement and gives way as more pressure is applied. It is a symptom of damage to the corticospinal tracts in the brain or spinal cord. It is usually accompanied by weakness in the affected limb (*see* spastic paralysis). *Compare* rigidity.

spastic paralysis weakness of a limb or limbs associated with increased reflex activity. This results in resistance to passive movement of the limb (*see* spasticity). It is caused by disease affecting the nerve fibres of the corticospinal tract, which in health not only initiate movement but also inhibit the stretch reflexes to allow the movements to take place. *See* cerebral palsy.

spatula *n.* an instrument with a blunt blade used to spread ointments or plasters and, particularly in dentistry, to mix materials.

special hospitals hospitals for the care of mentally ill patients who are also dangerous and must therefore be kept securely. There are four in the UK: Broadmoor, Rampton, Moss Side, and Carstairs. Most (but not all) patients are there compulsorily under a hospital order made by a court according to the *Mental Health Act.

Specialist in Community Medicine (SCM) *see* community physician.

special school (in Britain) an education establishment for handicapped children. The discovery and assessment (*ascertainment*) of those needing to attend a special school may occur long before school age (2 years or younger); the responsibility for deciding who attends a special school lies with the local education authority. Special schools exist for each of the following 11 groups of handicapped children: the blind, the partially sighted, the deaf, those with partial hearing, the delicate (those with such medical handicaps as congenital heart disease or cystic fibrosis), the educationally subnormal, the mentally handicapped (in which learning potential is limited and independent living may prove impossible), the maladjusted (those with behavioral difficulties), the physically handicapped (by such conditions as poliomyelitis, muscular dystrophy, or limb absence from thalidomide), the epileptic, and those with speech defects. Some special schools cater for combinations of two or more of these handicaps. Special education for the blind and for those with other severe handicaps may start as early as 2 years, deaf children requiring special education from the date of discovery.

species *n.* the smallest unit used in the classification of living organisms. Members of the same species are able to interbreed and produce fertile offspring. Similar species are grouped together within one *genus.

specific 1. *n.* a medicine that has properties especially useful for the treatment of a particular disease. **2.** *adj.* (of a disease) caused by a particular microorganism that causes no other disease. **3.** *adj.* of or relating to a species.

specificity *n.* (in screening tests) *see* sensitivity.

spectinomycin *n.* an *antibiotic used to treat various infections, particularly gonorrhoea. It is administered by injection; side-effects may include nausea, dizziness, fever, and rash. Trade name: **Trobicin.**

spectrograph *n.* an instrument (a *spectrometer or *spectroscope) that produces a photographic record (*spec-trogram*) of the intensity and wavelength of electromagnetic radiations.

spectrometer *n.* any instrument for measuring the intensity and wavelengths of visible or invisible electromagnetic radiations. *See also* spectroscope.

spectrophotometer *n.* an instrument (a spectrometer) for measuring the intensity of the wavelengths of the components of light (visible or ultraviolet).

spectroscope *n.* an instrument used to split up light or other radiation into components of different wavelengths. The simplest spectroscope uses a prism, which splits white light into the rainbow colours of the visible spectrum.

specular reflection (in *ultrasonics) the reflection of sound waves from the surface of an internal structure, which can be used to produce a picture of the surface as an echogram (*see* echography). A specular reflection contrasts with vaguer diffuse echoes produced by minor differences in tissue density.

speculum *n.* (*pl.* **specula**) a metal instrument for inserting into and holding open a cavity of the body, such as the vagina, rectum, or nasal orifice, in order that the interior may be examined (see illustration).

speech therapy the rehabilitation of patients who are unable to speak coherently because of congenital causes, accidents, or illness (e.g. stroke). Speech therapists have special training in this field but are not medically registered.

sperm *n.* *see* spermatozoon.

sperm- (spermi(o)- spermo-) *prefix denoting* sperm or semen.

spermat- (spermato-) *prefix denoting* **1.** sperm. **2.** organs or ducts associated with sperm.

spermatic artery either of two arteries that originate from the abdominal aorta

Cusco's

Fergusson's

Sims's

Vaginal specula

and travel downwards to supply the testes.

spermatic cord the cord, consisting of the *vas deferens, nerves, and blood vessels, that runs from the abdominal cavity to the testicle in the scrotum. The *inguinal canal, through which the spermatic cord passes, becomes closed after the testes have descended.

spermatid *n.* a small cell produced as an intermediate stage in the formation of spermatozoa. Spermatids become embedded in *Sertoli cells in the testis. They are transformed into spermatozoa by the process of spermiogenesis (*see* spermatogenesis).

spermatocele *n.* a cystic swelling in the scrotum containing sperm. The cyst arises from the epididymis (the duct conveying sperm from the testis) and can be felt as a lump above the testis. Needle *aspiration of the cyst reveals a milky opalescent fluid containing sperm. Treatment is by surgical removal.

spermatocyte *n.* a cell produced as an intermediate stage in the formation of spermatozoa (*see* spermatogenesis). Spermatocytes develop from spermatogonia in the walls of the seminiferous tubules of the testis; they are known as either *primary* or *secondary spermatocytes* according to whether they are undergoing the first or second division of meiosis.

spermatogenesis *n.* the process by which mature spermatozoa are produced in the testis (see illustration). *Spermatogonia, in the outermost layer of the seminiferous tubules, multiply throughout reproductive life. Some of them divide by meiosis into *spermatocytes, which produce haploid *spermatids. These are transformed into mature spermatozoa by the process of *spermiogenesis*. The whole process takes 70–80 days.

spermatogonium *n.* (*pl.* **spermatogonia**) a cell produced at an early stage in the formation of spermatozoa (*see* spermatogenesis). Spermatogonia first appear in the testis of the fetus but do not multiply significantly until after puberty. They act as stem cells in the walls of the seminiferous tubules, dividing continuously by mitosis and giving rise to *spermatocytes.

spermatorrhoea *n.* the involuntary discharge of semen without orgasm. Semen is usually produced by ejaculation at orgasm and does not normally discharge at other times. If, however, the mechanism of ejaculation is lost, spermatorrhoea may occur.

Spermatogenesis

A spermatozoon

spermatozoon (sperm) *n.* (*pl.* **spermatozoa**) a mature male sex cell (*see* gamete). The tail of a sperm enables it to swim, which is important as a means for reaching and fertilizing the ovum (although muscular movements of the womb may assist its journey from the vagina). *See also* acrosome, fertilization.

spermaturia *n.* the presence of spermatozoa in the urine. Spermatozoa are occasionally seen on microscopic examination of the urine and their presence is not abnormal. If present in large numbers, the urine becomes cloudy, usually towards the end of micturition. Abnormal ejaculation into the bladder on orgasm (retrograde ejaculation) may occur after *prostatectomy or other surgical procedures or in neurological conditions that destroy the ability of the bladder neck to close on ejaculation.

sperm count an estimate of the concentration of spermatozoa in ejaculated semen, which is used as a measure of male fertility. Between 300 million and 500 million spermatozoa in the total ejaculate is normal; less than 60 million is usually accompanied by *sterility.

spermicide *n.* an agent that kills spermatozoa. Creams and jellies containing chemical spermicides are used – in conjunction with a *diaphragm – as contraceptives. —**spermicidal** *adj.*

spermiogenesis n. the process by which spermatids become mature spermatozoa within the seminiferous tubules of the testis. *See* spermatogenesis.

spheno- *prefix denoting* the sphenoid bone. Examples: *sphenomaxillary* (relating to the sphenoid and maxillary bones); *sphenopalatine* (relating to the sphenoid bone and palate).

sphenoid bone a bone forming the base of the cranium behind the eyes. It consists of a *body*, containing air spaces continuous with the nasal cavity (*see* paranasal sinus); two *wings* that form part of the orbits; and two *pterygoid processes* projecting down from the point where the two wings join the body. *See* skull.

spherocyte n. an abnormal form of red blood cell (*erythrocyte) that is spherical rather than disc-shaped. In blood films spherocytes appear smaller and stain more densely than normal red cells. Spherocytes tend to be removed from the blood as they pass through the spleen, resulting in anaemia. *See also* spherocytosis.

spherocytosis n. the presence in the blood of abnormally shaped red cells (*spherocytes). Spherocytosis may occur as a hereditary disorder (*hereditary spherocytosis*) or in certain haemolytic *anaemias.

sphincter n. a specialized ring of muscle that surrounds an orifice. Contractions of the sphincter partly or completely close the orifice. Sphincters are found, for example, around the anus (*anal sphincter*) and at the opening between the stomach and duodenum (*pyloric sphincter*).

sphincter- *prefix denoting* a sphincter.

sphincterectomy n. **1.** the surgical removal of any sphincter muscle. **2.** surgical removal of part of the iris in the eye at the border of the pupil.

sphincterotomy n. surgical division of any sphincter muscle.

sphingomyelin n. a *phospholipid that contains sphingosine, a fatty acid, phosphoric acid, and choline. Sphingomyelins are found in large amounts in brain and nerve tissue.

sphingosine n. a lipid alcohol that is a constituent of sphingomyelin and cerebrosides.

sphygmo- *prefix denoting* the pulse.

sphygmocardiograph n. an apparatus for producing a continuous record of both the heart beat and the subsequent pulse in one of the blood vessels. The recording can be shown on a moving tape or on an electronic screen.

sphygmograph n. an apparatus for producing a continuous record of the pulse in one of the blood vessels, showing the strength and rate of the beats.

sphygmomanometer n. an instrument for measuring *blood pressure in the arteries. It consists of an inflatable cuff connected via a rubber tube to a column of mercury with a graduated scale. The cuff is applied to a limb (usually the arm) and inflated to exert pressure on a large artery until the blood flow stops. The pressure is then slowly released and, with the aid of a stethoscope to listen to the pulse, it is possible to determine both the systolic and diastolic pressures (which can be read on the scale).

sphygmophone n. a device to record the heart beat or pulse in the form of amplified sound waves played through a loudspeaker or earphones.

sphygmoscope n. a device for showing the heart beat or pulse as a visible signal, especially a continuous wave signal on a cathode-ray tube.

spica n. a bandage wound spirally around an injured limb. At each turn it

spicule

is given a twist so that the slack material is taken up at the overlap.

spicule *n.* a small splinter of bone.

spina bifida (rachischisis) a developmental defect in which the newborn baby has part of the spinal cord and its coverings exposed through a gap in the backbone. The symptoms may include paralysis of the legs, incontinence, and mental retardation from the commonly associated brain defect, *hydrocephalus. Spina bifida is associated with abnormally high levels of *alpha-fetoprotein in the amniotic fluid surrounding the embryo. The condition can be diagnosed at about the 16th week of pregnancy by a test on the amniotic fluid (*see* amniocentesis), so making termination of the pregnancy possible. *See also* neural tube defects.

spinal accessory nerve *see* accessory nerve.

spinal anaesthesia 1. suppression of sensation in part of the body by the injection of a local anaesthetic into the space surrounding the spinal cord. There are two types used for surgery: *subarachnoid* and *epidural.* In the latter the anaesthetic is injected into the outer lining of the cord. The injection site for subarachnoid spinal anaesthetics is in the lumbar region of the vertebral column, the needle being inserted between the vertebrae (anywhere between the second and fifth). For epidural anaesthetics, the sacral region may also be used. The extent of the area anaesthetised depends upon the amount and strength of local anaesthetic injected. Spinal anaesthesia is useful in patients whose condition makes them unsuitable for a general anaesthetic, perhaps because of chest infection; for certain obstetric procedures; or in circumstances where a skilled anaesthetist is not readily available to administer a general anaesthetic. The technique is more commonly used in Scandinavia and the USA than in Britain. **2.** loss of sensation in part of the body as a result of injury or disease to the spinal cord. The area of the body affected depends upon the site of the lesion: the lower it is in the cord the less the sensory disability.

spinal column *see* backbone.

spinal cord the portion of the central nervous system enclosed in the vertebral column, consisting of nerve cells

Transverse section through the spinal cord

580

and bundles of nerves connecting all parts of the body with the brain. It contains a core of grey matter surrounded by white matter (see illustration). It is enveloped in three layers of membrane, the *meninges, and extends from the medulla oblongata in the skull to the level of the second lumbar vertebra. From it arise 31 pairs of *spinal nerves.

spinal nerves the 31 pairs of nerves that leave the spinal cord and are distributed to the body, passing out from the vertebral canal through the spaces between the arches of the vertebrae. Each nerve has two *roots, an anterior, carrying motor nerve fibres, and a posterior, carrying sensory fibres. Immediately after the roots leave the spinal cord they merge to form a mixed spinal nerve on each side.

spindle *n.* a collection of fibres seen in a cell when it is dividing. The fibres radiate from the two ends (*poles*) and meet at the centre (the *equator*) giving a structure shaped like two cones placed base to base. It plays an important part in chromosome movement in *mitosis and *meiosis and is also involved in division of the cytoplasm.

spine *n.* **1.** a sharp process of a bone. **2.** the vertebral column (*see* backbone). —**spinal** *adj.*

spino- *prefix denoting* **1.** the spine. **2.** the spinal cord.

spinocerebellar degeneration any of a group of inherited disorders of the cerebellum and corticospinal tracts in the brain. They are characterized by *spasticity of the limbs and cerebellar *ataxia.

spiral bandage a bandage wound round a part of the body, overlapping the previous section at each turn.

spiral organ *see* organ of Corti.

Spirillum *n.* a genus of highly motile

Origins of the spinal nerves (one side only)

rigid spiral-shaped bacteria usually found in fresh and salt water containing organic matter. They bear tufts of flagella at one or both ends of the cell. Most species are saprophytes, but *S. minus* causes *rat-bite fever.

spiro- *prefix denoting* **1.** spiral. **2.** respiration.

spirochaete *n.* any one of a group of spiral-shaped bacteria that lack a rigid cell wall and move by means of muscular flexions of the cell. The group includes the species *Borrelia, *Leptospira, and *Treponema.

spirograph *n.* an instrument for recording breathing movements. The record (a tracing) obtained is called a *spirogram.* —**spirography** *n.*

spirometer *n.* an instrument for measuring the volume of air inhaled and exhaled. It is used in tests of *ventilation. —**spirometry** *n.*

spironolactone *n.* a synthetic *corticosteroid that inhibits the activity of the hormone *aldosterone and is used to treat heart failure, high blood pressure, and fluid retention (oedema). It is administered by mouth; side-effects may include headache, stomach upsets, and drowsiness. Trade name: **Aldactone**.

Spitz-Holter valve a one-way valve used to drain cerebrospinal fluid in order to control *hydrocephalus. The device is inserted into the ventricles of the brain and passes via a subcutaneous tunnel to drain into the right atrium.

splanch- (splanchno-) *prefix denoting* the viscera.

splanchnic *adj.* relating to the viscera, e.g. splanchnic *mesoderm. *Compare* somatic (def. 2).

splanchnic nerves the series of nerves in the sympathetic system that are distributed to the blood vessels and viscera, passing forwards and downwards from the chain of sympathetic ganglia near the spinal cord to enter the abdomen and branch profusely.

splanchnocranium *n.* the part of the skull that is derived from the *pharyngeal arches, i.e. the mandible (lower jaw).

splanchnopleure *n.* the wall of the embryonic gut, which consists of a layer of endoderm with a layer of mesoderm outside it. The yolk sac is a continuation of this structure. *Compare* somatopleure.

spleen *n.* a large dark-red ovoid organ situated on the left side of the body below and behind the stomach. It is enclosed within a fibrous capsule that extends into the spongy interior – the *splenic pulp* – to form a supportive framework. The pulp consists of aggregates of *lymphoid tissue (*white pulp*) within a meshwork of *reticular fibres packed with red blood cells (*red pulp*). The spleen is a major component of the *reticuloendothelial system, producing lymphocytes in the newborn and containing *phagocytes, which remove worn-out red blood cells and other foreign bodies from the bloodstream. It also acts as a reservoir for blood and, in the fetus, as a source of red blood cells. Anatomical name: **lien**. —**splenic** *adj.*

splen- (spleno-) *prefix denoting* the spleen. Example: *splenorenal* (relating to the spleen and kidney).

splenectomy *n.* surgical removal of the spleen. This is sometimes necessary in the emergency treatment of bleeding from a ruptured spleen and in the treatment of some blood diseases.

splenitis *n.* inflammation of the spleen. *See also* perisplenitis.

splenium *n.* the thickest part of the *corpus callosum, rounded and protruding backwards over the thalami, the pineal body, and the midbrain.

splenomegaly *n.* enlargement of the spleen. It commonly occurs in *malaria, *schistosomiasis, and other disorders caused by parasites; in infections; in blood disorders, including some forms of anaemia and lack of platelets (*thrombocytopenia); in *leukaemia; and in *Hodgkin's disease. *See also* hypersplenism.

splenorenal anastomosis a method of treating *portal hypertension by joining the splenic vein to the left renal vein. *Compare* portacaval anastomosis.

splint *n.* a rigid support to hold broken bones in position until healing has occurred.

spondyl- (spondylo-) *prefix denoting* a vertebra or the spine.

spondylitis *n.* inflammation of the synovial joints of the backbone. *Ankylosing spondylitis* is a rheumatic disease involving the backbone and sacroiliac joints (*see* sacroiliitis) and sometimes also causing arthritis in the shoulder and hip. The resultant pain and stiffness of the backbone are treated by analgesics and regular daily exercises. In severe cases the spine becomes completely rigid, through fusion of its joints, and *kyphosis results. *See also* ankylosis.

spondylolisthesis *n.* a forward shift of one vertebra upon another, due to a defect of the joints that normally bind them together. This may be congenital or develop after injury. The majority of cases in which pain is present are treated with rest and a surgical belt or corset; in a small minority, showing severe disability or pressure on nerve roots, surgical fusion may be required.

spondylosis *n.* degeneration of the intervertebral discs in the cervical, thoracic, or lumbar regions of the backbone. Symptoms include pain and restriction of movement. Spondylosis produces a characteristic appearance on X-ray, including narrowing of the space occupied by the disc and the presence of *osteophytes; these features of the disease (*radiological spondylosis*) may not be accompanied by any signs and symptoms. Pain is relieved by wearing a collar (when the neck region is affected) or a surgical belt (for the lower spine), which prevents movement. Very severe cases sometimes require surgical fusion.

spondylosyndesis *n.* surgical fusion of the intervertebral joints of the backbone.

spongioblast *n.* a type of cell that forms in the early stages of development of the nervous system, giving rise to *astrocytes and *oligodendrocytes.

spongioblastoma *n. see* glioblastoma.

spontaneous *adj.* arising without apparent cause or outside aid. The term is applied in medicine to certain conditions, such as pathological fractures, that arise in the absence of outside injury; also to recovery from a disease without the aid of specific treatment.

sporadic *adj.* describing a disease that occurs only occasionally or in a few isolated places. *Compare* endemic, epidemic.

spore *n.* a small reproductive body produced by plants and microorganisms. Some kinds of spores function as dormant stages of the life cycle, enabling the organism to survive adverse conditions. Other spores are the means by which the organism can spread vegetatively. *See also* endospore.

sporicide *n.* an agent that kills spores (e.g. bacterial spores). Some disinfectants that liberate chlorine are sporicides, but most germicides are ineffective since spores are very resistant to chemical action. —**sporicidal** *adj.*

sporocyst *n.* the second-stage larva of a parasitic *fluke, found within the tissues of a freshwater snail. A sporocyst develops from a first stage larva (*see* miracidium) and gives rise either to the next larval stage (*see* redia) or daughter sporocysts. The latter develop directly into the final larval stage (*see* cercaria) without the intermediate redia stage.

sporogony *n.* the formation of *sporozoites during the life cycle of a sporozoan. The contents of the zygote, formed by the fusion of sex cells, divide repeatedly and eventually release a number of sporozoites. *Compare* schizogony.

sporotrichosis *n.* a chronic infection of the skin and superficial lymph nodes that is caused by the fungus *Sporotrichum schenckii* and results in the formation of abscesses and ulcers.

Sporozoa *n.* a group of parasitic Protozoa that includes *Plasmodium*, the malaria parasite. Most sporozoans do not have cilia or flagella. Sporozoan life cycles are complex and usually involve both sexual and asexual stages. Some sporozoans are parasites of invertebrates, and the parasites are passed to new hosts by means of spores. Sporozoans that parasitize vertebrates are transmitted from host to host by invertebrates, which act as intermediate hosts. For example, the mosquito *Anopheles* is the intermediate host of *Plasmodium*.

sporozoite *n.* one of the many cells formed as a result of *sporogony during the life cyle of a sporozoan. In *Plasmodium* sporozoites are formed by repeated divisions of the contents of the *oocyst inside the body of the mosquito. The released sporozoites ultimately pass into the insect's salivary glands and await transmission to a human host at the next blood meal.

spotted fever *see* cerebrospinal fever, Rocky Mountain spotted fever, typhus.

sprain *n.* injury to a ligament, caused by sudden overstretching. As the ligament is not severed it gradually heals, but this may take several months. Sprains should be treated by cold compresses (ice-packs) at the time of injury, and later by restriction of activity.

Sprengel's deformity a congenital abnormality of the scapula (shoulder blade), which is small and positioned high in the shoulder. It is caused by failure of the normal development of this bone.

sprue (psilosis) *n.* deficient absorption of food due to disease of the small intestine. *Tropical sprue* is seen in people from temperate regions who stay in tropical climates for weeks or months. It is characterized by diarrhoea (usually *steatorrhoea), inflamed tongue (glossitis), anaemia, and weight loss; the lining of the small intestine is inflamed and atrophied, probably because of infection. Treatment with antibiotics and *folic acid is usually effective, but the condition often improves spontaneously on return to a temperate climate. *See also* coeliac disease (nontropical sprue), malabsorption.

spud *n.* a blunt needle used for removing foreign bodies embedded in the cornea of the eye.

spur *n.* a sharp projection, especially one of bone.

sputum *n.* saliva mixed with mucus coughed up from the respiratory tract. A sputum-productive cough occurs in many conditions in which examination of the sputum for microorganisms, cells, and other substances may help diagnosis.

squalene *n.* an unsaturated hydrocarbon (a terpene), synthesized in the body, from which *cholesterol is derived.

squama *n.* (*pl.* **squamae**) **1.** a thin plate of bone. **2.** a scale, such as any of the scales from the cornified layer of the *epidermis.

squamo- *prefix denoting* **1.** the squamous portion of the temporal bone. **2.** squamous epithelium.

squamous bone *see* temporal bone.

squamous epithelium *see* epithelium.

squint *n. see* strabismus.

stadium *n.* a stage in the course of a disease; for example, the *stadium invasioni* is the period between exposure to infection and the onset of symptoms.

stage *vb.* (in oncology) to determine the presence and site of metastases from a primary tumour in order to plan treatment. In addition to clinical examination, a variety of imaging and surgical techniques may be employed to provide a more accurate assessment.

stagnant loop syndrome a condition in which a segment of the small intestine (e.g. a jejunal *diverticulum) is out of continuity with the rest of the intestine or in which progress of contents through the small intestine is delayed by an obstruction (such as a *stricture or *Crohn's disease) that allows an overgrowth of bacteria, causing *malabsorption and the passing of fatty stools (see steatorrhoea).

stain 1. *n.* a dye used to colour tissues and other specimens for microscopical examination. In an *acid stain* the colour is carried by an acid radical and the stain is taken up by parts of the specimen having a basic (alkaline) reaction. In a *basic stain* the colour, carried by a basic radical, is attracted to parts of the specimen having an acidic reaction. *Neutral stains* have neither acidic nor basic affinities. A *contrast stain* is used to give colour to parts of a tissue not affected by a previously applied stain. A *differential stain* allows different elements in a specimen to be distinguished by staining them in different colours. **2.** *vb.* to treat a specimen for microscopical study with a stain.

stammering (stuttering) *n.* halting articulation with interruptions to the normal flow of speech and repetition of the initial consonants of words or syllables. It usually first appears in childhood and the symptoms are most severe when the stammerer is under any psychological stress. It is not a symptom of organic disease and it will usually respond to the re-education of speech by a trained therapist. Medical name: **dysphemia.** —**stammerer** *n.*

standard deviation (in statistics) a measure of the scatter of observations about their arithmetic *mean, which is calculated from the square root of the *variance* of the readings in the series. The arithmetic sum of the amounts by which each observation varies from the mean must be zero, but if these variations are squared before being summated, a positive value is obtained: the mean of this value is the variance. In practice a more reliable estimate of variance is obtained by dividing the sum of the squared deviations by one *less* than the total number of observations. *See also* significance.

standard error (of a *mean) the extent to which the means of several different samples would vary if they were taken repeatedly from the same population. Differences between means are said to have statistical *significance when they are greater than twice the standard error of those means, since the probability of this difference or a larger one occurring by chance is less than 5%.

stanolone *n.* a synthetic male sex hormone with *anabolic activity, used to treat wasting diseases, such as osteoporosis and anorexia, and breast cancer. It is administered by mouth. Trade name: **Anabolex.**

St Anthony's fire a popular name for inflammation of the skin associated with ergot poisoning. *See* ergotism.

stapedectomy *n.* surgical removal of the third ear ossicle (stapes): part of the treatment for deafness due to *otosclerosis.

stapes *n.* a stirrup-shaped bone in the middle *ear that articulates with the incus and is attached to the membrane of the fenestra ovalis. *See* ossicle.

staphylectomy *n.* surgical removal of the uvula (the back of the soft palate).

Staphylococcus *n.* a genus of Gram-positive nonmotile spherical bacteria occurring in grapelike clusters. Some species are saprophytes; others parasites. Many species produce *exotoxins.

staphyloma

The species *S. aureus* is commonly present on skin and mucous membranes; it causes boils and internal abscesses. *S. pyogenes albus* and *S. pyogenes aureus* are associated with most suppurative infections. Other species produce toxins causing *food poisoning.

staphyloma *n.* abnormal bulging of the cornea or sclera (white) of the eye. *Anterior staphyloma* is a bulging scar in the cornea to which a part of the iris is attached. It is usually the site of a healed corneal ulcer that has penetrated right through the cornea; the iris blocks the hole and prevents the further leakage of fluid from the front chamber of the eye. In *ciliary staphyloma* the sclera bulges over the ciliary body as a result of high pressure inside the eyeball. A bulging of the sclera at the back of the eye (*posterior staphyloma*) occurs in some severe cases of short-sightedness.

staphylorrhaphy (palatorrhaphy, uraniscorrhaphy) *n.* surgical suture of a cleft palate.

starch *n.* the form in which *carbohydrates are stored in many plants and a major constituent of the diet. Starch consists of linked glucose units and occurs in two forms, α-*amylose* and *amylopectin*. In α-*amylose* the units are in the form of a long unbranched chain; in amylopectin they form a branched chain. The presence of starch can be detected using iodine: α-amylose gives a blue colour with iodine; amylopectin a red colour. Starch is digested by means of the enzyme *amylase. *See also* dextrin.

Starling's law a law stating that a muscle, including the heart muscle, responds to increased stretching at rest by an increased force of contraction when stimulated.

starvation *n. see* malnutrition.

stasis *n.* stagnation or cessation of flow; for example, of blood or lymph whose flow is obstructed or of the intestinal contents when onward movement (peristalsis) is hindered.

-stasis *suffix denoting* stoppage of a flow of liquid; stagnation. Example: *haemostasis* (of blood).

static reflex the reflex maintenance of muscular tone for posture.

status asthmaticus an attack of *asthma lasting for more than 24 hours. This causes great distress and there is a risk of death from respiratory failure or exhaustion. Treatment with corticosteroid drugs may be life-saving and artificial respiration may be needed. Sedation is risky, and these cases require skilled care.

status epilepticus the occurrence of repeated epileptic fits without any recovery of consciousness between them. Its control is a medical emergency, since prolonged status epilepticus causes a serious imbalance of the salts (electrolytes) in the body, which may lead to the patient's death. During each fit, the breathing is arrested and the body is deprived of oxygen, resulting in further damage to the brain cells.

status lymphaticus enlargement of the thymus gland and other parts of the lymphatic system, formerly believed to be a predisposing cause to sudden death in infancy and childhood associated with hypersensitivity to drugs or vaccines.

steapsin *n. see* lipase.

stearic acid *see* fatty acid.

steat- (steato-) *prefix denoting* fat; fatty tissue.

steatoma *n. see* sebaceous cyst. The term is also used for any tumour of a sebaceous gland.

steatopygia *n.* the accumulation of large quantities of fat in the buttocks.

In the Hottentots of Africa this is a normal condition, thought to be an adaptation that allows fat storage without impeding heat loss from the rest of the body.

steatorrhoea *n.* the passage of abnormally increased amounts of fat in the faeces (more than 5 g/day) due to reduced absorption of fat by the intestine (*see* malabsorption). The faeces are pale, smell offensive, may look greasy, and are difficult to flush away.

stellate fracture a star-shaped fracture of the kneecap caused by a direct blow. The bone may be either split or severely shattered; if the fragments are displaced, the bone may need to be surgically removed (*patellectomy*).

stellate ganglion a star-shaped collection of sympathetic nerve cell bodies in the root of the neck, from which sympathetic nerve fibres are distributed to the face and neck and to the blood vessels and organs of the thorax.

Stellwag's sign apparent widening of the distance between the upper and lower eyelids (the palpebral fissure) due to retraction of the upper lid and protrusion of the eyeball. It is a sign of exophthalmic *goitre.

steno- *prefix denoting* **1.** narrow. Example: *stenocephaly* (narrowness of the head). **2.** constricted.

stenopaeic *adj.* (in ophthalmology) describing an optical device consisting of an opaque disc punctured with a fine slit or hole (or holes), which is placed in front of the eye in the same position as glasses and enables sharper vision in cases of gross long- or short-sightedness or astigmatism. It reduces distortion in the image formed on the retina because it confines the light reaching the eye to one or more fine beams. The same principle is used in the pin-hole camera.

stenosis *n.* the abnormal narrowing of a passage or opening, such as a blood vessel or heart valve. *See* aortic, mitral, pulmonary, and pyloric stenosis.

stenostomia (stenostomy) *n.* the abnormal narrowing of an opening, such as the opening of the bile duct.

Stensen's duct the long secretory duct of the *parotid salivary gland.

stent *n.* a splint left inside the lumen of a duct at operation to aid healing of an anastomosis by draining the contents away. *J-stents* or *double J-stents* are those with a 'pig-tail' curve on one or both ends of the splint to prevent extrusion. Stents are increasingly used in the ureter to overcome obstruction by draining the renal pelvis into the bladder.

sterco- *prefix denoting* faeces.

stercobilin *n.* a brownish-red pigment formed during the metabolism of the *bile pigments biliverdin and bilirubin, which are derived from haemoglobin. Stercobilin is subsequently excreted in the urine or faeces.

stercolith *n.* a stone formed of dried compressed faeces.

stercoraceous *adj.* composed of or containing faeces.

stereognosis *n.* the ability to recognize the three-dimensional shape of an object by touch alone. This is a function of the *association areas of the parietal lobe of the brain. *See also* agnosia.

stereoisomers *n.* compounds having the same molecular formula but different three-dimensional arrangements of their atoms. The atomic structures of stereoisomers are mirror images of each other.

stereoscopic vision perception of the shape, depth, and distance of an object as a result of having *binocular vision. The brain receives two distinct images from the eyes, which it interprets as a single three-dimensional image.

stereotaxy *n.* a relatively recent surgical procedure in which a deep-seated area in the brain is operated upon after its position has been established very accurately by three-dimensional measurements. The operation may be performed using an electrical current or by heat, cold, or mechanical techniques. *See also* leucotomy.

stereotypy *n.* the constant repetition of a complex action, which is carried out in the same way each time. It is seen in *catatonia and infantile *autism; sometimes it is an isolated symptom in mental *subnormality. It is more common in patients who live in institutions where they are bored and unstimulated. It can prevent a patient from carrying on normal life, and sometimes causes physical injury to the patient. Drugs, such as *phenothiazines, and behaviour therapy are sometimes used in treating the condition.

sterile *adj.* **1.** (of a living organism) barren; unable to reproduce its kind (*see* sterility). **2.** (of inanimate objects) completely free from bacteria, fungi, viruses, or other microorganisms that could cause infection.

sterility *n.* inability to have children, due either to *infertility or (in someone who has been fertile) to a surgical operation (*see* sterilization). Sterility may be an incidental result of an operation done for other reasons, such as removal of the womb (*hysterectomy) for cancer.

sterilization *n.* **1.** a surgical operation or any other process that induces *sterility in men or women; for example, by cutting the vasa deferentia in men (*see* vasectomy) and the Fallopian tubes in women (*see* salpingectomy) or by *castration. **2.** any means of rendering objects, wounds, etc., free of bacteria that would otherwise cause disease.

Surgical instruments and dressings can be sterilized by being subjected to steam in an *autoclave. *Disinfectants and *antiseptics are chemicals used to destroy bacteria.

stern- (sterno-) *prefix denoting* the sternum. Example: *sternocostal* (relating to the sternum and ribs).

sternebra *n.* (*pl.* **sternebrae**) one of the four parts that fuse during development to form the body of the sternum.

sternocleidomastoid muscle *see* sternomastoid muscle.

sternohyoid *n.* a muscle in the neck, arising from the sternum and inserted into the hyoid bone. It depresses the hyoid bone.

sternomastoid muscle (sternocleidomastoid muscle) a long muscle in the neck, extending from the mastoid process to the sternum and clavicle. It serves to rotate the neck and flex the head.

sternomastoid tumour a small painless nonmalignant swelling in the lower half of the *sternomastoid muscle, appearing a few days after birth. It occurs when the neck of the fetus is in an abnormal position in the womb, which interferes with the blood supply to the affected muscle, and it is most common after breech births. The tumour may cause a slight tilt of the head towards the tumour and turning of the face to the other side. This can be corrected by physiotherapy aimed at increasing all movements of the body, but without stretching the neck.

sternotomy *n.* surgical division of the breastbone (sternum), performed to allow access to the heart and its major vessels.

sternum *n.* (*pl.* **sterna**) the breastbone: a flat bone, 15–20 cm long, extending from the base of the neck to just below the diaphragm and forming the front part of the skeleton of the thorax. The sternum articulates with the collar bones (*see* clavicle) and the costal cartilages of the first seven pairs of ribs. It consists of three sections: the middle and longest section – the *body* or *gladiolus* – is attached to the *manubrium at the top and the *xiphoid (or ensiform) process at the bottom. The manubrium slopes back from the body so that the junction between the two parts forms an angle (*angle of Louis* or *sternal angle*). —**sternal** *adj.*

sternutator *n.* an agent that produces sneezing.

steroid *n.* one of a group of compounds having a common structure based on the *steroid nucleus*, which consists of three six-membered carbon rings and one five-membered carbon ring. The naturally occurring steroids include the male and female sex hormones (*androgens and *oestrogens), the hormones of the adrenal cortex (*see* corticosteroid), *progesterone, *bile salts, and *sterols. Synthetic steroids have been produced for therapeutic purposes.

sterol *n.* one of a group of *steroid alcohols. The most important sterols are *cholesterol and *ergosterol.

stertor *n.* a snoring type of noisy breathing heard in deeply unconscious patients.

steth- (stetho-) *prefix denoting* the chest.

stethograph *n.* an instrument for recording chest movements during breathing. —**stethography** *n.*

stethometer *n.* an instrument for measuring the expansion of the chest during breathing.

stethoscope *n.* an instrument used for listening to sounds within the body, such as those in the heart and lungs (*see* auscultation). A simple stethoscope usually consists of a diaphragm or an open bell-shaped structure (which is applied to the body) connected by rubber or plastic tubes to shaped earpieces for the examiner. More complicated devices may contain electronic amplification systems to aid diagnosis.

sthenia *n.* a state of normal or greater than normal strength. *Compare* asthenia. —**sthenic** *adj.*

stibophen *n.* a sodium-containing salt of antimony used to treat *schistosomiasis. It is administered by injection; side-effects may include digestive upsets, slow heart rate, and anaemia.

stigma *n.* (*pl.* **stigmata**) **1.** a mark that characterizes a particular disease, such as the café-au-lait spots characteristic of neurofibromatosis. **2.** any spot or lesion on the skin.

stilboestrol *n.* a synthetic female sex hormone (*see* oestrogen) used to relieve menstrual disorders and symptoms of the menopause, to treat prostate and breast cancer, and to suppress lactation. It is administered by mouth or injection; side-effects are those of other synthetic oestrogens.

stilet (stylet, stylus) *n.* **1.** a slender probe. **2.** a wire placed in the lumen of a catheter to give it rigidity while the instrument is passed along a body canal (such as the urethra).

stillbirth *n.* birth of a fetus that shows no evidence of life (heart beat, respiration, or independent movement) at any time later than 28 weeks after conception. The number of such births expressed per 1000 births (live and still) is known as the *stillbirth rate*. Viability is deemed to start at the 28th week of pregnancy and a fetus born dead before this time is known as an *abortion or miscarriage. There is no reason why a child born alive before the 28th week should not survive if properly nurtured, though the small size will greatly increase the risk of neonatal death (*see* infant mortality rate).

Still's disease

Still's disease chronic arthritis developing in children before the age of 16. There are several different forms of arthritis affecting children, and some authorities confine the diagnosis of Still's disease to the following: a disease of childhood marked by arthritis (often involving several joints) with a swinging fever and a transitory red rash. There is often severe illness affecting the entire body and the condition may be complicated by enlargement of the spleen and lymph nodes and inflammation of the pericardium and iris.

stimulant *n.* an agent that promotes the activity of a body system or function. *Amphetamine and *caffeine are stimulants of the central nervous system.

stimulus *n.* (*pl.* **stimuli**) any agent that provokes a response, or particular form of activity, in a cell, tissue, or other structure, which is said to be *sensitive* to that stimulus.

stippling *n.* a spotted or speckled appearance, such as is seen in the retina in certain eye diseases or in abnormal red blood cells stained with basic dyes.

stirrup *n.* (in anatomy) *see* stapes.

stitch *n.* **1.** a sharp localized pain, commonly in the abdomen, associated with strenuous physical activity (such as running), especially shortly after eating. It is a form of cramp. **2.** *see* suture.

stock culture *see* culture.

Stokes-Adams syndrome (Adams-Stokes syndrome) attacks of temporary loss of consciousness that occur when blood flow ceases due to ventricular *fibrillation or *asystole. This syndrome may complicate *heart block. It is treated by means of a battery-operated *pacemaker.

stoma *n.* (*pl.* **stomata**) **1.** (in anatomy) the mouth or any mouthlike part. **2.** (in surgery) the artificial opening of a tube (e.g. the colon or ileum) that has been brought to the abdominal surface (*see* colostomy, ileostomy). *Stoma therapists* are nurses specially trained in the care of these artificial openings and the appliances used with them. —**stomal** *adj.*

stomach *n.* a distensible saclike organ that forms part of the alimentary canal between the oesophagus (gullet) and the duodenum (see illustration). It communicates with the former by means of the *cardiac orifice* and with the latter by the *pyloric sphincter*.
The stomach lies just below the diaphragm, to the right of the spleen and partly under the liver. Its function is to continue the process of digestion that begins in the mouth. *Gastric juice, secreted by gastric glands in the mucosa, contains hydrochloric acid and the enzyme *pepsin, which contribute to chemical digestion. This – together with the churning action of the muscular layers of the stomach – reduces the food to a semiliquid partly digested mass that passes on to the duodenum.

stomachic *n.* an agent that stimulates the secretory activity of the stomach, used as a tonic to improve the appetite.

stomat- (stomato-) *prefix denoting* the mouth.

stomatitis *n.* inflammation of the mucous lining of the mouth.

stomatology *n.* the branch of medicine concerned with diseases of the mouth.

stomodeum *n.* the site of the embryonic mouth, marked by a depression lined with ectoderm from which the teeth develop. The membrane separating it from the foregut breaks down by the end of the first month of pregnancy. *Compare* proctodeum.

-stomy (-ostomy) *suffix denoting* a surgical opening into an organ or part. Example: *colostomy* (into the colon).

stone *n. see* calculus.

oesophagus

cardia

fundus

antrum

body

pylorus

greater omentum

rugae

gastric pits

gastric gland

muscularis
mucosa

mucosa

adipose tissue

submucosa

blood vessel

circular muscle

connective tissue

muscularis externa

longitudinal
muscle

serosa

Regions of the stomach seen from the front (above); layers of the stomach wall (below)

stool *n.* *faeces discharged from the anus.

stop needle a surgical needle with a shank that has a protruding collar to stop it when the needle has been pushed a prescribed distance into the tissue. A stop needle has the eye at the tip.

strabismus (heterotropia) *n.* squint: any abnormal alignment of the two eyes. The strabismus is most commonly horizontal – *convergent strabismus* (*esotropia*) or *divergent strabismus* (*exotropia*) – but it may be vertical (*hypertropia*, in which the eye looks upwards, or *hypotropia*, in which it looks downwards). In rare cases both eyes look towards the same point but one is twisted clockwise or anticlockwise in relation to the other (*cyclotropia*). Double vision is always experienced, but the image from the deviating eye usually becomes ignored. In cyclotropia the image is not separated from the normal one but tilted across it. Most strabismus is *concomitant*, i.e. the abnormal alignment of the two eyes remains fairly constant, in whatever direction the person is looking. This is usual with childhood squints. Strabismus acquired by injury or disease is usually *incomitant*, i.e. the degree of misalignment varies in different directions of gaze. *See also* cover test, heterophoria.

strain 1. *n.* excessive stretching or working of a muscle, resulting in pain and swelling of the muscle. *Compare* sprain. **2.** *n.* a group of organisms, such as bacteria, obtained from a particular source or having special properties distinguishing them from other members of the same species. **3.** *vb.* to damage a muscle by overstretching.

strangulated *adj.* describing a part of the body whose blood supply has been interrupted by compression of a blood vessel, as may occur in a loop of intestine trapped in a *hernia.

strangulation *n.* the closure of a passage, such as the main airway to the lungs (resulting in the cessation of breathing), a blood vessel, or the gastrointestinal tract.

strangury *n.* severe pain in the urethra referred from the base of the bladder and associated with an intense desire to pass urine. It occurs when the base of the bladder is irritated by a stone or an indwelling catheter. It is also noted in patients with an invasive cancer of the base of the bladder or severe *cystitis or *prostatitis, when the strong desire to urinate is accompanied by the painful passage of a few drops of urine.

stratum *n.* a layer of tissue or cells, such as any of the layers of the *epidermis of the skin (the *stratum corneum* is the outermost layer).

streak *n.* (in anatomy) a line, furrow, or narrow band. *See also* primitive streak.

Streptobacillus *n.* a genus of Gram-negative aerobic nonmotile rodlike bacteria that tend to form filaments. The single species, *S. moniliformis*, is a normal inhabitant of the respiratory tract of rats but causes *rat-bite fever in man.

Streptococcus *n.* a genus of Gram-positive nonmotile spherical bacteria occurring in chains. Most species are saprophytes; some are pathogenic. Many pathogenic species are *haemolytic*, i.e. they have the ability to destroy red blood cells in blood agar. This provides a useful basis for classifying the many different strains. Strains of *S. pyogenes* (the β-haemolytic streptococci) are associated with many infections, including *scarlet fever, and produce many *exotoxins. Strains of *S. viridans* (the α-haemolytic streptococci) are associated with bacterial *endocarditis. The species *S. pneumoniae* (formerly *Diplococcus pneumoniae*) – the *pneumococcus* – is associated with pneumonia. It occurs in pairs, surrounded by a capsule (*see* quellung reaction). *See also* Lancefield classification, streptokinase.

streptodornase *n.* an enzyme produced by some haemolytic bacteria of the genus *Streptococcus* that is capable of liquefying pus. *See also* streptokinase.

streptokinase *n.* an enzyme produced by some haemolytic bacteria of the genus *Streptococcus* that is capable of liquefying blood clots. It is injected to treat blockage of blood vessels, including infarction and pulmonary embolism. It is also used in combination with streptodornase, applied topically or taken by mouth or injection, to liquefy pus and relieve inflammation. Side-effects may include digestive upsets, fever, and haemorrhage.

streptolysin *n*. an *exotoxin that is produced by *Streptococcus pyogenes* and destroys red blood cells.

Streptomyces *n*. a genus of aerobic mouldlike bacteria. Most species live in the soil, but some are parasites of animals, man, and plants; in man they cause *Madura foot. They are important medically as a source of such antibiotics as *streptomycin, *actinomycin, *chloramphenicol, and *neomycin.

streptomycin *n*. an *antibiotic, derived from the bacterium *Streptomyces griseus*, that is effective against a wide range of bacterial infections; it is administered by mouth or intramuscular injection. Streptomycin is an important drug in tuberculosis therapy but is usually given in conjunction with other drugs (e.g. *isoniazid) because bacteria soon become resistant to it. Side-effects causing ear and kidney damage may develop in some patients.

stress *n*. any factor that threatens the health of the body or has an adverse effect on its functioning, such as injury, disease, or worry. The existence of one form of stress tends to diminish resistance to other forms. Constant stress brings about changes in the balance of hormones in the body.

stretch receptor a cell or group of cells found between muscle fibres that responds to stretching of the muscle by transmitting impulses to the central nervous system through sensory nerves. Stretch receptors are part of the *proprioceptor system necessary for the performance of coordinated muscular activity.

stretch reflex (myotatic reflex) the reflex contraction of a muscle in response to its being stretched.

stria *n*. (*pl*. **striae**) (in anatomy) a streak, line, or thin band. The *striae gravidarum* are the lines that appear on the skin of the abdomen of pregnant women, due to stretching and rupture of the elastic fibres. Pinkish during pregnancy, they become white after delivery. The *stria terminalis* is a white band that separates the thalamus from the ventricular surface of the caudate nucleus in the brain.

striated muscle a tissue comprising the bulk of the body's musculature. It is also known as *skeletal muscle*, because it is attached to the skeleton and is responsible for the movement of bones, and *voluntary muscle*, because it is under voluntary control. Striated muscle is composed of parallel bundles of multinucleate fibres (each containing many *myofibrils*), which reveal cross-

Structure of striated muscle

banding when viewed under the microscope. This effect is due to the alternation of *actin* and *myosin* protein filaments within each myofibril (see illustration). When muscle contraction takes place, the two sets of filaments slide past each other, so reducing the length of each unit (*sarcomere*) of the myofibril. The sliding is caused by a series of cyclic reactions resulting in a change in orientation of projections on the myosin filaments; each projection is first attached to an actin filament but contracts and releases it to become reattached at a different site.

stricture *n.* a narrowing of any tubular structure in the body, such as the oesophagus (gullet), bowel, ureter, or urethra. A stricture may result from inflammation, muscular spasm, growth of a tumour within the affected part, or from pressure on it by neighbouring organs. For example, a *urethral stricture* is a fibrous narrowing of the urethra, usually resulting from injury or inflammation. The patient has increasing difficulty in passing urine and may develop *retention. The site and length of the stricture is assessed by *urethrography and urethroscopy, and treatment is by periodic dilatation of the urethra using *sounds, *urethrotomy, or *urethroplasty.

stridor *n.* the noise heard on breathing in when the trachea or larynx is obstructed. It tends to be louder and harsher than *wheeze.

strobila *n.* (*pl.* **strobilae**) the entire chain of segments that make up the body of an adult *tapeworm.

stroke (apoplexy) *n.* a sudden attack of weakness affecting one side of the body. It is the consequence of an interruption to the flow of blood to the brain. The primary disease is in the heart or blood vessels and the effect on the brain is secondary. The flow of blood may be prevented by clotting (*thrombosis*), a detached clot that lodges in an artery (*embolus*), or rupture of an artery wall (*haemorrhage*). A stroke can vary in severity from a passing weakness or tingling in a limb to a profound paralysis, coma, and death. *See also* cerebral haemorrhage.

stroma *n.* **1.** the supportive tissue of an organ, as opposed to the functional tissue (*parenchyma*). **2.** the spongy framework of protein strands within a red blood cell in which the blood pigment haemoglobin is packed.

Strongyloides *n.* a genus of small slender nematode worms that live as parasites in the small intestines of mammals. *S. stercoralis* infects the human small intestine (*see* strongyloidiasis); its larvae, which are passed out in the stools, develop quickly into infective forms.

strongyloidiasis (strongyloidosis) *n.* an infestation of the small intestine with the parasitic nematode worm *Strongyloides stercoralis*, common in humid tropical regions. Larvae, present in soil contaminated with human faeces, penetrate the skin of a human host and may produce an itching rash. They migrate to the lungs, where they cause tissue destruction and bleeding, and then via the windpipe and gullet to the intestine. Adult worms burrow into the intestinal wall and may cause ulceration, diarrhoea, abdominal pain, nausea, anaemia, and weakness. Treatment involves use of the drugs thiabendazole and *dithiazanine.

strontium *n.* a yellow metallic element, absorption of which causes bone damage when its atoms displace calcium in bone. The radioactive isotope *strontium-90*, which emits beta rays, is used in radiotherapy for the *contact therapy of skin and eye tumours. Symbol: Sr.

struma *n.* (*pl.* **strumae**) a swelling of the thyroid gland (*see* goitre). *Riedel's struma* is a rare chronic inflammation of the thyroid (*see* thyroiditis), which becomes firm and enlarged and is eventually destroyed.

strychnine *n.* a poisonous alkaloid produced in the seeds of the East Indian tree *Strychnos nux-vomica*. In small doses it was formerly widely used in 'tonics'. Poisoning causes painful muscular spasms similar to those of tetanus; the back becomes arched (the posture known as *opisthotonus*) and death is likely to occur from spasm in the respiratory muscles.

Student's t test *see* significance.

stupe *n.* any piece of material, such as a wad of cottonwool, soaked in hot water (with or without medication) and used to apply a poultice.

stupor *n.* a condition of near unconsciousness, with apparent mental inactivity and reduced ability to respond to stimulation.

Sturge-Weber syndrome *see* angioma.

stuttering *n.* *see* stammering.

St. Vitus' dance an archaic name for Sydenham's *chorea.

stye *n.* acute inflammation of a gland at the base of an eyelash, caused by bacterial infection. The gland becomes hard and tender and a pus-filled cyst develops at its centre. Styes are treated by bathing in warm water or removal of the eyelash involved. Medical name: **hordeolum**.

stylet *n.* *see* stilet.

stylo- *prefix denoting* the styloid process of the temporal bone. Example: *stylomastoid* (relating to the styloid and mastoid processes).

styloglossus *n.* a muscle that extends from the tongue to the styloid process of the temporal bone. It serves to draw the tongue upwards and backwards.

stylohyoid *n.* a muscle that extends from the styloid process of the temporal bone to the hyoid bone. It serves to draw the hyoid bone backwards and upwards.

styloid process 1. a long slender downward-pointing spine projecting from the lower surface of the *temporal bone of the skull. It provides attachment for muscles and ligaments of the tongue and hyoid bone. **2.** any of various other spiny projections; occurring, for example, at the lower ends of the ulna and radius.

stylus *n.* **1.** a pencil-shaped instrument, commonly used for applying external medication; for example, to apply silver nitrate to warts. **2.** *see* stilet.

styptic *n.* *see* haemostatic.

sub- *prefix denoting* **1.** below; underlying. Examples: *subcostal* (below the ribs); *sublingual* (below the tongue); *submandibular* (below the mandible). **2.** partial or slight.

subacute *adj.* describing a disease that progresses more rapidly than a *chronic condition but does not become *acute.

subacute combined degeneration of the cord the neurological disorder complicating a deficiency of *vitamin B_{12} and pernicious anaemia. There is selective damage to the motor and sensory nerve fibres in the spinal cord, resulting in *spasticity of the limbs and a sensory *ataxia. It may also be accompanied by damage to the peripheral nerves and the optic nerve and by dementia. It is treated by giving vitamin B_{12} injections.

subarachnoid haemorrhage bleeding into the subarachnoid space surrounding the brain, which causes severe headache with stiffness of the neck. The usual source of such a haemorrhage is a cerebral *aneurysm that has burst. The diagnosis is confirmed by finding blood-stained cerebrospinal fluid at *lumbar puncture. Identification of the site of the aneurysm, upon which decisions about treatment will be based, is achieved by cerebral *angiography.

subarachnoid space the space between the arachnoid and pia *meninges of the brain and spinal cord, containing circulating cerebrospinal fluid and large blood vessels. Several large spaces within it are known as *cisternae*.

subclavian artery either of two arteries supplying blood to the neck and arms. The right subclavian artery branches from the innominate artery; the left subclavian arises directly from the aortic arch.

subclinical *adj.* describing a disease that is suspected but is not sufficiently developed to produce definite signs and symptoms in the patient.

subconscious *adj.* **1.** describing mental processes of which a person is not aware. **2.** (in psychoanalysis) denoting the part of the mind that includes memories, motives, and intentions that are momentarily not present in consciousness but can more or less readily be recalled to awareness. *Compare* unconscious.

subcutaneous *adj.* beneath the skin. A *subcutaneous injection* is given beneath the skin. *Subcutaneous tissue* is loose connective tissue, often fatty, situated under the dermis.

subdural *adj.* below the dura mater (the outermost of the meninges); relating to the space between the dura mater and arachnoid. *See also* haematoma.

subinvolution *n.* failure of a part of the body to return to its normal size after being enlarged. In *uterine subinvolution* the womb does not revert to its normal size during the six weeks following childbirth. *Compare* hyperinvolution.

sublimation *n.* the replacement of socially undesirable means of gratifying

motives or desires by means that are socially acceptable. *See also* defence mechanism, repression.

subliminal *adj.* subconscious: beneath the threshold of conscious perception.

sublingual gland one of a pair of *salivary glands situated in the lower part of the mouth, one on either side of the tongue. The sublingual glands are the smallest salivary glands; each gland has about 20 ducts, most of which open into the mouth directly above the gland.

subluxation *n.* partial *dislocation of a joint, so that the bone ends are misaligned but still in contact.

submandibular gland (submaxillary gland) one of a pair of *salivary glands situated below the parotid glands. Their ducts (*Wharton's ducts*) open in two papillae under the tongue, on either side of the frenulum.

submaxillary gland *see* submandibular gland.

submentovertical (SMV) *adj.* (in radiology) denoting a horizontal view of the base of the skull.

submucosa *n.* the layer of loose connective (*areolar) tissue underlying a mucous membrane; for example, in the wall of the intestine. —**submucosal** *adj.*

subnormality *n.* a state of arrested or incomplete development of the mind. *Mental subnormality* is essentially an administrative concept, describing the state of those whose intellectual powers have failed to develop to such an extent that they are in need of care and protection. This depends in part on social circumstances, for a person who is subnormal in a demanding culture may manage well in a simpler environment. It is also known as *mental retardation, mental deficiency*, and *amentia*. *Intellectual subnormality* is a scientific concept, denoting the state of those whose intellectual powers fall below some point on a standardized *intelligence test. Mildly subnormal people (with an IQ of approximately 50–70) often make a good adjustment to life after special help with education. The moderately and severely subnormal (with an IQ of approximately 20–50) usually need much more help; most are permanently dependent on other people. The profoundly subnormal (with an IQ less than about 20) usually need constant attention. There are very many causes of intellectual subnormality, including *Down's syndrome, inherited metabolic disorders, brain injury, and gross psychological deprivation; some are preventable or treatable. Good education alters the course of the handicap, but many patients need residential care in local authority homes or in hospitals.

subphrenic abscess a collection of pus in the space below the diaphragm, usually on the right side, between the liver and diaphragm. Causes include postoperative infection (particularly after the stomach or bowel have been opened) and perforation of an organ (e.g. perforated peptic ulcer). Prompt treatment by antibiotics may be effective, but more frequently the abscess requires surgical drainage.

substitution *n.* **1.** (in psychoanalysis) the replacement of one idea by another: a form of *defence mechanism. **2.** *symptom substitution* is the supposed process whereby removing one psychological symptom leads to another symptom appearing if the basic psychological cause has not been removed. It is controversial whether this happens.

substitution therapy treatment by providing a less harmful alternative to a drug or remedy that a patient has been receiving. It is used when the patient has become addicted to a drug or is placing too much reliance upon a particular remedy. The patient is weaned off the 'hard' drug to which he has become addicted by the gradual substitution of a nonaddictive drug with a similar or a sedative effect.

substrate *n.* the specific substance or substances on which a given *enzyme acts. For example, starch is the substrate for salivary amylase; RNA is the substrate for ribonuclease.

subsultus *n.* abnormal twitching or tremor of muscles, such as may occur in feverish conditions.

subtertian fever a form of *malaria resulting from repeated infection by *Plasmodium falciparum* and characterized by continuous fever.

subthalamic nucleus a collection of grey matter, shaped like a biconvex lens, lying beneath the *thalamus and close to the *corpus striatum, to which it is connected by nerve tracts. It has connections with the cerebral cortex and several other nuclei nearby.

succus *n.* any juice or secretion of animal or plant origin.

succus entericus (intestinal juice) the clear alkaline fluid secreted by the glands of the small intestine. It contains mucus and digestive enzymes, including *enteropeptidase, *erepsin, *lactase, and *sucrase.

succussion *n.* a splashing noise heard when a patient who has a large quantity of fluid in a body cavity, such as the pleural cavity, moves suddenly or is deliberately shaken.

sucrase *n.* an enzyme, secreted by glands in the small intestine, that catalyses the hydrolysis of sucrose into its components (glucose and fructose).

sucrose *n.* a carbohydrate consisting of glucose and fructose. Sucrose is the principal constituent of cane sugar and sugar beet; it is the sweetest of the natural dietary carbohydrates. The increasing consumption of sucrose in the last 50 years has coincided with an increase in the incidence of dental caries, diabetes, coronary heart disease, and obesity.

suction *n.* the use of reduced pressure to remove unwanted fluids or other material through a tube for disposal. Suction is often used to clear secretions from the airways of newly born infants to aid breathing. During surgery, suction tubes are used to remove blood from the area of operation.

sudamen *n.* (*pl.* **sudamina**) a white blister caused by sweat collecting in the sweat ducts or in the layers of the skin.

Sudan stains a group of azo compounds used for staining fats. The group includes *Sudan I*, *Sudan II*, *Sudan III*, *Sudan IV*, and *Sudan black*.

Sudek's atrophy rapid development of *osteoporosis in a hand or foot, resulting from injury, infection, or malignancy.

sudor *n.* *see* sweat.

sudorific *n.* *see* diaphoretic.

suffocation *n.* cessation of breathing as a result of drowning, smothering, etc., leading to unconsciousness or death (*see* asphyxia).

suffusion *n.* the spreading of a flush across the skin surface, caused by changes in the local blood supply.

sugar any *carbohydrate that dissolves in water, is usually crystalline, and has a sweet taste. Sugars are classified chemically as *monosaccharides or *disaccharides. Table sugar is virtually 100% pure *sucrose and contains no other nutrient; brown sugar is less highly refined sucrose. Sugar is used as both a sweetening and preserving agent. *See also* fructose, glucose, lactose.

suggestion *n.* (in psychology) the process of changing a person's beliefs, attitudes, or emotions by telling him that they will change. It is sometimes used as a synonym for *hypnosis. *See also* autosuggestion.

suicide *n.* self-destruction as a deliberate act. Distinction is usually made between *attempted suicide*, when death is averted although the person concerned intended to kill himself (or herself), and *parasuicide, when the attempt is made for reasons other than actually killing oneself. In the UK deliberate overdosing is the commonest cause of admission to hospital medical wards and it is estimated that some 85% of attempted suicides are happy to have survived. Death by suicide in the UK declined by some 36% in the period 1963–75, contrary to the general trend in other Western countries. This fall is claimed to have resulted from the work of the *Samaritans, a voluntary suicide-prevention organization that grew into a nationwide service over this period.

sulcus *n.* (*pl.* **sulci**) **1.** one of the many clefts or infoldings of the surface of the brain. The raised outfolding on each side of a sulcus is termed a *gyrus*. **2.** any of the infoldings of soft tissue in the mouth, for example between the cheek and the alveolus.

sulphacetamide *n.* a drug of the *sulphonamide group that is used in eye drops to treat such infections as conjunctivitis. Transient irritation may occur with higher doses. Trade names: **Albucid, Ocusol**.

sulphadimidine *n.* *see* sulphonamide.

sulphadoxine *n.* *see* sulphonamide.

sulpha drug *see* sulphonamide.

sulphafurazole *n.* *see* sulphonamide.

sulphaguanidine *n.* *see* sulphonamide.

sulphamethizole *n.* *see* sulphonamide.

sulphamethoxazole *n.* a drug of the *sulphonamide group. It is taken by mouth and is effective in the treatment of infections of the respiratory tract (including bronchitis), the urinary and gastrointestinal tracts, and the skin. The drug is frequently administered in a combined preparation with trimethoprim (*see* co-trimoxazole (Bactrim, Septrin)). Trade name: **Gantanol**.

sulphaphenazole *n. see* sulphonamide.

sulphasalazine *n.* a drug of the *sulphonamide group, used in the treatment of ulcerative colitis. It is given by mouth or in the form of suppositories. The most common side-effects are nausea, loss of appetite, and raised temperature. Trade name: **Salazopyrin**.

sulphinpyrazone *n.* a *uricosuric drug given by mouth for the treatment of chronic gout. The main side-effects are nausea and abdominal pain; the drug may also activate a latent duodenal ulcer and it should not be taken by patients with impaired kidney function. Trade name: **Anturan**.

sulphomyxin *n.* an antibiotic, similar to *polymyxin B, given by local application or intramuscular injection to treat infections of the skin, mucous membranes, eyes, and ears caused by *Pseudomonas*. Common side-effects include flushing, dizziness, blurred vision, and weakness.

sulphonamide (sulpha drug) *n.* one of a group of drugs, derived from sulphanilamide (a red dye), that prevent the growth of bacteria (i.e. they are bacteriostatic). Sulphonamides are usually given by mouth and are effective against a variety of infections. Most of them, including *sulphamethoxazole and *sulphaphenazole*, are rapidly absorbed from the stomach and small intestine and should be taken at frequent intervals. Some, such as *sulphadoxine* (used for leprosy and malaria) and *sulphametopyrazine* are long-acting and need be taken only once a day. Others, including *sulphaguanidine*, are poorly absorbed and are therefore used to treat infections of the gastrointestinal tract, such as bacillary dysentery and gastroenteritis. Prolonged use of these sulphonamides may lead to the development of resistant stains of microorganisms in the gut. Many sulphonamides are rapidly excreted and very soluble in the urine and are used to treat infections of the urinary tract; examples are *sulphadimidine, sulphafurazole*, and *sulphamethizole*.

A variety of side-effects may occur with sulphonamide treatment, including nausea, vomiting, headache, and loss of appetite. In acute infections these are unimportant compared with the benefit produced by the drugs. More severe effects include *cyanosis, blood disorders, skin rashes, and fever. Sulphonamides should be avoided in jaundice and kidney disease and in patients allergic to these drugs. In general, patients treated with sulphonamides should avoid exposure to direct sunlight.

sulphone *n.* one of a group of drugs closely related to the *sulphonamides in structure and therapeutic actions. Sulphones possess powerful activity against the bacteria that cause leprosy and tuberculosis. The best known sulphone is *dapsone.

sulphonylurea *n.* one of a group of drugs, derived from a sulphonamide, that reduce the level of glucose in the blood. These drugs are given by mouth and are used in the treatment of diabetes mellitus. They include *chlorpropamide, *tolazamide, and *tolbutamide.

sulphur *n.* a nonmetallic element that is active against fungi and parasites. It is a constituent of ointments and other preparations used in the treatment of skin disorders and infections (such as psoriasis and dermatitis).

sulphuric acid a powerful corrosive acid, H_2SO_4, widely used in industry. Swallowing the acid causes severe burning of the mouth and throat and difficulty in breathing, speaking, and swallowing. The patient should drink large quantities of milk or water or white of egg; gastric lavage should not be delayed. Skin or eye contact should be treated by flooding the area with water.

sulthiame *n.* an *anticonvulsant drug used in the treatment of severe forms of epilepsy. The drug is given by mouth and mild side-effects may develop in some patients, including muscular incoordination, loss of appetite, and headache. Trade name: **Ospolot**.

sunburn *n.* damage to the skin by prolonged or unaccustomed exposure to the sun's rays. Sunburn may vary from reddening of the skin to the development of large painful fluid-filled blisters, which may cause shock if they cover a large area (*see* burn). Fair-skinned people are more susceptible to sunburn than others.

sunstroke *n. see* heatstroke.

super- *prefix denoting* **1.** above; overlying. **2.** extreme or excessive.

superciliary *adj.* of or relating to the eyebrows (supercilia).

superego *n.* (in psychoanalysis) the part of the mind that functions as a moral conscience or judge. It is also responsible for the formation of ideals for the *ego. The superego is the result of the incorporation of parental injunctions into the child's mind.

superfecundation *n.* the fertilization of two or more ova of the same age by spermatozoa from different males. *See* superfetation.

superfetation *n.* the fertilization of a second ovum some time after the start of pregnancy, resulting in two fetuses of different maturity in the same womb.

superficial *adj.* (in anatomy) situated at or close to a surface. Superficial

blood vessels are those close to the surface of the skin.

superinfection *n.* an infection arising during the course of another infection and caused by a different microorganism, which is usually resistant to the drugs used to treat the primary infection. The infective agent may be a normally harmless inhabitant of the body that becomes pathogenic when other harmless types are removed by the drugs or it may be a resistant variety of the primary infective agent.

superinvolution *n. see* hyperinvolution.

superior *adj.* (in anatomy) situated uppermost in the body in relation to another structure or surface.

supernumerary *n.* (in dentistry) an additional tooth.

supination *n.* the act of turning the hand so that the palm is uppermost. *Compare* pronation.

supinator *n.* a muscle of the forearm that extends from the elbow to the shaft of the radius. It supinates the forearm and hand.

supine *adj.* **1.** lying on the back or with the face upwards. **2.** (of the forearm) in the position in which the palm of the hand faces upwards. *Compare* prone.

supplementary benefit *see* National Assistance Act (1945).

suppository *n.* a medicinal preparation in solid form suitable for insertion into the rectum or vagina. *Rectal suppositories* may contain simple lubricants (e.g. glycerin); drugs that act locally in the rectum or anus (e.g. corticosteroids, local anaesthetics); or drugs that are absorbed and act at other sites (e.g. *bronchodilators). *Vaginal suppositories* are used to treat some gynaecological disorders (*see* pessary).

suppression *n.* **1.** the cessation or complete inhibition of any physiological activity. **2.** treatment that removes the outward signs of an illness or prevents its progress. **3.** (in psychology) a *defence mechanism by which a person consciously and deliberately ignores an idea that is unpleasant to him.

suppuration *n.* the formation of pus.

supra- *prefix denoting* above; over. Examples: *supraclavicular* (above the clavicle); *suprahyoid* (above the hyoid bone); *suprarenal* (above the kidney).

supraorbital *adj.* of or relating to the area above the eye orbit.

supraorbital reflex the closing of the eyelids when the supraorbital nerve is struck, due to contraction of the muscle surrounding the orbit (orbicularis oculi muscle).

suprarenal glands *see* adrenal glands.

supravital staining the application of a *stain to living tissue, particularly blood cells, removed from the body.

suramin *n.* a nonmetallic drug used in the treatment of *trypanosomiasis. It is usually given by slow intravenous injection. Side-effects, which vary in intensity and frequency and are related to the nutritional state of the patient, include nausea, vomiting, shock, and loss of consciousness.

surfactant *n.* a wetting agent: a substance, such as a detergent, that reduces surface tension. A surfactant is secreted by the cells (*pneumocytes) lining the alveoli of the lungs to prevent the alveolar walls from sticking together. In its absence, as in the immature lungs of premature babies and in some diseases, the lungs tend to collapse. *See* atelectasis, respiratory distress syndrome.

surgeon *n.* a qualified medical practitioner who specializes in surgery. *See* doctor.

surgery *n.* the branch of medicine that treats injuries, deformities, or disease by operation or manipulation. *See also*
cryosurgery, microsurgery. —**surgical** *adj.*

surgical neck the constriction of the shaft of the *humerus, below the head. It is frequently the point at which fracture of the humerus occurs.

surgical spirit methylated spirit, usually with small amounts of castor oil and oil of wintergreen: used to sterilize the skin before surgery, injections, etc.

surrogate *n.* (in psychology) a person or object in someone's life that functions as a substitute for another person. In the treatment of sexual problems, when the patient does not have a partner to cooperate in treatment, a surrogate provided by the therapist acts as a sexual partner who gives service to the patient up to and including intercourse. According to psychoanalysts, people and objects in dreams can be surrogates for important individuals in a person's life.

susceptibility *n.* lack of resistance to disease. It is partly a reflection of general health but is also influenced by vaccination or other methods of increasing resistance to specific diseases.

suspensory bandage a bandage arranged to support a hanging part of the body. Examples include a sling used to hold an injured lower jaw in position and a bandage used to support the scrotum in various conditions of the male genital organs.

suspensory ligament a ligament that serves to support or suspend an organ in position. For example, the suspensory ligament of the lens is a fibrous structure attached to the ciliary processes (*see* ciliary body) by means of which the lens of the eye is held in position.

sustentaculum *n.* any anatomical structure that supports another structure. —**sustentacular** *adj.*

suture

suture 1. *n.* (in anatomy) a type of immovable joint, found particularly in the skull, characterized by a minimal amount of connective tissue between the two bones. The cranial sutures include the *coronal suture*, between the frontal and parietal bones; the *lambdoidal suture*, between the parietal and occipital bones; and the *sagittal suture*, between the two parietal bones (see illustration). **2.** *n.* (in surgery) the closure of a wound or incision with material such as silk or catgut, to facilitate the healing process. There is a wide variety of suturing techniques developed to meet the differing circumstances of injuries to and incisions in the body tissues (see illustration). **3.** *n.* the material – silk, catgut, nylon, or wire – used to sew up a wound. **4.** *vb.* to close a wound by suture.

Types of surgical suture

Sutures of the skull (internal surface of the vault)

suxamethonium *n.* a drug that relaxes voluntary muscle (*see* muscle relaxant). It is administered by intravenous injection and is used mainly to produce muscle relaxation during surgery carried out under general anaesthesia and to reduce muscular movements during *electroconvulsive therapy. Trade name: **Scoline**.

swab *n.* a pad of absorbent material (such as cotton), sometimes attached to a stick or wire, used for cleaning out or applying medication to wounds, oper-

ation sites, or body cavities. In operations, gauze swabs are used to clean blood from the site; such swabs are always carefully counted and contain a *radio-opaque 'tag' to facilitate identification should it by mischance remain in the body after operation.

swallowing (deglutition) *n.* the process by which food is transferred from the mouth to the oesophagus (gullet). Voluntary raising of the tongue forces food backwards towards the pharynx. This stimulates reflex actions in which the larynx is closed by the epiglottis and the nasal passages are closed by the soft palate, so that food does not enter the trachea (windpipe). Lastly, food moves down the oesophagus by *peristalsis and gravity.

sweat *n.* the watery fluid secreted by the *sweat glands. Its principal constituents in solution are sodium chloride and urea. The secretion of sweat is a means of excreting nitrogenous waste; at the same time it has a role in controlling the temperature of the body – the evaporation of sweat from the surface of the skin has a cooling effect. Therefore an increase in body temperature causes an increase in sweating. Other factors that increase the secretion of sweat include pain, nausea, nervousness, and drugs (*diaphoretics). Sweating may be reduced by colds, diarrhoea, and certain drugs. Anatomical name: **sudor**.

sweat gland a simple coiled tubular *exocrine gland that lies in the dermis of the *skin. A long duct carries its secretion (*sweat) to the surface of the skin. Sweat glands occur over most of the surface of the body; they are particularly abundant in the armpits, on the soles of the feet and palms of the hands, and on the forehead.

sycosis *n.* inflammation of the hair follicles caused by bacterial infection. It commonly affects the beard area (*sycosis barbae*) and may cause intense itching. The infection usually spreads unless treated by allowing the beard to grow and applying antibiotic ointments.

symbiosis *n.* an intimate and obligatory association between two different species of organism (*symbionts*) in which there is mutual aid and benefit. *Compare* commensal, mutualism, parasite.

symblepharon *n.* a condition in which the eyelid adheres to the eyeball. It is usually the result of acid or alkali burns to the conjunctiva lining the eyelid and eyeball.

symbolism *n.* (in psychology) the process of representing an object or an idea by something else. Typically an abstract idea is represented by a simpler and more tangible image. Psychoana-lytic theorists hold that conscious ideas frequently act as symbols for unconscious thoughts and that this is particularly evident in dreaming, in *free association, and in the formation of psychological symptoms. According to this theory, a symptom (such as difficulty in swallowing) might be a symbolic representation of an unconscious idea (such as a fantasy of oral intercourse). —**symbolic** *adj.*

symmelia *n.* a developmental abnormality in which the legs appear to be fused.

symmetry *n.* (in anatomy) the state of opposite parts of an organ or parts at opposite sides of the body corresponding to each other.

sympathectomy *n.* the surgical *division of sympathetic nerve fibres. It is done to minimize the effects of normal or excessive sympathetic activity. Most often it is used to improve the circulation to part of the body; less commonly to inhibit excess sweating or to relieve the *photophobia induced by an abnormally dilated pupil of the eye.

sympathetic nervous system one of the two divisions of the *autonomic nervous system, having fibres that leave the central nervous system, via a chain of ganglia close to the spinal cord, in the thoracic and lumbar regions. Its nerves are distributed to the blood vessels, sweat glands, salivary glands, heart, lungs, intestines and other abdominal organs, and the genitals, whose functions it governs by reflex action, in balance with the *parasympathetic nervous system.

sympathin *n.* the name given by early physiologists to the substances released from sympathetic nerve endings, now known to be a mixture of *adrenaline and *noradrenaline.

sympathoblast *n.* one of the small cells formed in the early development of nerve tissue that eventually become the neurones of the sympathetic nervous system.

sympatholytic *n.* a drug that opposes the effects of the sympathetic nervous system. Drugs such as *guanethidine and *methyldopa block the transmission of impulses along adrenergic nerves; they are used to treat high blood pressure. Drugs such as *phentolamine, *phenoxybenzamine, and *tolazoline block alpha-adrenergic receptors, causing – in particular – dilation of peripheral blood vessels; they are used for disorders of the circulation or to lower the blood pressure. Other sympatholytic drugs are *beta blockers, which selectively block the beta-adrenergic receptors and principally affect the heart.

sympathomimetic *n.* a drug that has the effect of stimulating the *sympathetic nervous system. The actions of sympathomimetic drugs are *adrenergic* (resembling those of *noradrenaline). *Alpha-adrenergic* drugs, e.g. *phenylephrine, constrict blood vessels in the skin and intestine and are used in nasal decongestants; *beta-adrenergic* drugs, e.g. *salbutamol, relax bronchial smooth muscle and are used as *bronchodilators. *Ephedrine and *isoprenaline are less selective and have both alpha- and beta-adrenergic effects; if used as bronchodilators, these drugs may have unwanted side-effects on the heart.

sympathy *n.* (in physiology) a reciprocal influence exercised by different parts of the body on one another.

symphysiectomy *n.* removal of a part of the bone at the front of the pelvis (pubic symphysis) in order to aid childbirth.

symphysiotomy (symphyseotomy) *n.* incision into the bone at the front of the pelvis (pubic symphysis) in order to enlarge the diameter of the birth passage and aid delivery.

symphysis *n.* **1.** a joint in which the bones are separated by fibrocartilage, which minimizes movement and makes the bony structure rigid. Examples are the *pubic symphysis* (the joint between the pubic bones of the pelvis) and the joints of the backbone, which are separated by intervertebral discs (see illustration). **2.** the line that marks the fusion of two bones that were separate at an early stage of development, such as the symphysis of the *mandible.

adjacent vertebrae

intervertebral disc

Symphysis between two vertebrae

sympodia (sirenomelia) *n.* a developmental abnormality in which there is fusion of the legs with absence of the feet.

symptom *n.* an indication of a disease or disorder noticed by the patient himself. A *presenting symptom* is one that leads a patient to consult a doctor. *Compare* sign.

symptomatology (semeiology) *n.* **1.** the branch of medicine concerned with the study of symptoms of disease. **2.** the symptoms of a disease, collectively.

syn- (sym-) *prefix denoting* union or fusion.

synalgia *n. see* referred pain.

synapse *n.* the minute gap across which *nerve impulses pass from one neurone to the next, at the end of a nerve fibre. Reaching a synapse, an impulse causes the release of a *neurotransmitter, which diffuses across the gap and triggers an electrical impulse in the next neurone. Some brain cells have more than 15,000 synapses. *See also* neuromuscular junction.

synarthrosis *n.* an immovable joint in which the bones are united by fibrous tissue. Examples are the cranial *sutures. *See also* gomphosis, schindylesis.

synchilia (syncheilia) *n.* congenital fusion of the lips.

synchondrosis *n.* a slightly movable joint (*see* amphiarthrosis) in which the surfaces of the bones are separated by hyaline cartilage, as occurs between the ribs and sternum. This cartilage may become ossified in later development, as between the *epiphyses and shaft of a long bone.

syncope (fainting) *n.* loss of consciousness induced by a temporarily insufficient flow of blood to the brain. It commonly occurs in otherwise healthy people and may be caused by an emotional shock, by standing for prolonged periods, or by injury and profuse bleeding. An attack comes on gradually, with lightheadedness, sweating, and blurred vision. Recovery is normally prompt and without any persisting ill-effects.

syncytiotrophoblast *n.* *see* plasmidotrophoblast.

syncytium *n.* (*pl.* **syncytia**) a mass of *protoplasm containing several nuclei. Muscle fibres are syncytia.

syndactyly *n.* congenital fusion of the fingers or toes. It varies in severity from no more than marked webbing of two or more fingers to virtually complete union of all the digits.

syndesm- (syndesmo-) *prefix denoting* connective tissue, particularly ligaments.

syndesmology *n.* the branch of anatomy dealing with joints and their components.

syndesmophyte *n.* a vertical outgrowth of bone from a vertebra, seen in ankylosing *spondylitis, *Reiter's syndrome, and *psoriatic arthritis. Fusion of syndesmophytes across the joints between vertebrae contributes to rigidity of the spine, seen in advanced cases of these diseases.

syndesmosis *n.* an immovable joint in which the bones are separated by connective tissue. An example is the articulation between the bases of the tibia and fibula (see illustration).

tibia_____   _____fibula

connective tissue

A syndesmosis

syndrome *n.* a combination of signs and/or symptoms that forms a distinct clinical picture indicative of a particular disorder.

synechia *n.* an adhesion between the iris and another part of the eye. An *anterior synechia* is between the iris and the cornea or the part of the sclera that normally hides the extreme outer edge of the iris from view. A *posterior synechia* is between the iris and the lens.

syneresis *n.* contraction of a blood clot. When first formed, a blood clot is a loose meshwork of fibres containing various blood cells. Over a period of time this contracts, producing a firm mass that seals the damaged blood vessels.

synergist *n.* **1.** a drug that interacts with another to produce increased activity, which is greater than the sum of the effects of the two drugs given separately. For example sodium aminosalicylate and streptomycin are used together to treat tuberculosis. Some synergists may have dangerous effects, as when MAO inhibitors enhance the effects of barbiturates. **2.** a muscle that acts with an *agonist in making a particular movement. —**synergism** *n.*

syngraft *n.* *see* isograft.

synoptophore *n.* *see* amblyoscope.

synostosis *n.* the joining by ossification of two adjacent bones. It occurs, for example, at the *sutures between the bones of the skull.

synovectomy *n.* surgical removal of the synovium of a joint. This is performed in cases of chronic synovitis, when other measures have been ineffective, in order to reduce pain in the joint and prevent further destruction.

synovia (synovial fluid) the thick colourless lubricating fluid that surrounds a joint or a bursa and fills a tendon sheath. It is secreted by the synovial membrane.

synovial joint *see* diarthrosis.

synovial membrane (synovium) the membrane, composed of mesothelium and connective tissue, that forms the sac enclosing a freely movable joint (*see* diarthrosis). It secretes the lubricating synovial fluid.

synovioma *n.* a benign or malignant tumour of the synovial membrane. Benign synoviomas occur on tendon sheaths; malignant synoviomas (*synovial sarcomas*) may occur where synovial tissue is not normally found, e.g. in the oesophagus.

synovitis *n.* inflammation of the membrane (synovium) that lines a joint capsule, resulting in pain and swelling (arthritis). It is caused by injury, infection, or rheumatic disease. Treatment depends on the underlying cause; to determine this, samples of the synovial fluid or membrane are taken for examination.

synovium *n.* *see* synovial membrane.

syphilide (syphilid) *n.* the skin rash that appears in the second stage of *syphilis, usually two months to two years after primary infection. Syphilides occur in crops that may last from a few days to several months. They denote a highly infectious stage of the disease.

syphilis *n.* a chronic venereal disease caused by the bacterium *Treponema pallidum*, resulting in the formation of lesions throughout the body. Bacteria usually enter the body during sexual intercourse, through the mucous membranes of the vagina or urethra, but they may rarely be transmitted through skin wounds or scratches. Bacteria may also pass from an infected pregnant woman across the placenta to the developing fetus, resulting in the disease being present at birth (*congenital syphilis*).

The primary symptom – a hard ulcer (*chancre) at the site of infection – forms 2–4 weeks after exposure. Neighbouring lymph nodes enlarge about two weeks later. Secondary stage symptoms appear about two months after infection and include fever, malaise, general enlargement of lymph nodes, and a faint red rash on the chest that persists for 1–2 weeks. After months, or even years, the disease enters its tertiary stage with widespread formation of tumour-like masses (*gummas). Tertiary syphilis may cause serious damage to the heart and blood vessels (*cardiovascular syphilis*) or to the brain and spinal cord (*neurosyphilis*), resulting in *tabes dorsalis, blindness, and *general paralysis of the insane.

Treatment with penicillin is fully effective if administered in the early weeks of the infection. Syphilis can be diagnosed by the *Wasserman reaction. *Compare* bejel. —**syphilitic** *adj.*

syring- (syringo-) *prefix denoting* a tube or long cavity, especially the central canal of the spinal cord.

syringe *n.* an instrument consisting of a piston in a tight-fitting tube that is attached to a hollow needle or thin tube. A syringe is used to give injections, remove material from a part of the body, or to wash out a cavity, such as the outer ear.

syringobulbia *n. see* syringomyelia.

syringocystadenoma (syringoma) *n.* a multiple benign tumour of the sweat glands, which shows as small hard swellings in the skin.

syringomyelia *n.* a disease of the spinal cord in which longitudinal cavities form within the cord in the cervical (neck) region. The centrally situated cavity (*syrinx*) is especially likely to damage the motor nerve cells and the nerve fibres that transmit the sensations of pain and temperature. Characteristically there is weakness and wasting of the muscles in the hands with a loss of awareness of pain and temperature. An extension of the cavitation into the lower brainstem is called *syringobulbia*. Cerebellar *ataxia, a partial loss of pain sensation in the face, and weakness of the tongue and palate may occur.

system *n.* (in anatomy) a group of organs and tissues associated with a particular physiological function, such as the *nervous system or *respiratory system.

systemic *adj.* relating to or affecting the body as a whole, rather than individual parts and organs.

systemic circulation the system of blood vessels that supplies all parts of the body except the lungs. It consists of the aorta and all its branches, carrying oxygenated blood to the tissues, and all the veins draining deoxygenated blood into the vena cava. *Compare* pulmonary circulation.

systole *n.* the period of the cardiac cycle during which the heart contracts. The term usually refers to *ventricular systole*, which lasts about 0.3 seconds. *Atrial systole* lasts about 0.1 seconds. —**systolic** *adj.*

systolic pressure *see* blood pressure.

T

tabes dorsalis (locomotor ataxia) a form of neurosyphilis occurring 5–20 years after the original venereal infection. The infecting organisms progressively destroy the sensory nerves. Severe stabbing pains in the legs and trunk, an unsteady gait, and loss of bladder control are common. Some patients have blurred vision caused by damage to the optic nerves. Penicillin is used to arrest the progression of this illness. *See also* syphilis, general paralysis of the insane.

tablet *n.* (in pharmacy) a small disc containing one or more drugs, made by compressing a powdered form of the drug(s). It is taken by mouth.

tabo-paresis *n.* a late effect of syphilitic infection of the nervous system in which the patient shows features of *tabes dorsalis and *general paralysis of the insane.

TAB vaccine

TAB vaccine a combined vaccine used to produce immunity against the diseases typhoid, paratyphoid A, and paratyphoid B.

tachy- *prefix denoting* fast; rapid.

tachycardia *n.* an increase in the heart rate above normal. *Sinus tachycardia* may occur normally with exercise or excitement or it may be due to illness, such as fever. *Arrhythmias may also produce tachycardia (*ectopic tachycardia*).

tachyphrasia *n.* rapid and voluble speech, such as that encountered in *mania.

tachyphrenia *n.* excessive rapidity of the mental processes, as in *mania.

tachyphylaxis *n.* a falling-off in the effects produced by a drug during continuous use or constantly repeated administration, common in drugs that act on the nervous system.

tachypnoea *n.* rapid breathing.

tactile *adj.* relating to or affecting the sense of touch.

taenia *n.* (*pl.* **taeniae**) a flat ribbon-like anatomical structure. The *taeniae coli* are the longitudinal ribbon-like muscles of the colon.

Taenia *n.* a genus of large tapeworms, some of which are parasites of the human intestine. The 4–10 m long beef tapeworm, *T. saginata*, is the commonest tapeworm parasite of man. Its larval stage (*see* cysticercus) develops within the muscles of cattle and other ruminants, and man becomes infected on eating raw or undercooked beef. *T. soleum*, the pork tapeworm, is 2–7 m long. Its larval stage may develop not only in pigs but also in man, in whom it may cause serious disease (*see* cysticercosis). *See also* taeniasis.

taeniacide (taenicide) *n.* an agent that kills tapeworms.

taeniafuge *n.* an agent, such as *dichlorophen, that eliminates tapeworms from the body of their host.

taeniasis *n.* an infestation with tapeworms of the genus *Taenia*. Man becomes infected with the adult worms following ingestion of raw or undercooked meat containing the larval stage of the parasite. The presence of a worm in the intestine may occasionally give rise to increased appetite, hunger pains, weakness, and weight loss. Worms are expelled from the intestine using various *anthelmintics, including niclosamide, dichlorophen, and quinacrine hydrochloride. *See also* cysticercosis.

Tagamet *n. see* cimetidine.

tal- (talo-) *prefix denoting* the ankle bone (talus).

talipes *n. see* club-foot.

talus (astragalus) *n.* the ankle bone. It forms part of the *tarsus, articulating with the tibia above, with the fibula to the lateral (outer) side, and with the calcaneus below.

tambour *n.* a recording drum consisting of an elastic membrane stretched over one end of a cylinder. It is used in various instruments for recording changes in air pressure.

tamoxifen *n.* a drug used in the treatment of advanced breast cancer. It combines with hormone receptors in the tumour to inhibit the effect of oestrogens. Side-effects are uncommon but include facial flushing, tumour pain, and hypercalcaemia. Trade name: **Nolvadex**.

tampon *n.* a pack of gauze, cotton wool, or other absorbent material used to plug a cavity or canal in order to absorb blood or secretions. A vaginal tampon is commonly used by women to absorb the menstrual flow.

tamponade *n.* **1.** the insertion of a tampon. **2.** abnormal pressure on a part of the body; for example, as caused by the presence of excessive fluid between the pericardium (sac surrounding the heart) and the heart.

tantalum *n.* a rare heavy metal used in surgery as it is easily moulded and does not corrode. For example, tantalum sutures and plates are used for repair of defects in the bones of the skull. Symbol: Ta.

tapetum *n.* **1.** a layer of specialized reflecting cells in the *choroid behind the retina of the eye. **2.** a band of nerve fibres that form the roof and wall of the lower posterior part of the *corpus callosum.

tapeworm *n.* any of a group of flatworms that have a long thin ribbon-like body and live as parasites in the intestines of man and other vertebrates. The body of a tapeworm consists of a head (*scolex*), a short neck, and a *strobila* made up of a chain of separate segments (*proglottides*). Mature proglottides, full of eggs, are released from the free end of the worm and pass out in the host's stools. Eggs are then ingested by an intermediate host, in whose tissues the larval stages develop (*see* plerocercoid, cysticercus, hydatid). Man is the primary host for some tapeworms (*see* Taenia, Hymenolepis). However, other genera are also medically important (*see* Diphyllobothrium, Dipylidium, Echinococcus).

tapotement *n.* a technique used in *massage in which a part of the body is struck rapidly and repeatedly with the hands. Tapotement of the chest wall in bronchitic patients often helps to loosen mucus within the air passages so that it can be coughed up.

tapping *n.* *see* paracentesis.

target cell (in haematology) an abnormal form of red blood cell (*erythro-cyte) in which the cell assumes the ringed appearance of a 'target' in stained blood films. Target cells are a feature of several types of anaemia, including those due to iron deficiency and abnormalities in haemoglobin structure.

target organ the specific organ or tissue upon which a hormone, drug, or other substance acts.

tars- (tarso-) *prefix denoting* **1.** the ankle; tarsal bones. **2.** the edge of the eyelid.

tarsal 1. *adj.* relating to the bones of the ankle and foot (*tarsus). **2.** *adj.* relating to the eyelid, esp. to its supporting tissue (tarsus). **3.** *n.* any of the bones forming the tarsus.

tarsalgia *n.* aching pain arising from the tarsus in the foot.

tarsal glands *see* meibomian glands.

tarsectomy *n.* **1.** surgical excision of the tarsal bones of the foot. **2.** surgical removal of a section of the tarsus of the eyelid.

tarsitis *n.* inflammation of the eyelid.

tarsoplasty *n.* *see* blepharoplasty.

tarsorrhaphy *n.* an operation in which the upper and lower eyelids are joined together, either completely or along part of their length. It is performed to protect the cornea or to allow a corneal injury to heal.

tarsus *n.* (*pl.* **tarsi**) **1.** the seven bones of the ankle and proximal part of the foot (see illustration). The tarsus articulates with the metatarsals distally and with the tibia and fibula proximally. **2.** the firm fibrous connective tissue that forms the basis of each eyelid.

tartar

Bones of the right ankle and foot

tartar *n.* an obsolete term for *calculus, the hard deposit that forms on the teeth.

tartar emetic *see* antimony potassium tartrate.

taste *n.* the sense for the appreciation of the flavour of substances in the mouth. The sense organs responsible are the *taste buds on the surface of the *tongue, which are stimulated when food dissolves in the saliva in the mouth. It is generally held that there are four basic taste sensations – sweet, bitter, sour, and salt – but two others – alkaline and metallic – are sometimes added to this list.

taste buds the sensory receptors concerned with the sense of taste (see illustration). They are located in the epithelium that covers the surface of the *tongue, lying in the grooves around the papillae, particularly the circumvallate papillae. Taste buds are also present in the soft palate, the epiglottis, and parts of the pharynx. When a taste cell is stimulated by the presence of a dissolved substance im-

pulses are sent via nerve fibres to the brain. From the anterior two-thirds of the tongue impulses pass via the facial nerve. The taste buds in the posterior third of the tongue send impulses via the glossopharyngeal nerve.

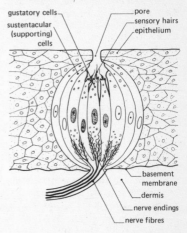

Structure of a taste bud

taurine *n.* an amino acid that is a constituent of the *bile salt taurocholate and also functions as a *neurotransmitter in the central nervous system.

taurocholic acid *see* bile acids.

taxis *n.* (in surgery) the returning to a normal position of displaced bones, organs, or other parts by manipulation only, unaided by mechanical devices.

Tay-Sachs disease (amaurotic familial idiocy) an inherited disorder of lipid metabolism (*see* lipidosis) in which abnormal accumulation of lipid in the brain leads to blindness, mental retardation, and death in infancy. The gene responsible for the disorder is *recessive, and the disease can now be largely prevented by genetic counselling in communities known to be affected.

TCP *Trade name.* a solution of trichlorphenol: an effective *antiseptic for minor skin injuries and irritations. It may also be used as a gargle for colds and sore throats.

tear gas any of the several kinds of gas used in warfare and by the police to produce temporary incapacitation. Most tear gases produce stinging pain in the eyes and streaming from the eyes and nose. *See also* CS gas.

tears *pl. n.* the fluid secreted by the lacrimal glands (*see* lacrimal apparatus) to keep the front of the eyeballs moist and clean. Tears contain *lysozyme, an enzyme that destroys bacteria. Irritation of the eye, and sometimes emotion, cause excessive production of tears. *See also* blinking.

technetium-131 *n.* an isotope of the artificial radioactive element technetium. It emits gamma radiation and is used as a *tracer for the examination of the brain and the thyroid gland in the technique of scintigraphy.

tectospinal tract a tract that conveys nerve impulses from the midbrain, across the midline as it descends, to the spinal cord in the cervical (neck) region. It contains important *motor neurones.

tectum *n.* the roof of the *midbrain, behind and above the *cerebral aqueduct. From the nerve tissue protrude two pairs of rounded swellings called the *superior* and *inferior colliculi*, which contain cells concerned with reflexes involving vision and hearing, respectively.

teeth *pl. n. see* tooth.

tegmen *n.* (*pl.* **tegmina**) a structure that covers an organ or part of an organ. For example the *tegmen tympani* is the bony roof of the middle ear.

tegmentum *n.* the region of the *midbrain below and in front of the *cerebral aqueduct. It contains the nuclei of several cranial nerves, the *reticular formation, and other ascending and descending nerve pathways linking the forebrain and the spinal cord.

teichopsia *n.* shimmering coloured lights, accompanied by blank spots in the visual field (*transient scotomata*), often seen by sufferers at the beginning of an attack of migraine.

tel- (tele-, telo-) *prefix denoting* 1. end or ending. 2. distance.

tela *n.* any thin weblike tissue, particularly the *tela choroidea*, a folded double layer of *pia mater containing numerous small blood vessels that extends into several of the *ventricles of the brain.

telangiectasis (*pl.* **telangiectases**) a localized collection of distended blood capillary vessels. It is recognized as a red spot, sometimes spidery in appearance, that blanches on pressure. Telangiectases may be found in the skin or the lining of the mouth, gastrointestinal, respiratory, and urinary passages. The condition in which multiple telangiectases occur is termed *telangiectasia*. It may be seen as an inherited condition associated with a bleeding tendency (*haemorrhagic telangiectasia*). Accessible bleeding telangiectases (e.g. in the nose) may be obliterated by cauterization.

telangiitis *n.* inflammation of the smallest blood vessels (*see* angiitis).

teleceptor *n.* a sensory *receptor that is capable of responding to distant stimuli. An example is the eye, which is capable of detecting changes and happenings at a great distance, unlike touch receptors, which require close contact.

telecurietherapy *n.* a form of *radiotherapy in which penetrating radiation is directed at a patient from a distance. Originally radium was used as the radiation source; today artificial radioactive isotopes, such as cobalt-60, are used.

telegony *n.* the unsubstantiated theory that mating with one male has an effect on the offspring of later matings with other males.

telencephalon *n. see* cerebrum.

teleradiography *n.* a form of *radiography in which the X-ray source is situated about 2 metres from the patient, which produces X-ray pictures with less distortion.

telocentric *n.* a chromosome in which the centromere is situated at either of its ends. —**telocentric** *adj.*

telodendron *n.* one of the branches into which the *axon of a neurone divides at its destination. Each telodendron finishes as a terminal *bouton*, which takes part in a *synapse or a *neuromuscular junction.

telophase *n.* the final stage of *mitosis and of each of the divisions of *meiosis, in which the chromosomes at each end of the cell become long and thin and the nuclear membrane reforms around them. The cytoplasm begins to divide.

temple *n.* the region of the head in front of and above each ear.

temporal *adj.* of or relating to the temple.

temporal arteritis *see* arteritis.

temporal artery a branch of the external carotid artery that supplies blood mainly to the temple and scalp.

temporal bone either of a pair of bones of the cranium. The *squamous* portion forms part of the side of the cranium. The *petrous* part contributes to the base of the skull and contains the middle and inner ears. Below it are the *mastoid process, *styloid process, and

zygomatic process (*see* zygomatic arch). *See also* skull.

temporalis *n.* a fan-shaped muscle situated at the side of the head, extending from the temporal fossa to the mandible. This muscle lifts the lower jaw, thus closing the mouth.

temporal lobe one of the main divisions of the *cerebral cortex in each hemisphere of the brain, lying at the side within the temple of the skull and separated from the frontal lobe by a cleft, the *lateral sulcus*. Areas of the cortex in this lobe are concerned with the appreciation of sound and spoken language.

temporal lobe epilepsy *see* epilepsy.

temporo- *prefix denoting* 1. the temple. 2. the temporal lobe of the brain.

temporomandibular joint the articulation between the *mandible and the *temporal bone: a hinge joint (*see* ginglymus).

temporomandibular joint syndrome a condition in which the patient has painful temporomandibular joints, tenderness in the muscles that move the jaw, clicking of the joints, and limitation of jaw movement.

tenaculum *n.* 1. a sharp wire hook with a handle. The instrument is used in surgical operations to pick up pieces of tissue or the cut end of an artery. 2. a band of fibrous tissue that holds a part of the body in place.

tendinitis *n.* inflammation of a tendon. It occurs most commonly after excessive overuse but is sometimes due to bacterial infection (e.g. *gonorrhoea), or a generalized rheumatic disease (e.g. *rheumatoid arthritis, ankylosing spondylitis). Treatment is by rest, achieved sometimes by splinting the adjacent joint, and corticosteroid injection into the tender area around the tendon. Tendinitis at the insertion of the supraspinatus muscle is a frequent cause of pain and restricted movement in the shoulder. *See also* tennis elbow. *Compare* tenosynovitis.

tendon *n.* a tough whitish cord, consisting of numerous parallel bundles of collagen fibres, that serves to attach a muscle to a bone. Tendons are inelastic but flexible; they assist in concentrating the pull of the muscle on a small area of bone. Some tendons are surrounded by *tendon sheaths* – these are tubular double-layered sacs lined with synovial membrane and containing synovial fluid. Tendon sheaths enclose the flexor tendons at the wrist and ankle, where they minimize friction and facilitate movement. *See also* aponeurosis. —**tendinous** *adj.*

tendon organ (Golgi tendon organ) a sensory *receptor found within a tendon that responds to the tension or stretching of the tendon and relays impulses to the central nervous system. Like stretch receptors in muscle, tendon organs are part of the *proprioceptor system.

tendovaginitis (tenovaginitis) *n.* inflammatory thickening of the fibrous sheath containing one or more tendons, usually caused by repeated minor injury. It usually occurs at the back of the thumb (*de Quervain's tendovaginitis*) and results in pain on wringing the wrists. Treatment is by rest, injection of cortisone into the tendon sheath, and, if these fail, surgical incision of the sheath.

tenesmus *n.* a sensation of the desire to defecate, which is continuous or recurs frequently, without the production of significant amounts of faeces (often small amounts of mucus or blood alone are passed). This uncomfortable symptom may be due to *proctitis, prolapse of the rectum, rectal tumour, or *irritable bowel syndrome.

tennis elbow a painful inflammation of the tendon at the outer border of the elbow, caused by overuse of the forearm muscles. Treatment is by rest, massage, and local corticosteroid injection. *See also* tendinitis.

teno- *prefix denoting* a tendon.

Tenon's capsule the fibrous tissue that lines the orbit and surrounds the eyeball.

tenoplasty *n.* surgical repair of a ruptured or severed tendon.

tenorrhaphy *n.* the surgical operation of uniting the ends of divided tendons by suture.

tenosynovitis (peritendinitis) *n.* inflammation of a tendon sheath, producing pain, swelling, and an audible creaking on movement. It may result from a bacterial infection or occur as part of a rheumatic disease causing *synovitis.

tenotomy *n.* surgical *division of a tendon. This may be necessary to correct a joint deformity caused by tendon shortening or to reduce the imbalance of forces caused by an overactive muscle in a spastic limb. *See also* scissor leg.

tenovaginitis *n. see* tendovaginitis.

tensor *n.* any muscle that causes stretching or tensing of a part of the body.

tent *n.* **1.** an enclosure of material (usually transparent plastic) around a patient in bed, into which a gas or vapour can be passed as part of treatment. An *oxygen tent* is relatively inefficient as a means of administering oxygen; a face mask or intranasal oxygen are used where possible. **2.** a piece of dried vegetable material, usually a seaweed stem, shaped to fit into an orifice, such as the cervical canal. As it absorbs moisture it expands, providing a slow but forceful means of dilating the orifice.

tentorium *n.* a curved infolded sheet of *dura mater that dips inwards from the skull and separates the cerebellum below from the occipital lobes of the cerebral hemispheres above.

terat- (terato-) *prefix denoting* a monster or congenital abnormality.

teratogen *n.* any substance, agent, or process that induces the formation of developmental abnormalities in a fetus. Known teratogens include such drugs as *thalidomide and alcohol; such infections as German measles and cytomegalovirus; and irradiation with X-rays and other ionizing radiation. *Compare* mutagen. —**teratogenic** *adj.*

teratogenesis *n.* the process leading to developmental abnormalities in the fetus.

teratology *n.* the study of developmental abnormalities and their causes.

teratoma *n.* a tumour composed of a number of tissues not usually found at that site. Teratomas most frequently occur in the testis and ovary, possibly derived from remnants of embryological cells that have the ability to differentiate into many types of tissue. *Malignant teratoma of the testis* is found in young men: it is most common in the undescended testis. Like *seminoma, it frequently occurs as a painless swelling of one testis (pain is not a good indication that the swelling is benign). Treatment is by *orchidectomy avoiding an incision into the scrotum. The tumour can spread to lymph nodes, lungs, and bone, treatment of which may involve the use of radiotherapy and drugs such as vinblastine, bleomycin, and platinum compounds. Teratomas often produce *alpha-fetoprotein, beta human chorionic gonadotrophin, or both; the presence of these substances in the blood is a useful indication of the amount of tumour and the effect of treatment.

terbutaline *n.* a *bronchodilator drug used in the treatment of asthma, bronchitis, and other respiratory disorders.

It may be given by mouth, injection, or inhalation; common side effects include nervousness and dizziness. Trade name: **Bricanyl**.

teres *n.* either of two muscles of the shoulder, extending from the scapula to the humerus. The *teres major* draws the arm towards the body and rotates it inwards; the *teres minor* rotates the arm outwards.

terpene *n.* any of a group of unsaturated hydrocarbons many of which are found in plant oils and resins and are responsible for the scent of these plants (e.g. mint). Larger terpenes include vitamin A, squalene, and the carotenoids.

Terramycin *n. see* oxytetracycline.

tertian fever *see* malaria.

tertigravida (trigravida) *n.* a woman who has been pregnant three times.

tertipara (tripara) *n.* a woman who has been pregnant at least three times and who has given birth to an infant capable of survival after each of three pregnancies.

tesla *n.* the *SI unit of magnetic flux density, equal to a density of 1 weber per square metre. Symbol: T.

testicle *n.* either of the pair of male sex organs within the scrotum. It consists of the *testis and its system of ducts (the vasa efferentia and epididymis).

testis *n.* (*pl.* **testes**) either of the pair of male sex organs that produce spermatozoa and secrete the male sex hormone *androgen under the control of *gonadotrophins from the pituitary gland. The testes of the fetus form within the abdomen but descend into the *scrotum in order to maintain a lower temperature that favours the production and storage of spermatozoa. The bulk of the testis is made up of long convoluted *seminiferous tubules* (see illustration), in which the spermatozoa develop (*see* spermatogenesis). The tubules also contain *Sertoli cells, which may nourish developing sperm cells. Spermatozoa pass from the testis to the *epididymis to complete their development. The *interstitial* (*Leydig*) *cells*, between the tubules, are the major producers of androgen.

tunica vaginalis

epididymis

tunica albuginea

seminiferous
tubules

vas deferens

Longitudinal section through a testis

test meal a standard meal given to stimulate secretion of digestive juices, which can then be withdrawn by tube and measured as a test of digestive function. A *fractional test meal* was a gruel preparation to stimulate gastric secretion, whose acid content was measured. This has been replaced by tests using histamine or pentagastrin as secretory stimulants. The *Lundh test meal* is a meal of oil and protein to stimulate pancreatic secretion, which is withdrawn from the duodenum and its trypsin content measured as a test of pancreatic function.

testosterone *n.* the principal male sex hormone (*see* androgen).

test-tube baby a baby born to a woman as a result of fertilization of one of her ova by her husband's sperm outside her body (*in vitro fertilization*). This technique, pioneered in Britain, resulted in the birth of a live baby girl in July 1978. It is useful when the woman has blocked Fallopian tubes or some similar defect in the reproductive system. The mother-to-be is given a short course of hormones, causing several ova to mature at the same time. Several ova are removed using a *laparoscope. The ova are mixed with sperm in a culture medium and incubated until the *blastocyst forms. The blastocyst is then implanted in the mother's womb and the pregnancy continues normally thereafter.

tetan- (tetano-) *prefix denoting* 1. tetanus. 2. tetany.

tetanolysin *n.* a toxin produced by tetanus bacilli in an infected wound, causing the local destruction of tissues.

tetanospasmin *n.* a toxin produced by tetanus bacilli in an infected wound. The toxin diffuses along nerves, causing paralysis, and may reach the spinal cord and brain, when it causes violent muscular spasms and the condition of lockjaw.

tetanus (lockjaw) *n.* an acute infectious disease, affecting the nervous system, caused by the bacterium *Clostridium tetani*. Infection occurs by contamination of wounds by bacterial spores. Bacteria multiply at the site of infection and produce a toxin that irritates nerves so that they cause spasmodic contraction of muscles. Symptoms appear 4–25 days after infection and consist of muscle stiffness, spasm, and subsequent rigidity, first in the jaw and neck then in the back, chest, abdomen, and limbs; in severe cases the spasm may affect the whole body, which is arched backwards (*see* opisthotonos). High fever, convulsions, and extreme pain are common. If respiratory muscles are affected, a *tracheostomy is essential to avoid death from asphyxia. Mortality is high in untreated cases but prompt treatment with penicillin and antitoxin is effective. An attack does not confer immunity. Immunization against tetanus is effective but temporary. —**tetanic** *adj.*

tetany *n.* spasm and twitching of the muscles, particularly those of the face, hands, and feet. Tetany is caused by a reduction in the blood calcium level, which may be due to underactive parathyroid glands, rickets, or *alkalosis.

tetra- *prefix denoting* four.

tetrachloroethylene *n.* an *anthelmintic drug used in the treatment of hookworm disease. It is given by mouth. Toxic side-effects are rare, but vertigo and headache frequently occur and patients with severe anaemia may collapse during treatment.

tetracycline *n.* **1.** one of a group of *antibiotic compounds derived from cultures of *Streptomyces* bacteria. These drugs, which include *chlortetracycline, doxycycline, *oxytetracycline, and tetracycline, are effective against a wide range of bacterial infections. They are usually given by mouth to treat various conditions, including respiratory-tract infections, syphilis, and acne. Side-effects such as nausea, vomiting, and diarrhoea are fairly common. In addition, suppression of normal intestinal bacteria may make the patient susceptible to infection with tetracycline-resistant organisms. Tetracyclines should not be administered after the fourth month of pregnancy and their use should be avoided in young children to prevent unsightly staining of the permanent teeth. **2.** a particular antibiotic of the tetracycline group. Trade names: **Achromycin, Steclin.**

tetrad *n.* (in genetics) **1.** the four cells resulting from meiosis after the second telophase. **2.** the four chromatids of a pair of homologous chromosomes (*see* bivalent) in the first stage of meiosis.

tetradactyly *n.* a congenital abnormality in which there are only four digits on a hand or foot.

tetrahydrocannabinol *n.* a derivative of marijuana that has antiemetic activity and also produces euphoria. These two properties are utilized in the prevention of chemotherapy-induced sickness.

tetrahydrozoline *n.* a drug that constricts blood vessels and is used as a nasal decongestant. *See* vasoconstrictor.

tetralogy of Fallot a form of congenital heart disease in which there is *pulmonary stenosis, enlargement of the right ventricle, a ventricular *septal defect, and in which the origin of the aorta lies over the septal defect. The affected child is blue (cyanosed) and frequently squats. The defect is corrected surgically.

tetraplegia *n. see* quadriplegia.

T-group *n.* a group of people who meet in order to increase their sensitivity and their skills in human relationships by discussing themselves and their relationships. Such groups are sometimes formed in the training of psychiatric staff (the *T* stands for *training*).

thalam- (thalamo-) *prefix denoting* the thalamus. Example: *thalamolenticular* (relating to the thalamus and lenticular nucleus of the brain).

thalamencephalon *n.* the structures, collectively, at the anterior end of the brainstem, comprising the *epithalamus, *thalamus, *hypothalamus, and subthalamus, all of which are concerned with the reception and processing of information entering from sensory nerve pathways.

thalamic syndrome a raised threshold to pain stimuli combined with a highly unpleasant burning quality to any pain that is experienced once the threshold is exceeded. It is caused by disease affecting the *thalamus.

thalamotomy *n*. an operation on the brain in which a lesion is made in a precise part of the *thalamus. It has been used to control psychiatric symptoms of severe anxiety and distress, in which cases the lesion is made in the dorsomedial nucleus of the thalamus, which connects with the frontal lobe. *See also* psychosurgery.

thalamus *n*. (*pl*. **thalami**) one of two egg-shaped masses of grey matter that lie deep in the cerebral hemispheres in each side of the forebrain. The thalami are relay stations for all the sensory messages that enter the brain, before they are transmitted to the cortex. All sensory pathways, except that for the sense of smell, are linked to nuclei within the thalamus, and it is here that the conscious awareness of messages as sensations – temperature, pain, touch, etc. – probably begins.

thalassaemia (Cooley's anaemia) *n*. a hereditary blood disease, widespread in the Mediterranean countries, Asia, and Africa, in which there is an abnormality in the protein part of the *haemoglobin molecule. The affected red cells cannot function normally, leading to anaemia. Other symptoms include enlargement of the spleen and abnormalities of the bone marrow. Individuals inheriting the disease from both parents are severely affected (*thalassaemia major*), but those inheriting it from only one parent are usually symptom-free. Patients with the major disease are treated with repeated blood transfusions. The disease can be detected by prenatal diagnosis.

thalassotherapy *n*. treatment by remedial bathing in sea water.

thalidomide *n*. a drug that was formerly used as a sedative. If taken during the first three months of pregnancy, it was found to cause fetal abnormalities involving limb malformation and has now been withdrawn.

thallium *n*. a leadlike element that has several dangerously poisonous compounds. The poison is cumulative and causes liver and nerve damage and bone destruction. The victim's hair is likely to fall out and does not grow again. Treatment is by administration of *chelating agents. Symbol: Tl.

thallium scan a method of studying myocardial *perfusion and diagnosing myocardial *ischaemia using an injection of the radioisotope thallium-201. Defects of perfusion, such as a recent infarct, emit little or no radioactivity and are seen as 'cold spots' when an image is formed using a gamma camera and computer. Exercise may be used to provoke 'cold spots' in the diagnosis of ischaemic heart disease.

theca *n*. a sheathlike surrounding tissue. For example, the *theca folliculi* is the outer wall of a *Graafian follicle.

theine *n*. the active volatile principle found in tea (*see* caffeine).

thenar *n*. **1.** the palm of the hand. **2.** the fleshy prominent part of the hand at the base of the thumb. *Compare* hypothenar. —**thenar** *adj*.

theobromine *n*. an alkaloid, occurring in cocoa, that has a weak diuretic action and dilates coronary and other arteries. It was formerly used to treat angina.

theophylline *n*. an alkaloid, occurring in the leaves of the tea plant, that has a diuretic effect and relaxes smooth muscles, especially of the bronchi. Theophylline preparations, particularly *aminophylline, are used mainly to control bronchial asthma.

therapeutics *n*. the branch of medicine that deals with different methods of treatment and healing (*therapy*), particularly the use of drugs in the cure of disease.

therm *n.* a unit of heat equal to 100,000 British thermal units. 1 therm = 1.055 × 10⁸ joules.

therm- (thermo-) *prefix denoting* **1.** heat. **2.** temperature.

thermoalgesia (thermalgesia) *n.* an abnormal sense of pain that is felt when part of the body is warmed. It is a type of *dysaesthesia and is a symptom of partial damage to a peripheral nerve or to the fibre tracts conducting temperature sensation to the brain.

thermoanaesthesia *n.* absence of the ability to recognize the sensations of heat and coldness. When occurring as an isolated sensory symptom it indicates damage to the spinothalamic tract in the spinal cord, which conveys the impulses of temperature to the thalamus.

thermocautery *n.* the destruction of unwanted tissues by heat (*see* cauterize).

thermocoagulation *n.* the coagulation and destruction of tissues by cautery.

thermography *n.* a technique for measuring and recording the heat produced by different parts of the body: by using photographic film sensitive to infrared radiation. The picture produced is called a *thermogram.* The heat radiated from the body varies in different parts according to the flow of blood through the vessels; thus areas of poor circulation produce less heat. On the other hand a tumour with an abnormally increased blood supply may be revealed on the thermogram as a 'hot spot'. The technique has been used in the diagnosis of tumours of the breast (*mammothermography*).

thermolysis *n.* (in physiology) the dissipation of body heat by such processes as the evaporation of sweat from the skin surface.

thermometer *n.* a device for registering temperature. A *clinical thermometer* consists of a sealed narrow-bore glass tube with a bulb at one end. It contains mercury, which expands when heated and rises up the tube. The tube is calibrated in degrees, and is designed to register temperatures between 35°C (95°F) and 43.5°C (110°F). An *oral thermometer* is placed in the mouth; a *rectal thermometer* is inserted into the rectum.

thermophilic *adj.* describing organisms, especially bacteria, that grow best at temperatures of 48–85°C. *Compare* mesophilic, psychrophilic.

thermophore *n.* any substance that retains heat for a long time, such as kaolin, which is often used in hot poultices.

thermoreceptor *n.* a sensory nerve ending that responds to heat or to cold. Such *receptors are scattered widely in the skin and in the mucous membrane of the mouth and throat.

thermotaxis *n.* the physiological process of regulating or adjusting body temperature.

thermotherapy *n.* the use of heat to alleviate pain and stiffness in joints and muscles and to promote an increase in circulation. *Diathermy provides a means of generating heat within the tissues themselves.

thiacetazone (thioparamizone) *n.* a drug used in the treatment of leprosy and (in combination with *isoniazid) tuberculosis. The drug is administered by mouth. Toxic effects, though infrequent, are severe and include anorexia, hepatitis, and exfoliative dermatitis.

thiamin *n. see* vitamin B₁.

Thiersch's graft (split-skin graft) a type of skin graft in which thin partial thicknesses of skin are cut in narrow strips and placed onto the wound area to be healed.

thioguanine *n.* a drug that prevents the growth of cancer cells and is used in the treatment of leukaemia. It is given by mouth and commonly reduces the numbers of white blood cells and platelets. Other side-effects include nausea, vomiting, loss of appetite, and jaundice. Trade name: **Lanvis**.

thioparamizone *n. see* thiacetazone.

thiopentone *n.* a short-acting *barbiturate. It is given by intravenous injection to produce general *anaesthesia or as a premedication prior to surgery. Possible complications of thiopentone anaesthesia include respiratory depression, laryngeal spasm, and thrombophlebitis. The drug is not used when respiratory obstruction is present. Trade name: **Pentothal**.

thiophilic *adj.* growing best in the presence of sulphur or sulphur compounds. The term is usually applied to bacteria.

thiopropazate *n.* a major *tranquillizer similar to *chlorpromazine in its actions and effects. It is given by mouth to treat agitated psychotic patients with anxiety states and to control nausea and vomiting. Trade name: **Dartalan**.

thioridazine *n.* a major *tranquillizer used in the treatment of a wide range of mental and emotional disturbances, including schizophrenia and senile dementia. The drug is given by mouth; side-effects include faintness, dizziness, dry mouth, and impairment of sexual function. Trade name: **Melleril**.

thiotepa *n.* a *cytotoxic drug. It is given by injection to treat cancer of the breast or ovary, lymphoma, and sarcoma. The most serious side-effects are on the blood-forming tissues, resulting in a reduction in white blood cells and platelets. Headache, nausea, and vomiting may also occur.

thiouracil *n.* a drug that is used in the treatment of overactivity of the thyroid gland (thyrotoxicosis). It is given by mouth; side-effects include fever, skin reactions, jaundice, and *agranulocytosis.

thorac- (thoraco-) *prefix denoting* the thorax or chest.

thoracectomy *n.* an operation in which the chest cavity is opened (thoracotomy) and a rib or part of a rib is removed.

thoracentesis *n. see* pleurocentesis.

thoracic cavity the chest cavity. *See* thorax.

thoracic duct one of the two main trunks of the *lymphatic system. It receives lymph from both legs, the lower abdomen, left thorax, left side of the head, and left arm and drains into the left innominate vein.

thoracic vertebrae the 12 bones of the *backbone to which the ribs are attached. They lie between the cervical (neck) and lumbar (lower back) vertebrae and are characterized by the presence of facets for articulation with the ribs. *See also* vertebra.

thoracocentesis *n. see* pleurocentesis.

thoracoplasty *n.* the surgical repair of abnormalities or defects of the thorax.

thoracotomy *n.* surgical opening of the chest cavity to inspect or operate on the heart, lungs, or other structures within.

thorascope *n.* an instrument used to inspect the *pleural cavity.

thorax *n.* the chest: the part of the body cavity between the neck and the diaphragm. The skeleton of the thorax is formed by the sternum, costal cartilages, ribs, and thoracic vertebrae of the backbone. It encloses the lungs, heart, oesophagus, and associated structures. *Compare* abdomen. —**thoracic** *adj.*

thorium-X *n.* the radioactive isotope radium-224, which emits alpha radiation and has several applications in *radiotherapy. *See also* radium.

threadworm *n. see* pinworm.

threonine *n.* an *essential amino acid. *See also* amino acid.

threshold *n.* (in neurology) the point at which a stimulus begins to evoke a response, and therefore a measure of the sensitivity of a system under particular conditions. A *thermoreceptor that responds to an increase in temperature of only two degrees is said to have a much lower threshold than one that will only respond to a change in temperature of ten degrees or more. In this example the threshold can be measured directly in terms of degrees.

thrill *n.* a vibration felt on placing the hand on the body. A heart murmur that is felt by placing the hand on the chest wall is said to be accompanied by a thrill.

-thrix *suffix denoting* a hair or hairlike structure.

thromb- (thrombo-) *prefix denoting* 1. a blood clot (thrombus). 2. thrombosis. 3. blood platelets.

thrombasthenia *n.* a hereditary blood disease in which the function of the *platelets is defective although they are present in normal numbers. The manifestations are identical to those of thrombocytopenic *purpura.

thrombectomy *n.* a surgical procedure in which a blood clot (thrombus) is removed from an artery or vein (*see* endarterectomy, phlebothrombosis).

thrombin *n.* a substance (*coagulation factor) that acts as an enzyme, converting the soluble protein fibrinogen to the insoluble protein fibrin in the final stage of *blood coagulation. Thrombin is not normally present in blood plasma, being derived from an inactive precursor, *prothrombin*.

thromboangiitis obliterans *see* Buerger's disease.

thrombocyte *n. see* platelet.

thrombocythaemia *n.* a disease in which there is an abnormal proliferation of the cells that produce blood *platelets (*megakaryocytes), leading to an increased number of platelets in the blood. This may result in an increased tendency to form clots within blood vessels (thrombosis); alternatively the function of the platelets may be abnormal, leading to an increased tendency to bleed. Treatment is by radiotherapy or by *cytotoxic drugs.

thrombocytopenia *n.* a reduction in the number of *platelets in the blood. This results in bleeding into the skin (*see* purpura), spontaneous bruising, and prolonged bleeding after injury. Thrombocytopenia may result from failure of platelet production or excessive destruction of platelets. —**thrombocytopenic** *adj.*

thrombocytosis *n.* an increase in the number of *platelets in the blood. It may occur in a variety of diseases, including chronic infections, cancers, and certain blood diseases and is likely to cause an increased tendency to form blood clots within vessels (thrombosis).

thromboembolism *n.* the condition in which a blood clot (thrombus), formed at one point in the circulation, becomes detached and lodges at another point. It is most commonly applied to the association of phlebothrombosis and *pulmonary embolism (*pulmonary thromboembolic disease*).

thromboendarterectomy *n. see* endarterectomy.

thromboendarteritis *n.* thrombosis complicating *endarteritis, seen in temporal *arteritis, *polyarteritis nodosa, and syphilis. It may cause death of part of the organ supplied by the affected artery.

thrombokinase *n. see* thromboplastin.

thrombolysis *n.* the dissolution of a blood clot (thrombus) by the infusion of an enzyme, such as *streptokinase, into the blood. It may be used in the treatment of *phlebothrombosis or *pulmonary embolism.

thrombolytic *adj.* describing an agent that breaks up blood clots (thrombi). *See* anticoagulant.

thrombophlebitis *n.* a condition in which thrombosis is associated with inflammation of a vein wall (*see* phlebitis).

thromboplastin (thrombokinase) *n.* a substance formed during the earlier stages of *blood coagulation. It acts as an enzyme, converting the inactive substance prothrombin to the enzyme *thrombin.

thrombopoiesis *n.* the process of blood *platelet production. Platelets are formed as fragments of cytoplasm shed from giant cells (*megakaryocytes) in the bone marrow by a budding process.

thrombosis *n.* a condition in which the blood changes from a liquid to a solid state and produces a blood clot (*thrombus*). Thrombosis may occur within a blood vessel in diseased states. Thrombosis in an artery obstructs the blood flow to the tissue it supplies: obstruction of an artery to the brain is one of the causes of a *stroke and thrombosis in an artery supplying the heart – *coronary thrombosis – results in a heart attack (*see* myocardial infarction). Thrombosis can also occur in a vein, and it may be associated with inflammation (*see* phlebitis, phlebothrombosis). The thrombus may become detached from its site of formation and carried in the blood to lodge in another part (*see* embolism).

thrombus *n.* a blood clot (*see* thrombosis).

thrush *n. see* candidiasis.

thym- (thymo-) *prefix denoting* the thymus.

thymectomy *n.* surgical removal of the thymus gland.

-thymia *suffix denoting* a condition of the mind. Example: *cyclothymia* (marked alternation of mood).

thymic aplasia failure of development of the *thymus gland. This was formerly thought to predispose to *hypersensitivity reactions and to infection and so to death in childhood (*see* status lymphaticus), a concept no longer held.

thymidine *n.* a compound containing thymine and the sugar ribose. *See also* nucleoside.

thymine *n.* one of the nitrogen-containing bases (*see* pyrimidine) occurring in the nucleic acids DNA and RNA.

thymitis *n.* inflammation of the thymus gland (the mass of lymphatic tissue behind the breastbone).

thymocyte *n.* a lymphocyte within the *thymus.

thymoma *n.* a benign or malignant tumour of the *thymus gland. It is sometimes associated with *myasthenia gravis, a chronic disease in which muscles tire easily. Surgical removal of the tumour may result in improvement of the muscle condition, but the response is often slow.

thymoxamine *n.* a drug that causes peripheral blood vessels to dilate (*see* vasodilator). It is administered by mouth in the treatment of Raynaud's disease and similar conditions. Side-effects include mild nausea, diarrhoea, headache, and flushing. The drug should be used with caution in patients with diabetes mellitus or heart disease. Trade name: **Opilon**.

thymus *n.* a bilobed organ in the root of the neck, above and in front of the heart. The thymus is enclosed in a capsule and divided internally by cross walls into many lobules, each full of lymphocytes (white blood cells associated with antibody production). In relation to body size the thymus is largest at birth. It doubles in size by puberty, after which it gradually shrinks, its functional tissue being replaced by fatty tissue. In infancy the thymus controls the development of *lymphoid tissue and immune response to microbes and foreign proteins (accounting for allergic response, autoimmunity, and rejection of organ transplants). Its function in the adult is unclear. —**thymic** *adj.*

thyro- *prefix denoting* the thyroid gland. Example: *thyroglossal* (relating to the thyroid gland and tongue).

thyrocalcitonin (calcitonin) *n.* a hormone, produced by certain cells in the thyroid gland, that lowers the levels of calcium and phosphate in the blood. Thyrocalcitonin is given by injection to treat hypercalcaemia and Paget's disease of the bone. *Compare* parathyroid hormone.

thyrocele *n.* a swelling of the thyroid gland. *See* goitre.

thyroglobulin *n.* a protein in the thyroid gland from which the *thyroid hormones (thyroxine and triiodotyrosine) are synthesized.

thyrohyoid *adj.* relating to the thyroid cartilage and hyoid bone. The *thyrohyoid ligaments* form part of the *larynx; contraction of the *thyrohyoid muscle* raises the larynx.

thyroid cartilage the main cartilage of the *larynx, consisting of two broad plates that join at the front to form a V-shaped structure. The thyroid cartilage forms the *Adam's apple* in front of the larynx.

thyroidectomy *n.* surgical removal of the thyroid gland. In *partial thyroidectomy*, only the diseased part of the gland is removed; in *subtotal thyroidectomy*, a method of treating *thyrotoxicosis, the surgeon removes 90% of the gland.

thyroid gland a large *endocrine gland situated in the base of the neck (see illustration). It consists of two lobes, one on either side of the trachea, that are joined by an *isthmus* (sometimes a third lobe extends upwards from the isthmus). The thyroid gland consists of a large number of closed follicles inside which is a jelly-like colloid, which contains the principle active substances that are secreted by the gland. The thyroid gland is concerned with regulation of the metabolic rate by the secretion of *thyroid hormone, which is stimulated by *thyroid-stimulating hormone from the pituitary gland and requires trace amounts of iodine. Thyroid extract is used in the treatment of thyroid deficiency diseases.

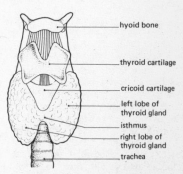

hyoid bone

thyroid cartilage

cricoid cartilage

left lobe of thyroid gland

isthmus

right lobe of thyroid gland

trachea

Position of the thyroid gland

thyroid hormone an iodine-containing substance, synthesized and secreted by the thyroid gland, that is essential for normal metabolic processes and mental and physical development. There are two thyroid hormones, *triio-*

dothyronine and thyroxine. Lack of these hormones gives rise to *cretinism in infants and *myxoedema in adults. Excessive production of thyroid hormones gives rise to *thyrotoxicosis.

thyroiditis *n.* inflammation of the thyroid gland. *Acute thyroiditis* is due to bacterial infection; *chronic thyroiditis* is commonly caused by an abnormal immune response (*see* autoimmunity) in which lymphocytes invade the tissues of the gland. *See* Hashimoto's disease, struma.

thyroid-stimulating hormone (thyrotrophin, TSH) a hormone, synthesized and secreted by the anterior pituitary gland under the control of *thyrotrophin-releasing hormone, that stimulates activity of the thyroid gland. Defects in TSH production lead to over- or under-secretion of *thyroid hormones. TSH may be given by injection to test thyroid gland function.

thyrotomy *n.* surgical incision of either the thyroid cartilage in the neck or of the thyroid gland itself.

thyrotoxicosis *n.* the syndrome due to excessive amounts of thyroid hormones in the bloodstream, causing a rapid heart beat, sweating, tremor, anxiety, increased appetite, loss of weight, and intolerance of heat. Causes include simple overactivity of the gland, a hormone-secreting benign tumour or carcinoma of the thyroid, and *Graves's disease* (exophthalmic goitre), in which there are additional symptoms including swelling of the neck (*goitre*) due to enlargement of the gland and protrusion of the eyes (*exophthalmos*). Treatment may be by surgical removal of the thyroid gland, administration of radioactive iodine to destroy part of the gland, or by the use of drugs (such as *carbimazole or *propylthiouracil) that interfere with the production of thyroid hormones. —**thyrotoxic** *adj.*

thyrotrophin *n. see* thyroid-stimulating hormone.

thyrotrophin-releasing hormone (TRH) a hormone-like substance from the hypothalamus (in the brain) that acts on the anterior pituitary gland to stimulate the release of *thyroid-stimulating hormone. TRH is given by intravenous injection to test thyroid gland function and to estimate reserves of thyroid-stimulating hormone in the pituitary.

thyroxine *n.* one of the hormones synthesized and secreted by the thyroid gland (*see* thyroid hormone). Thyroxine can be administered by mouth to treat underactivity of the thyroid gland (*see* cretinism, myxoedema).

tibia *n.* the shin bone: the inner and larger bone of the lower leg (see illustration). It articulates with the *femur above, with the *talus below, and with the *fibula to the side (at both ends); at the lower end is a projection, the medial *malleolus, forming part of the articulation with the talus.

Right tibia and fibula

tibialis *n.* either of two muscles in the leg, extending from the tibia to the metatarsal bones of the foot. The *tibialis anterior* turns the foot inwards and flexes the toes backwards. Situated behind it, the *tibialis posterior* extends the toes and inverts the foot.

tibio- *prefix denoting* the tibia. Example: *tibiofibular* (relating to the tibia and fibula).

tic *n.* a repeated and largely involuntary movement varying in complexity from the twitch of a muscle to elaborate well-coordinated actions. Tics most often become prominent when the individual is exposed to emotional stress.

tic douloureux *see* neuralgia.

tick *n.* a bloodsucking parasite belonging to the order of arthropods (Acarina) that also includes the *mites. Tick bites can cause serious skin lesions and occasionally paralysis (*see* Ixodes, Amblyomma), and certain tick species transmit *typhus and *relapsing fever. Dimethyl phthalate is used as a tick repellent. There are two families: Argasidae (soft ticks), including *Ornithodoros*, with mouthparts invisible from above and no hard shield (*scutum*) on the dorsal surface; and Ixodidae (hard ticks), including *Dermacentor, Haemaphysalis*, and *Rhipicephalus*, with clearly visible mouthparts and a definite scutum.

tick fever any infectious disease transmitted by ticks, especially *Rocky Mountain spotted fever.

Tietze's syndrome (costochondritis) a painful swelling of a rib in the region of the chest, over the junction of bone and cartilage. The cause is unknown and the condition usually resolves without treatment, but in some cases local injections of corticosteroids are required.

time sampling (in psychology) a way of recording behaviour in which the presence or absence of particular kinds of behaviour is noted during each of several fixed prearranged periods of time. *See also* event sampling.

tincture *n.* an alcoholic extract of a drug derived from a plant.

tinea *n. see* ringworm.

tinnitus *n.* any noise (buzzing, ringing, etc.) in the ear. The many causes include wax (*cerumen) in the ear; damage to the eardrum; diseases of the inner ear, such as *otosclerosis and *Menière's disease; drugs such as aspirin and quinine, and abnormalities of the auditory nerve and its connections within the brain.

tintometer *n.* an instrument for measuring the depth of colour in a liquid. The colour can then be compared with those on standard charts so that the concentration of a particular compound in solution can be estimated.

tissue *n.* a collection of cells specialized to perform a particular function. The cells may be of the same type (e.g. in nervous tissue) or of different types (e.g. in connective tissue). Aggregations of tissues constitute organs.

tissue culture the culture of living tissues, removed from the body, in a suitable medium supplied with nutrients and oxygen.

titre *n.* (in immunology) the extent to which a sample of blood serum containing antibody can be diluted before losing its ability to cause agglutination of the relevant antigen. It is used as a measure of the amount of antibody in the serum.

titubation *n.* a rhythmical nodding movement of the head, sometimes involving the trunk. Occasionally the use of this term is extended to include a stumbling gait.

tobacco *n.* the dried leaves of the plant *Nicotiana tabacum* or related species, used in smoking and as snuff. Tobacco contains the stimulant but poisonous alkaloid *nicotine, which enters the bloodstream during smoking. The volatile tarry material also released during smoking contains chemicals known to produce cancer in animals.

toco- *prefix denoting* childbirth or labour.

tocopherol *n. see* vitamin E.

Todd's paralysis (Todd's palsy) transient paralysis of a part of the body that has previously been involved in a focal epileptic fit (*see* epilepsy). It is thought to be due to the exhaustion of the cells of the motor cortex of the brain.

Tofranil *n. see* imipramine.

tolazamide *n.* a drug administered by mouth in the treatment of maturity-onset diabetes. Side-effects include nausea, loss of appetite, diarrhoea, weakness, and lethargy. Trade name: **Tolanase.** *See also* sulphonylurea.

tolazoline *n.* a *vasodilator drug, given by mouth for the treatment of peripheral vascular disorders, such as *Raynaud's disease. Side-effects include flushing, nausea, vomiting, diarrhoea, and a fall in blood pressure on standing. The drug should not be given to patients with peptic ulcers or heart disease. Trade name: **Priscol.**

tolbutamide *n.* a drug given by mouth in the treatment of diabetes mellitus. It is believed to act directly on the pancreas to stimulate insulin production and is particularly effective in elderly patients with mild diabetes. Side-effects are similar to those of the *sulphonamides and include skin reactions and transient jaundice. Trade names: **Pramidex, Rastinon.**

tolerance *n.* the reduction or loss of the normal response to a drug or other substance that usually provokes a reaction in the body. *Drug tolerance* may develop after taking a particular drug over a long period of time. In such cases increased doses are necessary to produce the desired effect. Some drugs that cause tolerance also cause *dependence. *See also* glucose tolerance test, immunological tolerance, tachyphylaxis.

tolnaftate *n.* an antiseptic applied topically as a cream, powder, or solution in the treatment of various fungal infections of the skin, including ringworm. It is not effective in candidiasis. Trade names: **Tinactin, Tinaderm.**

toluidine blue a dye used in microscopy for staining *basophilic substances in tissue specimens.

-tome *suffix denoting* a cutting instrument. Example: *microtome* (instrument for cutting microscopical sections).

tomo- *prefix denoting* **1.** section or sections. **2.** surgical operation.

tomography *n.* the technique of using X-rays or ultrasound waves to produce an image of structures at a particular depth within the body, bringing them into sharp focus while deliberately blurring structures at other depths. The visual record of this technique is called a *tomogram* (*see also* orthopantomogram). *See* computerized axial tomography, positron emission tomography.

tomotocia *n.* the delivery of a baby by cutting open the mother's abdomen and womb (*see* Caesarean section).

-tomy (-otomy) *suffix denoting* a surgical incision into an organ or part. Example: *gastrotomy* (into the stomach).

tone *n. see* tonus.

tongue *n.* a muscular organ attached to the floor of the mouth. It consists of a *body* and a *root*, which is attached by muscles to the hyoid bone below, the styloid process behind, and the palate above. It is covered by mucous mem-

tonic

brane, which is continuous with that of the mouth and pharynx. On the undersurface of the tongue a fold of mucous membrane, the *frenulum linguae*, connects the midline of the tongue to the floor of the mouth. The surface of the tongue is covered with minute projections (*papillae*), which give it a furred appearance (see illustration). *Taste buds are arranged in grooves around the papillae, particularly the fungiform and circumvallate papillae. The tongue has three main functions. It helps in manipulating food during mastication and swallowing; it is the main organ of taste; and it plays an important role in the production of articulate speech. Anatomical name: **glossa**.

The upper surface of the tongue

tonic 1. *adj.* **a.** relating to normal muscle tone. **b.** marked by continuous tension (contraction), e.g. a tonic muscle *spasm. 2. *n.* a medicinal substance taken to increase vigour and liveliness and produce a feeling of well-being.

tonicity *n.* 1. the normal state of slight contraction, or readiness to contract, of healthy muscle fibres. 2. the effective osmotic pressure of a solution. *See* hypertonic, hypotonic, osmosis.

tono- *prefix denoting* 1. tone or tension. 2. pressure.

tonofibril *n.* a tiny fibre occurring in bundles in the cytoplasm of cells that lie in contact, as in epithelial tissue. Tonofibrils are concerned with maintaining contact between adjacent cells. *See* desmosome.

tonography *n.* measurement of the pressure within the eyeball in such a way as to allow a record to be made on a chart of variations in pressure occurring over periods of several minutes at a time.

tonometer *n.* an instrument for measuring pressure in a part of the body, e.g. the eye (*see* ophthalmotonometer).

tonsil *n.* a mass of *lymphoid tissue on either side of the back of the mouth. It is concerned with protection against infection. The term usually refers to either of the *palatine tonsils*, but below the tongue is another pair, the *lingual tonsils*. *See also* adenoids (pharyngeal tonsils).

tonsillectomy *n.* surgical removal of the tonsils.

tonsillitis *n.* inflammation of the tonsils due to bacterial or viral infection, causing a sore throat, fever, and difficulty in swallowing. If tonsillitis due to streptococcal infection is not treated (by antibiotics) it may lead to *rheumatic fever or *nephritis.

tonsillotomy *n.* surgical incision of a tonsil or removal of part of a tonsil.

tonus (tone) *n.* the normal state of partial contraction of a resting muscle, maintained by reflex activity.

tooth *n.* (*pl.* teeth) one of the hard structures in the mouth used for cutting and chewing food. Each tooth is embedded in a socket in part of the jawbone (mandible or maxilla) known as the *alveolar bone* (or *alveolus*), to which it is attached by the *periodontal

membrane. The exposed part of the tooth (*crown*) is covered with *enamel and the part within the bone (*root*) is coated with *cementum; the bulk of the tooth consists of *dentine enclosing the *pulp (see illustration). The group of embryological cells that gives rise to a tooth is known as the *tooth germ*.
There are four different types of tooth (*see* canine, incisor, premolar, molar). *See also* dentition.

tooth extraction *see* extraction.

topagnosis *n.* inability to identify a part of the body that has been touched. It is a symptom of disease in the parietal lobes of the brain. The normal ability to localize touch is called *topognosis*.

topectomy *n.* an obsolete operation for the control of psychiatric symptoms by excising selected areas of the cerebral cortex. *See also* psychosurgery.

tophus *n.* (*pl.* **tophi**) a hard deposit of crystalline uric acid and its salts in the skin, cartilage (especially of the ears), or joints; a feature of *gout.

topical *adj.* local: used for the route of administration of a drug that is applied directly to the part being treated (e.g. to the skin or eye).

topo- *prefix denoting* place; position; location.

topography *n.* the study of the different regions of the body, including the description of its parts in relation to the surrounding structures. —**topographical** *adj.*

tormina *n. see* colic.

torpor *n.* a state of sluggishness and diminished responsiveness: a characteristic of certain mental disorders and a symptom of certain forms of poisoning or metabolic disorder.

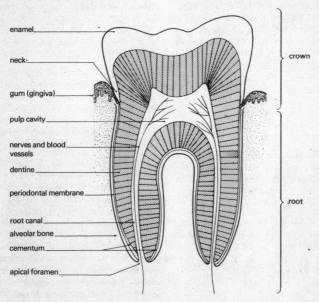

enamel
neck
gum (gingiva)
pulp cavity
nerves and blood vessels
dentine
periodontal membrane
root canal
alveolar bone
cementum
apical foramen
crown
root

Section of a molar tooth

torsion *n.* twisting. Abnormal twisting of a testis within the scrotum or of a loop of bowel in the abdomen may impair blood and nerve supplies to these parts and cause severe damage.

torticollis (wryneck) *n.* an irresistible turning movement of the head that becomes more persistent, so that eventually the head is held continually to one side. The spasm of the muscles is often painful and the patient is sensitive about his appearance. It may be caused by a birth injury to the sternomastoid muscle (*see* sternomastoid tumour). Relief may be obtained by cutting the motor nerve roots of the spinal nerves in the neck region.

toruloma *n.* a tumour-like lesion in the lungs resulting from *cryptococcosis.

torulosis *n. see* cryptococcosis.

tourniquet *n.* a device to press upon an artery and prevent flow of blood through it, usually a cord, rubber tube, or tight bandage tightened around a limb. Tourniquets are no longer recommended as a first-aid measure to stop bleeding from a wound because of the danger of reducing the supply of oxygen to other tissues (direct pressure on the wound itself is considered less harmful). However, a temporary tourniquet to increase the distension of veins when a sample of blood is being taken does no harm.

tow *n.* the teased-out short fibres of flax, hemp or jute, used in swabs for cleaning, in *packs or *stupes for the application of poultices, and for a variety of other purposes.

Towne's projection a *posteroanterior X-ray film to show the entire skull and mandible.

tox- (toxi-, toxo-, toxic(o)-) *prefix denoting* **1.** poisonous; toxic. **2.** toxins or poisoning.

toxaemia *n.* blood poisoning that is caused by toxins formed by bacteria growing in a local site of infection. It produces generalized symptoms, including fever, diarrhoea, and vomiting. *Compare* pyaemia, sapraemia, septicaemia.

toxaemia of pregnancy an illness of unknown cause affecting pregnant women. It includes the conditions of *pre-eclampsia and *eclampsia.

toxic *adj.* having a poisonous effect; potentially lethal.

toxicity *n.* the degree to which a substance is poisonous. *See also* LD_{50}.

toxicology *n.* the study of poisonous materials and their effects upon living organisms. —**toxicologist** *n.*

toxicosis *n.* the deleterious effects of a toxin; poisoning: includes any disease caused by the toxic effects of any substances.

toxin *n.* a poison produced by a living organism, especially by a bacterium (*see* endotoxin, exotoxin). In the body toxins act as *antigens, and special *antibodies (*antitoxins*) are formed to neutralize their effects.

Toxocara *n.* a genus of large nematode worms that are intestinal parasites of vertebrates. *T. canis* and *T. cati*, the common roundworms of dogs and cats respectively, have life cycles similar to that of the human roundworm, *Ascaris lumbricoides. See* toxocariasis.

toxocariasis (visceral larva migrans) *n.* an infestation with the larvae of the dog and cat roundworms, *Toxocara canis* and *T. cati*. Man, who is not the normal host, becomes infected on swallowing eggs of *Toxocara* present on hands or in food and drink contaminated with the faeces of infected domestic pets. The larvae, which migrate around the body, cause destruction of various tissues; the liver becomes enlarged and the lungs inflamed (*see* pneumonitis). Symptoms may include fever, joint and muscle pains, vomiting, an irritating rash, and convulsions. Larvae can also lodge in the retina of the eye where they cause inflammation and *granuloma. The disease, widely distributed throughout the world, primarily affects children. There is no satisfactory treatment.

toxoid *n.* a preparation of the poisonous material (toxin) that is produced by dangerous infective organisms, such as those of tetanus and diphtheria, and has been rendered harmless by chemical treatment while retaining its antigenic activity. Toxoids are used in *vaccines.

Toxoplasma *n.* a genus of crescent-shaped sporozoans that live as parasites within the cells of various tissues and organs of vertebrate animals, especially birds and mammals, and complete their life cycle in a single host. *T. gondii* infects sheep, cattle, dogs, and man, sometimes provoking an acute illness (*see* toxoplasmosis).

toxoplasmosis *n.* a disease of mammals and birds due to the protozoan *Toxoplasma gondii*, which is transmitted to man via undercooked meat, contaminated soil, or by direct contact. Generally symptoms are mild but severe infection of lymph nodes can occur. *Congenital toxoplasmosis*, in which a woman infected during pregnancy transmits the organism to her fetus, can produce blindness or mental retardation in the newborn. Severe cases are treated with sulphonamides and pyrimethamine.

trabecula *n.* (*pl.* **trabeculae**) **1.** any of the bands of tissue that pass from the outer part of an organ to its interior, dividing it into separate chambers. For example, trabeculae occur in the penis. **2.** any of the thin bars of bony tissue in spongy *bone. —**trabecular** *adj.*

trabeculectomy *n.* an operation for glaucoma, one part of which is the removal of a small segment of tissue

from part of the wall of *Schlemm's canal. This area is known as the *trabecular meshwork*.

tracer *n.* a substance that is introduced into the body and whose progress can subsequently be followed so that information is gained about metabolic processes. Radioactive tracers, giving off radiation that can be detected on a *scintigram or with a *gamma camera, are used for a variety of purposes, such as the investigation of thyroid disease or possible brain tumours.

trache- (tracheo-) *prefix denoting* the trachea.

trachea *n.* the windpipe: the part of the air passage between the *larynx and the main *bronchi, i.e. from just below the Adam's apple, passing behind the notch of the *sternum (breastbone) to behind the angle of the sternum. The upper part of the trachea lies just below the skin, except where the thyroid gland is wrapped around it. —**tracheal** *adj.*

tracheal tugging a sign that is indicative of an *aneurysm of the aortic arch: a downward tug is felt on the windpipe when the finger is placed in the midline at the root of the neck.

tracheitis *n.* inflammation of the *trachea, usually secondary to bacterial or viral infection in the nose or throat. Tracheitis causes soreness in the chest and a painful cough and is often associated with bronchitis. In babies it can cause asphyxia, particularly in *diphtheria. Treatment includes appropriate antibacterial drugs, humidification of the inhaled air or oxygen, and mild sedation to relieve exhaustion due to persistant coughing.

tracheostomy (tracheotomy) *n.* a surgical operation in which a hole is made into the *trachea through the neck to relieve obstruction to breathing, as in diphtheria. A curved metal, plastic, or rubber tube is usually inserted through the hole and held in position

tracheotomy

by tapes tied round the neck. It may be possible for the patient to speak by occluding the opening with his fingers. The tube must be kept clean and unblocked. It often helps breathing if secretions are sucked out of the bronchial tree.

tracheotomy *n. see* tracheostomy.

trachoma *n.* a chronic contagious eye disease – a severe form of *conjunctivitis – caused by the virus-like organism *Chlamydia trachomatis*; it is common in tropical regions. The conjunctiva of the eyelids becomes inflamed, leading to discharge of pus. If untreated, the conjunctiva becomes scarred and shrinks, causing the eyelids to turn inwards so that the eyelashes scratch the cornea (*trichiasis); blindness usually follows. Treatment with tetracyclines is effective.

tract *n.* **1.** a group of nerve fibres passing from one part of the brain or spinal cord to another, forming a distinct pathway, e.g. the spinothalamic tract, pyramidal tract, and corticospinal tract. **2.** an organ or collection of organs providing for the passage of something, e.g. the digestive tract.

traction *n.* the application of a pulling force as a means of counteracting the natural tension in the tissues surrounding a broken bone. This tension makes correct alignment of the fragments difficult. Considerable force, exerted with weights, ropes, and pulleys, may be necessary to ensure that a broken femur is kept correctly positioned during the early stages of healing.

tractotomy *n.* a neurosurgical operation for the relief of intractable pain. The nerve fibres that carry painful sensation to consciousness travel from the spinal cord through the brainstem in the spinothalamic tracts. This procedure is designed to sever the tracts within the medulla oblongata. *See also* cordotomy.

tragus *n.* the projection of cartilage in the *pinna of the outer ear that extends back over the opening of the external auditory meatus.

Training Opportunities Scheme *see* Employment Service Division.

Training Services Division *see* Employment Service Division.

trance *n.* a state in which reaction to the environment is diminished although awareness is not impaired. It can be caused by hypnosis, meditation, catatonia, hysteria, drugs (such as hallucinogens), and religious ecstasy.

tranquillizer *n.* a drug that produces a calming effect, relieving anxiety and tension. *Major tranquillizers*, such as the phenothiazines (e.g. *chlorpromazine, and *trifluoperazine), and *haloperidol, are used to treat severe mental disorders (psychoses), including schizophrenia and mania. *Minor tranquillizers*, such as the benzodiazepines (e.g. *chlordiazepoxide and *diazepam) and *meprobamate, are used to treat neuroses and to relieve anxiety and tension due to various causes. Some drowsiness and dizziness are side-effects of most tranquillizers, and abnormal muscle action and movements sometimes occur with major tranquillizers at high doses. Minor tranquillizers sometimes cause *dependence with prolonged use.

trans- *prefix denoting* through or across. Example: *transurethral* (through the urethra).

transaminase *n.* an enzyme that catalyses the transfer of an amino group from an amino acid to an α-keto acid in the process of *transamination. Examples are *glutamic oxaloacetic transaminase (GOT), catalysing the transamination of glutamate and oxaloacetate to α-ketoglutarate and aspartate, and *glutamic pyruvic transaminase (GPT), converting glutamate and pyruvate to α-ketoglutarate and alanine.

transamination *n.* a process involved in the metabolism of amino acids in which amino groups ($-NH_2$) are transferred from amino acids to certain α-keto acids, with the production of a second keto acid and amino acid. The reaction is catalysed by enzymes (*see* transaminase), which require pyridoxal phosphate as a coenzyme.

transcription *n.* the process in which the information contained in the *genetic code is transferred from DNA to RNA: the first step in the manufacture of proteins in cells. *See* messenger RNA, translation.

transduction *n.* the transfer of DNA from one bacterium to another by means of a *bacteriophage (phage). Some bacterial DNA is incorporated into the phage. When the host bacterium is destroyed the phage infects another bacterium and introduces the DNA from its previous host, which may become incorporated into the new host's DNA.

transection *n.* **1.** a cross section of a piece of tissue. **2.** cutting across the tissue of an organ (*see also* section).

transferase *n.* an enzyme that catalyses the transfer of a group (other than hydrogen) between a pair of substrates.

transference *n.* (in psychoanalysis) the process by which a patient comes to feel and act towards the therapist as though he were somebody from the patient's past life, especially a powerful parent. The patient's transference feelings may be of love or of hatred, but they are inappropriate to the actual person of the therapist. *Countertransference* is the reaction of the therapist to the patient, which is similarly based on his own past relationships.

transferrin (siderophilin) *n.* a *glycoprotein, found in the blood plasma, that is capable of binding iron and thus acts as a carrier for iron in the bloodstream.

transfer RNA a type of RNA whose function is to attach the correct amino acid to the protein chain being synthesized at a *ribosome. *See also* translation.

transfusion *n.* **1.** the injection of a volume of blood obtained from a healthy person (the *donor*) into the circulation of a patient (the *recipient*) whose blood is deficient in quantity or quality, through accident or disease. Direct transfusion from one person to another is rarely performed; usually bottles of carefully stored blood of different *blood groups are kept in *blood banks for use as necessary. During transfusion the blood is allowed to drip, under gravity, through a needle inserted into one of the recipient's veins. Blood transfusion is routine during major surgical operations in which much blood is likely to be lost. **2.** the administration of any fluid, such as plasma or saline solution, into a patient's vein by means of a *drip.

transillumination *n.* the technique of shining a bright light through part of the body to examine its structure. Transillumination of the sinuses of the skull is a means of detecting abnormalities.

translation *n.* (in cell biology) the manufacture of proteins in a cell, which takes place at the ribosomes. The information for determining the correct sequence of amino acids in the protein is carried to the ribosomes by *messenger RNA, and the amino acids are brought to their correct position in the protein by *transfer RNA.

translocation *n.* (in genetics) a type of chromosome mutation in which part of a chromosome is transferred to another part of the same chromosome or to a different chromosome. This changes the order of the genes on the chromosomes and can lead to serious genetic disorders, e.g. chronic myeloid leukaemia.

transmethylation *n.* the process whereby an amino acid donates its terminal methyl (–CH₃) group for methylation of other compounds. Methionine is the principal methyl donor in the body and the donated methyl group may subsequently be involved in the synthesis of such compounds as choline or creatinine or in detoxification processes.

transmigration *n.* the act of passing through or across, e.g. the passage of blood cells through the intact walls of capillaries and venules (*see* diapedesis).

transplantation *n.* the implantation of an organ or tissue (*see* graft) from one part of the body to another or from one person (the donor) to another (the recipient). Skin and bone grafting are examples of transplantation techniques in the same individual. A kidney transplant involves the grafting of a healthy kidney from a donor to replace the diseased kidney of the recipient. Heart transplants have also been carried out with limited success and a few liver transplants have also been attempted. Transplanting organs or tissues between individuals is a difficult procedure because of the natural rejection processes in the recipient of the graft. Special treatment (e.g. with *immunosuppresive drugs) is needed to prevent graft rejection.

transposition *n.* the abnormal positioning of a part of the body such that it is on the opposite side to its normal site in the body. For example, it may involve the heart (*see* dextrocardia).

transposition of the great vessels a congenital abnormality of the heart in which the aorta arises from the right ventricle and the pulmonary artery from the left ventricle. Life is impossible unless there is an additional abnormality, such as a septal defect, that permits the mixing of blood between the pulmonary and systemic (aortic) circulations. Few of those untreated survive infancy and childhood, but the defect may be improved or corrected surgically.

transsexualism *n.* the condition of one who firmly believes that he (or she) belongs to the sex opposite to his (or her) biological gender. The roots of such a belief usually go back to childhood. Children with such beliefs are treated with encouragement to engage in the activities appropriate to their biological sex and to work through their difficulties in psychotherapy. Adults with such beliefs can seldom be persuaded to change them; surgical sex reassignment is sometimes justifiable, to make the externals of the body conform to the individual's view of himself (or herself). —**transsexual** *adj.*, *n.*

transudation *n.* the passage of a liquid through a membrane, especially of blood through the wall of a capillary vessel. The liquid is called the *transudate*.

transurethral resection (TUR) *see* resection.

transverse *adj.* (in anatomy) situated at right angles to the long axis of the body of an organ.

transverse process the long projection from the base of the neural arch of a *vertebra.

transvestitism *n.* the condition in which sexual pleasure is obtained by dressing in the clothes of the opposite sex. It may occur in both heterosexual and homosexual people and may be directly related to masturbatory or other sexual behaviour. Treatment may be by behavioural techniques such as *aversion therapy, but is not always needed. *See also* perversion. —**transvestite** *n.*

tranylcypromine *n.* an antidepressant drug – one of the *MAO inhibitors – given by mouth for the treatment of severe mental depressive states. Common side-effects include restlessness, insomnia, giddiness, and a fall in blood pressure. Trade name: **Parnate**.

trapezium *n.* a bone of the wrist (*see* carpus). It articulates with the scaphoid bone behind and with the first metacarpal in front.

trapezius *n.* a flat triangular muscle covering the back of the neck and shoulder. It is important for movements of the scapula and it also draws the head backwards to either side.

Left trapezius muscle

trapezoid bone a bone of the wrist (*see* carpus). It articulates with the second metatarsal bone in front, with the scaphoid bone behind, and with the trapezium and capitate bones on either side.

trauma *n.* **1.** a physical wound or injury, such as a fracture or blow. **2.** (in psychology) an emotionally painful and harmful event. Theorists have speculated that some events (such as birth) are always traumatic. Symptoms of neurosis may follow an overwhelmingly stressful event, such as battle or serious injury. —**traumatic** *adj.*

traumatic fever a fever resulting from a serious injury.

traumatology *n.* accident surgery: the branch of surgery that deals with wounds and disabilities arising from injuries.

travel sickness (motion sickness) nausea, vomiting, and headache caused by motion during travel by sea, road, or air. The symptoms are due to overstimulation of the balance organs in the *inner ear by repeated small changes in the position of the body and are aggravated by movements of the horizon. *Antihistamine drugs provide effective treatment.

trematode *n. see* fluke.

tremor *n.* a rhythmical alternating movement that may affect any part of the body. The *physiological tremor* is a feature of the normal mechanism for maintaining posture. It may be more apparent in states of fatigue or anxiety. *Essential tremor* is slower and particularly affects the hands. It can be embarrassing and inconvenient but it is not accompanied by any other symptoms. A similar tremor may also occur in several members of one family or in elderly people. Tremor is a prominent symptom of *parkinsonism. An *intention tremor* occurs when a patient with disease of the cerebellum tries to touch an object. The closer the object is approached the wilder become the movements.

trench foot (immersion foot) blackening of the toes and the skin of the foot due to death of the superficial tissues and caused by prolonged immersion in cold water.

Trendelenburg position a special operating-table posture for patients undergoing surgery of the pelvis or for patients suffering from shock. The patient is laid on his back with the pelvis higher than the head, inclined at an angle of about 45°.

trephine *n.* a surgical instrument used to remove a circular area of tissue, usually from the cornea of the eye or from bone (the latter for microscopical examination). It consists of a hollow tube with a serrated cutting edge.

Treponema *n.* a genus of anaerobic spirochaete bacteria. All species are parasitic and some cause disease in animals and man: *T. carateum* causes *pinta, T. pallidum *syphilis, and *T. pertenue *yaws.

treponematosis *n.* any infection caused by spirochaete bacteria of the genus *Treponema. See* pinta, syphilis, yaws.

triad *n.* (in medicine) a group of three united or closely associated structures or three symptoms or effects that occur together. A *portal triad* in a portal canal of the liver consists of a branch of the portal vein, a branch of the hepatic artery, and an interlobular bile tubule.

triamcinolone *n.* a synthetic corticosteroid hormone with uses similar to *cortisone; it reduces inflammation but does not cause salt and water retention. It is administered by mouth and common side-effects include dizziness, headache, somnolence, muscle weakness, and a fall in blood pressure, particularly on the sudden withdrawal of treatment. Trade names: **Adcortyl, Ledercort**.

triamterene *n.* a *diuretic that is given by mouth and produces an effect within two hours. It causes the loss of sodium and chloride from the kidneys and is used in the treatment of various forms of fluid retention (oedema). Common side-effects include nausea, vomiting, weakness, reduced blood pressure, and digestive disorders. Trade name: **Dytac**.

triangle *n.* (in anatomy) a three-sided structure or area; for example, the *femoral triangle.

triangular bandage a piece of material cut or folded into a triangular

shape and used for making an arm sling or holding dressings in position.

Triatoma *n.* a genus of bloodsucking bugs (*see* reduviid). *T. infestans* is important in transmitting *Chagas' disease in Argentina, Uruguay, and Chile.

triaziquone *n.* a drug used in the treatment of various forms of cancer and administered by mouth, injection, or directly into the tumour. It has toxic actions on normal tissues, particularly the bone marrow; other side-effects include nausea, vomiting, loss of hair, and skin reactions. Trade name: **Trenimon**.

triceps *n.* a muscle with three heads of origin, particularly the *triceps brachii*, which is situated on the back of the upper arm and contracts to extend the forearm. It is the *antagonist of the *brachialis.

trich- (tricho-) *prefix denoting* hair or hairlike structures.

trichiasis *n.* a condition in which the eyelashes rub against the eyeball, producing discomfort and sometimes ulceration of the cornea. It may result from inflammation of the eyelids, which makes the lashes grow out in abnormal directions, or when scarring of the conjunctiva (lining membrane) turns the eyelid inwards. It accompanies all forms of *entropion.

Trichinella *n.* a genus of minute parasitic nematode worms. The adults of *T. spiralis* live in the small intestine of man, where the females release large numbers of larvae. These bore through the intestinal wall and can cause disease (*see* trichinosis). The parasite can also develop in pigs and rats.

trichiniasis *n. see* trichinosis.

trichinosis (trichiniasis) *n.* a disease of cold and temperate regions caused by larvae of the nematode worm *Trichinella spiralis*. Man contracts trichinosis after eating imperfectly cooked mea infected with the parasite's larval cysts. Larvae, released by females in the intestine, penetrate the intestinal wall and cause diarrhoea and nausea. They migrate around the body and may cause fever, vertigo, delirium, and pains in the limbs. The larvae eventually settle within cysts in the muscles, and this may result in pain and stiffness. Trichinosis, rarely a serious disease, is treated with thiabendazole.

trichloracetic acid an *astringent used in solution for a variety of skin conditions. It is also applied topically to produce sloughing, especially for the removal of warts.

trichobezoar *n.* hairball; a mass of swallowed hair in the stomach. It may be the patient's own hair or animal hairs. *See* bezoar.

Trichocephalus *n. see* whipworm.

trichoglossia *n.* hairiness of the tongue, due to the growth of fungal organisms infecting its surface.

trichology *n.* the study of hair.

Trichomonas *n.* a genus of parasitic flagellate protozoans that move by means of a wavy membrane, bearing a single flagellum, projecting from the body surface. *T. vaginalis* often infects the vagina, where it may cause severe irritation and a foul-smelling discharge (*see* vaginitis), and sometimes also the male *urethra; it can be transmitted during sexual intercourse. *Metronidazole is used in treatment. *T. hominis* and *T. tenax*, which live in the large intestine and mouth respectively, are not believed to cause disease.

trichomoniasis *n.* **1.** an infection of the digestive system by the protozoan *Trichomonas hominis*, causing dysentery. **2.** an infection of the vagina due to the protozoan *Trichomonas vaginalis*, causing inflammation of genital tissues with vaginal discharge. It can be transmitted to males in whom it causes

urethral discharge. Treatment with *metronidazole is effective.

trichomycosis *n.* any hair disease caused by infection with a fungus.

Trichophyton *n.* a genus of fungi, parasitic to man, that frequently infect the skin, nails, and hair and cause *favus and *ringworm.

trichorrhexis *n.* a condition in which the hairs break easily. It may be due to a hereditary condition or it may occur as a consequence of repeated physical or chemical injury. The latter condition may follow the use of heat or bleach on the hair or be caused by persistent rubbing.

trichosis *n.* any abnormal growth or disease of the hair.

Trichosporon *n.* a genus of fungi, parasitic to man, that infect the scalp and beard (*see* piedra).

trichotillomania *n.* loss of hair caused by a person persistently and neurotically rubbing or pulling it.

trichromatic *adj.* describing or relating to the normal state of colour vision, in which a person is sensitive to all three of the primary colours (red, green, and blue) and can match any given colour by a mixture of these three. *Compare* dichromatic, monochromat.

trichuriasis *n.* an infestation of the large intestine by the whipworm, *Trichuris trichiura*; it occurs principally in humid tropical regions. Man acquires the infection by eating food contaminated with the worms' eggs. Symptoms, including bloody diarrhoea, anaemia, weakness, and abdominal pain, are evident only in heavy infestations. Trichuriasis can be treated with various anthelmintics, including thiabendazole and piperazine salts.

Trichuris *n. see* whipworm.

triclofos *n.* a *sedative and *hypnotic, given by mouth, usually as a syrup. It is

tricuspid valve

used to induce sleep or as a daytime sedative, particularly in children. Prolonged administration may lead to *dependence. It is similar in its actions and effects to *chloral hydrate. Trade name: **Tricloryl**.

tricuspid valve the valve in the heart between the right atrium and right ventricle. It consists of three cusps that channel the flow of blood from the atrium to the ventricle and prevent any backflow.

tridactyly *n.* a congenital abnormality in which there are only three digits on a hand or foot.

trifluoperazine *n.* a major *tranquillizer with uses and effects similar to those of *chlorpromazine. Common side-effects include drowsiness, dizziness, dryness of mouth, muscular spasm and tremor, and amenorrhoea. Trade names: **Stelazine, Terfluzine**.

trifocal lenses lenses in which there are three segments. The upper provides a clear image of distant objects; the lower is used for reading and close work; and the middle one for the intermediate distance. Musicians sometimes find the middle segment useful for reading the score during performance.

trigeminal nerve the fifth and largest *cranial nerve (V), which is split into three divisions: the ophthalmic, maxillary, and mandibular nerves (see illustration). The motor fibres are responsible for controlling the muscles involved in chewing, while the sensory fibres relay information about temperature, pain, and touch from the whole front half of the head (including the mouth) and also from the meninges.

trigeminal neuralgia (tic douloureux) *see* neuralgia.

trigeminy *n.* a condition in which the heart beats can be subdivided into groups of three. The first beat is nor-

The trigeminal nerve

mal, but the second and third are premature beats (*see* ectopic beat).

trigger finger an impairment in the ability to extend a finger, resulting either from a nodular thickening in the flexor tendon or a narrowing of the flexor tendon sheath. On unclenching the fist, the affected finger (usually the third or fourth) at first remains bent and then, on overcoming the resistance, suddenly straightens ('triggers'). Treatment is by incision of the tendon sheath.

triglyceride *n.* a lipid or neutral *fat consisting of glycerol combined with three fatty-acid molecules. Triglycerides are synthesized from the products of digestion of dietary fat: they are the form in which fat is stored in the body.

trigone *n.* a triangular region or tissue, such as the triangular region of the wall of the bladder that lies between the openings of the two ureters and the urethra.

trigonitis *n.* inflammation of the trigone (base) of the urinary bladder. This can occur as part of a generalized *cystitis or it can be associated with inflammation in the urethra, prostate, or neck of the womb. The patient experiences an intense desire to pass urine frequently; treatment includes the clearing of any underlying infection by antibiotic administration.

trigonocephaly *n.* a deformity of the skull in which the vault of the skull is sharply angled just in front of the ears, giving the skull a triangular shape. —**trigonocephalic** *adj.*

trigravida *n. see* tertigravida.

triiodothyronine *n.* one of the hormones synthesized and secreted by the thyroid gland. *See* thyroid hormone.

trimeprazine *n.* an *antihistamine drug (a *phenothiazine derivative) that also possesses sedative properties. Given by mouth, it is mainly used in the treatment of pruritus (itching) and as a preoperative medication, especially in children. Common side-effects include drowsiness, dizziness, dryness of mouth, muscular tremor and incoordination, and confusion. Trade name: **Vallergan**.

trimester *n.* (in obstetrics) any one of the three successive three-monthly periods (the *first*, *second*, and *third trimesters*) into which a pregnancy may be divided.

trimethoprim *n.* an antiseptic that is active against a range of microorganisms. It is used mainly in the treatment of chronic urinary-tract infections and malaria and is often administered, by mouth, in a combined preparation with sulphamethoxazole (*see* co-trimoxazole (Bactrim, Septrin)). Long-term treatment may cause depression of the bone marrow function.

trimipramine *n.* a tricyclic *antidepressant drug that also possesses sedative properties. It is given by mouth or by injection for the treatment of acute or chronic mental depression. Common side-effects include drowsiness, dizziness, dry mouth, and a fall in blood pressure. Trade name: **Surmontil**.

trinitrophenol *n. see* picric acid.

triose *n.* a carbohydrate with three carbon units: for example, glyceraldehyde.

tripara *n. see* tertipara.

triploid *adj.* describing cells, tissues, or individuals in which there are three complete chromosome sets. *Compare* haploid, diploid. —**triploid** *n.*

triquetrum (triquetral bone) *n.* a bone of the wrist (*see* carpus). It articulates with the ulna behind and with the pisiform, hamate, and lunate bones in the carpus.

trismus *n.* spasm of the jaw muscles, keeping the jaws tightly closed. This is the characteristic symptom of *tetanus but it also occurs less dramatically with overuse of the *phenothiazine drugs and in disorders of the *basal ganglia.

trisomy *n.* a condition in which there is one extra chromosome present in each cell in addition to the normal (diploid) chromosome set. A number of chromosome disorders are due to trisomy, including *Down's syndrome and *Klinefelter's syndrome. —**trisomic** *adj.*

tritanopia *n.* a rare defect of colour vision in which affected persons are insensitive to blue light and confuse blues and greens. *Compare* deuteranopia, protanopia.

tritium *n.* an isotope of hydrogen that emits beta particles (electrons) during its decay. It has been used as a *tracer in the investigation of diseases of the heart and the lungs. Symbol: T or ^{3}H.

trocar *n.* an instrument used to draw off fluids from a body cavity (such as the peritoneal cavity). It comprises a metal tube containing a removable shaft with a sharp three-cornered point; the shaft is withdrawn after the trocar has been inserted into the cavity.

trochanter *n.* either of the two protuberances that occur below the neck of the *femur.

troche *n.* a medicinal lozenge, taken by mouth, used to treat conditions of the mouth or throat and also of the alimentary canal.

trochlea *n.* an anatomical part having the structure or function of a pulley; for example the groove at the lower end of the *humerus or the fibrocartilaginous ring in the frontal bone (where it forms part of the orbit), through which the tendon of the superior oblique eye muscle passes. —**trochlear** *adj.*

trochlear nerve the fourth *cranial nerve (IV), which supplies the superior oblique muscle, one of the muscles responsible for movement of the eyeball in its socket. The action of the trochlear nerve is coordinated with that of the *oculomotor and *abducens nerves.

trochoid joint (pivot joint) a form of *diarthrosis (freely movable joint) in which a bone moves round a central axis, allowing rotational movement. An example is the joint between the atlas and axis vertebrae.

Trombicula *n.* a genus of widely distributed mites – the harvest mites. The six-legged parasitic larvae (chiggers) are common in fields during the autumn and frequently attack man, remaining attached to the skin for several days while feeding on the lymph and digested skin tissues. Their bite causes intense irritation and a severe dermatitis. Various repellents, e.g. benzyl benzoate, can be applied to clothing. *Trombicula* larvae are responsible for transmitting scrub typhus in southeast Asia.

trometamol *n.* a *diuretic that also reduces the acidity of body fluids. It is given by intravenous injection in conditions of acidosis to adjust the pH of the blood to normal levels. Trade name: **Tham-E**.

troph- (tropho-) *prefix denoting* nourishment or nutrition.

trophoblast *n.* the tissue that forms the wall of the *blastocyst. At implantation it forms two layers, an inner cellular layer (*cytotrophoblast*) and an outer syncytial layer (*plasmidotrophoblast*), which forms the outermost layer of the placenta and attains direct contact with the maternal bloodstream.
Trophoblast sampling is a new screening technique for the prenatal diagnosis of congenital disorders, such as Down's syndrome and thalassaemia, as early as the ninth week of pregnancy. Still being developed, the technique involves the extraction of cells of the trophoblast, by suction through a flexible tube inserted through the cervix of the uterus, and their subsequent examination for genetic abnormalities.

trophozoite *n.* a stage in the life cycle of the malarial parasite (*Plasmodium*) that develops from a merozoite in the red blood cells. The trophozoite, which has a ring-shaped body and a single nucleus, grows steadily at the expense of the blood cell; eventually its nucleus and cytoplasm undergo division to form a *schizont containing many merozoites.

-trophy *suffix denoting* nourishment, development, or growth. Example: *dystrophy* (defective development).

-tropic *suffix denoting* **1.** turning towards. **2.** having an affinity for; influencing. Example: *inotropic* (muscle).

tropical medicine the study of diseases more commonly found in tropical regions than elsewhere, such as *malaria, *trypanosomiasis, *schistosomiasis, and *leishmaniasis.

tropical ulcer (Naga sore) a skin disease prevalent in wet tropical regions. A large open sloughing sore usually develops at the site of a wound or abrasion. The ulcer, commonly located on the feet and legs, is often infected with spirochaetes and bacteria and may extend deeply and cause destruction of muscles and bones. Treatment involves the application of mild antiseptic dressings and intramuscular doses of *penicillin. Skin grafts may be necessary in more serious cases. The exact cause of the disease has not yet been determined.

tropocollagen n. the molecular unit of *collagen. It consists of a helix of three collagen molecules: this arrangement confers on the fibres structural stability and resistance to stretching.

troxidone n. an *anticonvulsant drug given by mouth, alone or in conjunction with other drugs, in the treatment of epilepsy. It is highly toxic and, in addition to producing nausea, vertigo, visual disturbances, and skin reactions, it can affect the bone marrow and cause anaemia. Trade name: **Tridione**.

truncus n. a *trunk: a main vessel or other tubular organ from which subsidiary branches arise.

truncus arteriosus the main arterial trunk arising from the fetal heart. It develops into the aorta and pulmonary artery.

trunk n. 1. the main part of a blood vessel, lymph vessel, or nerve, from which branches arise. 2. the body excluding the head and limbs.

truss n. a device for applying pressure to a hernia to prevent it from protruding. It usually consists of a pad attached to a belt with straps or spring strips and it is worn under the clothing.

trypanocide n. an agent that kills trypanosomes and is therefore used to treat infestations caused by these parasites (see trypanosomiasis). The main trypanocides are arsenic-containing compounds.

Trypanosoma n. a genus of parasitic protozoans that move by means of a long trailing flagellum and a thin wavy membrane, which project from the body surface. Trypanosomes undergo part of their development in the blood of a vertebrate host. The remaining stages occur in invertebrate hosts, which then transmit the parasites back to the vertebrates. *T. rhodesiense* and *T. gambiense*, which are transmitted through the bite of *tsetse flies, cause *sleeping sickness in Africa. *T. cruzi*, carried by *reduviid bugs, causes Chagas' disease in South America.

trypanosomiasis n. any disease caused by the presence of parasitic protozoans of the genus *Trypanosoma*. The two most important diseases are *Chagas' disease (South American trypanosomiasis) and *sleeping sickness (African trypanosomiasis).

tryparsamide n. a drug used in the treatment of trypanosomiasis (sleeping sickness). Usually given by injection, it penetrates the cerebrospinal fluid and is highly active against the infective organism (*Trypanosoma gambiense*). Trade name: **Tryparsam**.

trypsin n. an enzyme that continues the digestion of proteins by breaking down peptones into smaller peptide chains (see peptidase). It is secreted by the pancreas in an inactive form, trypsinogen, which is converted in the duodenum to trypsin by the action of the enzyme enteropeptidase.

trypsinogen n. see trypsin.

tryptophan n. an *essential amino acid. See also amino acid.

tsetse n. a large bloodsucking fly of tropical Africa belonging to the genus *Glossina*. Tsetse flies, which have slender forwardly projecting biting mouthparts, feed during the day on man and other mammals. They transmit the blood parasites that cause *sleeping sickness. *G. palpalis* and *G. tachinoides*, which are found along river banks, transmit *Trypanosoma gambiense*; *G. morsitans*, *G. swynnertoni*, and *G. pallidipes*, which are found in savannah country, transmit *T. rhodesiense*.

TSH *see* thyroid-stimulating hormone.

tsutsugamushi disease *see* scrub typhus.

tubal pregnancy (oviducal pregnancy) *see* ectopic pregnancy.

tube *n.* (in anatomy) a long hollow cylindrical structure, e.g. a *Fallopian tube.

tuber *n.* (in anatomy) a thickened or swollen part. The *tuber cinereum* is a part of the brain situated at the base of the hypothalamus, connected to the stalk of the pituitary gland.

tubercle *n.* **1.** (in anatomy) a small rounded protuberance on a bone. For example, there are two tubercles at the upper end of the humerus. **2.** the specific nodular lesion of *tuberculosis.

tubercular *adj.* having small rounded swellings or nodules, not necessarily caused by tuberculosis.

tuberculid *n.* a papular lesion in the skin, probably due to an allergic reaction to tuberculosis infection.

tuberculin *n.* a protein extract from cultures of tubercle bacilli, used to test whether a person has suffered from or been in contact with tuberculosis. In the *Mantoux test* a quantity of tuberculin is injected beneath the skin and a patch of inflammation appearing in the next 18–24 hours is regarded as a positive reaction, meaning that a degree of immunity is present.

tuberculoma *n.* a mass of cheeselike material resembling a tumour, seen in some cases of *tuberculosis. Tuberculomas are found in a variety of sites, including the lung or brain, and a single mass may be the only clinical evidence of disease. Treatment is by surgical excision, together with antituberculous drugs.

tuberculosis *n.* an infectious disease caused by the bacillus *Mycobacterium tuberculosis* (first identified by Koch in 1882) and characterized by the formation of nodular lesions (*tubercles*) in the tissues.

In *pulmonary tuberculosis* – formerly known as *consumption* and *phthisis* (wasting) – the bacillus is inhaled into the lungs where it sets up a primary tubercle and spreads to the nearest lymph nodes (the *primary complex*). Natural immune defences may heal it at this stage; alternatively the disease may smoulder for months or years and fluctuate with the patient's resistance. Many people become infected but show no symptoms. They can, however, act as carriers, transmitting the bacillus by coughing and sneezing. Symptoms of the active disease include fever, night sweats, weight loss, and the spitting of blood. In some cases the bacilli spread from the lungs to the bloodstream, setting up millions of tiny tubercles throughout the body (*miliary tuberculosis*), or migrate to the meninges to cause tuberculous *meningitis. Bacilli entering by the mouth, usually in infected cows' milk, set up a primary complex in abdominal lymph nodes, leading to *peritonitis, and sometimes spread to other organs, joints, and bones (*see* Pott's disease).

Tuberculosis is curable by the antibiotics streptomycin, isoniazid (INH), and para-aminosalicylic acid (PAS). Preventive measures in the UK include the detection of carriers by X-ray screening of vulnerable populations and inoculation with *BCG vaccine of those with no immunity to the disease (the *tuberculin test identifies which people require vaccination).

tuberose *see* tuberous.

tuberosity *n.* a large rounded protuberance on a bone. For example, there is a tuberosity at the upper end of the tibia.

tuberous (tuberose) *adj.* knobbed; having nodules or rounded swellings.

tuberous sclerosis (epiloia) a congenital disorder in which the brain, skin, and other organs are studded with small plaques or tumours. Symptoms include epilepsy and mental retardation.

tubo- *prefix denoting* a tube, especially a Fallopian tube or auditory tube (meatus).

tuboabdominal *adj.* relating to or occurring in a fallopian tube and the abdomen.

tubocurarine *n.* a drug given by intravenous injection to produce relaxation of voluntary muscles before surgery and in such conditions as tetanus, encephalitis, and poliomyelitis (*see* muscle relaxant). Toxic side-effects are usually only seen with overdosage, when respiratory failure due to paralysis of respiratory muscles may occur. Trade name: **Tubarine**.

tubo-ovarian *adj.* relating to or occurring in a Fallopian tube and an ovary.

tubotympanal *adj.* relating to the tympanic cavity and the *Eustachian tube.

tubule *n.* (in anatomy) a small cylindrical hollow structure. *See also* renal tubule, seminiferous tubule.

tularaemia (rabbit fever) *n.* a disease of rodents and rabbits, caused by the bacterium *Pasteurella tularense*, that is transmitted to man by deer flies (*see* Chrysops), by direct contact with infected animals, by contamination of wounds, or by drinking contaminated water. Symptoms include an ulcer at the site of infection, enlarged lymph nodes, headache, aching pains, loss of weight, and a fever lasting several weeks. Treatment with chlorampheni-

col, streptomycin, or tetracycline is effective.

tulle gras a soft dressing consisting of open-woven silk (or other material) impregnated with a waterproof soft paraffin wax.

tumbu fly a large non-bloodsucking fly, *Cordylobia anthropophaga*, widely distributed in tropical Africa. The female fly lays her eggs on ground contaminated with urine or excreta or on clothing tainted with sweat or urine. The maggots are normally parasites of rats, but if they come into contact with man they penetrate the skin, producing boil-like swellings (*see also* myiasis). The maggots can be gently eased out by applying oil to the swellings.

tumefaction *n.* the process in which a tissue becomes swollen and tense by accumulation within it of fluid under pressure.

tumescence *n.* a swelling, or the process of becoming swollen, usually because of an accumulation of blood or other fluid within the tissues.

tumid *adj.* swollen.

tumor *n.* swelling: one of the classical signs of *inflammation in a tissue, the other three being *calor (heat), *rubor (redness), and *dolor (pain). The swelling of an inflamed area is due to the leakage from small blood vessels of clear protein-containing fluid, which accumulates between the cells.

tumour *n.* any abnormal swelling in or on a part of the body. The term is usually applied to an abnormal growth of tissue, which may be *benign or *malignant. *Compare* cyst.

Tunga *n.* a genus of sand fleas found in tropical America and Africa. The fertilized female of *T. penetrans*, the chigoe or jigger, burrows beneath the skin of the foot, where it becomes enclosed in a swelling of the surrounding tissues and causes intense itching and inflammation. Surgical removal of the fleas is recommended.

tunica *n.* a covering or layer of an organ or part; for example, a layer of the wall of a blood vessel (*see* adventitia, intima, media). The *tunica albuginea* is a fibrous membrane comprising one of the covering tissues of the ovary, penis, and testis.

tunnel *n.* (in anatomy) a canal or hollow groove. *See also* carpal tunnel.

TUR (transurethral resection) *see* resection.

turbinate bone *see* nasal concha.

turbinectomy *n.* the surgical removal of one of the bones forming the nasal cavity (nasal conchae, or turbinate bones).

turgescence *n.* a swelling, or the process by which a swelling arises in tissues, usually by the accumulation of blood or other fluid under pressure.

turgor *n.* a state of being swollen or distended.

Turner's syndrome a genetic defect in women in which there is only one X chromosome instead of the usual two. Affected women are infertile: they have female external genitalia but no ovaries and therefore no menstrual periods (*see* amenorrhoea). Characteristically they are short, mentally retarded, and have a webbed neck; other developmental defects are common.

turricephaly *n. see* oxycephaly.

tussis *n.* the medical name for *coughing.

twilight state a condition of disturbed consciousness in which the individual can still carry out some normal activities but is impaired in his awareness and has no memory of what he has done. It is encountered after epileptic attacks, in alcoholism, and in organic states of confusion. It may be associated with other symptoms, such as physical and mental slowing, episodes of rage, and hallucinations. Twilight states last only for a short time. commonly a few hours.

twins *n.* two individuals who are born at the same time and of the same parents. *Fraternal* (or *dizygotic*) *twins* are the result of the simultaneous fertilization of two egg cells; they may be of different sexes and are no more alike than ordinary siblings. *Identical* (or *monozygotic*) *twins* result from the fertilization of a single egg cell that subsequently divides to give two separate fetuses. They are of the same sex and otherwise genetically identical; any differences in their appearance are due to environmental influences. *See also* Siamese twins.

tylosis *n.* the development of a callus on the skin (*see* callosity).

tympan- (tympano-) *prefix denoting* **1.** the eardrum. Example: *tympanectomy* (surgical excision of). **2.** the middle ear.

tympanic cavity *see* middle ear.

tympanic membrane (eardrum) the membrane at the inner end of the external auditory meatus, separating the outer and middle ears. It is formed from the outer wall of the lining of the tympanic cavity and the skin that lines the external auditory meatus. When sound waves reach the ear the tympanum vibrates, transmitting these vibrations to the malleus – one of the auditory *ossicles in the middle ear – to which it is attached.

tympanites (meteorism) *n.* distension of the abdomen with air or gas: the abdomen is resonant (drumlike) on *percussion. Causes include intestinal obstruction, *irritable bowel syndrome, and *aerophagy.

tympanoplasty *n. see* myringoplasty.

tympanotomy *n. see* myringotomy.

tympanum *n.* the *middle ear (tympanic cavity) and/or the eardrum (*tympanic membrane).

typhlitis *n.* inflammation of the caecum: formerly a common diagnosis of the condition now recognised as appendicitis.

typhlosis *n.* an obsolete term for *blindness.

typho- *prefix denoting* 1. typhoid fever. 2. typhus.

typhoid fever an infection of the digestive system by the bacterium *Salmonella typhi*, causing general weakness, high fever, a rash of red spots on the chest and abdomen, chills, sweating, and in serious cases inflammation of the spleen and bones, delirium, and erosion of the intestinal wall leading to haemorrhage. It is transmitted through food or drinking water contaminated by the faeces or urine of patients or carriers. In most cases recovery occurs naturally but treatment with ampicillin or chloramphenicol reduces the severity of symptoms. Vaccination with *TAB provides temporary immunity. *Compare* paratyphoid fever.

typhus (spotted fever) *n.* any one of a group of infections caused by *rickettsiae and characterized by severe headache, a widespread rash, prolonged high fever, and delirium. They all respond to treatment with chloramphenicol or tetracyclines. *Epidemic typhus* (also known as *classical* or *louse-borne typhus*) is caused by infection with *Rickettsia prowazeki* transmitted by lice. It was formerly very prevalent in overcrowded insanitary conditions (as during wars and famines), with a mortality rate approaching 100%. *Endemic typhus* (*murine* or *flea-borne typhus*) is a disease of rats due to *Rickettsia mooseri*; it can be transmitted to man by rat fleas, causing a mild typhus fever. There are in addition several kinds of *tick typhus* (in which the rickettsiae are transmitted by ticks), including *Rocky Mountain spotted fever, and typhus transmitted by mites (*see* rickettsial pox, scrub typhus).

tyramine *n.* an amine naturally occurring in cheese. It has a similar effect in the body to that of *adrenaline. This effect can be dangerous in patients taking *MAO inhibitors (antidepressants), in whom blood pressure may become very high. Cheese is therefore not advised when such drugs are prescribed.

Tyroglyphus *n. see* Acarus.

tyrosine *n. see* amino acid.

tyrosinosis *n.* an inborn defect of metabolism of the amino acid tyrosine causing excess excretion of parahydroxyphenylpyruvic acid in the urine, giving it abnormal reducing power.

tyrothricin *n.* an *antibiotic derived from the bacterium *Bacillus brevis*. It is used, alone or in combination with other drugs, mainly in the treatment of infections of the mouth, throat, skin, wounds and burns; it is applied topically as it is very toxic if taken into the body. Trade name: **Hydrotricine**.

U

ubiquinone *n.* a *coenzyme that acts as an electron transfer agent in the mitochondria of cells (*see* electron transport chain).

ulcer *n.* a break in the skin or in the mucous membrane lining the alimentary tract that fails to heal and is often accompanied by inflammation. Ulcers in the skin include *varicose ulcers* complicating *varicose veins, due to defective circulation; *bedsores (decubitus ulcers), due to pressure; and *rodent ulcers, due to malignant growth. For ulcers of the alimentary tract, *see*

ulcerative colitis

aphtha, duodenal ulcer, gastric ulcer, peptic ulcer.

ulcerative colitis inflammation and ulceration of the colon and rectum. *See* colitis.

ulcerative gingivitis acute painful gingivitis with ulceration, in which the tissues of the gums are rapidly destroyed. Occurring mainly in debilitated patients, it is associated with anaerobic microorganisms (*see* Borrelia, Fusobacterium) and is accompanied by an unpleasant odour. Treatment is with *metronidazole and a careful and thorough regime of oral hygiene supplemented with oxidizing mouthwashes. In the past ulcerative gingivitis has been called *Vincent's angina*; in its severe form it is known as *noma.

ule- (ulo-) *prefix denoting* **1.** scars; scar tissue. **2.** the gums.

ulna *n.* the inner and longer bone of the forearm (see illustration). It articulates with the humerus and radius above and with the radius and indirectly with the wrist bones below. At its upper end is the *olecranon process and *coronoid process; at the lower end is a cone-shaped *styloid process*. —**ulnar** *adj.*

ulnar artery a branch of the brachial artery arising at the elbow and running deep within the muscles of the medial side of the forearm. It passes into the palm of the hand, where it unites with the arch of the radial artery and gives off branches to the hand and fingers.

ulnar nerve one of the major nerves of the arm. It originates in the neck, from spinal roots of the last cervical and first thoracic divisions, and runs down the inner side of the upper arm to behind the elbow. In the forearm it supplies the muscles with motor nerves; lower down it divides into several branches that supply the skin of the palm and fourth and fifth fingers.

Right ulna and radius (front view)

ultra- *prefix denoting* **1.** beyond. **2.** an extreme degree (e.g. of large or small size).

ultracentrifuge *n.* a *centrifuge that works at extremely high speeds of rotation: used for separating large molecules, such as proteins.

ultrafiltration *n.* filtration under pressure. In the kidney, blood is subjected to ultrafiltration to remove the unwanted water, urea, and other waste material that goes to make up urine.

ultramicroscope *n.* a microscope for examining particles suspended in a gas or liquid under intense illumination from one side. Light is scattered or reflected from the particles, which can be seen through the eyepiece as bright objects against a dark background.

ultramicrotome *n.* an instrument for cutting extremely thin sections of tissue (not more than 0.1 μm thick) for electron microscopy. *See also* microtome.

ultrasonics *n.* the study of the uses and properties of sound waves of very high frequency (*see* ultrasound). —**ultrasonic** *adj.*

ultrasonography *n.* the use of *ultrasound to produce pictures of structures within the body.

ultrasonotomography (**echotomography**) *n.* the use of *ultrasound to examine the internal structure of the body by producing images of the reflections from different depths. A picture of the structures within a 'slice' of the body can be built up, much in the same way as X-rays can be employed to produce a tomogram (*see* tomography).

ultrasound (**ultrasonic waves**) *n.* sound waves of extremely high frequency (above 20,000 Hz), inaudible to the human ear. Ultrasound can be used to examine the structure of the inside of the body, in the same way that X-rays can be used to build up pictures but with the advantages that the patient is not submitted to potentially harmful radiation and that structures not opaque to X-rays can be seen. The vibratory effect of these sound waves can also be used in the treatment of various disorders of deep tissues, and even to break up stones in the kidney or elsewhere. *See also* echography.

ultraviolet rays invisible short-wavelength radiation beyond the violet end of the visible spectrum. Sunlight contains ultraviolet rays, which are responsible for the production of both suntan and – on overexposure – sunburn. The dust and gases of the earth's atmosphere absorb most of the ultraviolet rays in sunlight (*see* ozone). If this did not happen, the intense ultraviolet radiation from the sun would be lethal to living organisms.

umbilical cord the strand of tissue connecting the fetus to the placenta. It contains two arteries that carry blood to the placenta and one vein that returns it to the fetus. It also contains remnants of the *allantois and *yolk sac and becomes ensheathed by the *amnion.

umbilicus (**omphalus**) *n.* the navel: a circular depression in the centre of the abdomen marking the site of attachment of the *umbilical cord in the fetus. —**umbilical** *adj.*

umbo *n.* a projecting centre of a round surface, especially the projection of the inner surface of the eardrum to which the malleus is attached.

unciform bone *see* hamate bone.

uncinate fits a form of temporal lobe *epilepsy in which hallucinations of taste and smell and inappropriate chewing movements are prominent features.

unconscious *adj.* **1.** in a state of unconsciousness. **2.** describing mental processes of which a person is not aware. **3.** (in psychoanalysis) denoting the part of the mind that includes memories, motives and intentions that are not accessible to awareness and cannot be made conscious without overcoming resistances. *Compare* subconscious.

unconsciousness *n.* a condition of being unaware of one's surroundings, as in sleep, or of being unresponsive to stimulation. An unnatural state of unconsciousness may be caused by factors that produce reduced brain activity, such as lack of oxygen, a blow on the head, poisoning, blood loss, and many diseases, or it may be brought about deliberately during general *anaesthesia. *See also* coma.

uncus *n.* any hook-shaped structure, especially a projection of the lower surface of the cerebral hemisphere that is composed of cortex belonging to the temporal lobe.

undecenoic acid an antifungal agent, applied to the skin in the form of powder, ointment, lotion, or aerosol spray for the treatment of such infections as athlete's foot. Trade name: **Mycota**.

undine *n.* a small rounded container, usually made of glass, for solutions used to wash out the eye. It has a small neck for filling and a long tapering spout with a narrow outlet to deliver a fine stream of fluid to the eye.

undulant fever *see* brucellosis.

ungual *adj.* relating to the fingernails or toenails (ungues).

unguentum (in pharmacy) *n.* an ointment.

unguis *n.* a fingernail or toenail. *See* nail.

uni- *prefix denoting* one.

unicellular *adj.* describing organisms or tissues that consist of a single cell. Unicellular organisms include the Protozoa, most bacteria, and some fungi.

unigravida *n. see* primigravida.

unilateral *adj.* (in anatomy) relating to or affecting one side of the body or one side of an organ or other part.

union *n.* (in a fractured bone) the successful result of healing of a fracture, in which the previously separated bone ends have become firmly united by newly formed bone. Failure of union (*non-union*) may result if the bone ends are not immobilized or from infection or bone diseases. *Compare* malunion.

unipara *n. see* primipara.

unipolar *adj.* (in neurology) describing a neurone that has one main process extending from the cell body. *Compare* bipolar.

urachus *n.* the remains of the cavity of the *allantois, which usually disappears during embryonic development. In the adult it normally exists in the form of a solid fibrous cord connecting the bladder with the umbilicus, but it may persist abnormally as a patent duct. —**urachal** *adj.*

uracil *n.* one of the nitrogen-containing bases (*see* pyrimidine) occurring in the nucleic acid RNA.

uraemia *n.* the presence of excessive amounts of urea and other nitrogenous waste compounds in the blood. These waste products are normally excreted by the kidneys in urine; their accumulation in the blood occurs in kidney failure and results in nausea, vomiting, lethargy, drowsiness, and eventually (if untreated) death. Treatment may require *haemodialysis on a kidney machine. —**uraemic** *adj.*

uramustine *n.* a *cytotoxic drug used in the treatment of various forms of cancer, particularly chronic lymphatic leukaemia. It is administered by intravenous injection and is highly toxic; common side-effects are nausea, vomiting and diarrhoea, and depression of bone marrow function. Trade name: **Uracil Mustard**.

uran- (urano-) *prefix denoting* the palate.

uraniscorrhaphy *n. see* staphylorrhaphy.

uranism *n.* lead poisoning. *See* lead¹.

urataemia *n.* the presence in the blood of sodium urate and other urates, formed by the reaction of uric acid with bases. In *gout, urataemia leads to deposition of urates in various parts of the body.

uraturia *n.* the presence in the urine of urates (salts of uric acid). Abnormally high concentrations of urates in urine occur in *gout.

urea *n.* the main breakdown product of protein metabolism. It is the chemical form in which unrequired nitrogen is excreted by the body in the urine. Urea is formed in the liver from ammonia and carbon dioxide in a series of enzyme-mediated reactions (the *urea cycle*). Accumulation of urea in the bloodstream together with other nitrogenous compounds is due to kidney failure and gives rise to *uraemia.

urease *n.* an enzyme that catalyses the hydrolysis of urea to ammonia and carbon dioxide.

urecchysis *n.* the escape of uric acid from the blood into spaces in the connective tissue.

ureter *n.* either of a pair of tubes, 25–30 cm long, that conduct urine from the pelvis of kidneys to the bladder. The walls of the ureters contain thick layers of smooth muscle, which contract to force urine into the bladder, between an outer fibrous coat and an inner mucous layer. —**ureteral, ureteric** *adj.*

ureter- (uretero-) *prefix denoting* the ureter(s). Example: *ureterovaginal* (relating to the ureters and vagina).

ureterectomy *n.* surgical removal of a ureter. This usually includes removal of the associated kidney as well (*see* nephroureterectomy). If previous nephrectomy has been performed to remove a kidney destroyed by *vesicoureteric reflux or because of a tumour of the renal pelvis, subsequent ureterectomy may be necessary to cure reflux into the stump of the ureter or tumour in the ureter, respectively.

ureteritis *n.* inflammation of the ureter. This usually occurs in association with inflammation of the bladder (*see* cystitis), particularly if caused by *vesicoureteric reflux. Tuberculosis of the urinary tract can also cause ureteritis, which progresses to *stricture formation.

ureterocele *n.* a cystic swelling of the wall of the ureter at the point where it passes into the bladder. It is associated with stenosis of the opening of the ureter and it may cause impaired drainage of the kidney with dilatation of the ureter and *hydronephrosis. If urinary obstruction is present, the ureterocele should be dealt with surgically.

ureteroenterostomy *n.* an artificial communication, surgically created, between the ureter and the bowel. In this form of urinary diversion, which bypasses the bladder, the ureters are attached to the sigmoid colon (*see* ureterosigmoidostomy).

ureterolithotomy *n.* the surgical removal of a stone from the ureter (*see* calculus). The operative approach depends upon the position of the stone within the ureter. If the stone occupies the lower portion of the ureter, it may be extracted by *cystoscopy, thus avoiding open surgery.

ureteroneocystostomy *n.* the surgical reimplantation of a ureter into the bladder. This is most commonly performed to cure *vesicoureteric reflux. The ureter is reimplanted obliquely through the bladder wall to act as a valve and prevent subsequent reflux. The operation is usually referred to as an *antireflux procedure* or simply *reimplantation of ureter*.

ureteronephrectomy *n. see* nephroureterectomy.

ureteroplasty *n.* surgical reconstruction of the ureter using a segment of bowel or a tube of bladder (*Boari flap*). This is necessary if a segment of ureter is damaged by disease or injury.

ureteropyelonephritis *n.* inflammation involving both the ureter and the renal pelvis (*see* ureteritis, pyelitis).

ureterosigmoidostomy *n.* the operation of implanting the ureters into the sigmoid colon (*see* ureterenterostomy).

This method of permanent urinary diversion may be used after *cystectomy or to bypass a diseased or damaged bladder. The urine is passed together with the faeces, and continence depends upon a normal anal sphincter. The main advantage of this form of diversion is the avoidance of an external opening and appliance to collect the urine; the disadvantages include possible kidney infection and acidosis.

ureterostomy *n.* the surgical creation of an external opening into the ureter. This usually involves bringing the ureter to the skin surface so that the urine can drain into a suitable appliance (*cutaneous ureterostomy*). The divided dilated ureter can be brought through the skin to form a spout, but ureters of a normal size need to be implanted into a segment of bowel used for this purpose (*see* ileal conduit) to avoid narrowing and obstruction.

ureterotomy *n.* surgical incision into the ureter. The commonest reason for performing this is to allow removal of a stone (*see* ureterolithotomy).

urethr- (urethro-) *prefix denoting* the urethra.

urethra *n.* the tube that conducts urine from the bladder to the exterior. The female urethra is quite short (about 3.5 cm) and opens just within the *vulva, between the clitoris and vagina. The male urethra is longer (about 20 cm) and runs through the penis. As well as urine, it receives the secretions of the male accessory sex glands (prostate and Cowper's glands and seminal vesicles) and spermatozoa from the *vas deferens; thus it also serves as the ejaculatory duct.

urethritis *n.* inflammation of the urethra. This may be due to gonorrhoea (*specific urethritis*), a nonspecific venereal infection (*nonspecific urethritis*), or to the presence of a catheter in the urethra. The symptoms are those of urethral discharge with painful or difficult urination (*dysuria). Treatment of urethritis due to infection is by administration of appropriate antibiotics after the causative organisms have been isolated from the discharge. Untreated or severe urethritis results in a urethral *stricture.

urethrocele *n.* **1.** a pouch formed from a weakened portion of the wall of the *urethra that encroaches on the vaginal canal. It may result from infection or from the pressure of the fetal head in prolonged labour. **2.** downward displacement (prolapse) of the female urethra through its external opening.

urethrography *n.* X-ray examination of the urethra, after introduction of a *radio-opaque fluid, so that its outline and any narrowing or other abnormalities may be observed in X-ray photographs (*urethrograms*). In *ascending urethrography* a radio-opaque jelly is injected up the urethra using a special syringe and penile clamp. In *descending urethrography* (*micturating cystourethrography, MCUG*), X-rays of the urethra can be taken during the passing of water-soluble contrast material previously inserted into the bladder.

urethroplasty *n.* surgical repair of a urethral *stricture. The operation entails the insertion of a flap or patch of skin from the scrotum or perineum into the urethra at the site of the stricture, which is laid widely open. The operation can be performed in one stage, although two stages are usual in the reconstruction of a posterior urethral stricture (*see* urethrostomy).

urethrorrhaphy *n.* surgical restoration of the continuity of the urethra. This may be required following laceration of the urethra.

urethrorrhoea *n.* a discharge from the urethra. This is a symptom of *urethritis.

urethroscope *n.* an *endoscope, consisting of a fine tube fitted with a light and lenses, for examination of the interior of the male urethra, including the prostate region. —**urethroscopy** *n.*

urethrostenosis *n.* a *stricture of the urethra.

urethrostomy *n.* the operation of creating an opening of the urethra in the perineum in men. This can be permanent, to bypass a severe *stricture of the urethra in the penis, or it can form the first stage of an operation to cure a stricture of the posterior section of the urethra (*urethroplasty).

urethrotomy *n.* the operation of cutting a *stricture in the urethra. It is usually performed with a *urethrotome*. This instrument, a type of *endoscope, consists of a sheath down which is passed a fine knife, which is operated by the surgeon viewing the stricture down an illuminated telescope.

-uria *suffix denoting* 1. a condition of urine or urination. Example: *polyuria* (passage of excess urine). 2. the presence of a specified substance in the urine. Example: *haematuria* (blood in).

uric acid a nitrogen-containing organic acid that is the end-product of nucleic acid metabolism and is a component of the urine. Crystals of uric acid are deposited in the joints of people suffering from *gout.

uricosuric drug a drug, such as *probenecid or *sulphinpyrazone, that increases the amount of *uric acid excreted in the urine. Uricosuric drugs are used to treat gout and other conditions in which the levels of uric acid in the blood are increased, as during treatment with some *diuretics. Uricosuric drugs are sometimes administered with certain antibiotics (such as penicillin) to maintain high blood levels since they inhibit their excretion.

uridine *n.* a compound containing uracil and the sugar ribose. *See also* nucleoside.

uridrosis *n.* the presence of excessive amounts of urea in the sweat; when the sweat dries, a white flaky deposit of urea may remain on the skin. The phenomenon occurs in *uraemia.

urin- (urino-, uro-) *prefix denoting* urine or the urinary system.

urinalysis *n.* the analysis of *urine, using physical, chemical and microscopical tests, to determine the proportions of its normal constituents and to detect alcohol, drugs, sugar, or other abnormal constituents.

urinary bladder *see* bladder.

urinary tract the entire system of ducts and channels that conduct urine from the kidneys to the exterior. It includes the ureters, the bladder, and the urethra.

urination (micturition) *n.* the periodic discharge of urine from the bladder through the urethra. It is initiated by voluntary relaxation of the sphincter muscle below the bladder and maintained by reflex contraction of the muscles of the bladder wall.

urine *n.* the fluid excreted by the kidneys, which contains many of the body's waste products. It is the major route by which the end-products of nitrogen metabolism – *urea, *uric acid, and *creatinine – are excreted. The other major constituent is sodium chloride. Over 100 other substances are usually present, but only in trace amounts. Biochemical analysis of urine is commonly used in the diagnosis of diseases (for example, there are high levels of urinary glucose in diabetes and of ketone bodies in ketonuria) and in *pregnancy tests.

uriniferous tubule *see* renal tubule.

urinogenital (urogenital) *adj.* of or relating to the organs and tissues concerned with excretion and reproduction, which are anatomically closely associated.

urinogenital sinus the duct in the embryo that receives the ureter and mesonephric and paramesonephric ducts and opens to the exterior. The innermost portion forms most of the bladder and the remainder forms the urethra with its associated glands. Part of it may also contribute towards the vagina.

urinometer *n.* a hydrometer for measuring the specific gravity of urine.

urobilinogen *n.* a colourless product of the reduction of the *bile pigment bilirubin. Urobilinogen is formed from bilirubin in the intestine by bacterial action. Part of it is reabsorbed and returned to the liver; part of it is excreted in the faeces (a trace may also appear in the urine). When exposed to air, urobilinogen is oxidized to a brown pigment, *urobilin*.

urocele *n.* a cystic swelling in the scrotum, containing urine that has escaped from the urethra. This may arise following urethral injury. Immediate treatment is to divert the urine by suprapubic *cystotomy, local drainage of the swelling, and antibiotic administration.

urochesia *n.* the passage of urine through the rectum. This may follow a penetrating injury involving both the lower urinary tract and the bowel.

urogenital *adj.* *see* urinogenital.

urography *n.* *see* pyelography.

urolith *n.* a stone in the urinary tract. *See* calculus.

urology *n.* the branch of medicine concerned with the study and treatment of diseases of the urinary tract. —**urological** *adj.* —**urologist** *n.*

uroporphyrin *n.* a porphyrin that plays an intermediate role in the synthesis of *protoporphyrin IX. It is excreted in significant amounts in the urine in porphyria.

urticaria (hives, nettle rash) *n.* an acute or chronic allergic reaction in which red round wheals develop on the skin, ranging in size from small spots to several inches across. These itch intensely and may last for hours or days; the cause is sensitivity to certain foods, such as shellfish or strawberries. Sometimes urticaria may affect areas other than the skin, causing swelling on the tongue and lips: this serious variety, *angioneurotic oedema*, needs urgent medical attention.

uter- (utero-) *prefix denoting* the womb (uterus). Examples: *uterocervical* (relating to the cervix (neck) of the womb); *uterovaginal* (relating to the womb and vagina); *uterovesical* (relating to the womb and bladder).

uterine *adj.* of or relating to the womb (uterus).

uterocele *n.* *see* hysterocele.

uterogestation *n.* the development of a fetus in the womb, i.e. a normal pregnancy. *Compare* ectopic pregnancy.

uterography *n.* *radiography of the womb.

utero-ovarian *adj.* relating to or occurring in the womb and an ovary.

uterosalpingography (hysterosalpingography) *n.* *radiography of the interior of the womb and the Fallopian tubes following injection of a *radio-opaque fluid.

uterus (womb) *n.* the part of the female reproductive tract that is specialized to allow the embryo to become implanted in its inner wall and to nourish the growing fetus from the maternal blood. The nonpregnant uterus is a pear-shaped organ, about 7.5 cm long. It is suspended in the pelvic cavity by means of peritoneal folds (ligaments) and fibrous bands. The upper part is connected to the two *Fallopian tubes and the lower part joins the vagina at the cervix. The uterus has an inner mucous lining (*endometrium) and a thick wall of smooth muscle (*myometrium). During childbirth the myometrium undergoes strong contractions to expel the fetus through the cervix and vagina. In the absence of pregnancy the endometrium undergoes periodic development and degeneration (*see* menstrual cycle). —**uterine** *adj.*

utricle (utriculus) *n.* **1.** the larger of the two membranous sacs within the vestibule of the ear: it forms part of the membranous *labyrinth. It is filled with fluid (endolymph) and contains a *macula. This responds to gravity and relays information to the brain about the position of the head. **2.** a small sac (the *prostatic utricle*) extending out of the urethra of the male into the substance of the prostate gland.

uvea (uveal tract) *n.* the vascular pigmented layer of the eye, which lies beneath the outer layer (sclera). It consists of the *choroid, *ciliary body, and *iris. —**uveal** *adj.*

uveal tract *see* uvea.

uveitis *n.* inflammation of any part of the uveal tract of the eye, either the iris (*iritis*), ciliary body (*cyclitis*), or choroid (*choroiditis*). Inflammation confined to the iris and ciliary body, which are commonly inflamed together, is called *anterior uveitis*; that confined to the choroid is termed *posterior uveitis*. In general, the causes of anterior and posterior uveitis are different; anterior uveitis (unlike choroiditis) is usually painful. All types may lead to visual impairment, and uveitis is an important cause of blindness. In most cases the disease appears to originate in the uveal

tract itself, but it may occur secondarily to disease of other parts of the eye, particularly of the cornea and sclera. Treatment consists of the use of drugs that suppress the inflammation, combined with measures to relieve the discomfort and more specific drug treatment if a specific cause of the uveitis is found. The drugs may be given as drops, injections, or tablets, often in combination.

uveoparotitis (uveoparotid fever) *n.* inflammation of the iris, ciliary body, and choroid regions of the eye (the uvea) and swelling of the parotid salivary gland: one of the more common varieties of the chronic disease *sarcoidosis.

uvula *n.* a small soft extension of the soft palate that hangs from the roof of the mouth above the root of the tongue. It is composed of muscle, connective tissue, and mucous membrane.

uvulectomy *n.* surgical removal of the uvula.

uvulitis *n.* inflammation of the uvula.

V

vaccination *n.* a means of producing immunity to a disease by using a *vaccine, or a special preparation of antigenic material, to stimulate the formation of appropriate antibodies. The name was applied originally only to treatment with vaccinia (cowpox) virus, which gives protection not only against cowpox itself but also against the related smallpox. However, it is now used synonymously with *inoculation* as a method of *immunization against any disease. Vaccination is often carried out in two or three stages, as separate doses are less likely to cause unpleasant side-effects. A vaccine is usually given by injection but may be introduced into the skin through light scratches; for some diseases, oral vaccines are available.

vaccine *n.* a special preparation of antigenic material that can be used to stimulate the development of antibodies and thus confer active *immunity against a specific disease or number of diseases. Many vaccines are produced by culturing bacteria or viruses under conditions that lead to a loss of their virulence but not of their antigenic nature. Other vaccines consist of specially treated toxins (*toxoids) or of dead bacteria that are still antigenic. Examples of live but attenuated (weakened) organisms in vaccines are those against tuberculosis, rabies, and smallpox. Dead organisms are used against cholera and typhoid; precipitated toxoids are used against diphtheria and tetanus. *See* immunization.

vaccinia *n. see* cowpox.

vaccinoid *adj.* resembling a local infection with vaccinia (cowpox) virus. A vaccinoid reaction is one of the possible results of vaccination against smallpox in individuals who already have partial immunity. The swelling, reddening, and blistering are considerably less than the so-called primary reaction that occurs after the inoculation of a person with no immunity against smallpox.

vacuole *n.* a space within the cytoplasm of a cell, formed by infolding of the cell membrane, that contains material taken in by the cell. White blood cells form vacuoles when they surround and digest bacteria and other foreign material.

vacuum extractor a suction cup that can be attached to the head of a fetus in order to aid delivery.

vagin- (vagino-) *prefix denoting* the vagina.

vagina *n.* the lower part of the female reproductive tract: a muscular tube, lined with mucous membrane, connecting the cervix of the uterus (womb) to the exterior. It receives the erect penis during coitus: semen is ejaculated into the upper part of the vagina and from there the sperms must pass through the cervix and womb in order to fertilize an ovum in the Fallopian tube. The wall of the vagina is sufficiently elastic to allow the passage of the newborn child. —**vaginal** *adj.*

vaginismus *n.* sudden and painful contraction of the muscles surrounding the vagina, usually in response to the *vulva or vagina being touched. Sexual intercourse may be impeded, and the condition may be associated with fear of or aversion to coitus. Other causative factors include vaginal injury or ulceration, dryness or shrinkage of the lining membrane of the vagina, and inflammation of the vagina or bladder. *See also* dyspareunia.

vaginitis *n.* inflammation of the vagina, which may be caused by infection (commonly with *Trichomonas vaginalis*), ill-fitting contraceptive devices, dietary deficiency, or poor hygiene. There is often irritation, increased vaginal discharge, and pain on passing urine. Vaginitis may indicate the presence of venereal disease. *Postmenopausal vaginitis* is caused by a deficiency of female sex hormones.

vaginoplasty (colpoplasty) *n.* a tissue-grafting operation on the vagina.

vaginoscope *n. see* colposcope.

vago- *prefix denoting* the vagus nerve.

vagotomy *n.* the surgical cutting of any of the branches of the vagus nerve. This is usually performed to reduce secretion of acid and pepsin by the stomach in order to cure a peptic ulcer. *Truncal vagotomy* is the cutting of the main trunks of the vagus nerve; in *selective vagotomy* the branches of the nerve to the gall bladder and pancreas are left intact. *Highly selective* or *proximal va-*

gotomy is the cutting of the branches of the vagus nerve to the body of the stomach, leaving the branches to the outlet (pylorus) intact: this makes additional surgery to permit emptying of the stomach contents unnecessary.

vagus nerve the tenth *cranial nerve (X), which supplies motor nerve fibres to the muscles of swallowing and parasympathetic fibres to the heart and organs of the chest cavity and abdomen. Sensory branches of the vagus carry impulses from the viscera and the sensation of taste from the mouth.

valgus *adj.* describing any deformity that displaces the hand or foot away from the midline. *See* club-foot (talipes valgus), knock knee (genu valgum).

validity *n.* an indication of the extent to which a clinical sign or test is a true indicator of disease. Reduced validity can arise if the tests produce different results when conducted several times on the same person under identical conditions (i.e. *reduced reproducibility*, *reliability*, or *repeatability*). This may be because the same observer gets different results on successive occasions (*intraobserver error*) or because a series of different observers fail to obtain the same result (*interobserver error*). Such errors may arise because of a true difference in observation and/or interpretation or because of a preconceived notion (often unconscious) by the observer, which influences either his judgment or the tone and manner with which he questions the patient. *Compare* intervention study.

valine *n.* an *essential amino acid. *See also* amino acid.

Valium *n. see* diazepam.

vallecula *n.* a furrow or depression in an organ or other part. On the undersurface of the cerebellum a vallecula separates the two hemispheres.

valve *n.* a structure found in some tubular organs or parts that restricts the flow of fluid within them to one direction only. Valves are important structures in the heart, veins, and lymphatic vessels. Such a valve consists of two or three *cusps fastened like pockets to the walls of the vessel. Blood flowing in the right direction flattens the cusps to the walls, but when flow is reversed the cusps become filled with blood or lymph and dilate to block the opening (see illustration). *See also* mitral valve, tricuspid valve, semilunar valve.

(A) cut vein showing the two cusps of a valve;
(B) action of a venous valve

valvotomy (valvulotomy) *n.* surgical cutting through a valve. The term is usually used to describe the operation to relieve obstruction caused by stenosed valves in the heart.

valvula *n.* (*pl.* **valvulae**) a small valve. The *valvulae conniventes* are circular folds of mucous membrane in the small intestine.

valvulitis *n.* inflammation of one or more valves, particularly the heart valves. This may be acute or chronic and is most often due to rheumatic fever (*see* endocarditis).

vancomycin *n.* an *antibiotic, derived from the bacterium *Streptomyces orientalis*, that is effective against most Gram-positive organisms (e.g. streptococci and staphylococci). It is given by intravenous infusion for infections due to strains that are resistant to other antibiotics. It usually has a low toxicity but may cause deafness or thrombophlebitis. Trade name: **Vancocin**.

van den Bergh's test a test to determine whether jaundice in a patient is due to *haemolysis or to disease of the liver or bile duct. A sample of serum is mixed with sulphanilic acid, hydrochloric acid, and sodium nitrite. The immediate appearance of a violet colour is called a *direct reaction* and indicates that the jaundice is due to liver damage or obstruction of the bile duct. If the colour appears only when alcohol is added, this is an *indirect reaction* and points to haemolytic jaundice.

vaporizer *n.* a piece of equipment for producing an extremely fine mist of liquid droplets by forcing a jet of liquid through a narrow nozzle with a jet of air. Vaporizers are used to produce aerosols of various medications for use in inhalation therapy.

Vaquez-Osler disease *see* polycythaemia vera.

variable *n.* (in biostatistics) a characteristic (e.g. morbidity, life style, or habit) relating to a single individual or group. *Qualitative variables* are descriptive characteristics, such as sex, race, or occupation; *quantitative variables* relate to a numerical scale and are subdivided into *discrete variables*, found only at fixed points (e.g. number of children), and *continuous variables*, found at any point on a scale (e.g. weight).

variance *n.* *see* standard deviation.

varicectomy *n.* *see* phlebectomy.

varicella *n.* *see* chickenpox.

varices *pl. n.* *see* varix.

varicocele *n.* a collection of dilated veins in the spermatic cord, more commonly affecting the left side of the scrotum than the right. It usually produces no symptoms apart from occasional aching discomfort. In some cases varicocele is associated with a poor sperm count (*see* oligospermia) sufficient to cause infertility. Surgical correction of the varicocele in such patients (*varicocelectomy*) usually results in a considerable improvement in the quality and motility of the sperm.

varicose veins veins that are distended, lengthened, and tortuous. The superficial veins (saphenous veins) of the legs are most commonly affected; other sites include the rectum (*haemorrhoids) and testes (*varicocele). There is an inherited tendency to varicose veins but obstruction to blood flow is responsible in some cases. Complications including thrombosis, *phlebitis, and haemorrhage may occur. Treatment includes elastic support and *sclerotherapy, but *avulsion (stripping) or excision (*phlebectomy) is required in some cases.

varicotomy *n.* incision into a varicose vein (*see* phlebectomy).

variola *n.* *see* smallpox.

varioloid 1. *n.* a mild form of smallpox in people who have previously had smallpox or have been vaccinated against it. **2.** *adj.* resembling smallpox.

varix *n.* (*pl.* **varices**) a single varicose vein.

varus *adj.* describing any deformity that displaces the hand or foot towards the midline. *See* bowleg (genu varum), club-foot (talipes varus).

vas *n.* (*pl.* **vasa**) a vessel or duct.

vas- (vaso-) *prefix denoting* **1.** vessels, especially blood vessels. **2.** the vas deferens.

vasa efferentia (*sing.* **vas efferens**) the many small tubes that conduct spermatozoa from the testis to the epididymis. They are derived from some of the excretory tubules of the embryonic *mesonephros.

vasa vasorum *pl. n.* the tiny arteries and veins that supply the walls of blood vessels.

vascular *adj.* relating to or supplied with blood vessels.

vascularization *n.* the development of blood vessels (usually capillaries) within a tissue.

vascular system *see* cardiovascular system.

vasculitis *n. see* angiitis.

vas deferens (*pl.* **vasa deferentia**) either of a pair of ducts that conduct spermatozoa from the *epididymis to the *urethra on ejaculation. It has a thick muscular wall the contraction of which assists in ejaculation.

vasectomy *n.* the surgical operation of cutting the duct (vas deferens) connecting the testis to the seminal vesicle and urethra. Vasectomy of both ducts causes sterility and is an increasingly popular means of birth control. Vasectomy does not affect sexual desire or potency.

vaso- *prefix. see* vas-.

vasoactive *adj.* affecting the diameter of blood vessels, especially arteries. Examples of vasoactive agents are emotion, pressure, carbon dioxide, and temperature. Some exert their effect directly, others via the *vasomotor centre in the brain.

vasoconstriction *n.* a decrease in the diameter of blood vessels, especially arteries. This results from activation of the *vasomotor centre in the brain, which brings about contraction of muscular walls of the arteries and hence an increase in blood pressure.

vasoconstrictor *n.* an agent that causes narrowing of the blood vessels and therefore a decrease in blood flow. Examples are *cyclopentamine, *methoxamine, and *phenylephrine. Vasoconstrictors are used to raise the blood pressure in disorders of the circulation, shock, or severe bleeding and to maintain blood pressure during surgery. Some vasoconstrictors (e.g. *xylometazoline) have a rapid effect when applied to mucous membranes and may be used to relieve nasal congestion. If the blood pressure rises too quickly headache and vomiting may occur. A vasoconstrictor is often added to local anaesthetic solutions used in dentistry to prolong their effectiveness.

vasodilatation *n.* an increase in the diameter of blood vessels, especially arteries. This results from activation of the *vasomotor centre in the brain, which brings about relaxation of the arterial walls and a consequent lowering of blood pressure.

vasodilator *n.* a drug that causes widening of the blood vessels and therefore an increase in blood flow. Vasodilators are used to lower blood pressure in cases of hypertension. *Coronary vasodilators*, such as *glyceryl trinitrate and *pentaerithrytol, increase the blood flow through the heart and are used to relieve and prevent angina. Large doses of coronary vasodilators cause such side-effects as flushing of the face, severe headache, and fainting. *Peripheral vasodilators*, such as *cyclandelate, *phenoxybenzamine, and *tolazoline, affect the blood vessels of the limbs and are used to treat conditions of poor circulation such as acrocyanosis, chilblains, and Raynaud's disease.

vaso-epididymostomy *n.* the operation of joining the vas deferens to the epididymis in a side-to-side manner in order to bypass an obstruction to the passage of sperm from the testis. The obstruction, which may be congenital or acquired, is usually present in the mid-portion or tail of the epididymis. Vaso-epididymostomy is therefore usually performed by anastomosing the head of the epididymis to a longitudinal incision in the lumen of the adjacent vas.

vasoligation *n.* the surgical tying of the vas deferens (the duct conveying sperm from the testis). This is performed to prevent infection spreading from the urinary tract causing recurrent *epididymitis. It is sometimes performed at the time of *prostatectomy to prevent the complication of epididymitis in the postoperative period.

vasomotion *n.* an increase or decrease in the diameter of blood vessels, particularly the arteries. *See* vasoconstriction, vasodilatation.

vasomotor *adj.* controlling the muscular walls of blood vessels, especially arteries, and therefore their diameter.

vasomotor centre a collection of nerve cells in the medulla oblongata that receives information from sensory receptors in the circulatory system (*see* baroreceptor) and brings about reflex changes in the rate of the heart beat and in the diameter of blood vessels, so that the blood pressure can be adjusted. The vasomotor centre also receives impulses from elsewhere in the brain, so that emotion (such as fear) may also influence the heart rate and blood pressure. The centre works through *vasomotor nerves of the sympathetic and parasympathetic systems.

vasomotor nerve any nerve, usually belonging to the autonomic nervous system, that controls the circulation of blood through blood vessels by its action on the muscle fibres within their walls or its action on the heart beat. The *vagus nerve slows the heart and reduces its output, but sympathetic nerves increase the rate and output of the heart and increase blood pressure by causing the constriction of small blood vessels at the same time.

vasopressin (antidiuretic hormone, ADH) *n.* a hormone, released by the pituitary gland, that increases the reabsorption of water by the kidney, thus preventing excessive loss of water from the body. Vasopressin also causes constriction of blood vessels. It is administered either nasally or by injection to treat *diabetes insipidus.

vasopressor *adj.* stimulating the contraction of blood vessels and therefore bringing about an increase in blood pressure.

vasospasm *n. see* Raynaud's disease.

vasotomy *n.* a surgical incision into the vas deferens (the duct conveying sperm from the testis). This is usually undertaken to allow catheterization of the vas and the injection of radio-opaque contrast material for X-ray examination (*vasography*), to test for patency of the duct in patients with *azoospermia.

vasovagal *adj.* relating to the action of impulses in the *vagus nerve on the circulation. The vagus reduces the rate at which the heart beats, and so lowers its output.

vasovagal attack excessive activity of the vagus nerve, causing slowing of the heart and a fall in blood pressure, which leads to fainting. *See* syncope.

vasovasostomy n. the surgical operation of reanastomosing the vas deferens after previous vasectomy: the reversal of vasectomy, undertaken to restore fertility.

vasovesiculitis n. inflammation of the *seminal vesicles and *vas deferens. This usually occurs in association with *prostatitis and causes pain in the perineum, groin, and scrotum and a high temperature. On examination the vasa and seminal vesicles are thickened and tender. Treatment includes administration of antibiotics.

vastus n. any of three muscles (*vastus intermedius*, *vastus lateralis*, and *vastus medialis*) that form part of the *quadriceps muscle of the thigh.

vectis n. a curved instrument used to assist the delivery of an infant.

vector n. an animal, usually an insect or a tick, that transmits parasitic microorganisms – and therefore the diseases they cause – from person to person or from infected animals to human beings. Mosquitoes, for example, are vectors of malaria, filariasis, and yellow fever.

vectorcardiography n. *see* electrocardiography.

vegetation n. (in pathology) an abnormal outgrowth from a membrane, fancied to resemble a vegetable growth. In ulcerative endocarditis, such outgrowths, consisting of *fibrin with enmeshed blood cells, are found on the membrane lining the heart valves.

vegetative adj. **1.** relating to growth and nutrition rather than to reproduction. **2.** functioning unconsciously; autonomic.

vehicle n. (in pharmacy) any substance that acts as the medium in which a drug is administered. Examples are sterile water, isotonic sodium chloride, and dextrose solutions.

vein n. a blood vessel conveying blood towards the heart. All veins except the *pulmonary vein carry deoxygenated blood from the tissues, via the capillaries, to the vena cava. The walls of veins consist of three tissue layers, but these are much thinner and less elastic than those of arteries (see illustration). Veins contain *valves that assist the flow of blood back to the heart. Anatomical name: **vena**. —**venous** adj.

Transverse section through a vein

velamen (velamentum) n. a covering membrane.

vellus n. the fine hair that occurs on the body before puberty is reached.

velum n. (in anatomy) a veil-like covering. The *medullary velum* is either of two thin layers of tissue that form part of the roof of the fourth ventricle of the brain.

vena n. (pl. **venae**) *see* vein.

vena cava either of the two main veins, conveying blood from the other veins to the right atrium of the heart. The *inferior vena cava*, formed by the union of the right and left common iliac veins, receives blood from parts of the body below the diaphragm. The *superior vena cava*, originating at the junction of the two innominate veins, drains blood from the head, neck, thorax, and arms.

vene- (veno-) *prefix denoting* veins.

venene n. a mixture of two or more *venoms: used to produce antiserum against venoms (*antivenene*).

venepuncture (venipuncture) n. the puncture of a vein for any therapeutic

subclavian	internal jugular
	external jugular
cephalic	superior vena cava
axillary	
hepatic	
brachial	
inferior vena cava	suprarenal
	renal
median cubital	testicular (ovarian)
	common iliac
basilic	external iliac
superficial palmar network	femoral
	great saphenous
popliteal	
small saphenous	
anterior tibial	
dorsal venous arch	

The principal veins of the body

purpose; for example, to extract blood for laboratory tests. *See also* phlebotomy.

venereal disease (VD) an infectious disease transmitted by sexual intercourse. The most important are *soft sore (chancroid), *gonorrhoea, and *syphilis.

venereology *n.* the study of venereal diseases, including syphilis and gonorrhoea.

venesection *n. see* phlebotomy.

veno- *prefix. see* vene-.

venoclysis *n.* the continuous infusion into a vein of saline or other solution.

venography (phlebography) *n.* X-ray examination to show up the course of veins in a particular region of the body. A *radio-opaque contrast medium is injected slowly into a vein and X-ray photographs (*venograms*) taken as the compound is carried towards the heart. Damage, obstruction, or abnormal communication with other vessels will be seen where the medium does not fill the vein properly or apparently leaks from it. *See also* angiography.

venom *n.* the poisonous material produced by snakes, scorpions, spiders, and other animals for injecting into their prey or enemies. Some venoms produce no more than local pain and swelling; others produce more general effects and can prove lethal.

venosclerosis *n. see* phlebosclerosis.

ventilation *n.* the passage of air into and out of the respiratory tract. The air that reaches only as far as the conducting airways cannot take part in gas exchange and is known as *dead space ventilation* – this may be reduced by performing a *tracheostomy. In the air sacs of the lungs (alveoli) gas exchange is most efficient when matched by adequate blood flow (*perfusion). Ventilation/perfusion imbalance (ventila-

tion of under-perfused alveoli or perfusion of under-ventilated alveoli) is an important cause of *anoxia and *cyanosis.

ventilator *n.* 1. a device to ensure a supply of fresh air. 2. equipment that is manually or mechanically operated to maintain a flow of air into and out of the lungs of a patient who is unable to breathe normally. *See also* respirator.

ventouse *n.* a cupping glass: a bell-shaped glass vessel from which the air can be removed, used for drawing blood to the surface of the skin. *See* cupping.

ventral *adj.* relating to or situated at or close to the front of the body or to the anterior part of an organ.

ventricle *n.* 1. either of the two lower chambers of the *heart, which have thick muscular walls. The left ventricle, which is thicker than the right, receives blood from the pulmonary vein via the left atrium and pumps it into the aorta. The right ventricle pumps blood received from the venae cavae (via the right atrium) into the pulmonary artery. 2. one of the four fluid-filled cavities within the brain (see illustration). The paired first and second ventricles (*lateral ventricles*), one in each cerebral hemisphere, communicate with the third ventricle in the midline between them. This in turn leads through a narrow channel, the *cerebral aqueduct*, to the fourth ventricle in the hindbrain, which is continuous with the spinal canal in the centre of the spinal cord. *Cerebrospinal fluid circulates through all the cavities. —**ventricular** *adj.*

ventricul- (ventriculo-) *prefix denoting* a ventricle (of the brain or heart).

ventricular folds *see* vocal cords.

ventriculitis *n.* inflammation in the ventricles of the brain, usually caused by infection. It may result from the

ventriculoatriostomy

frontal lobe
lateral ventricle
foramen of Monro
(interventricular
foramen)
fourth ventricle
third ventricle
cerebral aqueduct

Ventricles of the brain (side view)

rupture of a cerebral abscess into the cavity of the ventricle or from the spread of a severe form of *meningitis from the subarachnoid space.

ventriculoatriostomy *n.* an operation for the relief of raised pressure due to the build-up of cerebrospinal fluid that occurs in *hydrocephalus. Using a system of catheters, the fluid is drained into the jugular vein in the neck.

ventriculography *n.* X-ray examination of the ventricles of the brain after the introduction of a contrast medium, such as air or radio-opaque material.

ventriculoscopy *n.* observation of the ventricles of the brain through a fibre-optic instrument. *See* endoscope, fibre optics.

ventriculostomy *n.* an operation to introduce a hollow needle (cannula) into one of the lateral ventricles (cavities) of the brain. This may be done to relieve raised intracranial pressure, to obtain cerebrospinal fluid from the ventricle for examination, or to introduce antibiotics or contrast material for X-ray examination.

ventro- *prefix denoting* 1. ventral. 2. the abdomen.

ventrofixation *n.* an operation to secure a retroverted womb to the wall of the abdomen.

ventrosuspension *n.* the stitching of the round ligaments of a displaced womb to the abdominal wall.

venule *n.* a minute vessel that drains blood from the capillaries. Many venules unite to form a vein.

verbigeration *n.* repetitive utterances of the same words over and over again. This is a kind of *stereotypy affecting speech and is most common in institutionalized schizophrenics.

vermicide *n.* a chemical agent used to destroy parasitic worms living in the intestine. *Compare* vermifuge.

vermiform appendix *see* appendix.

vermifuge *n.* any drug or chemical agent used to expel worms from the intestine. *See also* anthelmintic.

vermis *n.* the central portion of the *cerebellum, lying between its two lateral hemispheres and immediately behind the pons and the medulla oblongata of the hindbrain.

vermix *n.* the vermiform *appendix.

vernier *n.* a device for obtaining accurate measurements of length, to 1/10th, 1/100th or smaller fractions of a unit. It consists of a fixed graduated main scale against which a shorter vernier scale slides. The vernier scale is graduated into divisions equal to nine-tenths of the smallest unit marked on the main scale. The vernier scale is often adjusted by means of a screw thread. A reading is taken by observing which of the markings on the scales coincide.

vernix caseosa the layer of greasy material that covers the skin of a fetus or newborn baby. It is produced by the oil-secreting glands of the skin and contains skin scales and fine hairs.

verruca *n. see* wart.

verrucous carcinoma an *indolent pre-invasive wartlike carcinoma of the oral cavity, which is associated with chewing tobacco.

version *n.* the changing of the position of a fetus in the womb. This may be done to facilitate delivery by applying manual pressure to the outside of the abdomen, by inserting the hand into the womb, or by combining both methods (*see* cephalic version, podalic version). In *spontaneous version* the position of the fetus alters because of the natural contractions of the womb muscles.

vertebra *n.* (*pl.* **vertebrae**) one of the 33 bones of which the *backbone is composed. Each vertebra typically consists of a *body*, or *centrum*, from the back of which arises an arch of bone (the *neural arch*) enclosing a cavity (the *vertebral canal*, or *foramen*) through which the spinal cord passes. The neural arch bears one *spinous process* and two *transverse processes*, providing anchorage for muscles, and four *articular processes*, with which adjacent vertebrae articulate (see illustration). Individual vertebrae are bound together by ligaments and *intervertebral discs. —**vertebral** *adj*.

vertebral column *see* backbone.

vertigo *n.* a disabling sensation in which the affected individual feels that either he himself or his surroundings are in a state of constant movement. It is most often a spinning sensation but there may be a feeling that the ground is tilting. It is a symptom of disease either in the *labyrinth of the inner ear or in the *vestibular nerve or its nuclei in the brainstem, which are involved in the sense of balance.

A typical thoracic vertebra (from above)

vesical *adj.* relating to or affecting a bladder, especially the urinary bladder.

vesicant (epispastic) *n.* an agent that causes blistering of the skin.

vesicle *n.* **1.** a very small blister in the skin, often no bigger than a pinpoint, that contains a clear fluid (serum). Vesicles occur in a variety of skin disorders, including eczema and herpes. **2.** (in anatomy) any small bladder, especially one filled with fluid. —**vesicular** *adj.*

vesico- *prefix denoting* the urinary bladder. Example: *vesicovaginal* (relating to the bladder and vagina).

vesicofixation *n. see* cystopexy.

vesicoureteric reflux the backflow of urine from the bladder into the ureters. This is due to defective valves (which normally prevent reflux). Infection is conveyed to the kidneys, causing recurrent attacks of acute *pyelonephritis and scarring of the kidneys in childhood. Children with urinary infection must be investigated for reflux by *cystoscopy; if the condition does not settle with antibiotic therapy corrective surgery must be performed.

vesicular breathing *see* breath sounds.

vesiculectomy *n.* surgical removal of a *seminal vesicle. This operation, which is rarely undertaken, may be performed for a tumour of the seminal vesicles.

vesiculitis *n.* inflammation of the seminal vesicles. *See* vasovesiculitis.

vesiculography *n.* X-ray examination of the seminal vesicles. This is usually performed by injecting radio-opaque contrast material into the exposed vasa deferentia. It can also be undertaken by inserting a catheter into the ejaculatory duct (which discharges semen from the vesicle into the vas deferens) via an *endoscope. This examination is rarely undertaken for the specific purpose of outlining the seminal vesicles; it is more commonly performed to test for the patency of the vas deferens in patients with *azoospermia.

vesiculopapular *adj.* describing a skin condition typified by having both vesicles (blisters) and papules (raised spots).

vesiculopustular *adj.* describing a skin condition that has both vesicles (blisters) and pustules (pus-filled blisters).

vessel *n.* a tube conveying a body fluid, especially a blood vessel or a lymphatic vessel.

vestibular glands the two pairs of glands that open at the junction of the vagina and vulva. The more posterior of the two are the *greater vestibular glands* (*Bartholin's glands*); the other pair are the *lesser vestibular glands*. Their function is to lubricate the entrance to the vagina during coitus.

vestibular nerve the division of the *vestibulocochlear nerve that carries impulses from the semicircular canals, utricle, and saccule of the inner ear to the brain, conveying information about the body's posture and movements in space and allowing coordination and balance.

vestibule *n.* (in anatomy) a cavity situated at the entrance to a hollow part. The vestibule of the ear is the cavity of the bony *labyrinth that contains the *saccule and *utricle – the organs of equilibrium.

vestibulocochlear nerve (acoustic nerve, auditory nerve) the eighth cranial nerve (VIII), responsible for carrying sensory impulses from the inner ear to the brain. It has two branches, the *vestibular nerve* and the *cochlear nerve*. The cochlear nerve carries impulses from the spiral *cochlea and is therefore the nerve of hearing, while the vestibular nerve serves equilibrium, carrying impulses from the semicircular canals, utricles, and saccules with information about posture, movement, and balance.

vestigial *adj.* existing only in a rudimentary form. The term is applied to organs whose structure and function have diminished during the course of evolution until only a rudimentary structure exists.

viable *adj.* capable of surviving. The term is applied to a fetus from about the 28th week of gestation at which stage it can survive.

Vibramycin *n. see* doxycycline.

vibrator *n.* a machine used to generate vibrations of different frequencies, which have a stimulating effect when applied to different parts of the body. A vibrator may also be used to loosen thick mucus in the sinuses or air passages.

Vibrio *n.* a genus of Gram-negative motile comma-shaped bacteria widely distributed in soil and water. Most species are saprophytic but some are parasites, including *V. cholerae*, which causes *cholera.

vibrissa *n.* (*pl.* **vibrissae**) a stiff coarse hair, especially one of the stiff hairs that lie just inside the nostrils.

vicarious *adj.* describing an action or function performed by an organ not normally involved in the function. For example, *vicarious menstruation* is a rare disorder in which monthly bleeding occurs from places other than the vagina, such as the sweat glands, breasts, nose, or eyes.

villus *n.* (*pl.* **villi**) one of many short finger-like processes that project from some membranous surfaces. Numerous *intestinal villi* line the small *intestine. Each contains a network of blood capillaries and a *lacteal. Their function is to absorb the products of digestion and they greatly increase the surface area over which this can take place. *Chorionic villi* are folds of the chorion (the outer membrane surrounding a fetus). They are particularly numerous in the *placenta, where they provide an extensive area for the exchange of oxygen, carbon dioxide, food, and waste products between maternal and fetal blood. *See also* arachnoid villus.

vinblastine *n.* a *cytotoxic drug that is given by intravascular injection mainly in the treatment of cancers of the lymphatic system, such as Hodgkin's disease. It is highly toxic, since it also acts on normal tissues; common side-effects include nausea, vomiting, diarrhoea, and depression of bone marrow function. Trade names: **Velban, Velbe**.

Vincent's angina an obsolete term for *ulcerative gingivitis.

vincristine *n.* a cytotoxic drug with uses and side-effects similar to those of vinblastine. Trade name: **Oncovin**.

vinculum *n.* (*pl.* **vincula**) a connecting band of tissue. The *vincula tendinum* are threadlike bands of synovial membrane that connect the flexor tendons of the fingers and toes to their point of insertion on the phalanges.

vindesine *n.* a cytotoxic drug with similarities to *vinblastine and vincristine. Additional side-effects include alopecia and peripheral neuropathy. Trade name: **Eldisine**.

vinyl ether a general anaesthetic, used mainly for inducing anaesthesia and for minor surgery under short anaesthesia. Both induction and recovery are more rapid than with ether. It is not used alone for long operations because of the dangers of overdosage and liver damage, but it is sometimes given in combination with nitrous oxide or ether. Trade name: **Vinethene**.

viomycin *n.* an *antibiotic derived from bacteria of the genus *Streptomyces*. It is given by intramuscular injection in the treatment of tuberculosis, particularly against strains that are resistant to other antibiotics (such as *streptomycin and *isoniazid). Side-effects, including ear and kidney damage, may occur in some patients. Trade name: **Viocin**.

viprynium *n.* a drug administered by mouth for the treatment of threadworm infestation. It has low toxicity but may cause nausea and vomiting. It stains the stools a red colour. Trade name: **Vanquin**.

viraemia *n.* the presence in the blood of virus particles.

virilism *n.* the development in a female of a combination of increased body hair, muscle bulk, and deepening of the voice (*masculinization) and male psychological characteristics.

virilization *n.* the induction in a female of increased body hair, muscle bulk, and deepening of the voice as a result of hormone imbalance or hormone therapy.

virology *n.* the science of viruses. *See also* microbiology.

virulence *n.* the disease-producing (pathogenic) ability of a microorganism. *See also* attenuation.

virus *n.* a minute particle that is capable of replication but only within living cells. Viruses are too small to be visible with a light microscope and too small to be trapped by filters. They infect animals, plants, and microorganisms (*see* bacteriophage). Each consists of a core of nucleic acid (DNA or RNA) surrounded by a protein shell. Some bear an outer lipid capsule. Viruses cause many diseases, including the common cold, influenza, measles, mumps, chickenpox, herpes, smallpox, polio, and rabies. Antibiotics are ineffective against them, but many viral diseases are controlled by means of vaccines. —**viral** *adj.*

viscera *pl. n.* (*sing.* **viscus**) the organs within the body cavities, especially the organs of the abdominal cavities (stomach, intestines, etc.). —**visceral** *adj.*

visceral arch *see* pharyngeal arch.

visceral cleft *see* pharyngeal cleft.

visceral pouch *see* pharyngeal pouch.

viscero- *prefix denoting* the viscera.

viscus *n. see* viscera.

visual acuity sharpness of vision. How well one sees things depends on how well they are illuminated and upon such factors as practice and motivation, but the essential requirements are a healthy retina and the ability of the eye to focus incoming light to form a sharp image on the retina. The commonest way of assessing visual acuity is the *Snellen chart, which measures the *resolving power* of the eye.

visual field the area in front of the eye in any part of which an object can be seen without moving the eye. With both eyes open and looking straight forward it is possible to see well-illuminated objects placed anywhere in front of the eyes, although the eyebrows and eyelids reduce the extent of the field somewhat. This is the *binocular visual field*. With only one eye open the field is *uniocular* and is restricted inwards by the nose. If the object is small or poorly illuminated it will not be seen until it is moved closer to the point at which the eye is actually looking, i.e. nearer to the centre of the visual field. Similarly, coloured objects are not seen so far away from the centre as are white objects of the same size and brightness. This is because the retina is not uniformly sensitive to light of different colours or intensities (*see* rod, cone): retinal sensitivity increases towards its centre (the *macula). Thus, while there is an absolute visual field beyond which things cannot be seen, no matter how large or bright they are, a relative field exists for objects of different brightness, size, and colour. *See also* campimetry, perimeter.

visual purple *see* rhodopsin.

vital capacity the maximum volume of air that a person can exhale afer maximum inhalation. It is usually measured on an instrument called a *spirometer*.

vital centre any of the collections of nerve cells in the brain that act as governing centres for different vital body functions – such as breathing, heart rate, blood pressure, temperature control etc. – making reflex adjustments according to the body's needs. Most lie in the hypothalamus and brainstem.

Vitallium *n. Trademark.* an alloy of chromium and cobalt that is used in instruments, prostheses, surgical appliances, and dentures.

vital staining (intravital staining) the process of staining a living tissue by injecting a stain into the organism. *Compare* supravital staining.

vital statistics *see* biostatistics.

vitamin *n.* any of a group of substances that are required, in very small amounts, for healthy growth and development: they cannot be synthesized in the body and are therefore essential constituents of the diet. Vitamins are divided into two groups, according to whether they are soluble in water or fat. The water-soluble group includes the vitamin B complex and vitamin C; the fat-soluble vitamins are vitamins A, D, E, and K. Lack of sufficient quantities of any of the vitamins in the diet results in specific vitamin deficiency diseases.

vitamin A (retinol) a fat-soluble vitamin that occurs preformed in foods of animal origin (especially milk products, egg yolk, and liver) and is formed in the body from the pigment β-carotene, present in some vegetable foods (for example cabbage, lettuce, and carrots). Retinol is essential for growth, vision in dim light, and the maintenance of soft mucous tissue. A deficiency causes stunted growth, *night blindness, *xerophthalmia, *keratomalacia, and eventual blindness. The recommended daily intake is 750 µg retinol equivalents for an adult (1 µg retinol equivalent = 1 µg retinol or 6 µg β-carotene).

vitamin B any one of a group of water-soluble vitamins that, although not chemically related, are often found together in the same kinds of food (milk, liver, cereals, etc.) and all function as *coenzymes. See vitamins B_1, B_2, B_6, B_{12}, biotin, folic acid, nicotinic acid, pantothenic acid.

vitamin B_1 (thiamin, aneurin) a vitamin of the B complex that is active in the form of *thiamin pyrophosphate*, a coenzyme in decarboxylation reactions in carbohydrate metabolism. A deficiency of vitamin B_1 leads to *beriberi. Good sources of the vitamin are cereals, beans, meat, potatoes, and nuts. The recommended daily intake is 1 mg for an adult.

vitamin B_2 (riboflavin) a vitamin of the B complex that is a constituent of the coenzymes *FAD (flavine adenine dinucleotide) and *FMN (flavine mononucleotide). Riboflavin is therefore important in tissue respiration. A deficiency of riboflavin causes a condition known as *ariboflavinosis, which is not usually serious. Good sources of riboflavin are liver, milk, and eggs. The recommended daily intake for an adult is 1.7 mg.

vitamin B_6 (pyridoxine) a vitamin of the B complex from which the coenzyme *pyridoxal phosphate, involved in the transamination of amino acids, is formed. The vitamin is found in most foods and a deficiency is therefore rare.

vitamin B_{12} (cyanocobalamin) a vitamin of the B complex. The form of vitamin B_{12} with coenzyme activity is *5-deoxyadenosyl cobalamin*, which is necessary for the synthesis of nucleic acids, the maintenance of *myelin in the nervous system, and the proper functioning of *folic acid, another B vitamin. The vitamin can be absorbed only in the presence of *intrinsic factor*, a protein secreted in the stomach. A deficiency of vitamin B_{12} affects nearly all the body tissues, particularly those containing rapidly dividing cells. The most serious effects of a deficiency are *pernicious anaemia and degeneration of the nervous system. Vitamin B_{12} is manufactured only by certain microorganisms and is contained only in foods of animal origin. Good sources are liver, fish, and eggs. The daily recommended adult intake is 3–4 µg.

vitamin C (ascorbic acid) a water-soluble vitamin that is essential in maintaining healthy connective tissues and the integrity of cell walls. It is necessary for the synthesis of collagen. A deficiency of vitamin C leads to *scurvy. The recommended daily intake is 30 mg for an adult; rich sources are citrus fruits and vegetables.

vitamin D a fat-soluble vitamin that enhances the absorption of calcium and phosphorus from the intestine and promotes their deposition in the bone. It occurs in two forms: *ergocalciferol* (*vitamin D₂, calciferol*), which is manufactured by plants when the sterol ergosterol is exposed to ultraviolet light, and *cholecalciferol* (*vitamin D₃*), which is produced by the action of sunlight on 7-dehydrocholesterol, a sterol widely distributed in the skin. A deficiency of vitamin D, either from a poor diet or lack of sunlight, leads to decalcified bones and the development of *rickets and *osteomalacia. Good sources of vitamin D are liver and fish oils. The recommended daily intake is 10 μg for a child up to five years and 2.5 μg thereafter. Vitamin D is toxic and large doses must therefore be avoided.

vitamin E any of a group of chemically related compounds (*tocopherols* and *tocotrienols*) that have antioxidant properties and are thought to stabilize cell membranes by preventing oxidation of their unsaturated fatty acid components. The most potent of these is α-*tocopherol*. Good sources of the vitamin are vegetable oils, eggs, butter, and wholemeal cereals. It is fairly widely distributed in the diet and a deficiency is therefore unlikely.

vitamin K a fat-soluble vitamin occurring in two main forms: *phytomenadione* (of plant origin) and *menaquinone* (of animal origin). It is necessary for the formation of *prothrombin in the liver, which is essential for blood clotting, and it also regulates the synthesis of other clotting factors. A dietary deficiency does not often occur as the vitamin is synthesized by bacteria in the large intestine and is widely distributed in green leafy vegetables and meat.

vitellus *n.* the yolk of an ovum.

vitiligo (leucoderma) *n.* a condition in which areas of skin lose their pigment and become white. There are no other changes, but the white patches, which appear anywhere, grow in size until much of the body is affected. The cause is unknown and treatment is unsatisfactory in Europeans.

vitrectomy *n.* the removal of the whole or part of the vitreous humour of the eye.

vitreous humour (vitreous body) the transparent jelly-like material that fills the chamber behind the lens of the eye.

viviparous *adj.* describing animal groups (including most mammals) in which the embryos develop within the body of the mother so that the young are born alive rather than hatch from an egg. —**viviparity** *n.*

vivisection *n.* a surgical operation on a living animal for experimental purposes.

vocal cords (vocal folds) the two folds of tissue which protrude from the sides of the *larynx to form a narrow slit (glottis) across the air passage (see illustration). Their controlled interference with the expiratory air flow produces audible vibrations that make up speech, song, and all other vocal noises. Alterations in the vocal cords themselves or in their nerve supply by disease interferes with phonation.

vocal fremitus *see* fremitus.

vocal resonance the sounds heard through the stethoscope when the patient speaks ("ninety nine"). These are normally just audible but become much louder (*bronchophony*) if the lung under the stethoscope is consolidated, when they resemble the sounds heard over the trachea and main bronchi. Vocal

- root of the tongue
- epiglottis
- vocal fold (true vocal cord)
- ventricular fold (false vocal cord)
- glottis
- larynx

The vocal cords

resonance is lost over pleural fluid except at its upper surface, when it has a bleating quality and is called *aegophony*. *See also* pectoriloquy.

volar *adj.* relating to the palm of the hand or the sole of the foot (the *vola*).

volsella (vulsella) *n.* surgical forceps with clawlike hooks at the ends of both blades.

volt *n.* the *SI unit of electric potential, equal to the potential difference between two points on a conducting wire through which a constant current of 1 ampere flows when the power dissipated between these points is 1 watt. Symbol: V.

voluntary admission entry of a patient into a psychiatric hospital with his (or her) agreement. *Compare* compulsory admission.

voluntary muscle *see* striated muscle.

volvulus *n.* twisting of part of the digestive tract, usually leading to partial or complete obstruction and sometimes reducing the blood supply, causing gangrene. A volvulus may untwist spontaneously or by manipulation, but surgical exploration is usually performed. *Gastric volvulus* is a twist of the stomach, usually in a hiatus *hernia. *Small-intestinal volvulus* is twisting of part of the bowel around an *adhesion. *Sigmoid volvulus* is a twist of the sig-

von Recklinghausen's disease

moid colon, usually when this loop is particularly long.

vomer *n.* a thin plate of bone that forms part of the nasal septum (*see* nasal cavity). *See also* skull.

vomica *n.* **1.** an abnormal cavity in an organ, usually a lung, sometimes containing pus. **2.** the abrupt expulsion from the mouth of a large quantity of pus or decaying matter originating in the throat or lungs.

vomit **1.** *vb.* to eject the contents of the stomach through the mouth (*see* vomiting). **2.** *n.* the contents of the stomach ejected during vomiting. Medical name: **vomitus**.

vomiting *n.* the reflex action of ejecting the contents of the stomach through the mouth. Vomiting is controlled by a special centre in the brain that may be stimulated by drugs (e.g. *apomorphine) acting directly on it; or by impulses transmitted through nervous pathways either from the stomach (e.g. after ingesting irritating substances, in gastritis and other stomach diseases), the intestine (e.g. in intestinal obstruction), or from the inner ear (in travel sickness). The stimulated vomiting centre sets off a chain of nerve impulses producing coordinated contractions of the diaphragm and abdominal muscles, relaxation of the muscle at the entrance to the stomach, etc., causing the stomach contents to be expelled. Medical name: **emesis**.

von Hippel-Lindau disease a syndrome in which *haemangioblastomas, particularly in the cerebellum, are associated with renal and pancreatic cysts, *angiomas in the retina, cancer of the kidney cells, and red birthmarks.

von Recklinghausen's disease **1.** a syndrome due to excessive secretion of *parathyroid hormone (hyperparathyroidism), characterized by loss of mineral from bones, which become weakened and fracture easily, and formation of kidney stones. Medical name: **osteitis fibrosa. 2.** *see* neurofibromatosis.

voyeurism *n.* the condition of obtaining sexual pleasure by watching other people undressing or enjoying sexual relations. *See also* perversion. —**voyeur** *n.*

vulsella *n. see* volsella.

vulv- (vulvo-) *prefix denoting* the vulva.

vulva *n.* the female external genitalia. Two pairs of fleshy folds – the *labia majora* and *labia minora* – surround the openings of the vagina and urethra and extend forward to the clitoris (see illustration). *See also* vestibular glands.

urethral opening
clitoris
labium minoris
vaginal opening
labium majus
anus

The vulva

vulvectomy *n.* surgical removal of the external genitals (vulva) of a woman.

vulvitis *n.* inflammation of the vulva, which is often accompanied by intense itching and burning pain. It may be caused by infection with the fungus *Candida albicans* or the bacterium *Neisseria gonococcus* or by ill-fitting underwear (which causes the lips of the vulva to rub together).

vulvovaginitis *n.* **1.** inflammation of the vulva and vagina (*see* vaginitis, vulvitis). **2.** *see* bartholinitis.

W

wafer *n.* a thin sheet made from moistened flour, formerly used to enclose a powdered medicine that is taken by mouth.

waiting list a list of the names of patients who are awaiting admission to hospital after having been assessed either as an out-patient or on a domiciliary consultation involving a specialist. In general the patients are offered places in the order in which their names were placed on the list, but in certain circumstances (e.g. if the condition is potentially dangerous or painful) the consultant may recommend urgent or even immediate admission. One of the facts recorded in relation to hospital admissions is the length of time between the name being placed on the list and the patient being admitted (*waiting time*). General practitioners may also request *direct admission* (immediate) for urgent cases who have not been seen by the consultant; such admission may be arranged by phone with the consultant or his deputy or channelled through the accident and emergency department of the hospital.

Walcher's position a position in which the patient lies on the back with the legs hanging down: sometimes adopted to aid childbirth.

Waldeyer's ring the ring of lymphoid tissue formed by the tonsils.

warfarin *n.* an *anticoagulant used mainly in the treatment of coronary or venous thrombosis to reduce the risk of embolism. It is given by mouth or injection. The principal toxic effect is local bleeding, usually from the gums and other mucous membranes. Warfarin has also been used as a rat poison. Trade names: **Coumadin, Marevan**.

wart *n.* a small (often hard) benign growth in the skin. Caused by a virus, warts are commoner in young people, usually occurring on the face, fingers, hands, elbows, and knees. There are several types. *Juvenile warts* occur profusely on the hands and face of children; *common warts* are larger, with a rougher surface, and occur on the hands. *Plantar warts* occur on the sole of the foot; they are subject to pressure and are therefore painful and may be covered by a thick callus. They spread rapidly in communities, such as schools. *Venereal warts* are found on the genitals or around the anus in both sexes. Warts usually disappear spontaneously but there is a wide range of treatments, including local application of chemicals, removal with a *curette, and *electrocautery. Medical name: **verruca**.

Wassermann reaction the most commonly used test for the diagnosis of *syphilis. A sample of the patient's blood is examined, using a *complement-fixation reaction, for the presence of antibodies to the organism *Treponema pallidum*. A positive reaction (WR+) indicates the presence of antibodies and therefore infection with syphilis.

water bed a bed with a flexible water-containing mattress. The surface of the bed adapts itself to the patient's posture, which leads to greater comfort and fewer bedsores.

waterbrash *n.* a sudden filling of the mouth with dilute saliva. This often accompanies dyspepsia, particularly if there is nausea.

Waters' projection a *posteroanterior X-ray film to show the maxillae, maxillary sinuses, and zygomatic bones.

watt *n.* the *SI unit of power, equal to 1 joule per second. In electrical terms it is the energy expended per second when a current of 1 ampere flows between two points on a conductor between which there is a potential difference of 1 volt. 1 watt = 10^7 ergs per second. Symbol: W.

weal *n. see* wheal.

weber *n.* the *SI unit of magnetic flux, equal to the flux linking a circuit of one turn that produces an e.m.f. of 1 volt when reduced uniformly to zero in 1 second. Symbol: Wb.

Weber-Christian disease *see* panniculitis.

Weber's test a hearing test in which a vibrating tuning fork is placed at the midpoint of the forehead. A normal individual hears it equally in both ears, but if one ear is affected by conductive *deafness the sound appears louder in the affected ear.

Wegener's granuloma a disease predominantly affecting the nasal passages, lungs, and kidneys, characterized by *granuloma formation in addition to arteritis. It is usually fatal but can be controlled (sometimes for years) with steroids and/or cyclophosphamide.

Weil-Felix reaction a diagnostic test for typhus. A sample of the patient's serum is tested for the presence of antibodies against the organism *Proteus vulgaris*. Although this relatively harmless organism is not the cause of typhus, it possesses certain antigens in common with the causative agent of the disease and can therefore be used instead of it in laboratory tests. Typhus is suspected if antibodies are found to be present.

Weil's disease *see* leptospirosis.

Welch's bacillus

Welch's bacillus *see* Clostridium.

wen *n. see* sebaceous cyst.

Wernicke's encephalopathy mental confusion or delirium occurring in combination with paralysis of the eye muscles, *nystagmus, and an unsteady gait. It is caused by a deficiency of vitamin B₁ (thiamin) and is most commonly seen in alcoholics and in patients with persistent vomiting. Treatment with thiamin relieves the symptoms.

Wertheim's hysterectomy an operation performed for cancer of the womb or ovary, in which the womb, Fallopian tubes, ovaries, upper vagina, broad ligaments, and regional lymph nodes are removed.

Wharton's duct the secretory duct of the submandibular *salivary gland.

Wharton's jelly the mesoderm tissue of the umbilical cord, which becomes converted to a loose jelly-like *mesenchyme surrounding the umbilical blood vessels.

wheal (weal) *n.* a temporary red or pale raised area of the skin, often accompanied by severe itching. Wheals may be caused by scratching or rubbing the skin and are sometimes the sign of a local or general allergy (*see* urticaria). *See also* dermographia.

wheeze *n.* low-pitched breathing sounds associated with *bronchospasm, such as occurs in asthma and byssinosis. *Compare* stridor.

whiplash injury damage to the ligaments, vertebrae, spinal cord, or nerve roots in the neck region, caused by sudden jerking back of the head and neck. At its most severe death or permanent paralysis (*quadriplegia or *paraplegia) may result. Sudden deceleration in a motor accident is the commonest cause. Immobilization using a special collar is the principal treatment.

Whipple's disease a rare disease, occurring only in males, in which absorption of digested food in the intestine is reduced. As well as symptoms and signs of *malabsorption there is usually skin pigmentation and arthritis. Diagnosis is made by *jejunal biopsy; microorganisms have been found in the mucosa, and the disease usually responds to prolonged antibiotic treatment.

Whipple's operation *see* pancreatectomy.

whipworm *n.* a small parasitic whip-like nematode worm, *Trichuris trichiura* (*Trichocephalus dispar*), that lives in the large intestine. Eggs are passed out of the body with the faeces and human infection (*see* trichuriasis) results from the consumption of water or food contaminated with faecal material. The eggs hatch in the small intestine but mature worms migrate to the large intestine.

white blood cell *see* leucocyte.

white leg (milk leg) a condition that may affect women after childbirth in which there is clotting and inflammation in a vein in the leg. The leg becomes pale, swollen, and tense and is painful; the condition resolves only slowly. Medical name: **phlegmasia alba dolens**.

white matter nerve tissue of the central nervous system that is paler in colour than the associated *grey matter because it contains more nerve fibres and thus larger amounts of the insulating material *myelin. In the brain the white matter lies within the grey layer of cerebral cortex; in the spinal cord it is between the arms of the X-shaped central core of grey matter.

whites *n. see* leucorrhoea.

whitlow (felon) *n.* an abscess affecting the pulp of the fingertip. *See also* paronychia.

whoop *n.* a noisy convulsive drawing in of the breath following the spasmodic coughing attack characteristic of *whooping cough.

whooping cough an acute contagious disease, primarily affecting children, due to infection of the mucous membranes lining the air passages by the bacterium *Haemophilus pertussis*. After an incubation period of 1–2 weeks catarrh, mild fever, coughing, and loss of appetite gradually develop and persist for 1–2 weeks. The cough becomes paroxysmal: series of short coughs are followed by involuntary drawing in of the breath, which produces the whooping sound. Bleeding from the nose and mouth and vomiting often occur after a paroxysm. This stage lasts about two weeks and the child is infectious throughout. Over the following 2–3 weeks symptoms slowly decline but the cough may persist for many weeks. Whooping cough is seldom serious but the child is susceptible to pneumonia and tuberculosis. Immunization reduces the incidence and severity of the disease: the vaccine is usually given in a combined form (*see* DPT vaccine). An attack usually also confers immunity. Medical name: **pertussis**.

Widal reaction an *agglutination test for the presence of antibodies against the *Salmonella* organisms that cause typhoid fever. It is thus a method of diagnosing the presence of the disease in a patient and also a means of identifying the organisms in infected material.

Wilms' tumour *see* nephroblastoma.

Wilson's disease an inborn defect of copper metabolism in which there is a deficiency of *caeruloplasmin (which normally forms a nontoxic complex with copper). The free copper may be deposited in the liver, causing jaundice and cirrhosis, or in the brain, causing mental retardation and symptoms resembling *parkinsonism. There is a characteristic brown ring in the cornea (the *Kayser-Fleischer ring*). If the excess copper is removed from the body by regular treatment with *penicillamine both mental and physical development may be normal. Medical name: **hepatolenticular degeneration**.

windigo *n.* a delusion of having been transformed into a *windigo*, a mythical monster that eats human flesh. It is often quoted as an example of a syndrome confined to one culture (that of some North American Indian tribes, such as the Cree).

windpipe *n. see* trachea.

wisdom tooth the third *molar tooth on each side of either jaw, which erupts normally around the age of 20.

witch hazel (hamamelis) a preparation made from the leaves and bark of the tree *Hamamelis virginiana*, used as an *astringent, especially for the treatment of sprains and bruises.

withdrawal *n.* **1.** (in psychology) the removal of one's interest from one's surroundings. *Thought withdrawal* is the experience of one's thoughts being removed from one's head, which is characteristic of *schizophrenia. **2.** *see* coitus interruptus.

withdrawal symptoms *see* dependence.

Wohlfahrtia *n.* a genus on non-blood-sucking flies. The females of *W. magnifica* and *W. vigil* deposit their parasitic maggots in wounds and the openings of the body. This causes *myiasis, particularly in children.

Wolffian body *see* mesonephros.

Wolffian duct the mesonephric duct (*see* mesonephros).

womb

womb *n. see* uterus.

wood point *see* tooth pick.

word blindness *see* alexia.

worm *n.* any member of several groups of soft-bodied legless animals, including flatworms, nematode worms, earthworms, and leeches, that were formerly thought to be closely related and classified as a single group – Vermes.

wormian bone one of a number of small bones that occur in the cranial sutures.

wound *n.* a break in the structure of an organ or tissue caused by an external agent. Bruises, grazes, tears, cuts, punctures, and burns are all examples of wounds.

wrist *n.* **1.** the joint between the forearm and hand. It consists of the proximal bones of the *carpus, which articulate with the radius and ulna. **2.** the whole region of the wrist joint, including the carpus and lower parts of the radius and ulna.

wrist drop paralysis of the muscles that raise the wrist, which is caused by damage to the *radial nerve. This may result from compression of the nerve against the humerus in the upper arm or from selective damage to the nerve, which is a feature of *lead poisoning.

wryneck *n. see* torticollis.

Wuchereria *n.* a genus of white threadlike parasitic worms (*see* filaria) that live in the lymphatic vessels. *W. bancrofti* is a tropical and subtropical species that causes *elephantiasis, lymphangitis, and chyluria. The immature forms concentrate in the lungs during the day. At night they become more numerous in the blood vessels of the skin, from which they are taken up by blood-sucking mosquitoes, acting as carriers of the diseases they cause.

X

xanthaemia (carotenaemia) *n.* the presence in the blood of the yellow pigment *carotene, from excessive intake of carrots, tomatoes, or other vegetables containing the pigment.

xanthelasma *n.* one or more yellow deposits of fatty material in the skin around the eyes. In elderly people it is quite common and of no more than cosmetic importance, but severe cases may be seen in certain disorders of fat metabolism.

xanthine *n.* a nitrogenous breakdown product of the purines adenosine and guanine. Xanthine is an intermediate product of the breakdown of nucleic acids to uric acid.

xanthinuria *n.* excess of the purine derivative *xanthine in the urine, usually the result of an inborn defect of metabolism. It is both rare and symptomless.

xantho- *prefix denoting* yellow colour.

xanthochromia *n.* yellow discoloration, such as may affect the skin (for example, in jaundice) or the cerebrospinal fluid (when it contains the breakdown products of haemoglobin from red blood cells that have entered it).

xanthoma *n.* (*pl.* **xanthomata**) a yellowish swelling, nodule, or plaque in the skin resulting from deposits of fat. The presence of xanthomata is usually accompanied by a raised blood *cholesterol level. There are several types; for example, *xanthoma palpebrarum*, in which the plaques appear on the eyelids in the elderly (*see* xanthelasma). *See also* xanthomatosis.

xanthomatosis *n.* the presence of multiple small fatty tumours in the skin, the eyes, and the internal organs due to an excess of fats in the blood (hyperlipidaemia). *See* xanthoma.

xanthophyll *n.* a yellow pigment found in green leaves. An example of a xanthophyll is *lutein*.

xanthopsia *n.* yellow vision: the condition in which all objects appear to have a yellowish tinge. It is sometimes experienced in digitalis poisoning.

X chromosome the sex chromosome present in both sexes. Women have two X chromosomes and men one. Genes for some important genetic disorders, including *haemophilia, are carried on the X chromosomes; these genes are described as *sex-linked. *Compare* Y chromosome.

xeno- *prefix denoting* different; foreign; alien.

xenodiagnosis *n.* a procedure for diagnosing infections transmitted by insect carriers. Uninfected insects of the species known to carry the disease in question are allowed to suck the blood of a patient suspected of having the disease. A positive diagnosis is made if the disease parasites appear in the insects. This method has proved invaluable for diagnosing Chagas' disease, using reduviid bugs (the carriers), since the parasites are not always easily detected in blood smears.

xenograft *n. see* heterograft.

xenophobia *n.* excessive fear of strangers and foreigners. *See* phobia.

Xenopsylla *n.* a genus of tropical and subtropical fleas, with some 40 species. The rat flea, *X. cheopis*, occasionally attacks man and can transmit plague from an infected rat population; it also transmits murine typhus and two tapeworms, *Hymenolepis nana* and *H. diminuta*.

xero- *prefix denoting* a dry condition.

xeroderma *n.* a mild form of the hereditary disorder *ichthyosis, in which the skin develops slight dryness and forms branlike scales.

xerophthalmia *n.* a progressive disease of the eye due to deficiency of vitamin A. The cornea and conjunctiva become dry, thickened, and wrinkled. This may progress to *keratomalacia and eventual blindness.

xerosis *n.* abnormal dryness of the conjunctiva, the skin, or the mucous membranes. Xerosis affecting the conjunctiva is due not to decreased production of tears but to changes in the membrane itself, which becomes thickened and grey in the area exposed when the eyelids are open.

xerostomia *n.* dryness of the mouth resulting from diminished secretion of saliva. The phenomenon may be caused by drugs or poisons or be associated with disease. *Compare* ptyalism.

xiphi- (xipho-) *prefix denoting* the xiphoid process of the sternum. Example: *xiphocostal* (relating to the xiphoid process and ribs).

xiphisternum *see* xiphoid process.

xiphoid process (xiphoid cartilage) the lowermost section of the breastbone (*see* sternum): a flat pointed cartilage that gradually ossifies until it is completely replaced by bone, a process not completed until after middle age. It does not articulate with any ribs. Also called: **ensiform process** *or* **cartilage**, **xiphisternum**.

X-rays *n.* electromagnetic radiation of extremely short wavelength (beyond the ultraviolet), with great penetrating powers in matter opaque to light. X-rays are produced when high-energy beams of electrons strike matter. They are used in diagnosis in the techniques of *radiography and also in certain forms of *radiotherapy. Great care is needed to avoid unnecessary exposure, because the radiation is harmful in large quantities to all living things. *See* radiation sickness.

xylene (dimethylbenzene) *n.* a liquid used for increasing the transparency of tissues prepared for microscopic examination after they have been dehydrated. *See* clearing.

xylometazoline *n.* a drug that constricts blood vessels (*see* vasoconstrictor). It is rapidly acting and long lasting and is applied topically as a nasal decongestant in the relief of the common cold and sinusitis. Toxic effects are rare. Trade name: **Otrivine**.

xylose *n.* a pentose sugar (i.e. one with five carbon atoms) that is involved in carbohydrate interconversions within cells.

Y

yawning *n.* a reflex action in which the mouth is opened wide and air is drawn into the lungs then slowly released. It is a result of drowsiness, fatigue, or boredom.

yaws (pian, framboesia) *n.* a tropical infectious disease caused by the presence of the spirochaete *Treponema pertenue* in the skin and its underlying tissues. Yaws occurs chiefly in conditions of poor hygiene. It is transmitted by direct contact with infected persons and their clothing and possibly also by flies of the genus *Hippelates*. The spirochaetes enter through abrasions on the skin. Initial symptoms include fever, pains, and itching, followed by the appearance of small tumours, each covered by a yellow crust of dried serum, on the hands, face, legs, and feet. These tumours may deteriorate into deep ulcers. The final stage of yaws, which may appear after an inter-val of several years, involves destructive and deforming lesions of the skin, bones, and periosteum (*see also* gangosa, goundou). Yaws, which commonly affects children, is prevalent in hot humid lowlands of equatorial Africa, tropical America, the Far East, and the West Indies. It responds well to treatment with *penicillin and other antibiotics.

Y chromosome a sex chromosome that is present in men but not in women; it is believed to carry the genes for maleness. *Compare* X chromosome.

yeast *n.* any unicellular fungus of the genus *Saccharomyces*. Yeasts reproduce asexually by budding and sexually by the formation of spores. They ferment carbohydrates, producing alcohol and carbon dioxide, and are important in brewing and breadmaking. Yeasts are a commercial source of proteins and of vitamins of the B complex.

yellow fever an infectious disease, caused by an *arbovirus, occurring in tropical Africa and the northern regions of South America. It is transmitted by mosquitoes, principally *Aëdes aegypti*. The virus causes degeneration of the tissues of the liver and kidneys. Symptoms, depending on severity of infection, include chill, headache, pains in the back and limbs, fever, vomiting, constipation, a reduced flow of urine (which contains high levels of albumin), and *jaundice. Yellow fever often proves fatal, but recovery from a first attack confers subsequent immunity. The disease can be prevented by vaccination.

yellow spot *see* macula (lutea).

yolk (deutoplasm) *n.* a substance, rich in protein and fat, that is laid down within the egg cell as nourishment for the embryo. It is absent (or nearly so) from the eggs of mammals (including man) whose embryos absorb nutrients from their mother.

yolk sac (vitelline sac) the membranous sac, composed of mesoderm lined with endoderm, that lies ventral to the embryo. Its initially wide communication with the future gut is later reduced to a narrow duct passing through the *umbilicus. It probably assists in transporting nutrients to the early embryo and is one of the first sites where blood cells are formed.

yttrium-90 *n.* an artificial radioactive isotope of the element yttrium, used in *radiotherapy. Yttrium-90, which emits beta rays, can be used in the form of 1 mm spheres scattered around a tumour or injected directly into a tumour in the form of a solution.

Z

zein *n.* a protein found in maize.

zinc chloride a *caustic substance having strong *astringent properties. It is used as a solution for cleansing wounds and ulcers and also as a mouth wash and deodorant; in paste form it is the main component of zinc dental cement. Toxic effects are essentially due to poisoning by ingestion.

zinc oxide a mild *astringent used in various skin conditions, usually mixed with other substances. It is applied as a cream, ointment, dusting powder, or as a paste, sometimes in the form of an impregnated bandage.

zinc sulphate an *astringent applied in a lotion for the treatment of ulcers of the skin and mouth and to assist wound healing. It is also used in eye drops and, occasionally, as an emetic.

zinc undecenoate (zinc undecylenate) an antifungal agent with uses similar to those of *undecenoic acid.

Zollinger-Ellison syndrome a rare disorder in which there is excessive secretion of gastric juice due to high levels of circulating *gastrin, which is produced by a pancreatic tumour (benign or malignant) or an enlarged pancreas. The high levels of stomach acid cause peptic ulcers, which may be multiple, in unusual sites (e.g. jejunum), or which quickly recur after *vagotomy or partial *gastrectomy. Treatment with a histamine-blocking drug, by removal of the tumour (if benign), or by total gastrectomy is usually effective.

zona pellucida the thick membrane that develops around the mammalian oocyte within the ovarian follicle. It is penetrated by at least one spermatozoon at fertilization and persists around the *blastocyst until it reaches the womb. *See* ovum.

zonula *n. see* zonule.

zonule (zonula) *n.* (in anatomy) a small band or zone; for example the *zonule of Zinn* (*zonula ciliaris*) is the suspensory ligament of the eye. —**zonular** *adj.*

zonulolysis *n.* dissolution of the suspensory ligament of the lens of the eye (the *zonule of Zinn*), which facilitates removal of the lens in cases of cataract. A small quantity of a solution of an enzyme that dissolves the zonule without damaging other parts of the eye is injected behind the iris a minute or two before the lens is removed.

zoo- *prefix denoting* animals.

zoonosis *n.* an infectious disease of animals that can be transmitted to man. *See* anthrax, brucellosis, cat-scratch fever, cowpox, glanders, Q fever, Rift Valley fever, rabies, rat-bite fever, toxoplasmosis, tularaemia, typhus.

zoophilism *n.* sexual attraction to animals, which may be manifest in stroking and fondling or in sexual intercourse (*bestiality*). —**zoophilic** *adj.*

zoophobia *n.* excessively strong fear of animals. *See* phobia.

zoopsia *n.* visual hallucinations of animals. These can occur in any condition causing hallucinations but are most typical of *delirium tremens.

zwitterion *n.* an ion that bears a positive and a negative charge. Amino acids can yield zwitterions.

zygoma *n. see* zygomatic arch, zygomatic bone.

zygomatic arch (zygoma) the horizontal arch of bone on either side of the face, just below the eyes, formed by connected processes of the zygomatic and temporal bones. *See* skull.

zygomatic bone (zygoma, malar bone) either of a pair of bones that form the prominent part of the cheeks and contribute to the orbits. *See* skull.

zygote *n.* the fertilized ovum before *cleavage begins. It contains both male and female pronuclei.

zygotene *n.* the second stage of the first prophase of *meiosis, in which the homologous chromosomes form pairs (bivalents).

zym- (zymo-) *prefix denoting* **1.** an enzyme. **2.** fermentation.

zymogen *n. see* proenzyme.

zymology *n.* the science of the study of yeasts and fermentation.

zymolysis *n.* the process of *fermentation or digestion by an enzyme.

zymosis *n.* **1.** the process of *fermentation, brought about by yeast organisms. **2.** the changes in the body that occur in certain infectious diseases, once thought to be the result of a process similar to fermentation. —**zymotic** *adj.*

zymotic disease an old name for a contagious disease, which was formerly thought to develop within the body following infection in a process similar to the fermentation and growth of yeast.

Appendix

Table 1. Base and Supplementary SI Units

physical quantity	name of unit	symbol for unit
length	metre	m
mass	kilogram	kg
time	second	s
electric current	ampere	A
thermodynamic temperature	kelvin	K
luminous intensity	candela	cd
amount of substance	mole	mol
* plane angle	radian	rad
* solid angle	steradian	sr

* supplementary units

Table 2. Derived SI Units with Special Names

physical quantity	name of unit	symbol for unit
frequency	hertz	Hz
energy	joule	J
force	newton	N
power	watt	W
pressure	pascal	Pa
electric charge	coulomb	C
electric potential difference	volt	V
electric resistance	ohm	Ω
electric conductance	siemens	S
electric capacitance	farad	F
magnetic flux	weber	Wb
inductance	henry	H
magnetic flux density (magnetic induction)	tesla	T
luminous flux	lumen	lm
illuminance (illumination)	lux	lx
absorbed dose	gray	Gy
activity	becquerel	Bq
dose equivalent	sievert	Sv

Table 3. Decimal Multiples and Submultiples to be used with SI Units

submultiple	prefix	symbol	multiple	prefix	symbol
10^{-1}	deci-	d	10^{1}	deca-	da
10^{-2}	centi-	c	10^{2}	hecto-	h
10^{-3}	milli-	m	10^{3}	kilo-	k
10^{-6}	micro-	μ	10^{6}	mega-	M
10^{-9}	nano-	n	10^{9}	giga-	G
10^{-12}	pico-	p	10^{12}	tera-	T
10^{-15}	femto-	f	10^{15}	peta-	P
10^{-18}	atto-	a	10^{18}	exa-	E

OXFORD

MORE OXFORD PAPERBACKS

Details of a selection of other books follow. A complete list of Oxford Paperbacks, including The World's Classics, Twentieth-Century Classics, OPUS, Past Masters, Oxford Authors, Oxford Shakespeare, and Oxford Paperback Reference, is available in the UK from the General Publicity Department, Oxford University Press (JN), Walton Street, Oxford OX2 6DP.

In the USA, complete lists are available from the Paperbacks Marketing Manager, Oxford University Press, 200 Madison Avenue, New York, NY 10016.

Oxford Paperbacks are available from all good bookshops. In case of difficulty, customers in the UK can order direct from Oxford University Press Bookshop, 116 High Street, Oxford, Freepost, OX1 4BR, enclosing full payment. Please add 10 per cent of published price for postage and packing.

THE OXFORD–DUDEN PICTORIAL ENGLISH DICTIONARY:
SCIENCE AND MEDICINE

Certain kinds of information are conveyed better visually than by written definitions. It is, for instance, easier to describe the features of a range of fold mountains or a peacock butterfly with a picture than with a verbal description.

Each double page of this dictionary explains the vocabulary of a particular subject by means of a picture illustrating it. The illustrations are clearly drawn and finely detailed. An alphabetical index is also provided for quick and easy reference. As a result, this volume of *The Oxford–Duden* brings clarity and immediacy to descriptions of a great many objects used in the major fields of Science and Medicine or encountered in the natural world. Subjects include Astronomy, Physical Geography, Dentistry, Agriculture, Mathematics, Chemistry, Forestry, Animals, Plants, and many more.

Oxford Paperback Reference

CONCISE SCIENCE DICTIONARY

Over 7,000 entries provide full coverage of terms and concepts in physics, chemistry, biology (including human biology), biochemistry, palaeontology, the earth sciences, and astronomy, plus commonly encountered terms from mathematics and computing sciences. It is written in a clear and explanatory style to provide both straightforward definitions and invaluable background information.

'an essential tool for all school and college libraries, and in fact for anyone wanting to understand a wide range of scientific words and matters' *New Scientist*

Oxford Paperback Reference